Diagnosis and Clinical Management of Bladder Cancer

Diagnosis and Clinical Management of Bladder Cancer

Editor: Jaime Allison

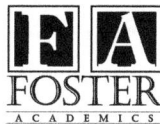

FA

FOSTER
ACADEMICS

www.fosteracademics.com

www.fosteracademics.com

FA
FOSTER
A C A D E M I C S

Cataloging-in-Publication Data

Diagnosis and clinical management of bladder cancer / edited by Jaime Allison.
       p. cm.
Includes bibliographical references and index.
ISBN 978-1-63242-740-3
1. Bladder--Cancer. 2. Bladder--Cancer--Diagnosis. 3. Bladder--Cancer--Treatment.
I. Allison, Jaime.
RC280.B5 D55 2019
616.994 62--dc23

© Foster Academics, 2019

Foster Academics,
118-35 Queens Blvd., Suite 400,
Forest Hills, NY 11375, USA

ISBN 978-1-63242-740-3 (Hardback)

Contents

Preface

In my initial years as a student, I used to run to the library at every possible instance to grab a book and learn something new. Books were my primary source of knowledge and I would not have come such a long way without all that I learnt from them. Thus, when I was approached to edit this book; I became understandably nostalgic. It was an absolute honor to be considered worthy of guiding the current generation as well as those to come. I put all my knowledge and hard work into making this book most beneficial for its readers.

Bladder cancer is a form of cancer that occurs in the tissues of the urinary bladder. Symptoms such as pain while urinating, blood in the urine and low back pain are usually present in this cancer. Some of the risk factors of bladder cancer are frequent bladder infections, smoking, exposure to certain chemicals, cancer in the family, etc. Transitional cell carcinoma is the most common type of bladder cancer, while adenocarcinoma and squamous cell carcinoma are other types. Cystoscopy and tissue biopsies are used to diagnose the condition while the staging is determined by bone and CT scans. The treatment of bladder cancer depends on the stage of the cancer and may involve a combination of surgery, chemotherapy, radiation therapy or immunotherapy. Surgical procedures such as urinary diversion, transurethral resections, complete or partial removal of the bladder may also be performed. The objective of this book is to give a general view of the different clinical aspects of bladder cancer including its concerns and challenges. It is a compilation of chapters that discuss the most vital concepts and emerging trends in the diagnosis and clinical management of bladder cancer. This book is a vital tool for all researching and studying this field.

I wish to thank my publisher for supporting me at every step. I would also like to thank all the authors who have contributed their researches in this book. I hope this book will be a valuable contribution to the progress of the field.

Editor

Risk Prediction Scores for Recurrence and Progression of Non-Muscle Invasive Bladder Cancer: An International Validation in Primary Tumours

Moniek M. Vedder[1], Mirari Márquez[2], Esther W. de Bekker-Grob[1], Malu L. Calle[3], Lars Dyrskjøt[4], Manoils Kogevinas[5], Ulrika Segersten[6], Per-Uno Malmström[6], Ferran Algaba[7], Willemien Beukers[8], Torben F. Ørntoft[4], Ellen Zwarthoff[8], Francisco X. Real[9,10], Nuria Malats[2], Ewout W. Steyerberg[1]*

1 Department of Public Health, Erasmus Medical Centre, Rotterdam, the Netherlands, 2 Genetic and Molecular Epidemiology Group, Spanish National Cancer Research Centre (CNIO), Madrid, Spain, 3 Systems Biology Department, University of Vic, Vic, Barcelona, Spain, 4 Department of Molecular Medicine, Aarhus University Hospital, Aarhus, Denmark, 5 Centre for Research in Environmental Epidemiology, Municipal Institute of Medical Research, Barcelona, Spain, 6 Department of Surgical Sciences, Uppsala University, Uppsala, Sweden, 7 Department of Pathology, Fundació Puigvert-University Autonomous, Barcelona, Spain, 8 Department of Pathology, Erasmus Medical Centre, Rotterdam, the Netherlands, 9 Epithelial Carcinogenesis Group, Spanish National Cancer Research Centre (CNIO), Madrid, Spain, 10 Department of Experimental and Health Sciences, Universitat Pompeu Fabra, Barcelona, Spain

Abstract

Objective: We aimed to determine the validity of two risk scores for patients with non-muscle invasive bladder cancer in different European settings, in patients with primary tumours.

Methods: We included 1,892 patients with primary stage Ta or T1 non-muscle invasive bladder cancer who underwent a transurethral resection in Spain (n = 973), the Netherlands (n = 639), or Denmark (n = 280). We evaluated recurrence-free survival and progression-free survival according to the European Organisation for Research and Treatment of Cancer (EORTC) and the Spanish Urological Club for Oncological Treatment (CUETO) risk scores for each patient and used the concordance index (c-index) to indicate discriminative ability.

Results: The 3 cohorts were comparable according to age and sex, but patients from Denmark had a larger proportion of patients with the high stage and grade at diagnosis (p<0.01). At least one recurrence occurred in 839 (44%) patients and 258 (14%) patients had a progression during a median follow-up of 74 months. Patients from Denmark had the highest 10-year recurrence and progression rates (75% and 24%, respectively), whereas patients from Spain had the lowest rates (34% and 10%, respectively). The EORTC and CUETO risk scores both predicted progression better than recurrence with c-indices ranging from 0.72 to 0.82 while for recurrence, those ranged from 0.55 to 0.61.

Conclusion: The EORTC and CUETO risk scores can reasonably predict progression, while prediction of recurrence is more difficult. New prognostic markers are needed to better predict recurrence of tumours in primary non-muscle invasive bladder cancer patients.

Editor: Georgios Gakis, Eberhard-Karls University, Germany

Funding: This research received funding from the European Community's Seventh Framework program FP7/2007-2011 under grant agreement 201663 (Uromol project, http://www.uromol.eu/). The funders had no role in study design, data collection and analysis, decision to publish, or preparation of the manuscript.

* E-mail: e.steyerberg@erasmusmc.nl

Introduction

Bladder cancer is the most common malignancy of the urinary tract and a major health issue [1]. Most patients with bladder cancer are diagnosed with non-muscle invasive disease (NMIBC: stage Ta or T1) [2]. After transurethral resection (TUR), recurrence of disease occurs in 30–60% of patients and, approximately, 10–15% develop progression to muscle-invasive disease in 5-year after diagnosis [3]. Therefore, regular cystoscopy is carried out for surveillances after TUR. To better target surveillance, risk scores for recurrence and progression prediction have been developed. The best known are the European

Organisation for Research and Treatment of Cancer (EORTC) [4] and the Spanish Urological Club for Oncological Treatment (CUETO) [5] risk scores; the latter focusing on BCG treated patients. Despite their potential usefulness in daily practice, few studies have externally validated these models [6–11] and no study focussed on primary NMIBC. In addition, since the EORTC score was based on a cohort of patients included in 7 clinical trials, the question arises whether these scores are still valid in a broader set of NMIBC patients for predictive purposes. The EORTC and CUETO scores were based on specimens evaluated by central pathologies and specialized pathologists, whereas the specimens

Table 1. Patient characteristics of 1,892 patients with non-muscle invasive bladder cancer in the participating cohorts.*

		Denmark (n = 280)		Netherlands (n = 639)		Spain (n = 973)	
Age	Mean (SD)	66.4	10.2	65.3	12.4	65.7	10.0
Gender	Male	219	78.2%	503	78.7%	850	87.4%
Stage	Ta	177	63.2%	432	67.6%	818	84.1%
	T1	103	36.8%	207	32.4%	155	15.9%
Grade	G1	78	27.9%	189	29.6%	419	43.1%
	G2	83	29.6%	283	44.3%	327	33.6%
	G3	119	42.5%	167	26.1%	227	23.3%
Carcinoma in situ	CIS	89	31.8%	52	8.1%	0	0.0%
	No CIS	189	67.5%	572	89.5%	0	0.0%
	Missing	2	0.7%	15	2.4%	973	100.0%
Tumour size	<3 cm	175	62.5%	238	37.2%	564	58.0%
	≥3 cm	73	26.1%	114	17.9%	133	13.6%
	Missing	32	11.4%	287	44.9%	276	28.4%
Number of tumours	1	82	29.3%	349	54.6%	647	66.5%
	>1	13	4.6%	178	27.9%	277	28.5%
	Missing	185	66.1%	112	17.5%	49	5.0%
Treatment	TUR alone	227	81.0%	140	21.9%	404	41.5%
	TUR+BCG	52	18.6%	108	16.9%	289	29.7%
	TUR+Chemo	0	0.0%	80	12.5%	212	21.8%
	TUR+Chemo+BCG	1	0.4%	29	4.5%	51	5.2%
	Other	0	0.0%	5	0.8%	17	1.7%
	Missing	0	0.0%	277	43.4%	0	0.0%
Status tumour**	Recurrence	209	74.6%	303	47.4%	327	33.6%
	Progression	66	23.6%	99	15.5%	93	9.6%
Vital status**	Alive	72	25.7%	321	50.2%	700	71.9%
	Cancer death	12	4.3%	51	8.0%	62	6.4%
	Other death	7	2.5%	90	14.1%	211	21.7%
	Missing	189	67.5%	177	27.7%	0	0.0%

*Numbers are totals (%), unless stated otherwise.
**At the end of follow-up.

Table 2. Distribution of patients over the risk groups for all patients (n = 1892) and BCG treated patients (n = 449).

Risk category	CUETO		EORTC	
	Recurrence	Progression	Recurrence	Progression
All patients (N = 1892)				
Low risk	1195 (63.2%)	1289 (68.1%)	383 (20.2%)	346 (18.3%)
Intermediate risk	421 (22.3%)	135 (7.1%)	1099 (58.1%)	929 (49.1%)
High risk*	276 (14.6%)	468 (24.7%)	410 (21.7%)	617 (32.6%)
BCG (N = 449)				
Low risk	226 (50.3%)	241 (53.7%)	48 (10.7%)	30 (6.7%)
Intermediate risk	136 (30.3%)	36 (8.0%)	257 (57.2%)	197 (43.9%)
High risk*	87 (19.4%)	172 (38.3%)	144 (32.1%)	222 (49.4%)

*The high risk group is the combined group from intermediate-high and high-risk EORTC and CUETO scores, because of low patient numbers.

included in the present study had been evaluated by routine pathology. In the present study, we investigated the external validity of these risk scores in patients with primary NMIBC across European centres in an everyday routine setting.

Methods

Study Population

We included 1,892 patients with primary NMIBC from three countries; Spain, Denmark, and the Netherlands. Patients from Spain were recruited between 1998 and 2001 from 18 general and University hospitals as part of the Spanish Bladder Cancer/ EPIdemiology of Cancer of the UROthelium (EPICURO) study [12]. All centres are outlined in Appendix table S1. Patients from Denmark were selectively included based on being at higher risk of progression from patient records of the Aarhus University Hospital between 1979 and 2007 [13]. For the Netherlands, we included consecutive patients from the Erasmus MC who underwent a TUR between 1990 and 2012. Patient and tumour characteristics and data on recurrence and progression after TUR of the primary NMIBC were extracted from hospital records till November 2012. All patients had histologically confirmed NMIBC and were treated according to the centres' usual procedures. At the Erasmus MC in the Netherlands, follow-up of patients was according to the EAU guidelines at the time, and risk-adapted according to the EORTC risk scores outcome. At the Aarhus University Hospital in Denmark, the common follow-up strategy for all patients was every three months. In Spain, protocols for the follow-up of bladder cancer patients were developed within each centre. For non-muscle invasive bladder cancers, follow-up for these patients consisted of bladder endoscopy every three months the first year, every six months the second year and then annually bladder endoscopy to complete five years of monitoring. White light cystoscopy was used in all centres participating in our study.

Disease progression was defined as cystoscopically detected tumour relapse with histological confirmation at tumour stage T2 or higher (progression to a muscle invasive tumour stage); it was assumed that a tumour progression always precedes death because of cancer. Patients that died because of bladder cancer without a progression were recorded as having had a progression at the time of death. Recurrence was defined as cystoscopically detected tumour relapse with histological confirmation. Data from the 3 cohorts were harmonized, anonymized, and combined in one data set for statistical analyses, stratified by cohort.

All Danish and Spanish patients gave their written informed consent, and the study was approved by the Central Denmark Region Committees on Biomedical Research Ethics (1994/2920) and by the Ethics Committees of each Spanish participating centre and the Institutional Review Board of the U.S. National Cancer Institute, NIH, USA. This observational study was exempted from formal ethical approval in the Netherlands. All data is anonymized before being used in this study.

Risk Scores

The EORTC scores for recurrence and progression were based on data from 2,596 patients diagnosed with Ta/T1 tumours from seven EORTC trials [4]. A limitation of the EORTC scores was the low number of patients treated with bacillus Calmette Guérin (BCG). Therefore, the CUETO group developed a scoring model in 1,062 BCG-treated patients [5]. The EORTC score incorporated the number of tumours (single, 2–7 or ≥8), tumour size (< 3 cm or ≥3 cm), prior recurrence rate (primary, ≤1 recurrence/ year, >1 recurrence/year), T stage (Ta or T1), concomitant carcinoma in situ (yes/no), and grade (1, 2, or 3). The CUETO

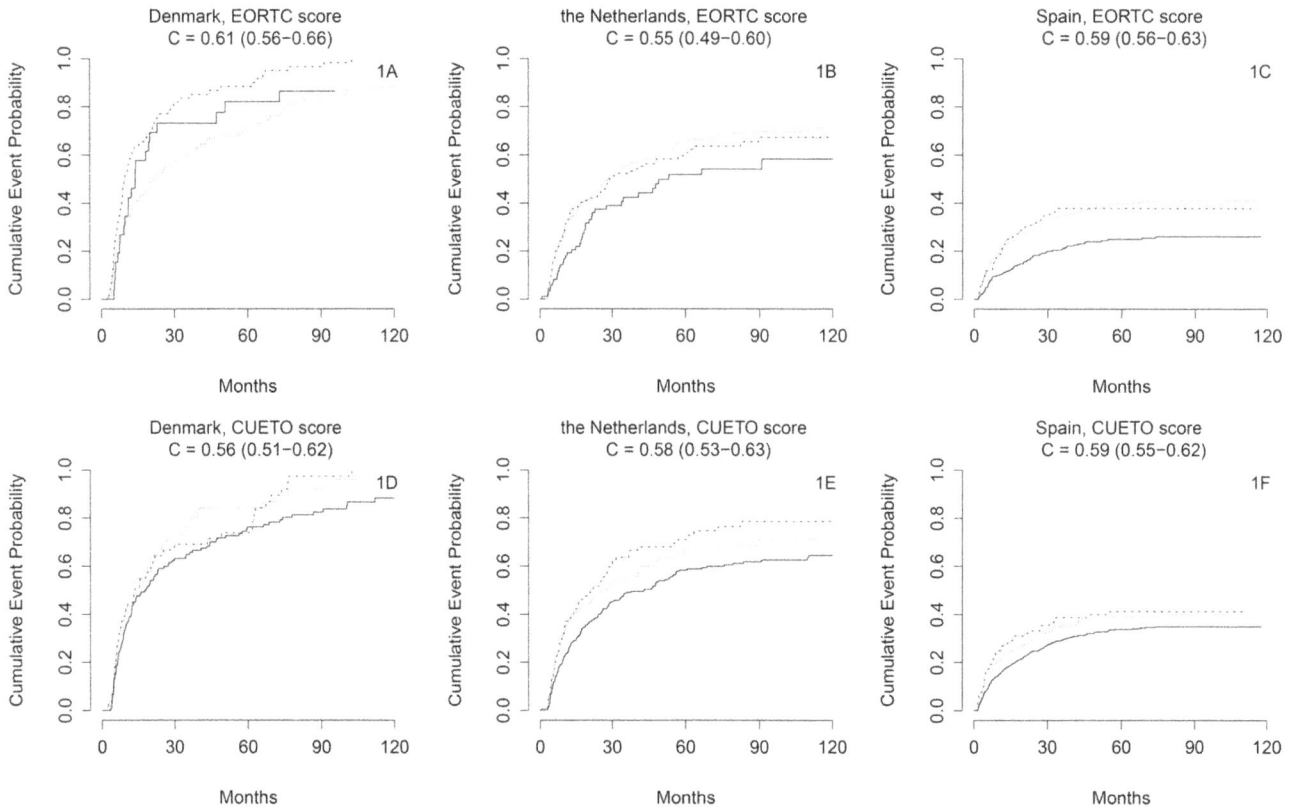

Figure 1. A–F. Kaplan-Meier estimates of recurrence of bladder cancer in a ten-year period from transurethral resection of a non-muscle invasive bladder tumour. Full line: low risk patients, dotted line: intermediate risk patients, dashed line: high risk patients. Number of patients per country: Denmark n = 280; The Netherlands n = 639; Spain n = 973.

model incorporated gender, age (<60, 60–70, >70 years), recurrent tumour (yes/no), number of tumours (≤3 or >3), T stage (Ta or T1), concomitant carcinoma in situ (yes/no), and grade (1, 2, or 3).

Validation

For all patients, we calculated risks for recurrence and progression according to the EORTC and CUETO scores based on the primary tumour. Standard pathologic procedures were followed in each cohort. Tumour grade was scored according to the 1973 system, and pathological stage was according to the 2002 staging system. The presence of concomitant carcinoma in situ was incomplete (CIS, n = 990, 52% missing), as well as data on the number of tumours (n = 346, 18% missing). We used a multiple imputation strategy [14] resulting in five sets of complete data to compute risk scores. We subsequently averaged these risk scores for each patient. Patient scores were then categorized into four risk groups, i.e. low, intermediate low, intermediate high, and high risk for recurrence or progression, as originally specified for the EORTC and CUETO scores. The two highest risk groups were combined because of low numbers. Observed recurrence-free survival (RFS) and progression-free survival (PFS) were calculated from the date of TUR of the primary tumour. An event for RFS was defined as recurrence or progression, if progression occurred as the first event during follow-up. Follow-up was censored at either the last date of follow-up, the date of death, or 120 months. We used standard Kaplan–Meier plots to visualize recurrence and progression patterns in relation to risk groups. This cause-specific analysis was not adjusted for the competing risk of death before

recurrence or progression, since we focused on the discriminative ability of the 2 risk scores (quantified by a concordance measure, c-index) [15]. We conducted subgroup analyses for patients receiving only BCG treatment after TUR. Furthermore, we refitted the scores with a Cox regression analysis stratified by cohort by recalculating risk scores with EORTC and CUETO coefficients based on our data, to obtain further insight in the validity of the scores. We used likelihood ratio statistics to determine the statistical significance of predictors. For comparability with the original EORTC and CUETO scores, we scaled the refitted regression coefficients by the inverse of the Cox regression coefficient for the original scores in our data. For example, the refitted score for T1 vs Ta in the EORTC model for recurrence was calculated as: multivariable coefficient for T1 vs Ta*1/(coefficient for EORTC score for recurrence). SPSS (version 20.0, SPSS Inc, Chicago, Illinois, USA) and R (Version R-2.15.2 for Windows, http://www.r-project.org/) were used for data analysis.

Results

Study Population

We included 1,892 patients; 280 patients from Denmark, 639 from the Netherlands, and 973 from Spain. During 10 years of follow-up, 209 (11%) patients died before a recurrence occurred, 839 (44%) patients had a recurrence and 258 (14%) a progression. Median follow-up for those without recurrence was 74 months. There were 98 patients (N = 90 from the Netherlands, N = 8 from Denmark) without follow-up because of loss to follow-up immediately after TUR. CIS (yes/no) and number of tumours was imputed in patients with missing data, based on 902 patients

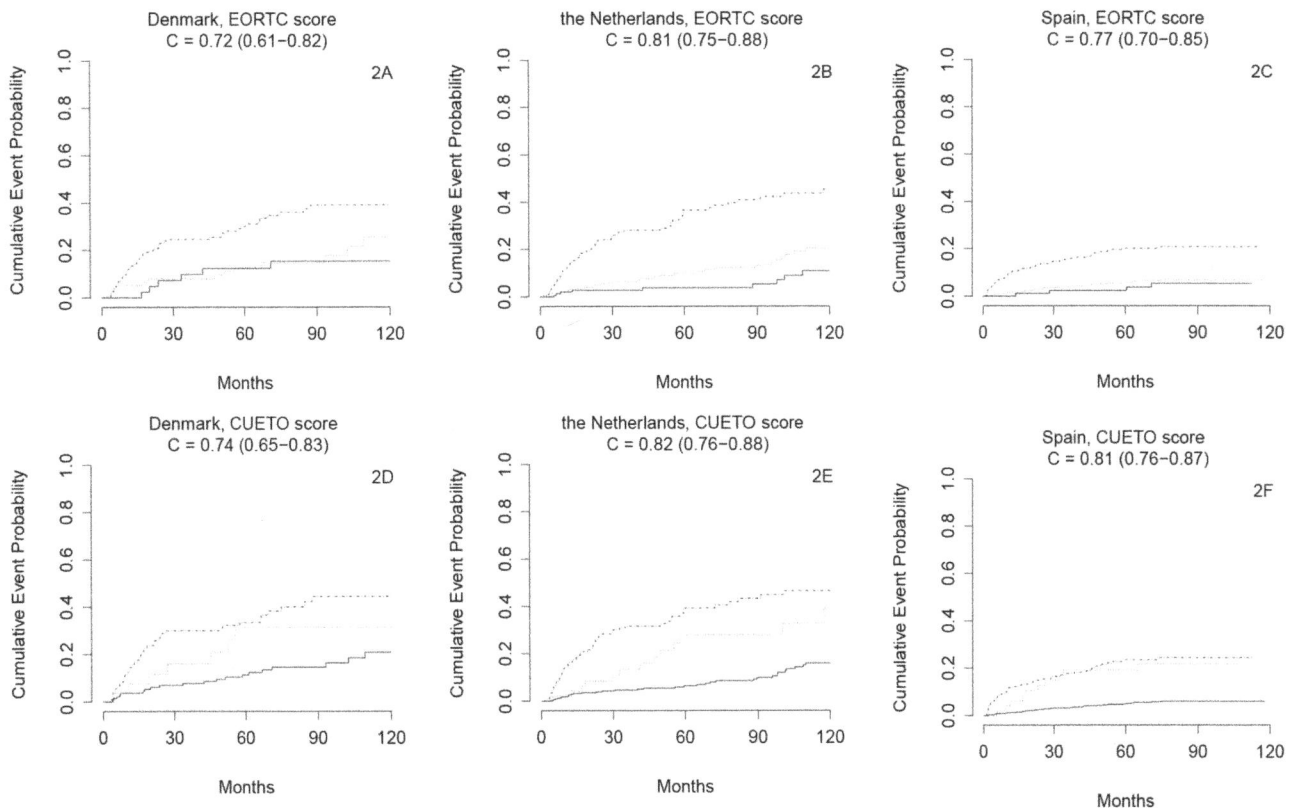

Figure 2. A–F. Kaplan-Meier estimates of progression of bladder cancer in a ten-year period from transurethral resection of a non-muscle invasive bladder tumour. Full line: low risk patients, dotted line: intermediate risk patients, dashed line: high risk patients. Number of patients per country: Denmark n = 280; The Netherlands n = 639; Spain n = 973.

with information on CIS and 1546 patients with information on the number of tumours, as well as complete information on tumour stage, grade, and size, and progression and recurrence free survival (time and yes/no). The mean age was 66 years and the majority was male (Table 1). We do not present totals over all cohorts because of the substantial differences in settings between cohorts. Danish patients presented a larger proportion of patients with high stage and grade (P<0.01), and relatively more recurrences and progressions. The distribution of patients over the risk groups is shown in table 2.

Validation

The EORTC score could not well separate low risk from high risk patients with respect to disease recurrence (Figures 1a–c, c-indices 0.55 to 0.61). Discrimination was somewhat better for progression (Figures 2a–c, c-indices 0.72 to 0.81). The CUETO score had a similar performance (figures 1d–f and 2d–f). Subgroup analyses in patients receiving BCG treatment (n = 449) showed poorer results (Figures S1a–f and S2a–f).

When we refitted the EORTC score for recurrence in Cox regression models, the prognostic effects of multiple tumours, tumour size, CIS and tumour grade were largely confirmed, but T1 tumours had no increased risk over Ta tumours (Results not shown). For progression, tumour size and CIS were less predictive than in the original EORTC score, while the effect for grade was stronger. For the CUETO score, gender was confirmed to be predictive of recurrence. While older age was not predictive of recurrence, we confirmed its value for predicting progression in the refitted CUETO score (p<0.01).

Discussion

The EORTC risk tables have become a standard of care with their inclusion in European guidelines [2]. The CUETO risk model was developed more recently, with a focus on patients treated with BCG. External validation of a prognostic model on a new dataset is crucial to assess its generalizability [16]. In our study, the EORTC and CUETO risk scores showed only modest discriminative ability for the recurrence of NMIBC, with c-indices of, at most, 0.61. Prediction of progression was better with c-indices ranging from 0.72 to 0.82. Our findings were consistent in the cohorts from Denmark, Spain and the Netherlands, and are in line with another external validation of the EORTC risk score [6] and with validation in primary bladder cancer cases [11].

Remarkably, the CUETO score was specifically developed for patients treated with BCG, but discriminated better in the overall population than in the selected BCG population. BCG treatment, which has become a common treatment to manage intermediate- and high-risk NMIBC [17], was used in 449 patients, of over 50% at low risk of recurrence and progression according to the CUETO risk scores. For the EORTC risk scores, we noted that BCG treatment was usually administered to higher risk patients with a relatively narrow distribution of risk scores. This homogeneity in risk may partly explain the poor discriminative ability of the scores in those treated with BCG [18]. More research in this specific group of patients needs to be done, also because of the lack of statistical power due to low numbers of BCG patients in the current study.

In the original study that presented the EORTC risk scores, prior recurrence rate was an important prognostic factor for both recurrence and progression [4]. In the clinical setting, we need to establish a surveillance plan already after TUR for the primary tumour. Therefore, it is of great importance that the EORTC risk score has predictive value also for these patients, who have not had one or multiple recurrences. We found that predicting recurrence was very difficult for primary tumours. The heterogeneity in recurrence risk becomes better known once one or more recurrences have been observed [19].

A possible explanation for the poor performance of the risk scores for the prediction of recurrence outside controlled trials is interobserver variability in bladder cancer staging and grading by pathologists. To partly overcome these issues, new methods for bladder cancer pathology have been introduced in 1998 [20] and 2004 [21]. The 1998 method has been shown to be an improvement over the 1973 method [22], which was used for our patients.

The poor predictability of recurrence may also relate to other factors, unrelated to the (observed) pathology of the disease. For example, detection of all primary tumours may be difficult at primary tumour presentation. Tumour tissue may be left behind, falsely leading to classification as a recurrent tumour. The quality of the TUR may be important but it could not be considered in our evaluation. Moreover, detection policies may vary between urologists with respect to surveillance intervals and treatment modalities (e.g. TUR vs ablation). Progression is a more robust end point, which may partly explain its better predictability with the EORTC and CUETO scores.

The retrospective analysis is a limitation of this study, and explains the presence of missing values in important variables such as CIS and tumour size. We used multiple imputation, which has been shown to be a reliable method to handle missing data [23][23]. We had no detailed information on treatments and surveillance policies, which may have changed over time. The treatment modalities may have led to a dilution of differences between the risk groups. On the other hand, a real life situation was considered with respect to the standard care of urologists. We furthermore note that a selected group of high risk patients was included from Denmark, which can be explained by the fact that patients originated form a specialised university medical centre. However, patients from Spain were a representative sample from standard primary NMIBC population in that country, and patients from the Netherlands, though originating from an academic centre, were similar to the general Dutch primary NMIBC patient population [24].

It is clear that the EORTC and CUETO scores need further improvement. Several markers have shown promising results, such as FGFR3 and Ki67, which improved c-indices for prediction of progression from 0.75 to 0.82 in one study [8]. Various other promising molecular and germline markers are available, which need further rigorous evaluation for their usefulness to predict recurrence and progression [25–26]. Future risk scores will again need external validation, considering discrimination and other aspects of predictive performance, such as calibration (correspondence between observed and predicted risks) and clinical usefulness (ability to make better decisions) [27–29].

We conclude that the discriminatory ability of currently available risk scores is poor for recurrence and moderate for progression in primary NMIBC. Since successful discrimination of low and high risk patients is essential to the right intensity of bladder cancer surveillance, new risk markers are urgently needed to improve risk classification in NMIBC patients.

Supporting Information

Figure S1   A–F. Kaplan-Meier estimates of recurrence of bladder cancer in a ten-year period from transurethral resection of a bladder tumour for patients with non-muscle invasive bladder cancer treated with BCG. Full line: low risk patients, dotted line: intermediate risk patients, dashed line: high risk patients. Number of patients per country: Denmark n = 52; The Netherlands n = 108; Spain n = 289.

Figure S2   A–F. Kaplan-Meier estimates of progression of bladder cancer in a ten-year period from transurethral resection of a bladder tumour for patients with non-muscle invasive bladder cancer treated with BCG. Full line: low risk patients, dotted line: intermediate risk patients, dashed line: high risk patients. Number of patients per country: Denmark n = 52; The Netherlands n = 108; Spain n = 289.

Table S1   Centres and members of the Spanish study group.

Acknowledgments

We would like to thank all who were involved in study design, funding, and data collection used for this analysis, specifically Debra Silverman, Nathaniel Rothman, Adonina Tardón, Alfredo Carrato, Josep Lloreta, and the rest of the Spanish Bladder Cancer/EPICURO Study investigators.

Author Contributions

Analyzed the data: MV NM ES. Contributed reagents/materials/analysis tools: MM WB EZ LD. Wrote the paper: MV EdB-G. Critical revision of the manuscript for important intellectual content: ES MV MM EdB-G MC LD MK US PUM FA WB TØ EZ FR NM. Obtained funding: TØ.

References

1. Ferlay J, Shin HR, Bray F, Forman D, Mathers C, et al. (2010) GLOBOCAN 2008 v2.0, Cancer Incidence and Mortality Worldwide: IARC CancerBase No. 10. Lyon, France: International Agency for Research on Cancer.
2. Babjuk M, Burger M, Zigeuner R, Shariat SF, van Rhijn BW, et al. (2013) EAU guidelines on non-muscle-invasive urothelial carcinoma of the bladder: update 2013. Eur Urol 64: 639–653.
3. Kirkali Z, Chan T, Manoharan M, Algaba F, Busch C, et al. (2005) Bladder cancer: epidemiology, staging and grading, and diagnosis. Urology 66: 4–34.
4. Sylvester RJ, van der Meijden AP, Oosterlinck W, Witjes JA, Bouffioux C, et al. (2006) Predicting recurrence and progression in individual patients with stage Ta T1 bladder cancer using EORTC risk tables: a combined analysis of 2596 patients from seven EORTC trials. Eur Urol 49: 466–465; discussion 475–467.
5. Fernandez-Gomez J, Madero R, Solsona E, Unda M, Martinez-Pineiro L, et al. (2009) Predicting nonmuscle invasive bladder cancer recurrence and progression in patients treated with bacillus Calmette-Guerin: the CUETO scoring model. J Urol 182: 2195–2203.

6. Hernandez V, De La Pena E, Martin MD, Blazquez C, Diaz FJ, et al. (2011) External validation and applicability of the EORTC risk tables for non-muscle-invasive bladder cancer. World J Urol 29: 409–414.
7. Buethe DD, Sexton WJ (2011) Bladder cancer: validating the EORTC risk tables in BCG-treated patients. Nat Rev Urol 8: 480–481.
8. van Rhijn BW, Zuiverloon TC, Vis AN, Radvanyi F, van Leenders GJ, et al. (2010) Molecular grade (FGFR3/MIB-1) and EORTC risk scores are predictive in primary non-muscle-invasive bladder cancer. Eur Urol 58: 433–441.
9. Rosevear HM, Lightfoot AJ, Nepple KG, O'Donnell MA (2011) Usefulness of the Spanish Urological Club for Oncological Treatment scoring model to predict nonmuscle invasive bladder cancer recurrence in patients treated with intravesical bacillus Calmette-Guerin plus interferon-alpha. J Urol 185: 67–71.
10. Fernandez-Gomez J, Madero R, Solsona E, Unda M, Martinez-Pineiro L, et al. (2011) The EORTC tables overestimate the risk of recurrence and progression in patients with non-muscle-invasive bladder cancer treated with bacillus

Calmette-Guerin: external validation of the EORTC risk tables. Eur Urol 60: 423–430.

11. Xylinas E, Kent M, Kluth L, Pycha A, Comploj E, et al. (2013) Accuracy of the EORTC risk tables and of the CUETO scoring model to predict outcomes in non-muscle-invasive urothelial carcinoma of the bladder. Br J Cancer 109: 1460–1466.

12. Porta N, Calle ML, Malats N, Gomez G (2012) A dynamic model for the risk of bladder cancer progression. Stat Med 31: 287–300.

13. Fristrup N, Ulhoi BP, Birkenkamp-Demtroder K, Mansilla F, Sanchez-Carbayo M, et al. (2012) Cathepsin E, maspin, Plk1, and survivin are promising prognostic protein markers for progression in non-muscle invasive bladder cancer. Am J Pathol 180: 1824–1834.

14. Rubin DB, Schenker N (1991) Multiple imputation in health-care databases: an overview and some applications. Stat Med 10: 585–598.

15. Harrel FEJ (2001) Regression Modeling Strategies: Springer-Verlag New York, Inc.

16. Justice AC, Covinsky KE, Berlin JA (1999) Assessing the generalizability of prognostic information. Ann Intern Med 130: 515–524.

17. Fahmy N, Lazo-Langner A, Iansavichene AE, Pautler SE (2013) Effect of anticoagulants and antiplatelet agents on the efficacy of intravesical BCG treatment of bladder cancer: A systematic review. Can Urol Assoc J 7: E740–749.

18. Vergouwe Y, Moons KG, Steyerberg EW (2010) External validity of risk models: Use of benchmark values to disentangle a case-mix effect from incorrect coefficients. Am J Epidemiol 172: 971–980.

19. Kompier LC, van der Aa MN, Lurkin I, Vermeij M, Kirkels WJ, et al. (2009) The development of multiple bladder tumour recurrences in relation to the FGFR3 mutation status of the primary tumour. J Pathol 218: 104–112.

20. Epstein JI, Amin MB, Reuter VR, Mostofi FK (1998) The World Health Organization/International Society of Urological Pathology consensus classification of urothelial (transitional cell) neoplasms of the urinary bladder. Bladder Consensus Conference Committee. Am J Surg Pathol 22: 1435–1448.

21. Montironi R, Lopez-Beltran A (2005) The 2004 WHO classification of bladder tumors: a summary and commentary. Int J Surg Pathol 13: 143–153.

22. Gonul II, Poyraz A, Unsal C, Acar C, Alkibay T (2007) Comparison of 1998 WHO/ISUP and 1973 WHO classifications for interobserver variability in grading of papillary urothelial neoplasms of the bladder. Pathological evaluation of 258 cases. Urol Int 78: 338–344.

23. Ambler G, Omar RZ, Royston P (2007) A comparison of imputation techniques for handling missing predictor values in a risk model with a binary outcome. Stat Methods Med Res 16: 277–298.

24. Dutch Cancer registration (2010) www.iknl.nl.Integraal Kankercentrum Nederland.

25. van Rhijn BW (2012) Combining molecular and pathologic data to prognosticate non-muscle-invasive bladder cancer. Urol Oncol 30: 518–523.

26. Shariat SF, Lotan Y, Vickers A, Karakiewicz PI, Schmitz-Drager BJ, et al. (2010) Statistical consideration for clinical biomarker research in bladder cancer. Urol Oncol 28: 389–400.

27. Steyerberg EW, Vickers AJ, Cook NR, Gerds T, Gonen M, et al. (2010) Assessing the performance of prediction models: a framework for traditional and novel measures. Epidemiology 21: 128–138.

28. Vickers AJ, Elkin EB (2006) Decision curve analysis: a novel method for evaluating prediction models. Med Decis Making 26: 565–574.

29. Vickers A (2010) Prediction models in urology: are they any good, and how would we know anyway? Eur Urol 57: 571–573; discussion 574.

2

Standardization of Diagnostic Biomarker Concentrations in Urine: The Hematuria Caveat

Cherith N. Reid[1], Michael Stevenson[2], Funso Abogunrin[3], Mark W. Ruddock[1], Frank Emmert-Streib[3], John V. Lamont[1], Kate E. Williamson[3]*

1 Molecular Biology, Randox Laboratories, Crumlin, Northern Ireland, 2 Department of Epidemiology and Public Health, Queens University Belfast; Belfast, Northern Ireland, 3 Centre for Cancer Research & Cell Biology, Queens University Belfast, Belfast, Northern Ireland

Abstract

Sensitive and specific urinary biomarkers can improve patient outcomes in many diseases through informing early diagnosis. Unfortunately, to date, the accuracy and translation of diagnostic urinary biomarkers into clinical practice has been disappointing. We believe this may be due to inappropriate standardization of diagnostic urinary biomarkers. Our objective was therefore to characterize the effects of standardizing urinary levels of IL-6, IL-8, and VEGF using the commonly applied standards namely urinary creatinine, osmolarity and protein. First, we report results based on the biomarker levels measured in 120 hematuric patients, 80 with pathologically confirmed bladder cancer, 27 with confounding pathologies and 13 in whom no underlying cause for their hematuria was identified, designated "no diagnosis". Protein levels were related to final diagnostic categories (p = 0.022, ANOVA). Osmolarity (mean = 529 mOsm; median = 528 mOsm) was normally distributed, while creatinine (mean = 10163 µmol/l, median = 9350 µmol/l) and protein (0.3297, 0.1155 mg/ml) distributions were not. When we compared AUROCs for IL-6, IL-8 and VEGF levels, we found that protein standardized levels consistently resulted in the lowest AUROCs. The latter suggests that protein standardization attenuates the "true" differences in biomarker levels across controls and bladder cancer samples. Second, in 72 hematuric patients; 48 bladder cancer and 24 controls, in whom urine samples had been collected on recruitment and at follow-up (median = 11 (1 to 20) months)), we demonstrate that protein levels were approximately 24% lower at follow-up (Bland Altman plots). There was an association between differences in individual biomarkers and differences in protein levels over time, particularly in control patients. Collectively, our findings identify caveats intrinsic to the common practice of protein standardization in biomarker discovery studies conducted on urine, particularly in patients with hematuria.

Editor: Bharat B. Aggarwal, The University of Texas M. D. Anderson Cancer Center, United States of America

Funding: Randox Laboratories undertook laboratory analyses on anonymised patient samples. Randox played no role in data analyses which were undertaken by MS, FES and KW (Queen's University Belfast). Randox employees contributed to the preparation of the manuscript but were not involved in the decision to publish which was taken by Queen's University Belfast. The funders, Randox Laboratories Ltd., played no role in the design of the case control study and were not involved in collection of patient data and samples.

Competing Interests: The following authors on the paper, MR, CR, JL and KW, are named inventors on British Patent Number 0916193.6 which protects the biomarkers in the algorithms. In addition, MR, CR and JL are employees of Randox Laboratories Ltd. who undertook the biomarker analyses using multianalyte biochip technology. Randox funded the salary of FA who recruited the patients over two years.

* E-mail: k.williamson@qub.ac.uk

Introduction

Advances in proteomics have enhanced our understanding of the urinary proteome [1–4] and subsequently encouraged biomarker discovery screens in a range of complex diseases [2,3], including bladder cancer [5,6]. Urine has the advantage of ease of access and is relatively stable thermodynamically [3]. Despite these encouraging developments, no biomarker or biomarker combination to date, has achieved widespread clinical application as a diagnostic assay. Perhaps this is partly attributable to the range of methodologies used to standardise urinary biomarker levels which introduces a lack of consistency in reported levels and inhibits cross study comparisons.

When we reviewed publications on biomarkers for urological pathologies to ascertain the 'correct' methodology to employ for urine normalization, we found inconsistency. As there is no standard methodology, the normalization method employed for any given study is still very much at the discretion of the project investigator, the accessibility of equipment and the available technical expertise. Further, insufficient research into the effects of different standardization approaches means that researchers are employing methods which may introduce bias. Thus there is the potential both for biased data and masking detection of valuable biomarkers secreted into urine at low levels [7].

Some researchers have reported biomarker levels in units per unit volume of urine [5,8,9]; others have standardized biomarker levels using urinary creatinine [10–13]. Most, however, have opted to use protein as their denominator [5,14–16]. Creatinine, the breakdown product of creatine phosphate during muscle metabolism, is filtered out of the blood into the urine by the kidney. Creatinine production is usually at a fairly constant rate when renal function, metabolism and muscle mass are stable, but can be dependent on age, sex, race and size [17]. Serum creatinine and the albumin:creatinine ratio in urine are in clinical use as biomarkers of kidney disease [18]. Osmolarity is a measure of the osmoles of solute per litre of solution and therefore reflects the concentrating ability of the kidneys. Protein is often used to normalize potential bladder cancer biomarkers [5,14–16]. Proteinuria is, however, synonymous with diabetes and renal diseases [7,18–20].

Potential biomarkers must proceed through rigorous validation before they progress through the phases that span discovery to clinical application [21]. However, in the absence of evidence-based guidelines for the standardization of urinary biomarkers, it is possible that potential biomarkers secreted at low levels into urine have not been identified. Urine standardization guidelines would complement those already established for Standards for Reporting of Diagnostic Accuracy (STARD) [22,23] and would ensure that promising biomarkers could be cross-referenced thus facilitating their more expeditious development. It is, however, conceivable that individual guidelines tailored to the specifics of different confounding factors may be required.

The aim of this study was to increase our understanding about the consequences and effects of different methods employed to standardize biomarker levels detected in urine collected from hematuric patients. We assessed the effects on three biomarkers previously reported to be associated with bladder cancer i.e., interleukin- 6 (IL-6) [24], IL-8 [25] and vascular endothelial growth factor (VEGF) [26]. Using data collected during a case control study [27], we characterized urinary creatinine, osmolarity and protein levels across patient groups with the following final diagnoses: no diagnosis (n = 13), confounding pathologies (n = 27) and bladder cancer (n = 80). We determined areas under the receiver operator characteristic (AUROC) for IL-6, IL-8 and VEGF both for uncorrected data and for data standardized using urinary creatinine, osmolarity or protein. In 72 hematuric patients, we compared the intra-patient variability of levels measured at recruitment and at follow-up. We assessed whether there was any association between the differences in levels of biomarkers on recruitment and those measured at follow-up and the differences similarly detected in levels of the standards in the same samples. We present findings that indicate urine volume standardization is preferable to the use of protein standardization because of the high incidence of proteinuria in the hematuric patient population.

Methods

Patient Samples

A case control study approved by the Research Ethics Committee, Faculty of Medicine, Queen's University Belfast (80/04) and the Office for Research Ethics Committees Northern Ireland (ORECNI 80/04); and reviewed by the Belfast City Hospital Trust review board and the Ulster Community and Hospital Trust Research Committee was conducted according to STARD guidelines [22,23]. Written consent was obtained from 181 patients with hematuria (103 patients with confirmed transitional cell carcinoma; and 78 controls); recruited between November 2006 and October 2008 [27]. All patients were white Caucasians except for one of black African origin. Dipstick analysis is a simple and fast analyses of urine undertaken by medical personnel to determine the levels of constituents in urine, including blood, protein, and white blood cells. Dipstick analyses were undertaken on urine samples collected from each of the patients using Aution Sticks 10EA, which were interpreted using PocketChem (Arkray factory, Inc. Japan). The dipstick results for protein were recorded. Approximately 250 mg/l (0.25 mg/ml) is the lower limit of sensitivity for urine dipstick testing [20]. Urine samples from each patient were then stored at −80°C for

a maximum of 12 months prior to triplicate analyses of urinary creatinine, osmolarity, protein, IL-6, IL-8 and VEGF.

First, we analysed data from 120/181 hematuric patients (96 males:24 females) with a mean age = 66 years. Eighty of these patients had pathologically confirmed transitional cell carcinoma of the bladder (TCCB) and 40 were controls. Of the controls, 27 had confounding pathologies, such as stones, inflammation or benign prostate enlargement. In 13 patients, even after detailed investigations, including cystoscopy and radiological imaging of the upper urinary tract, no underlying cause for their hematuria was identified. The diagnosis for these patients is referred to as "no diagnosis".

In our second set of analyses, we compared standards and biomarker levels across time in 72/181 patients (60 males: 12 females) with a mean age = 69 years. Urine samples were collected from these 72 patients both at the time of recruitment and at a second visit (median interval = 11 months (range 1 to 20 months)). It was not possible to collect longitudinal samples from all 181 patients recruited to the study because many patients had significant distances to travel to hospital. The characteristics of these 72 patients were representative of the 120 patients previously analysed. Forty-eight of these patients had TCCB. Sixteen of the 24 controls had confounding pathologies and 8 had a final diagnosis of no diagnosis.

Creatinine, Osmolarity, Protein, IL-6, IL-8 and VEGF Analyses

Scientists, blinded to patient data, completed triplicate analyses of urine samples at Randox Laboratories Ltd. Creatinine levels (μmol/L) and osmolarity (mOsm) were measured using a Daytona RX Series Clinical Analyser (Randox) and a Löser Micro-Osmometer (Type 15) (Löser Messtechnik, Germany), respectively [28,29]. Total protein levels (mg/ml) in urine were determined by Bradford assay $A_{595\ nm}$ (Hitachi U2800 spectrophotometer) using Bovine Serum Albumin (BSA) as standard. IL-6, IL-8 and VEGF (pg/ml) levels in urine (sensitivity = 1.6, 7.9 and 14.6 pg/ml, respectively) were measured [30] using Randox Biochip Array Technology (Randox Evidence © and Investigator ©), which are multiplex systems for protein analysis [31].

SDS PAGE Analyses

Urine samples (2.5 μl/lane) from each patient were investigated for protein using SDS PAGE (16%) analysis. The gels were stained with Coomassie Blue for 1 h and then de-stained in methanol/acetic acid/water (2:1:7) until clear. Protein bands, observed for each patient, were quantified using Quantiscan © software.

Statistical Analyses

Using data from the 120 hematuric patients, we assessed the distribution of the three standards by visual comparison of histograms and boxplots and interpretation of means, medians, skewness and kurtosis. We explored correlations and then used linear regression to determine the extent to which one standard could predict another. To determine the relationship between protein levels measured in urine and protein categories defined using dipstick analyses, we examined a scatter plot of protein levels (mg/ml) against dipstick protein categories to ascertain the range of protein levels within each dipstick category i.e. "+", "++", "+++" and "++++". We used one-way ANOVA to determine whether protein levels were related to final diagnoses categories. To ascertain their diagnostic potential, we compared the area under the receiver operating characteristic (AUROC) determined for the standardized and uncorrected biomarker levels. We divided the average measurement for each of the three biomarkers by the average osmolarity, creatinine or protein level measured in the same patient's urine sample and then $\log_{10}$ transformed the data.

Urine samples were obtained from 72 patients on two visits; one on recruitment and a second at follow-up (median = 11 (1 to 20 months)). To assess the agreement between the levels of the standards on recruitment and at follow-up, we constructed Bland Altman plots and undertook paired t-test analyses. In addition, we were interested to ascertain whether there were significant associations between differences in individual biomarkers levels over time and differences in standard levels over time. For each biomarker we divided the mean biomarker level measured at follow-up by the mean biomarker level measured on recruitment, and then computed the $\log_{10}$ of this value. Similarly, for each standard we divided the mean level measured at follow-up by the mean level measured at recruitment and then computed the $\log_{10}$ of this value. To compare these ratios we undertook regression analyses inserting log differences of each biomarker into the dependent box and log differences of creatinine, osmolarity and protein sequentially into the independent box.

Statistical analyses were completed using SPSS v17.

Results

Osmolarity (mean = 529 mOsm; median = 528 mOsm) was normally distributed while creatinine (mean = 10163 µmol/l, median = 9350 µmol/l) and protein (mean = 0.3297 mg/ml; median = 0.1155 mg/ml) distributions were not. This is substantiated by skewness and kurtosis values for osmolarity (0.1; −0.5), creatinine (2.2; 8.8), and protein (3.1; 10.6) (Figure 1). Measurements for osmolarity, creatinine, and protein ranged from 103 to 1047 mOsm; 1329 to 44542 µmol/l (1.3 to 44.5 mmol); and zero to 3.36 mg/ml, respectively. Two patients had extreme creatinine levels (Figure 1B). These levels, 44542 and 39077 µmol/l respectively, were measured in a 40 year-old male with stone disease and a 58 year-old male with non-muscle invasive TCCB. All other measurements were <24000 µmol/l. Extreme creatinine levels have been reported previously [12]. There was a modest relationship between osmolarity and creatinine in that 51.9% of the variation in creatinine was accounted for by osmolarity (linear regression; R Square = 0.519) (Figure 2). In this study we report 49% false positives and <1% false negatives in dipstick analyses based on our findings that 25/51 patients deemed dipstick positive had protein levels <0.25 mg/ml; and that 4/62 patients with measured protein levels >0.25 mg/ml were deemed dipstick negative (Figure 3).

Urinary protein levels were related to final diagnoses categories (ANOVA; p = 0.022). Protein levels in urine from bladder cancer patients were higher than in those with no diagnosis (p = 0.073)(Table 1). In contrast, osmolarity and creatinine levels were not significantly related to final diagnoses (ANOVA p = 0.851 and 0.630, respectively).

The ranges and median levels for the biomarkers were: IL-6 (pg/ml) (n = 119)(range = 1.2 to 900.0; median = 3.0), IL-8 (pg/ml) (n = 119)(range 7.90 to 2900.0; median = 117.3) and VEGF (pg/ml)(n = 119)(range = 14.6 to 1500.0; median = 107.6). AUROCs for uncorrected biomarker levels and those standardized using osmolarity or creatinine were very similar. The lowest AUROCs were consistently recorded following protein standardization (Figure 4).

Median protein levels were lower at follow-up (0.08 mg/ml) when compared to levels on recruitment levels (0.10 mg/ml). Osmolarity and creatinine were constant. Mean osmolarity = 519, 521 mOsm; mean creatinine = 9835, 9941 µmol/l, respectively on recruitment and at follow-up. Median osmolarity = 527, 515 mOsm; median creatinine = 9086, 8832 µmol/l, respectively on recruitment and at follow-up. Bland Altman plots illustrated that protein levels decreased by approximately 24% between recruitment and follow-up (mean $\log_e$difference = −0.24 (95% Confidence Interval (CI) 2.18 to −2.66). In contrast, osmolarity and creatinine were stable with little variation across the scale in the Bland Altman plots (Figure 5). Protein levels decreased between recruitment and follow-up (Paired T-test; p<0.10) (Table 2).

When we studied longitudinal ratios there were significant associations between the differences in logarithms (base 10) between all three biomarkers and protein. These associations between the biomarkers and protein ratios were stronger in the control sub-population (n = 24) than in the bladder cancer sub-population (n = 48). In the control sub-population, IL-6 = −0.55+0.739 protein, R Square = 0.318 (p = 0.004); IL-8 = −0.231+0.848 protein, R Square = 0.318 (p = 0.004); and VEGF = −0.075+0.477 protein, R Square = 0.322 (p = 0.004). In the bladder cancer sub-population, IL-6 = −0.130+1.099 protein, R Square = 0.285 (p = <0.0001); IL-8 = −0.216+0.928 protein, R Square = 0.278 (p = <0.0001); and VEGF = −0.111+0.569 protein, R Square = 0.165 (p = 0.0001). There were no significant associations when recruitment levels were subtracted from follow-up levels of biomarkers and the differences similarly determined in either osmolarity or creatinine in the same samples (Figure 6).

We analysed the urine from each patient using PAGE. The levels of protein in the urine that we observed on the gel, following equal loading (2.5 µl, i.e. no standardization or normalization), did not reflect the level of the biomarker in the same urine sample. Therefore high levels of protein observed on the PAGE gel did not correlate with high levels of the biomarkers. For example, IL-8 levels did not significantly correlate with the band density frequently observed at approximately 64–66 kDa (Figure 7).

Discussion

We have presented evidence that the high prevalence of proteinuria in hematuric patients introduces a caveat with respect to using protein as the standardiser of urinary biomarker levels. The origin of proteins shed into the urine of patients with proteinuria is dependent on the specific disorder that the patient has [7]. Further, drugs which are often prescribed for hematuric patients, including nonsteroidal anti-inflammatory and occasionally angiotensin-converting enzyme (ACE) drugs, can cause increases or decreases in proteinuria [32]. In certain renal diseases large proteins such as albumin leak into urinary space and the amount of secreted protein very much depends on the specific disease [7]. Dipstick protein analyses detects predominantly albumin. Proteinuria is classified as selective when albumin is the major protein constituent [7]. Albumin is detected as a dense band at approximately 64 to 66 kDa observed on the SDS PAGE gel indicating that the corresponding patients have selective proteinuria. In contrast, the patient with a dense band around 13 kDa may have non-selective proteinuria. There was a significant correlation r = 0.802 (Pearson correlation; p<001) between the density of the albumin band quantified using Quantiscan © software and $\log_{10}$ average protein levels, but this, on its own, would not justify the classification of patients with proteinuria as having albuminuria.

This study has therefore demonstrated in three ways the caveats of protein normalization in patients with hematuria. These being that protein levels are not homogeneous across diagnostic groupings in hematuric patients; that there is intra-patient

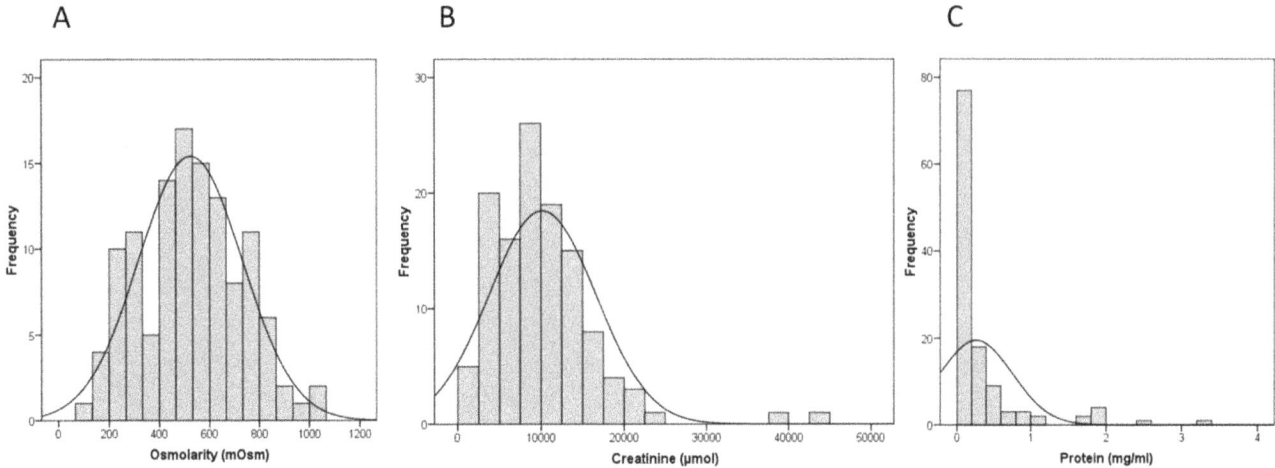

Figure 1. Creatinine, Osmolarity and Protein distributions. Triplicate levels of the standards were measured in 120 hematuric patients and then averaged. (A) Osmolarity was normally distributed; (B) creatinine and (C) protein had skewed distributions.

variability in protein levels in urine over time; and that protein standardization reduced AUROCs in biomarkers previously demonstrated to be elevated in bladder cancer patients [24–26]. First, we have demonstrated that urinary protein levels were higher in patients with bladder cancer compared to those with no final diagnosis and that protein *per se* is associated with final diagnosis. Second, we found that standardization using protein resulted in the lowest AUROCs for each of the three bladder cancer diagnostic biomarkers. The latter indicates that biomarker differences between controls and bladder cancer patients can be attenuated following protein standardization. Third, we observed that protein levels were generally lower on follow-up, perhaps indicative of successful treatment. However, there were significant associations between the differences determined in each of in the biomarkers when recruitment levels were subtracted from follow-up levels and the differences similarly determined in protein in the

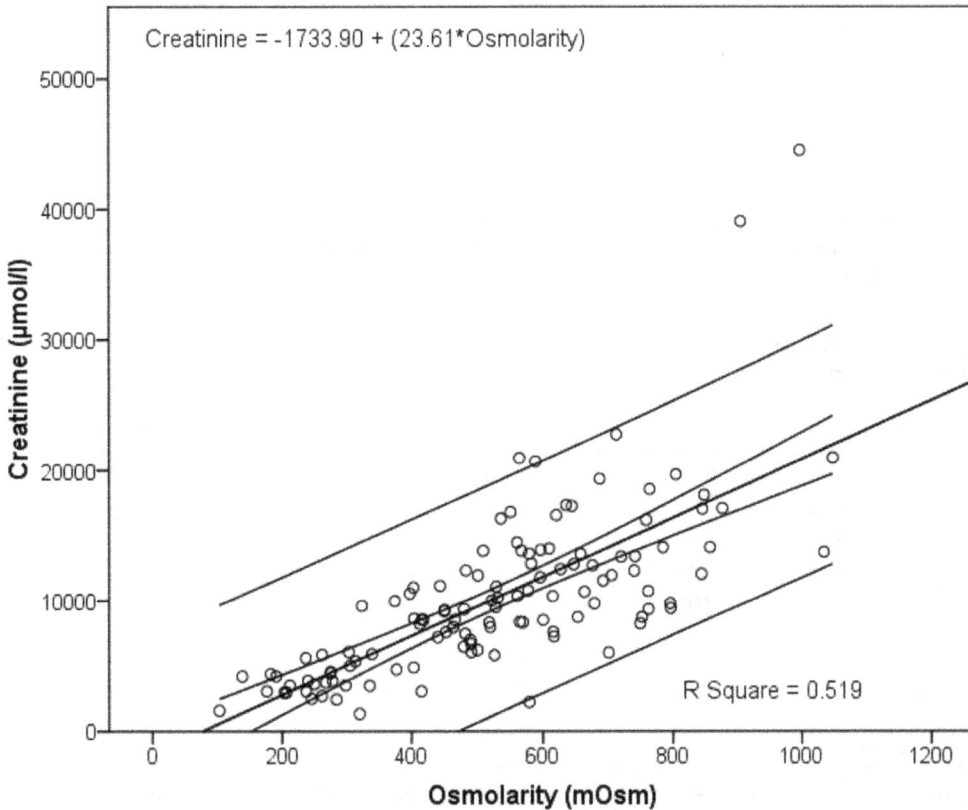

Figure 2. Relationship between osmolarity and creatinine. Triplicate levels of osmolarity and creatinine were measured in urine from 119 hematuric patients. There was a modest relationship between osmolarity and creatinine (R Square = 0.519).

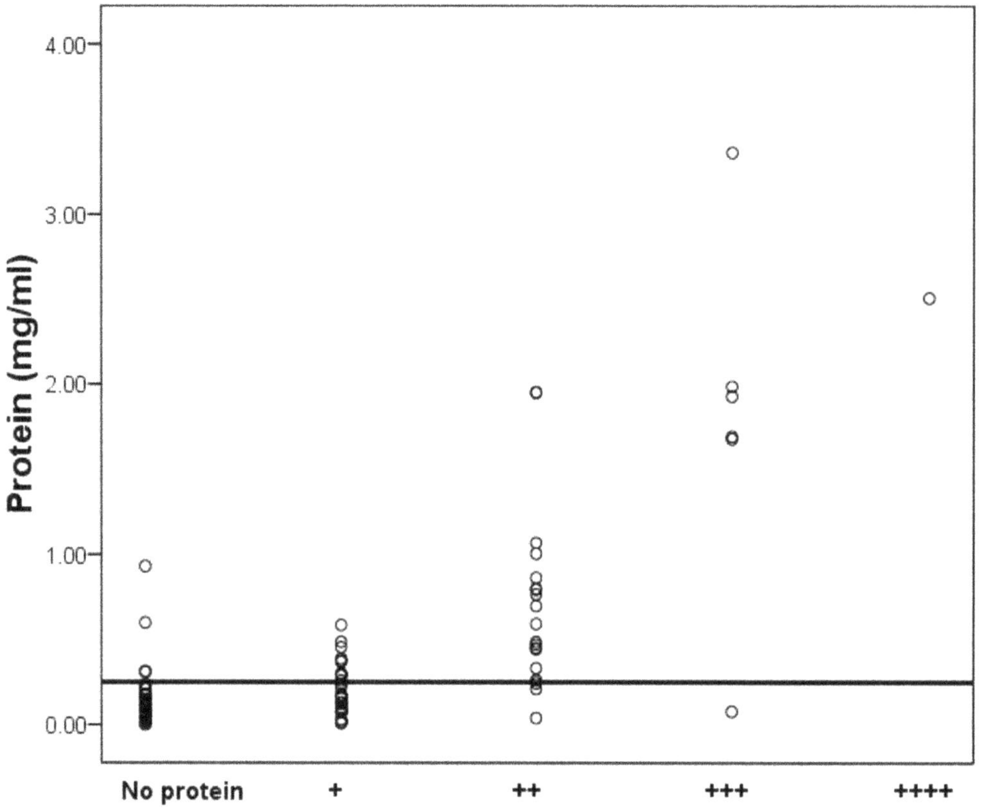

Figure 3. Comparison between measured protein levels and protein dipstick analyses. Total protein levels (mg/ml) in urine were determined by Bradford assay $A_{595\ nm}$ (Hitachi U2800 spectrophotometer) using Bovine Serum Albumin as standard. Dipstick analyses were undertaken using Aution Sticks 10EA. Analyses were interpreted using PocketChem (Arkray factory, Inc. Japan). Protein levels were plotted against dipstick results with the Y –axis reference line indicating the usual lower limit of sensitivity for urine dipstick testing (0.25 mg/ml).

same samples. This was most evident in controls. These findings suggest that after treatment and/or recovery, protein levels decreased in the control sub-population to a greater extent than in the cancer patients. This finding would only arise if controls were not healthy and controls in some case control studies would be healthy and therefore protein concentration would not be

expected to be lower at the end of the study. The latter associations would support the use of protein normalization, particularly in controls. However, in light of other findings, particularly considering that the lowest AUROCs were determined following protein normalization and the high prevalence

Table 1. Comparison of protein levels across final diagnostic categories.

	(I) final diagnostic category	(J) final diagnostic category	Mean Difference (I–J)	Std. Error	Sig.	95% CI Lower bound	95% CI Upper bound
Dunnett T3	no diagnosis	confounding pathologies	−.33166	.20616	.316	−.8650	.2017
		bladder cancer	−.46508	.18809	.073	−.9667	.0366
	confounding pathologies	no diagnosis	.33166	.20616	.316	−.2017	.8650
		bladder cancer	−.13342	.12194	.621	−.4352	.1684
	bladder cancer	no diagnosis	.46508	.18809	.073	−.0366	.9667
		Confounding pathologies	.13342	.12194	.621	−.1684	.4352

Urinary protein levels measured in 120 patients with hematuria were related to final diagnostic categories in (ANOVA; p = 0.022). Subsequently, we carried out a one way ANOVA with post-hoc Dunnett T3 analyses using log_{10} transformed protein data. Higher protein levels were measured in urine from patients diagnosed with bladder cancer in comparison to those with no diagnosis (p = 0.073). There were no significant differences between the protein levels measured in patients with confounding pathologies and levels measured in the urines from bladder cancer patients (p = 0.621) or between patients with no diagnosis and patients with confounding pathologies (p = 0.316).

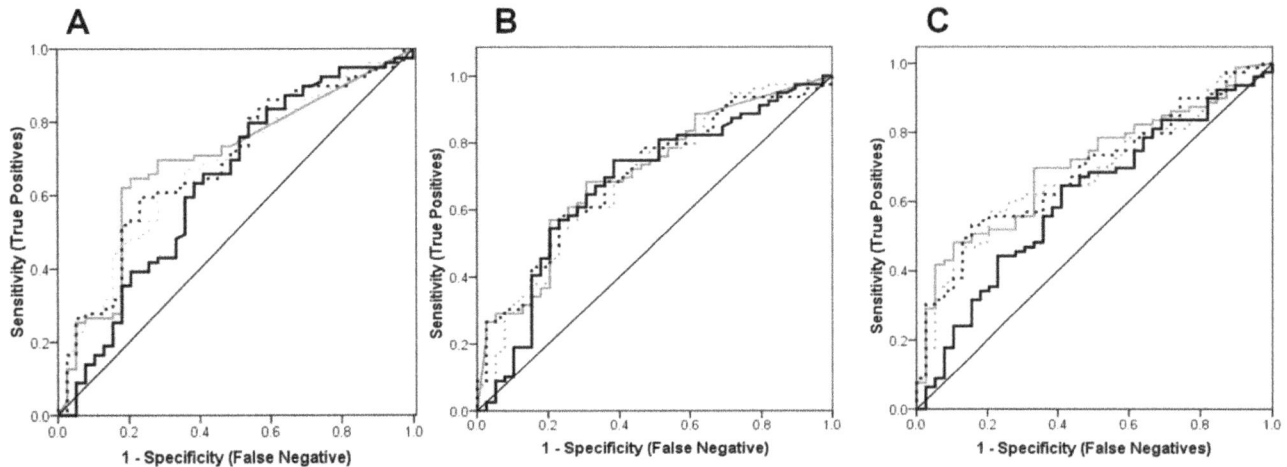

Figure 4. AUROC for IL-6, IL-8 and VEGF. The lowest area under receiver operating characteristic (AUROC) were determined after protein normalization as represented by the solid black curve which was always closest to the diagonal reference line i.e., IL-6 = 0.634 (0.523 to 0.745); IL-8 = 0.677 (0.570 to 0.784); and VEGF = 0.609 (0.501 to 0.716). The AUROCs for uncorrected biomarker levels (thick grey curve), and those standardized using osmolarity (dashed black curve) or creatinine (dashed grey curve) were very similar for individual biomarkers : (A) IL-6 = 0.693 (0.592 to 0.794), 0.683 (0.582 to 0.784) and 0.678 (0.578 to 0.779), respectively; (B) IL-8 = 0.706 (0.608 to 0.804), 0.701 (0.603 to 0.799) and 0.694 (0.592 to 0.795), respectively; and (C) VEGF = 0.705 (0.610 to 0.799), 0.687 (0.591 to 0.783) and 0.680 (0.583 to 0.777), respectively. Figures in brackets are 95% Confidence Intervals.

of proteinuria in this patient population, this approach could bias true biomarker levels.

These observations demonstrate that it is not appropriate to use protein standardization of urine samples in hematuric patient populations where proteinuria is often a co-morbidity. However, our findings cannot be extrapolated to patients who have proteinuria who are nonhematuric. Proteinuria has widespread causes including ureteric calculi, minimal change glomerulo-nephritis, diabetes, malaria and congestive heart failure [7,33]. Many of these pathologies present with hematuria [27].

Interestingly, differences in protein levels between recruitment and follow-up accounted for a significant amount of the differences in biomarker levels at the same time-points. Further this relationship was strongest in the control samples. This reflects a close relationship between a disease status indicator, i.e. proteinuria, and IL-6, IL-8 and VEGF levels in Patients with hematuria.

The persistent trend for researchers to normalize biomarker levels using protein [5,14–16] perhaps stems from the concept of equal loading in Western blot experiments, which has been carried through, to biomarker studies and then more recently, to proteomic screens. It is interesting that Chen *et al* (2010) achieved higher AUROCs for novel potential bladder cancer- biomarkers using urine volumes rather than protein normalized samples [5]. Our data suggest that in hematuric populations in which there is a high incidence of proteinuria, urine volume is likely to be more accurate, and indeed a simpler approach to standardization, than applying protein as a denominator. The consequences of normalizing using protein in this study were that biomarker levels in patients with proteinuria were proportionately reduced. This approach therefore introduced bias. It might be prudent to consider proteinuria as a contraindication to protein based standardization of urine in proteomic studies conducted in patients

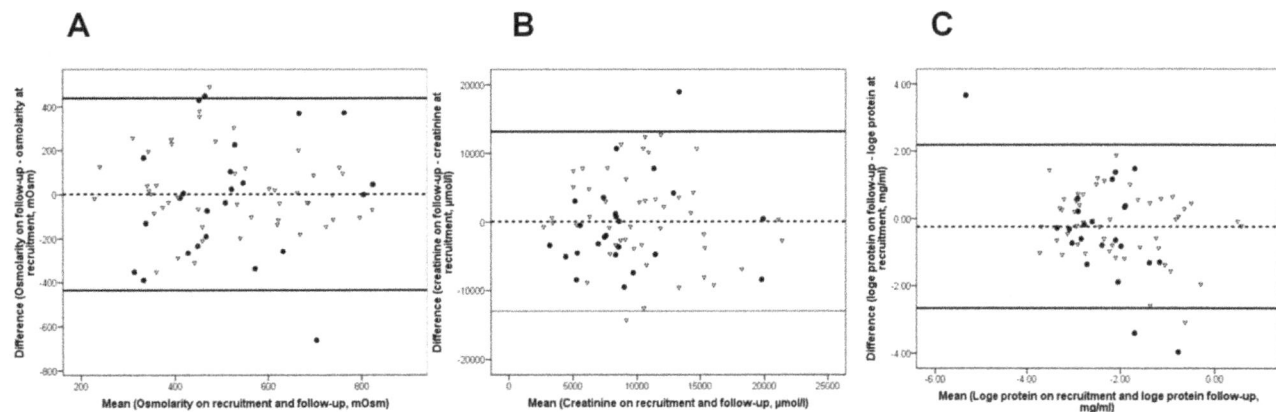

Figure 5. Bland Altman plots for osmolarity, creatinine and protein. Bland Altman plots for (A) osmolarity; (B) creatinine; and (C) protein ($\log_e$) were plotted to determine the agreement between the levels of each standard measured on recruitment and those measured at follow-up. The hashed line (mean of the mean differences) demonstrates that protein levels decreased by approximately 24% at follow-up. Osmolarity and creatinine levels did not significantly change. Solid lines, 95% CI limits. Open triangles (bladder cancer); closed black circles (controls).

Table 2. Paired t-test comparing standard levels measured on recruitment and at follow-up.

		Mean	Std. Deviation	Std. Error Mean	95% CI Lower	95% CI Upper	t	df	Sig. (2-tailed)
Pair 1	$\log_{10}$ protein on recruitment – $\log_{10}$ protein at follow-up	.10451	.52658	.06206	−.01923	.22825	1.684	71	.097
Pair 2	creatinine on recruitment – creatinine at follow-up	−87.45193	6531.78735	775.18054	−1633.50077	1458.59692	−.113	70	.911
Pair 3	osmol arity on recruitment- osmolarity at follow-up	−1.75926	218.40565	25.73935	−53.08207	49.56355	−.068	71	.946

Urine samples were obtained on two visits; one on recruitment and a second at follow-up (median = 11 (1 to 20 months)) from 72 patients who had presented with hematuria. The mean difference between log10 protein levels decreased over time (p = 0.097).

with hematuria. In other biomarker applications different confounding pathologies may play a role and our findings might not apply [7].

This is the first time that the effects of biomarker standardization have been compared across four methodologies simultaneously, i.e. uncorrected levels, creatinine, osmolarity and protein. Standardization of the urinary biomarker levels using protein, attenuated the data reducing both sensitivity and specificity of the biomarkers IL-6, IL-8 and VEGF. In this study, urinary creatinine and osmolarity levels in patients were constant in patients over time. Since creatinine and osmolarity did not differ significantly across disease pathologies frequently diagnosed in hematuric patients, our data suggest that creatinine or osmolarity could be used to normalize for urinary protein biomarkers. Further, osmolarity levels measured in this study predicted creatinine levels supporting the notion that osmolarity and creatinine levels in urine are interchangeable. However differences in IL-6, IL-8 and VEGF measured on recruitment and at follow-up were not significantly associated with differences in either of these standards. In this study we did not evaluate the efficacy of standardization based on 24 hour urine collections which might be more accurate than the state measurements used in this study. This study provides no justification for normalization using either creatinine or osmolarity when they are determined as state measurements. Uncorrected IL-6, IL-8 and VEGF AUROC analyses were very similar to those normalized using osmolarity and creatinine. Therefore, it makes more sense to use uncorrected biomarker levels for biomarker studies in hematuric patients.

Our study provides evidence that urinary diagnostic biomarkers should be standardized by urine volume in hematuric patients where there is a high incidence of proteinuria. Since proteinuria is a common condition in patients with hypertension, ureteric calculi, minimal change glomerulo-nephritis, diabetes, malaria and congestive heart failure, our findings may have implications for a wide range of biomarker discovery, biomarker validation and quantitative proteomic studies investigating complex diseases.

Author Contributions

Conceived and designed the experiments: CNR FA JL KW. Performed the experiments: CNR MR. Analyzed the data: MS FES KW. Contributed reagents/materials/analysis tools: JL. Wrote the paper: CNR FA MR KW.

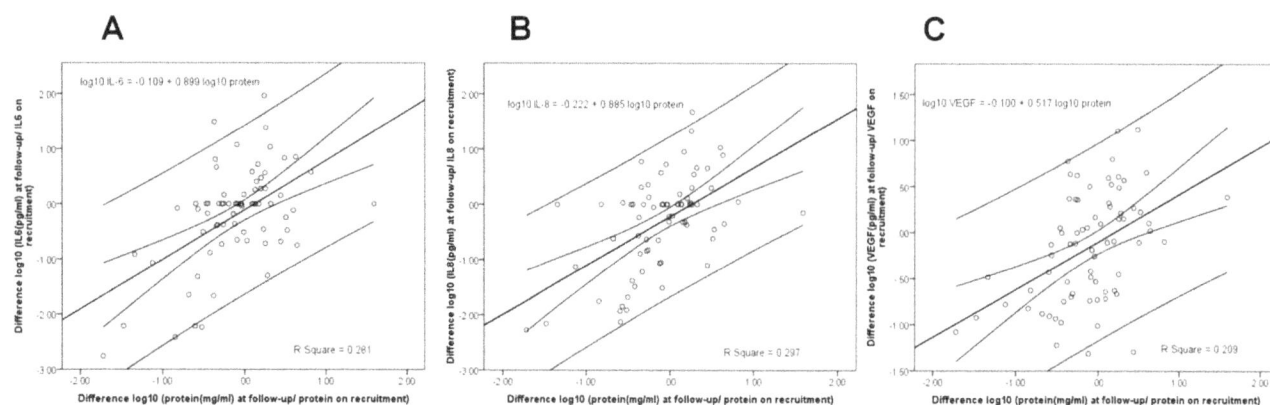

Figure 6. Regression analyses to determine the relationship between differences in standards and biomarkers over time. Scatter plots, based on data from 72 hematuric patients, plotting the differences between biomarker levels on recruitment and follow-up against the differences between protein levels on recruitment and follow-up for (A) IL-6, (B) IL-8 and (C) VEGF. The regression line and 95% confidence interval show significant associations (p<0.0001 for all biomarkers). Differences in biomarker levels across time were associated with differences in protein levels.

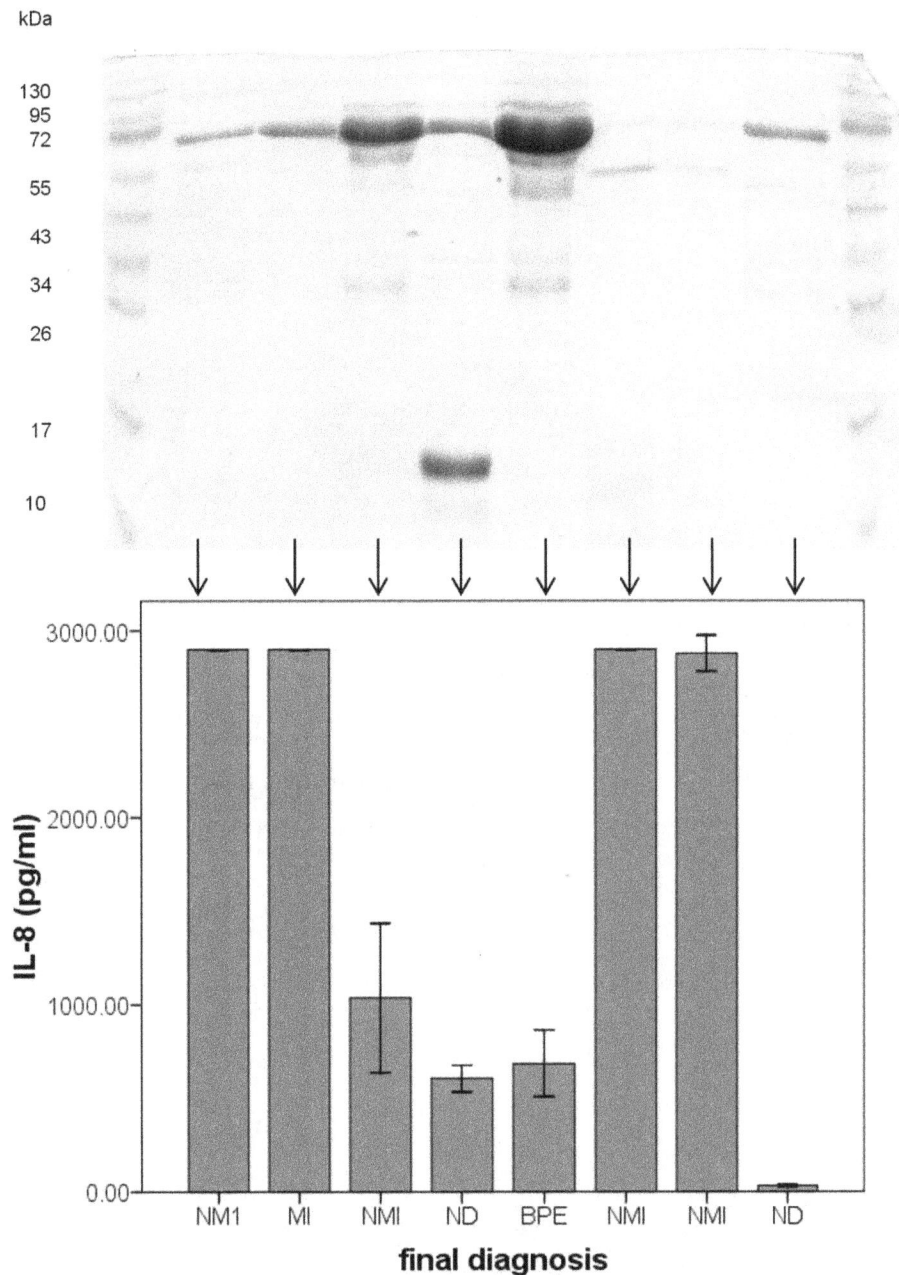

Figure 7. SDS PAGE on urine samples. SDS PAGE was carried out on urine from each patient. A dense band was frequently observed at approximately 64–66 kDa. This band represents albumin. Eight representative samples demonstrate the diverse relationship between this albumin band on the SDS PAGE and corresponding IL-8 levels measured in urine from the same patient sample. Corresponding IL-8 levels are illustrated in the 95% confidence limit error bar chart directly below each lane. The density of the albumin band was not always indicative of the IL-8 levels. Four patients had non-muscle invasive bladder cancer (NMI), one patient had muscle invasive bladder cancer (MI), two patients had no diagnosis (ND), and one patient had benign prostate enlargement.

References

1. Adachi J, Kumar C, Zhang Y, Olsen JV, Mann M (2006) The human urinary proteome contains more than 1500 proteins, including a large proportion of membrane proteins. Genome Biol 7(9): R80.
2. Pisitkun T, Johnstone R, Knepper MA (2006) Discovery of urinary biomarkers. Mol Cell Proteomics 5: 1760–1771.
3. Hu S, Loo JA, Wong DT (2006) Human body fluid proteome analysis. Proteomics 6: 6326–6353.
4. Nagaraj N, D'Souza RC, Cox J, Olsen JV, Mann M (2010) Feasibility of large-scale phosphoproteomics with higher energy collisional dissociation fragmentation. J Proteome Res 9: 6786–6794.
5. Chen YT, Chen CL, Chen HW, Chung T, Wu CC, et al (2010) Discovery of novel bladder cancer biomarkers by comparative urine proteomics using iTRAQ technology. J Proteome Res 9: 5803–5815.
6. Iwaki H, Kageyama S, Isono T, Wakabayashi Y, Okada Y, et al. (2004) Diagnostic potential in bladder cancer of a panel of tumor markers (calreticulin,

gamma -synuclein, and catechol-o-methyltransferase) identified by proteomic analysis. Cancer Sci 2004, 95: 955–961.

7. Julian BA, Suzuki H, Suzuki Y, Tomino Y, Spasovski G, et al. (2009) Sources of Urinary Proteins and their Analysis by Urinary Proteomics for the Detection of Biomarkers of Disease. Proteomics Clin Appl 2009, 3: 1029–1043.

8. Margel D, Pesvner-Fischer M, Baniel J, Yossepowitch O, Cohen IR (2011) Stress proteins and cytokines are urinary biomarkers for diagnosis and staging of bladder cancer. Eur Urol 59: 113–119.

9. Svatek RS, Herman MP, Lotan Y, Casella R, Hsieh JT, et al. (2006) Soluble Fas–a promising novel urinary marker for the detection of recurrent superficial bladder cancer. Cancer 106: 1701–1707.

10. Urquidi V, Kim J, Chang M, Dai Y, Rosser CJ, et al. (2012) CCL18 in a multiplex urine-based assay for the detection of bladder cancer. PLoS One 7: e37797.

11. Sanchez-Carbayo M, Urrutia M, Silva JM, Romani R, Garcia J, et al, (2000) Urinary tissue polypeptide-specific antigen for the diagnosis of bladder cancer. Urology 55: 526–532.

12. Miller RC, Brindle E, Holman DJ, Shofer J, Klein NA, et al. (2004) Comparison of specific gravity and creatinine for normalizing urinary reproductive hormone concentrations. Clin Chem 50: 924–932.

13. Garde AH, Hansen AM, Kristiansen J, Knudsen LE (2004) Comparison of uncertainties related to standardization of urine samples with volume and creatinine concentration. Ann Occup Hyg 48: 171–179.

14. Pesic I, Stefanovic V, Muller GA, Muller CA, Cukuranovic R, et al (2011) Identification and validation of six proteins as marker for endemic nephropathy. J Proteomics 74: 1994–2007.

15. Lokeshwar VB, Obek C, Pham HT, Wei D, Young MJ, et al. (2000) Urinary hyaluronic acid and hyaluronidase: markers for bladder cancer detection and evaluation of grade. J Urol 163: 348–356.

16. Smalley DM, Sheman NE, Nelson K, Theodorescu D (2008) Isolation and identification of potential urinary microparticle biomarkers of bladder cancer. J Proteome Res 7: 2088–2096.

17. Barr DB, Wilder LC, Caudill SP, Gonzalez AJ, Needham LL, et al. (2005) Urinary creatinine concentrations in the U.S. population: implications for urinary biologic monitoring measurements. Environ Health Perspect 2005, 113: 192–200.

18. Goldstein SL (2011) Acute kidney injury biomarkers: renal angina and the need for a renal troponin I. BMC Med 9: 135.

19. Seegmiller JC, Sviridov D, Larson TS, Borland TM, Hortin GL, et al. (2009) Comparison of urinary albumin quantification by immunoturbidimetry, competitive immunoassay, and protein-cleavage liquid chromatography-tandem mass spectrometry. Clin Chem 55: 1991–1994.

20. Barratt J, Topham P (2007) Urine proteomics: the present and future of measuring urinary protein components in disease. CMAJ 177: 361–368.

21. Lee JW (2009) Method validation and application of protein biomarkers: basic similarities and differences from biotherapeutics. Bioanalysis 1: 1461–1474.

22. Bossuyt PM, Reitsma JB, Bruns DE, Gatsonis CA, Glasziou PP, et al. (2003) Standards for Reporting of Diagnostic Accuracy: Towards complete and accurate reporting of studies of diagnostic accuracy: the STARD initiative. Standards for Reporting of Diagnostic Accuracy. Clin Chem 49: 1–6.

23. Bossuyt PM, Reitsma JB, Bruns DE, Gatsonis CA, Glasziou PP, et al. (2003) Standards for Reporting of Diagnostic Accuracy: The STARD statement for reporting studies of diagnostic accuracy: explanation and elaboration. Clin Chem 49: 7–18.

24. Leibovici D, Grossman HB, Dinney CP, Millikan RE, Lerner S, et al. (2005) Polymorphisms in inflammation genes and bladder cancer: from initiation to recurrence, progression, and survival. J Clin Oncol 23(24): 5746–5756.

25. Sheryka E, Wheeler MA, Hausladen DA, Weiss RM (2003) Urinary interleukin-8 levels are elevated in subjects with transitional cell carcinoma. Urology 62: 162–166.

26. Eissa S, Salem AM, Zohny SF, Hegazy MG (2007) The diagnostic efficacy of urinary TGF-beta1 and VEGF in bladder cancer: comparison with voided urine cytology. Cancer Biomark 3: 275–285.

27. Abogunrin F, O'Kane HF, Ruddock MW, Stevenson M, Reid CN, et al. (2011) The impact of biomarkers in multivariate algorithms for bladder cancer diagnosis in patients with hematuria. Cancer 18: 2641–2650.

28. Henry RJ (1974) Clinical Chemistry, Principles and Techniques. New York: Harper and Row. 525p.

29. Bazari H (2007). Approach to the patient with renal disease. In: Goldman L, Ausiello D, editors. Cecil Medicine. Philadelphia: Saunders Elsevier. chap 115.

30. Sertic J, Slavicek J, Bozina N, Malenica B, Kes P, et al. (2007) Cytokines and growth factors in mostly atherosclerotic patients on hemodialysis determined by biochip array technology. Clinical Chemistry and Laboratory Medicine : CCLM/FESCC 45: 1347–1352.

31. Fitzgerald SP, Lamont JV, McConnell RI, Benchikh el O (2005) Development of a high-throughput automated analyzer using biochip array technology. Clin Chem 51: 1165–1176.

32. Kashif W, Siddiqi N, Dincer AP, Dincer HE, Hirsch S (2003) Proteinuria: how to evaluate an important finding. Cleve Clin J Med 70: 535–7, 541–4, 546–7.

33. Perkovic V, Verdon C, Ninomiya T, Barzi F, Cass A, et al. (2008) The relationship between proteinuria and coronary risk: a systematic review and meta-analysis. PLoS Med 5: e207.

3

Reference miRNAs for miRNAome Analysis of Urothelial Carcinomas

Nadine Ratert[1,2], Hellmuth-Alexander Meyer[1,3], Monika Jung[1], Hans-Joachim Mollenkopf[4], Ina Wagner[4], Kurt Miller[1], Ergin Kilic[5], Andreas Erbersdobler[6], Steffen Weikert[1], Klaus Jung[1,2]*

1 Department of Urology, University Hospital Charité, Berlin, Germany, 2 Berlin Institute for Urologic Research, Berlin, Germany, 3 Institute of Physiology, University Hospital Charité, Berlin, Germany, 4 Max Planck Institute for Infection Biology, Berlin, Germany, 5 Institute of Pathology, University Hospital Charité, Berlin, Germany, 6 Institute of Pathology, University Rostock, Rostock, Germany

Abstract

Background/Objective: Reverse transcription quantitative real-time PCR (RT-qPCR) is widely used in microRNA (miRNA) expression studies on cancer. To compensate for the analytical variability produced by the multiple steps of the method, relative quantification of the measured miRNAs is required, which is based on normalization to endogenous reference genes. No study has been performed so far on reference miRNAs for normalization of miRNA expression in urothelial carcinoma. The aim of this study was to identify suitable reference miRNAs for miRNA expression studies by RT-qPCR in urothelial carcinoma.

Methods: Candidate reference miRNAs were selected from 24 urothelial carcinoma and normal bladder tissue samples by miRNA microarrays. The usefulness of these candidate reference miRNAs together with the commonly for normalization purposes used small nuclear RNAs RNU6B, RNU48, and Z30 were thereafter validated by RT-qPCR in 58 tissue samples and analyzed by the algorithms geNorm, NormFinder, and BestKeeper.

Principal Findings: Based on the miRNA microarray data, a total of 16 miRNAs were identified as putative reference genes. After validation by RT-qPCR, miR-101, miR-125a-5p, miR-148b, miR-151-5p, miR-181a, miR-181b, miR-29c, miR-324-3p, miR-424, miR-874, RNU6B, RNU48, and Z30 were used for geNorm, NormFinder, and BestKeeper analyses that gave different combinations of recommended reference genes for normalization.

Conclusions: The present study provided the first systematic analysis for identifying suitable reference miRNAs for miRNA expression studies of urothelial carcinoma by RT-qPCR. Different combinations of reference genes resulted in reliable expression data for both strongly and less strongly altered miRNAs. Notably, RNU6B, which is the most frequently used reference gene for miRNA studies, gave inaccurate normalization. The combination of four (miR-101, miR-125a-5p, miR-148b, and miR-151-5p) or three (miR-148b, miR-181b, and miR-874,) reference miRNAs is recommended for normalization.

Editor: Bernard W. Futscher, The University of Arizona, United States of America

Funding: This study was partly supported by grants from the Foundation for Urological Research (BFIU_2010), the SONNENFELD-Stiftung (89838210), and the Federal Ministry of Education and Research (MedSys). The funders had no role in study design, data collection and analysis, decision to publish, or preparation of the manuscript.

Competing Interests: The authors have declared that no competing interests exist.

* E-mail: klaus.jung@charite.de

Introduction

MicroRNAs (miRNAs) belong to a class of small noncoding RNAs of 19 to 24 nucleotides that are known to regulate signaling pathways for various cell functions. Not surprisingly, changes in miRNA expression have been associated with several diseases, including cancer [1,2]. It has been shown that different tumors have specific miRNA expression profiles and that miRNA profiles correlate with patient diagnosis, prognosis, and responses to treatment [3]. Thus, analyzing the differential expression of the microRNAome [4], defined as the entirety of all miRNAs in a cell, is of scientific and practical significance.

Several methods such as bead-based flow cytometry, microarray, deep sequencing, and real-time quantitative PCR (RT-qPCR) allow fast, high-throughput, and sensitive profiling of miRNAs. RT-qPCR

produces specific, sensitive, and reproducible quantification of nucleic acids. To overcome experimental variations in RT-qPCR analyses (RNA isolation, cDNA synthesis, PCR runs), relative quantification of miRNAs of interest based on the normalization to reference genes is the approach of choice to prevent errors within a dataset [5]. This approach complies with normalization procedures used in mRNA expression studies and is summarized in the recent MIQE guidelines [6]. Suitable reference genes should be expressed constitutively and be independent of biological changes, diseases or treatments. The use of multiple rather than single reference genes has been recommended for RT-qPCR data normalization [7,8]. The computional programs geNorm [9] and NormFinder [10] are based on this principle. These tools allow identifying the most stable reference genes from a panel of putative reference genes for normalization. Moreover, several studies in addition to our own experiments have shown that the use of inappropriate reference genes in the relative quantification of gene expression can result in biased expression profiles [11–13]. As there are no universal reference genes [14,15], it is strongly recommended that researchers test for the most suitable reference genes specific to the tissues and experimental conditions used.

Because of our general interest on miRNAomes in urological tumors and the increasing incidence of urothelial cancer [16], we performed a literature search in PubMed. The MeSH term "microRNAs" was combined with the search string ["micro-RNAs" OR "microRNA" OR "miRNA" OR "miRNAs"] and in combination with the MeSH term "urinary bladder neoplasms". Fifty-eight articles published until May 2012 were identified, of which 27 investigated miRNA expression. Specifically, 20 publications reported miRNA expression by RT-qPCR and used small nuclear, nucleolar or ribosomal RNAs as well as mRNAs for normalization, namely RNU6B (15 times) [17–31], RNU48 (6 times) [17,18,32–35], RNU43 (1 time) [30], RNU44 (1 time) [18], beta-actin (1 time) [36], and 18srRNA (1 time) [32] without confirming their validity for normalization. Thus, no systematic study has been performed to identify suitable miRNA reference genes in urothelial carcinoma while corresponding studies have been performed for other cancer entities, including urological tumors [13,37–40].

Bladder cancer is the fourth most common cancer in Western industrialized countries [16]. Approximately 90% of all urothelial neoplasms are classified as urothelial carcinoma. Although surgical techniques and treatments have improved over time, bladder cancer is still a common cancer with a high mortality. To date, mechanisms of urothelial carcinogenesis have not been fully elucidated. However, miRNA expression patterns have been linked to clinical outcomes in urothelial carcinoma [18,24]. Therefore, single miRNA biomarkers or biomarker signatures of multiple miRNAs may improve risk stratification of patients and may supplement the histological diagnosis of urological tumors including bladder cancer [24,41–43]. In addition, miRNAs and their regulated genes represent interesting drug targets because miRNAs can influence the expression of multiple genes and thereby affect numerous points in disease pathways [22,44–46]. The significance of miRNAs in the regulation of signal transduction in bladder cancer was recently summarized [47]. Improved knowledge in this field will contribute to enhanced prognosis and selection of treatment strategies. However, as mentioned above, accurate quantification of miRNA expression by RT-qPCR and thus reliable expression data require proper normalization strategies. Computer programs based on various algorithms including geNorm [9], NormFinder [10], and BestKeeper [48] have been developed to rank putative reference genes according to their expression stability and indicate the best reference gene or combination of reference genes for accurate normalization.

In the present study, we aimed to systematically identify suitable reference genes for normalizing RT-qPCR assays of miRNA expression in urothelial carcinoma tissue. Using miRNA microarray analyses, we first identified invariant miRNAs that showed stable expression in both nonmalignant and malignant bladder tissue samples as candidate reference miRNAs. RT-qPCR analyses were subsequently performed for validating these miRNAs from the microarray experiments and the above mentioned small RNAs RNU6B, RNU48, and Z30 as putative reference genes. Appropriate reference miRNAs were identified by geNorm, NormFinder, and BestKeeper, and the results of unsuitable normalization are illustrated with invalid normalizers.

Materials and Methods

Patients and Tissue Samples

All bladder cancer patients went through radical cystectomy or transurethral resection at the University Hospital Charité in Berlin between 2008 and 2009 and gave written informed consent for the use of representative tissue specimens for research purposes. The study was approved by the Ethic Committee of the University Hospital Charité (File: EA1/153/07). The samples were collected immediately after surgery in liquid nitrogen and stored at $-80°C$ until further analysis. Tumor staging was performed in conformity with the International Union Against Cancer [49] and histological grading in accordance with the WHO/ISUP criteria of 2004 [50]. In total, 58 urothelial samples were included in this study. Seventeen samples were from nonmalignant bladder tissue (15 male, 2 female patients; median age 68, range 47–80 years), 20 samples were from low-grade papillary urothelial carcinoma (18 male, 2 female patients; median age 68, range 50–86 years), and 21 samples were from high-grade tumors (14 male, 7 female patients; median age 73, range 48–82 years).

Isolation of RNA and Characterization of Quantity and Quality

Frozen histologic sections were prepared, stained with hematoxylin/eosin, and examined by uropathologists (A.E., E.K.). Only tissue specimens with more than 80% tumor cells were included in the study as tumor samples. Tissue cryotome sections (approximately 20–30 mg of tissue, wet weight) were treated with 350 μl of lysis buffer and total RNA including miRNAs was isolated using the miRNeasy Mini Kit (Qiagen, Hilden, Germany) with 30 to 50 μl of elution buffer according to the manufacturer's protocol. An additional DNase I digestion step on the RNA binding silica gel membrane of the spin column was performed. RNA concentration and the 260 nm to 280 nm absorbance ratios were measured on the NanoDrop 1000 spectrophotometer (NanoDrop Technologies, Wilmington, DE, USA). The quality of isolated RNA was determined by the RNA integrity number (RIN) with a Bioanalyzer 2100 (Agilent Technologies, Santa Clara, CA, USA). Only samples with RIN values >5 were used. The RNA samples (medians: 693 ng/μl; 830 ng/mg tissue) isolated from nonmalignant as well as from low-grade and high-grade tumor tissue samples showed comparable median 260/280 absorbance ratios (2.02, 2.03, and 2.03) and RIN values (6.7, 5.9, and 6.3; Kruskal-Wallis test, P = 0.171).

Microarray-based miRNA Analysis

Microarray analyses of eight samples each from nonmalignant tissue and low and high grade tumor specimens were performed. One-color hybridizations on human catalog 8-plex 15 K microRNA microarrays (AMADID 019118) from Agilent encoding probes for 723 human and 76 viral microRNAs from the Sanger database v10.1 were used. All reaction steps were carried out as previously described in detail [51]. After hybridization, microarrays were washed, scanned, and processed according to the supplier's protocol. The raw data were normalized using Genespring GX11 Software (Agilent) with default parameters (threshold raw signal to 1.0, percent shift to 90th percentile as normalization algorithm and no baseline transformation). All microarray data have been deposited in the NCBI GEO database with accession number GSE36121. Further data analysis is described in the Results section.

Quantitative Real-time PCR

RT-qPCR analyses of miRNAs were carried out with TaqMan microRNA assays (Applied Biosystems, Foster City, CA, USA) according to the manufacturer's protocol and the MIQE guidelines [6] (Table S1) as previously described [13]. The reverse transcription of miRNAs from total RNA (10 ng) was performed with miRNA-specific stem-loop primers, 10 nmol dNTP mix, 2.6 U of RNase Inhibitor, 33.5 U of MultiScribe RT enzyme, and 1 × RT Buffer (Applied Biosystems). The generated cDNAs were stored at 20°C until analysis. The qPCR measurements were executed in white 96-well PCR plates (cat.no. 04729692001 with sealing foils) with a 10 µl of final volume containing 1 µl of RNA-specific cDNA, 1× TaqMan Universal PCR Master Mix No AmpErase UNG, and gene-specific TaqMan MiRNA real-time PCR assay solution on the Light Cycler 480 Instrument (Roche Diagnostics GmbH, Mannheim, Germany; software version 1.5.0) (Table S2). The reaction was performed at 95°C for 10 min, followed by 45 cycles of 95°C for 15 s, and 60°C for 60 s. All samples were measured in triplicate; each PCR run included a no-template control and two inter-plate calibrators. All no-template controls were negative. To assess the specific amplification efficiencies, we created calibration curves from dilution series of miRNA-specific cDNAs or small nuclear RNAs (Methods S1). The efficiency was determined from the slope of the log regression plot of Cq values versus log input of cDNA. Efficiencies were in the range between 81% and 88%. All data were corrected to the PCR efficiency and to the inter-run calibrators. For that purpose, the software qBase^{PLUS} (Biogazelle NV, Zwijnaarde, Belgium) was used, employing a generalized and universally applicable quantification model based on efficiency correction, error propagation, and multiple reference gene normalization [52]. The intra-run precision for the finally considered candidate reference miRNAs miR-29c, miR-101, miR-125a-5p, miR-148b, miR-151-3p, miR-151-5p, miR-181a, miR-181b, miR-324-3p, miR-424, and miR-874 as well as the investigated small nuclear RNU6B, RNU48, and Z30 ranged from 0.15% to 0.35% for mean Cq values between 21.93 to 26.65. The between-run precision (n = 42) measured for the control miR-21 was found to be 1.62% (mean Cq ± standard deviation: 28.35±0.46).

Data Analysis

Statistical analyses were performed using GraphPad Prism Version 5.04 (GraphPad Software Inc., La Jolla, CA, USA). Non-parametric tests (Mann-Whitney U test; Kruskal-Wallis test with Dunn's multiple comparison test) were used to analyze significant differences between independent groups. The Spearman correlation coefficients were applied to calculate the relationships between the miRNAs as well as between the clinical variables and the expression of candidate reference miRNAs. P values <0.05 (two-tailed) were considered statistically significant.

The assessment of the putative reference genes for normalization was evaluated by the computer programs geNorm [9] using the improved version geNorm^{Plus} as an implementation of the software qBase^{PLUS} (Biogazelle, Belgium) [52], NormFinder [10], and BestKeeper [48].

Results

Selection of Candidate Reference miRNAs by Microarray Analysis

To identify putative reference miRNAs in the miRNA microarray data obtained from the eight samples of each tissue group, the following criteria were used: (a) miRNAs had to be detected in Genespring GX11 software as "present" in all

Table 1. Candidate reference miRNAs selected from microarray analysis.[†]

miRNA[&]	ID according miRBase version[#]	Selection criterion[§]
hsa-miR-15a	hsa-miR-15a (v10.1)	R
	hsa-miR-15a-5p (v18)	
hsa-miR-20b	hsa-miR-20b (v10.1)	R
	hsa-miR-20b-5p (v18)	
hsa-miR-29c	hsa-miR-29c (v10.1)	R
	hsa-miR-29c-3p(v18)	
hsa-miR-101	hsa-miR-101 (v10.1)	N
	hsa-miR-101-3p (v18)	
hsa-miR-107	hsa-miR-107 (v10.1)	N
	hsa-miR-107 (v18)	
hsa-miR-125a-5p	hsa-miR-125a-5p (v10.1)	N
	hsa-miR-125a-5p (v18)	
hsa-miR-148b	hsa-miR-148b (v10.1)	R
	hsa-miR-148b-3p (v18)	
hsa-miR-151-3p	hsa-miR-151-3p (v10.1)	R
	hsa-miR-151-3p (v18)	
hsa-miR-151-5p	hsa-miR-151-5p (v10.1)	N
	hsa-miR-151-5p (v18)	
hsa-miR-181a	hsa-miR-181a (v10.1)	R
	hsa-miR-181a-5p (v18)	
hsa-miR-181b	hsa-miR-181b (v10.1)	R
	hsa-miR-181b-5p (v18)	
hsa-miR-324-3p	hsa-miR-324-3p (v10.1)	N
	hsa-miR-324-3p (v18)	
hsa-miR-424	hsa-miR-424 (v10.1)	N
	hsa-miR-424-5p (v18)	
hsa-miR-513a-5p	hsa-miR-513a-5p (v10.1)	R
	hsa-miR-513a-5p (v18)	
hsa-miR-874	hsa-miR-874 (v10.1)	N
	hsa-miR-874 (v18)	
hsa-miR-939	hsa-miR-939 (v10.1)	N
	hsa-miR-939 (v18)	

[†]The TaqMan MicroRNA Assay ID, miRBase accession number, and the sequence for each miRNA are compiled in Table S2.
[&]miRNAs marked in Italics were not included in further analyses because their low expression level was beyond the dynamic range of the assay (>35Cq) (further details see text).
[#]The miRNA ID from the miRBase version 10.1 and 18, respectively.
[§]Symbols "N" and "R" indicate the selection of the candidate reference miRNAs based on normalized or raw microarray data as described in the text.

examined 24 samples to filter out signals that did not reach a minimum of intensity, (b) the absolute fold change between the nonmalignant and the two cancerous groups had to be lower than 1.2-times with (c) no significant differences (P>0.05) between the groups. Based on the total of 723 human miRNA species located on the Agilent microarray chip according to the miRBase version 10.1, we identified 101 miRNAs that were flagged as "present" in all of the examined groups (Table S3). Eight of these miRNAs showed absolute fold changes lower than 1.2-times and had no significant differences between the groups (Table 1, indicated by

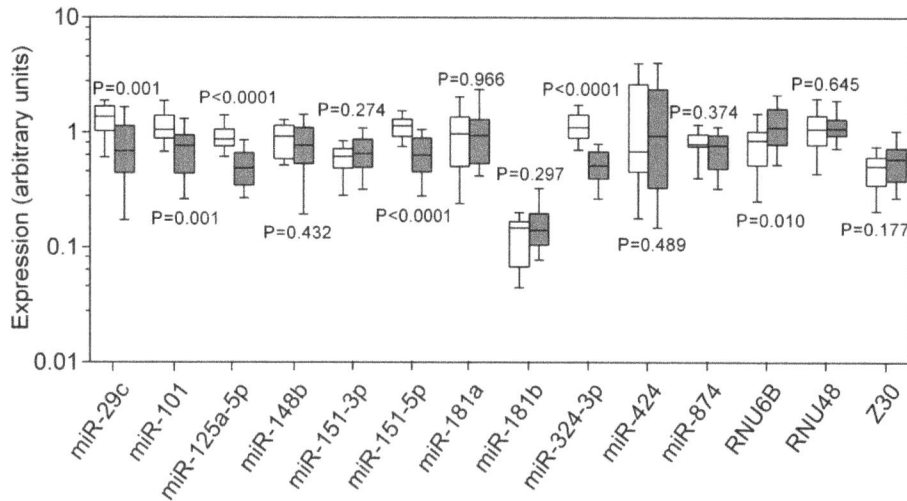

Figure 1. Expression of candidate reference genes in human nonmalignant and malignant bladder tissue samples. RT-qPCR analyses were performed from 17 nonmalignant bladder tissue samples and 41 samples from low-grade and high-grade papillary urothelial carcinoma. Expression levels of the candidate reference genes are given as arbitrary units. Boxes (blank, nonmalignant samples; black, malignant samples) represent lower and upper quartiles with median as horizontal line; whiskers depict the 10 and 90 percentiles. Significances are illustrated as *P* values of the Mann-Whitney *U* test.

the symbol "N"). To avoid normalization artifacts of the microarray data, we also used raw microarray expression data. Thus, with the criteria mentioned above, we revealed a second set of eight candidate reference miRNAs (Table 1, indicated by symbol "R"). Taking these sets together, 16 putative reference miRNAs were included in further analyses (Table 1; Table S2).

Validation of Candidate Reference Genes by RT-qPCR

To increase the statistical power to find suitable reference miRNAs, in addition to the 24 analyzed samples in the microarray experiments, we included nine nonmalignant and 25 malignant tissue samples as described in the section "Patients and tissue samples" to validate the aforementioned 16 candidate reference miRNAs in more detail by RT-qPCR. Furthermore, the set of candidate reference miRNAs was extended by the small RNAs RNU6B, RNU48, and Z30 that were commonly used for expression normalization in the literature as stated in the Introduction. First, to determine if reliable quantification of these putative normalizers is feasible by RT-qPCR, three RNA pools were prepared containing equal amounts of RNA from the samples used in the microarray analysis. miR-15a, miR-20b, miR-107, miR-513a-5p, and miR-939 showed Cq values >35 in the pools and were excluded from further analyses because accurate quantification would be questionable. By this preselection, 11 putative reference miRNAs (Table 1: miR-29c, miR-101, miR-125a-5p, miR-148b, miR-151-3p, miR-151-5p, miR-181a, miR-181b, miR-324-3p, miR-424, and miR-874) as well as RNU6B, RNU48, and Z30 were further investigated and showed Cq values ranging from 22 (RNU48) to 28 (miR-324-3p).

In the second step, all 14 reference candidates were separately measured in the 58 samples (Figure 1). The expression levels significantly differed for miR-29c (P=0.0012), miR-101 (P=0.0007), miR-125a-5p (P<0.0001), miR-151-5p (P<0.0001), miR-324-3p (P<0.0001), and RNU6B (P=0.0101) between nonmalignant and malignant samples. The remaining eight miRNAs, namely miR-148b, miR-151-3p, miR-181a, miR-181b, miR-424, miR-874, RNU48, and Z30, revealed no significant differences between nonmalignant and malignant samples

(P>0.05). We followed the general recommendation of the geNorm program and included all these putative reference miRNAs and small RNAs in further analyses for reassessing their potential contribution as normalizers. However, miR-151-3p was excluded due to the fact that miR-151-3p and miR-151-5p are mature miRNAs of the same pre-miRNA and miR-151-5p exhibited higher expression in examined samples.

Association between the Candidate Reference miRNAs and Clinical Variables

The correlation between the putative reference miRNAs and the correlation of these miRNAs with age, sex, and tumor characteristics were determined. Spearman rank correlations are summarized in Table S4. Classifying miRNA pairs with coefficients ≥0.60 as co-expressed, we identified this characteristic co-expression feature among the four miRNAs miR-101, miR-125a-5p, miR-151-5p and miR-324-3p as well as between miR-148 and miR-151-3p, and between miR-181a and miR-181b. The correlation between miR-101, miR-151-5p, and miR-324-3p was remarkable.

The expression of the 11 miRNAs and three small RNAs was not associated with age (Spearman rank correlation from r_S −0.23 to 0.177, P values from 0.083 to 0.974), sex (Mann-Whitney U test, P values from 0.062 to 0.851), or tumor stage (Ta, T1, T2, T3; Kruskal-Wallis test, P values from 0.092 to 0.826, except for miR-29c, which had P=0.044). Differences in expression between low-grade and high-grade tumors were found for miR-29c (down-regulated, P=0.005), miR-874 (down-regulated, P=0.019), miR-181a (up-regulated, P=0.031), and miR-181b (up-regulated, P=0.0008), while all other miRNAs were not differentially expressed (P values from 0.092 to 0.826).

Identification of Suitable Reference miRNAs using geNorm, NormFinder, and BestKeeper

To identify suitable reference genes for the normalization of miRNA expression, we applied the aforementioned three computer programs geNorm, NormFinder, and BestKeeper. GeNorm, an implementation of the new software qBase^PLUS, automatically returns the average expression stability value M and the average

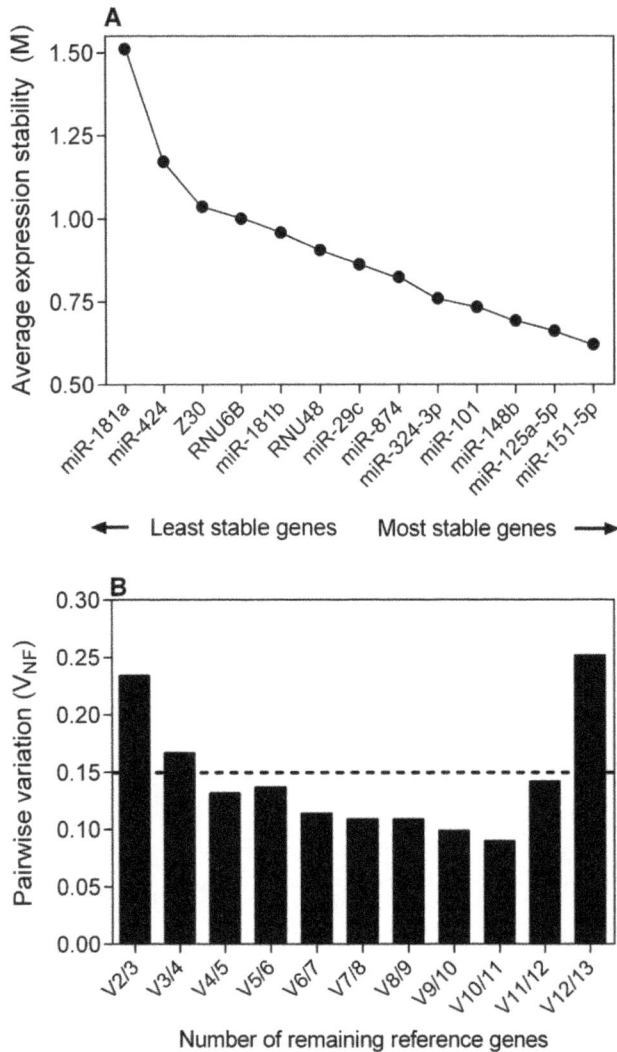

Figure 2. geNorm analysis of RT-qPCR-based candidate reference genes. (A) The geNorm analysis shows the calculation of the average expression stability value M of all candidate reference genes determined by RT-qPCR. Genes with the highest M value have the least stable expression, while the genes with the lowest M value have the most stable expression. The x-axis presents the ranking of reference genes in order of increasing stability from left to right. (B) Calculation of the optimal number of reference genes for normalization. geNorm calculates a normalization factor assessing the optimal number of reference genes for generating that factor. The normalization factor is calculated from at least two genes taking into account the variable V as the average pairwise variation (V_{NF}) between two sequential normalization factors. The thin broken line illustrates the cut-off value V_{NF} <0.15. In this experiment, the optimal number of reference genes was four (V4/5). geNorm shows the variation of the normalization factor of four genes as the best combination (miR-101, miR-148b; miR-125a-5p, and miR-151-5p) in relation to five genes as shown in (A) and in the following order. All the results are presented according to the output files of the geNorm program.

pairwise variation V of a particular gene with all other control genes. The highest M value indicates the gene with the least stable expression. Figure 2A and Table 2 indicate the M values and the resulting ranking order of all investigated candidate reference miRNAs and small RNAs based on expression stability. miR-181a (M = 1.511) showed the highest M value, whereas miR-151-5p (M = 0.622) and miR-125a-5p (M = 0.663) showed the lowest M

values. Consequently, miR-181a had the least stable expression while miR-125a-5p and miR-151-5p had the most stable expression. Additionally, geNorm calculates a normalization factor (V_{NF} value), which is a criterion for the optimum number of reference genes (Figure 2B). The program recommends V_{NF} values less than 0.15 for proper normalization. When this cut-off value is achieved, it is not necessary to include any additional reference genes. As illustrated in Figure 2B, the four miRNAs miR-101, miR-148b, miR-125a-5p, and miR-151-5p (V_{NF} value 0.14) were recommended as an optimum reference miRNA set for normalization; the best combination of two reference miRNAs was miR-125a-5p and miR-151-5p, and the best single reference miRNA was miR-151-5p. After excluding the potentially deregulated reference miRNAs mentioned above, geNorm analysis was repeated. However, under these conditions, geNorm calculated a V_{NF} value >0.15 and therefore did not recommend a normalization set.

Similar to geNorm, NormFinder identified genes with the lowest M values as the most stably expressed reference targets (Table 2). NormFinder ranked the four best reference genes for normalization as miR-148, miR-874, miR-181b, and Z30. Z30 and miR-125a-5p were recommended as the best combination, and miR-148b was recommended as the best single normalizer (Table 2).

BestKeeper considers all genes in all observed groups. First, BestKeeper determines the geometric mean and coefficient of variance. Genes with a standard deviation greater than 1 were assumed to be inconsistent. In the second step, the inter-gene relationships were examined by pairwise correlation analysis. This calculation is used to determine whether the gene expression exhibits a similar behavior. Candidate reference genes that highly correlate with each other are included in the BestKeeper-Index calculation. The program provides only an analysis of ten candidate reference genes simultaneously. Therefore, we excluded the reference targets with the lowest M values as determined by geNorm (miR-181a) and NormFinder (miR-424) and also excluded miR-29c (rank 9 by geNorm; rank 11 by NormFinder). Under these conditions, BestKeeper ranked RNU48 as the best reference gene, followed by miR-874, miR-151-5p, and Z30.

The comparison of the summarized data in Table 2 shows that the results provided by NormFinder and BestKeeper displayed slight differences from the geNorm analysis but did have some overlap. While geNorm recommended miR-101, miR-125a-5p, miR-148b, and miR-151-5p for proper normalization, NormFinder indicated miR-148b as the best reference miRNA and miR-125a-5p as a part of the best combination. Additionally, BestKeeper identified miR-151-5p within the four most stably expressed miRNAs. As stated in the Introduction, the small nucleolar RNU6B is commonly used for miRNA expression normalization and in our study was ranked 10th by geNorm, 12th by NormFinder, and 9th by BestKeeper (Table 2). Thus, RNU6B seems to be a rather inappropriate reference gene for the miRNA expression normalization in studies on bladder cancer.

Influence of Reference miRNA Selection on the Accuracy of Relative Quantification

To illustrate the impact of reference gene selection on miRNA expression analysis, we applied different normalization strategies for the relative quantification of miR-200a and miR-20a (Figure 3A–B). A preliminary evaluation of the miRNA microarray data showed a strong up-regulation of miR-200a (fold change 22.1) and a less robust, but significant up-regulation of miR-20a (fold change 2.78) in the tumor samples compared to the nonmalignant tissue samples. Different normalization approaches

Table 2. Ranking of candidate reference miRNAs and small RNAs in human nonmalignant and malignant bladder tissues according to their stability value using geNorm, NormFinder, and BestKeeper algorithms.

Gene name	geNorm		NormFinder		BestKeeper	
	Stability value[&]	Rank	Stability value[&]	Rank	SD [±x-fold][#]	Rank
miR-101	0.734	4	0.215	8	0.69	10
miR-125a-5p	0.663	2	0.192	6	0.62	5
miR-148b	0.693	3	0.086	1	0.65	8
miR-151-5p	0.622	1	0.230	9	0.60	3
miR-181a	1.511	13	0.209	7	–	
miR-181b	0.959	9	0.155	3	0.62	6
miR-29c	0.863	7	0.246	10	–	
miR-324-3p	0.76	5	0.291	11	0.64	7
miR-424	1.172	12	0.371	13	–	
miR-874	0.824	6	0.102	2	0.53	2
RNU6B	1.001	10	0.349	12	0.67	9
RNU48	0.906	8	0.173	5	0.51	1
Z30	1.037	11	0.171	4	0.61	4
Best gene	miR-151-5p		miR-148b		RNU48	
Best combination	miR-101, miR-125a-5p, miR-148b, miR-151-5p		Z30, miR-125a-5p		–	

[&]High expression stability is indicated by low stability value.
[#]SD [±x-fold]: standard deviation of the absolute regulation coefficients. SD >1 can be considered inconsistent.

were used based on the recommendations by geNorm, NormFinder, and BestKeeper as described above. As shown in Figure 3, we normalized the expression of miR-200a and miR-20a using the geNorm recommended reference miRNAs as follows: (a) the combination of four reference miRNAs that were suggested to be necessary for reliable normalization (geometric mean of miR-101, miR-125a-5p, miR-148b, and miR-151-5p; Table 2); (b) the three best ranked miRNAs according to their M values (miR-125a-5p, miR-148b, and miR-151-5p); and (c) the best combination of two miRNAs (miR-125a-5p and miR-151-5p). The NormFinder recommended approaches were the following: (d) the best two reference gene combination (miR-125a-5p and Z30); (e) the three best ranked reference miRNAs (miR-148b, miR-181b, and miR-874), and (f) the best single miRNA miR-148b. Based on the BestKeeper recommendation, we also used (g) the calculated best single reference gene RNU48. In addition, we performed normalization with (h) RNU6B, which was estimated by all three programs to have low usefulness as a reference gene but is frequently used in expression studies. Regardless of the normalization approach, miR-200a was found to be up-regulated (Figure 3A). However, the expression pattern of miR-20a was different depending on the normalization approach (Figure 3B). Using the reference miRNAs recommended by geNorm or NormFinder, miR-20a appeared to be up-regulated in tumor samples, whereas normalization with RNU6B or RNU48 as recommended by BestKeeper did not show up-regulation of this miRNA. Thus, although all reference miRNA suggestions by geNorm and NormFinder were obviously suited to be appropriate for normalization, we recommend the use of more than two reference miRNAs preferring the use of four miRNAs (miR-101, miR-148b, miR-125a-5p, and miR-151-5p) as recommended by geNorm or the combination of three miRNAs (miR-148b, miR-181b, and miR-874) suggested by NormFinder. The two-miRNA combinations or single miRNAs should be cautiously considered

as alternative normalization approaches only if limited sample material is available for analysis.

Discussion

The selection of suitable reference genes as normalizers for relative quantification of mRNA and miRNA expression is essential to avoid erroneous expression results and to improve the comparability of gene expression data between different studies. Different models such as the global mean normalization [5], panels of miRNAs [37] or small RNAs [53] have been suggested for the normalization of miRNA expression data. D'haene et al. [54] recently reported that the side-by-side comparison of small nuclear RNA normalization with global mean normalization indicated that small nuclear RNAs are less efficient in reducing the technical variation and do not reveal in accurate expression differences. In addition, the recommended global mean normalization method [5] that is also included in the algorithm of the qBase[PLUS] software requires a large number of genes, for example in microarray, deep sequencing, bead-based or TaqMan array card analyses. Thus, the global normalization approach is not feasible in RT-qPCR studies because only a few miRNAs are generally measured. In this case, the normalization of miRNA RT-qPCR data with suitable miRNA reference markers can be considered as the method of choice [55].

Studies to identify and validate suitable reference miRNAs have been performed for several cancers [13,37–40]. As discussed in the Introduction, it is therefore quite astonishing that no miRNA expression studies in bladder cancer have used endogenous miRNAs for normalization. Only nuclear, nucleolar, and ribosomal RNAs as well as mRNAs have been used. However, the different lengths of these RNAs compared to miRNAs result in different physico-chemical properties with different isolation efficiencies and degradation [56,57]. miRNAs are more stable

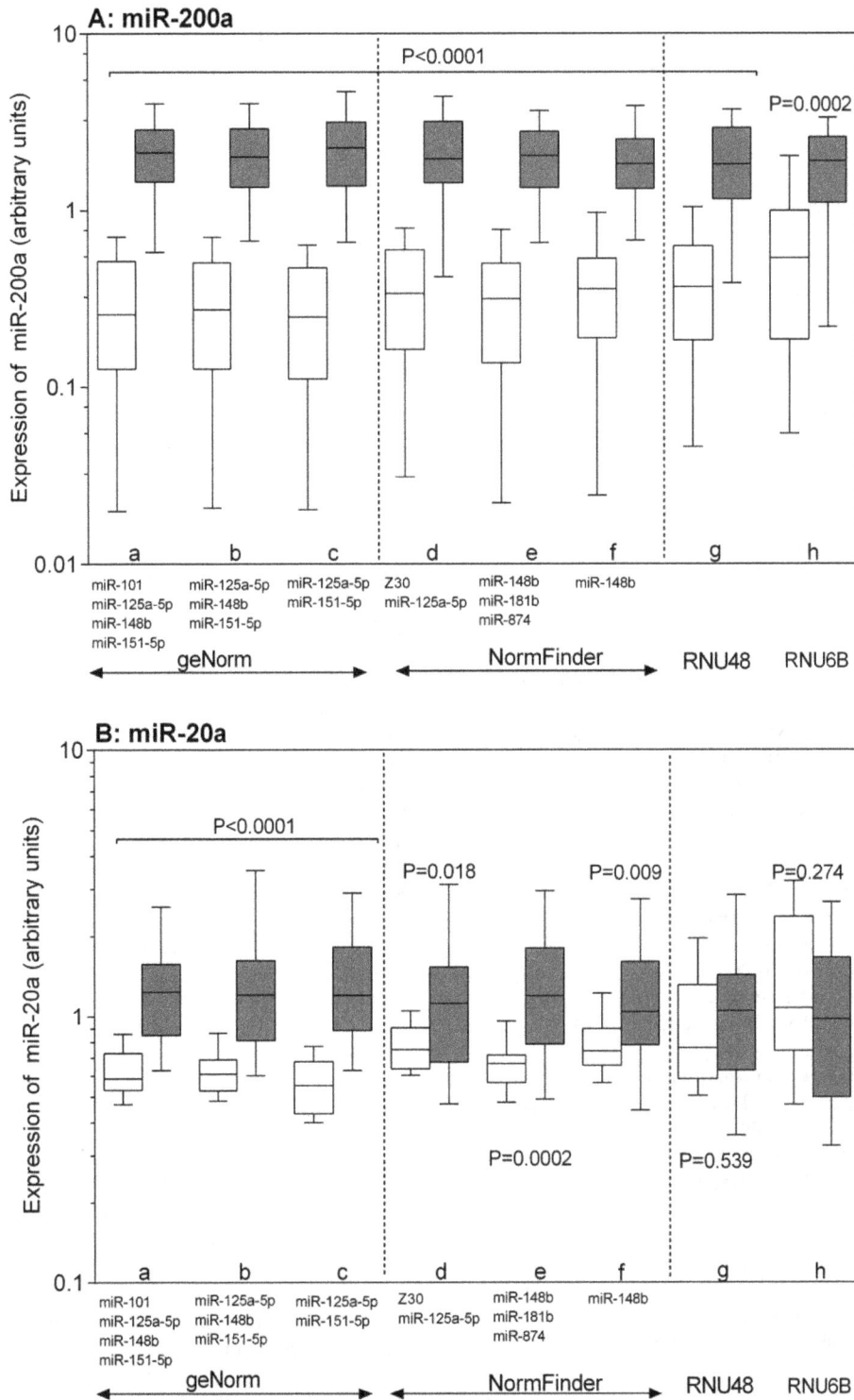

Figure 3. Effects of different normalization approaches on the expression of miR-200a and miR-20a. The relative expression of (A) miR-200a and (B) miR-20a as highly and moderately differentially expressed miRNAs, respectively was calculated using the following normalization strategies recommended by geNorm (a–c), NormFinder (d–f), BestKeeper (g), and RNU6B (h). The geNorm approaches were: (a) the four-reference-miRNA combination recommended as necessary number of reference miRNAs (miR-101, miR-125a-5p, miR-148b, miR-151-5p); (b) the three best ranked miRNAs according to their M values (miR-125a-5p, miR-148b, and miR-151-5p) and (c) the best two-gene-reference combination (miR-125a-5p, miR-151-5p). NormFinder normalization approaches were: (d) the best two reference gene combination (miR-125a-5p, Z30); (e) the three best ranked reference genes (miR-148b, miR-181b, miR-874); (f) the best single miRNA, miR-148b. BestKeeper normalization approach was (g) RNU48; (j) RNU6B as the most frequently recommended normalizer in bladder cancer studies. Values are given as arbitrary units; boxes (blank, nonmalignant tissue; black, malignant tissue) represent lower and upper quartiles with medians as horizontal line; whiskers depict the 10–90 percentiles. Significances are illustrated as *P* values of the Mann-Whitney *U* test.

than mRNAs or small RNAs like RNU6B, and they can therefore be more accurately detected in tissues [57]. In addition, different techniques of reverse transcription used for miRNAs and the other RNAs make the latter less suitable for normalization. Furthermore, as previously shown for mRNAs, the tissue-specific expression of miRNAs is also reflected in the behavior of putative endogenous reference genes [14,15]. Thus, RT-qPCR-based miRNA expression studies optimally require normalization by reference miRNAs. Previous reports from our group have demonstrated the importance of suitable reference miRNAs in avoiding biased results in miRNA expression studies in other urological tumors [13,39]. These data strongly support the need for determining appropriate endogenous reference miRNAs to allow stringent normalization of miRNA expression patterns in urothelial carcinoma.

To the best of our knowledge, the present study is the first systematic investigation of suitable normalizers for relative quantification of miRNA expression in bladder cancer. In this study, we combined different strategies for identifying suitable reference miRNAs. A four step approach was used. First, to obtain an overview of the miRNAome in bladder cancer tissue, miRNA microarray analyses for nonmalignant and malignant bladder samples were performed to identify invariant miRNAs as stably-expressed candidate reference miRNAs within the data set. Second, these candidate reference miRNAs were validated by RT-qPCR, in addition to RNU6B, RNU48, and Z30, the most frequently reported reference genes for miRNA expression studies in bladder cancer. Third, the statistical algorithms geNorm, NormFinder, and BestKeeper were applied to identify the most useful endogenous reference miRNAs for relative quantification. Finally, the impact of different normalization approaches was illustrated for two deregulated miRNAs in bladder cancer tissue to emphasize the importance of an appropriate normalization approach.

The starting point of the present study was miRNA microarray analysis. According to the criteria for the microarray data evaluation and the measurability criterion for subsequent RT-qPCR analysis (Cq values <35), 11 invariant miRNAs were identified to be putative reference miRNAs. Since miR-151-3p and miR-151-5p derive from the same pre-miRNA and miR-151-5p exhibited slightly higher expression in examined samples, we included only miR-151-5p in further analysis. A data search in the miRNA bladder cancer studies mentioned in the Introduction showed that miR-29c, one of these 11 invariant, stably expressed miRNAs, was found to be down-regulated in two microarray studies [19,36]. Our subsequent RT-qPCR confirmed this observation (Figure 1). Although we did not eliminate this miRNA from the subsequent analysis for the validation of suitable reference miRNAs through geNorm, NormFinder, and Best-Keeper, miR-29c was never recommended as a reference miRNA by one of these evaluation tools in our following analyses. This finding also indicates the usefulness of the software packages in the search for suitable reference genes.

The putative reference miRNAs identified by the microarray analyses, except miR-151-3p as mentioned, were included with the additional RNAs RNU6B, RNU48, and Z30 in the geNorm, NormFinder, and BestKeeper analysis. Differences in expression observed in the subsequent RT-qPCR measurements between nonmalignant, low-grade, and high-grade tumor samples as well as co-expressions of genes did not exclude candidate reference genes. However, as comprehensively described in the Results section, geNorm, NormFinder, and BestKeeper did not always recommend the same reference miRNAs for normalization (Table 2). The lack of agreement between geNorm and NormFinder results has been described previously [15]. The reasons for these

differences in the ranking order of the putative reference miRNAs might be due to the different calculation models on which the tools are based. NormFinder is an ANOVA-based model, geNorm uses a pairwise comparison model, and BestKeeper determines the optimal reference genes by employing the pairwise correlation analysis on all pairs of candidate reference genes. While the geNorm approach is theoretically robust with regard to inter-sample variations arising from sources such as differing RNA input and quality, it has been shown to prefer co-regulated genes in the selection as normalizers [10]. In this study, geNorm also recommended co-regulated reference miRNAs (miR-101 with miR-125a-5p, miR-151-5p) but miR-324-3p was never recommended as normalizer despite its strong correlation with miR-101 and miR-151-5p.

The differences between the recommended reference miRNAs by the three programs prompted us to validate their suitability in clinical samples (Figure 3A–B). The importance of selecting suitable reference genes for accurate miRNA expression data has been shown not only in mRNA but also in miRNA expression studies [13,37,39,40]. We tested the suitability of the different approaches with miR-200a, a highly up-regulated miRNA, and miR-20a, which is up-regulated less robustly (Figure 3A, B). The results clearly demonstrated that RNUB6, which is the most frequent normalizer used in previous miRNA expression studies in bladder cancer, and RNU48, which was recommended by BestKeeper, were unable to confirm the small expression changes, e.g. for miR-20a. The poor quality of RNU6B as a reference gene has already been reported in miRNA expression studies in renal cell carcinoma and prostate cancer [13,58], where its altered expression stability depended on the degradation of the RNA as compared with miRNAs [13]. In contrast, all geNorm and NormFinder recommendations for single and multiple reference miRNA combinations proved to be suitable normalization approaches in the present study for revealing not only strongly but also less robustly deregulated miRNA expression levels between nonmalignant and malignant urothelial tumor samples. However, we recommend the combination of four (miR-101, miR-125a-5p, miR-148b, and miR-151-5p) or three (miR-148b, miR-181b, and miR-874) reference miRNAs. Although the normalization with the best single (NormFinder) or the best two (geNorm) reference miRNAs in our study gave comparable results to the larger gene sets, the use of multiple reference miRNAs is critical in achieving more reliable expression data [7–10].

In summary, the present study was the first systematic investigation to identify suitable reference miRNAs in a transparent and comprehensive manner for the relative quantification of the microRNAome in urothelial carcinoma. It was based on a four-step approach with microarray analyses, RT-qPCR validation, reference miRNA selection through computer software, and proof of principle with different miRNA expression levels. Starting with 16 putative reference miRNAs from the microarray analysis and three additional small RNAs from the literature, we validated several combinations of reference miRNAs for miRNA expression studies in bladder cancer. We believe that these are robust methods that will allow future studies on the functional roles of miRNAs as regulators in signal transduction and metabolic pathways that are associated with small expression changes.

Supporting Information

Table S1   Description of the experimental details of the RT-qPCR analyses according to the checklist of the MIQE guidelines.

Table S2 TaqMan assays for microRNAs and small nuclear and nucleolar RNAs.

Table S3 List of the 101 miRNAs from the microarray for the identification of candidate reference miRNAs.

Table S4 Spearman rank correlation coefficients (r_s) between the candidate reference genes.

Methods S1 qPCR validation experiments according to the MIQE guidelines with respect to the calibration curves and the dynamic range of measurements.

Acknowledgments

The technical assistance of Silke Rabenhorst is highly appreciated. The authors also would like to thank the staff of the Departments of Urology and Pathology, University Hospital Charité for their help collecting samples. We especially thank two anonymous reviewers for critical comments that were very helpful for improving the manuscript.

Author Contributions

Conceived and designed the experiments: NR MJ HJM AE SW KJ. Performed the experiments: NR MJ HJM IW EK AE. Analyzed the data: NR MJ HAM KJ. Contributed reagents/materials/analysis tools: HJM HAM. Wrote the paper: NR HAM KJ. Provided cancer specimens and clinical information: KM EK AE SW. Critical revision and final approval of manuscript: NK HAM MJ HJM IW KM EK AE SW KJ.

References

1. Calin GA, Croce CM (2006) MicroRNA signatures in human cancers. Nat Rev Cancer 6: 857–866.
2. Zhang B, Pan X, Cobb GP, Anderson TA (2007) microRNAs as oncogenes and tumor suppressors. Dev Biol 302: 1–12.
3. Gottardo F, Liu CG, Ferracin M, Calin GA, Fassan M, et al. (2007) Micro-RNA profiling in kidney and bladder cancers. Urol Oncol 25: 387–392.
4. Liu CG, Calin GA, Meloon B, Gamliel N, Sevignani C, et al. (2004) An oligonucleotide microchip for genome-wide microRNA profiling in human and mouse tissues. Proc Natl Acad Sci U S A 101: 9740–9744.
5. Mestdagh P, Van VP, De WA, Muth D, Westermann F, et al. (2009) A novel and universal method for microRNA RT-qPCR data normalization. Genome Biol 10: R64.
6. Bustin SA, Benes V, Garson JA, Hellemans J, Huggett J, et al. (2009) The MIQE guidelines: minimum information for publication of quantitative real-time PCR experiments. Clin Chem 55: 611–622.
7. Bustin SA (2002) Quantification of mRNA using real-time reverse transcription PCR (RT-PCR): trends and problems. J Mol Endocrinol 29: 23–39.
8. Tricarico C, Pinzani P, Bianchi S, Paglierani M, Distante V, et al. (2002) Quantitative real-time reverse transcription polymerase chain reaction: normalization to rRNA or single housekeeping genes is inappropriate for human tissue biopsies. Anal Biochem 309: 293–300.
9. Vandesompele J, De PK, Pattyn F, Poppe B, Van RN, et al. (2002) Accurate normalization of real-time quantitative RT-PCR data by geometric averaging of multiple internal control gene. Genome Biol 3: RESEARCH0034.
10. Andersen CL, Jensen JL, Orntoft TF (2004) Normalization of real-time quantitative reverse transcription-PCR data: a model-based variance estimation approach to identify genes suited for normalization, applied to bladder and colon cancer data sets. Cancer Res 64: 5245–5250.
11. Dheda K, Huggett JF, Chang JS, Kim LU, Bustin SA, et al. (2005) The implications of using an inappropriate reference gene for real-time reverse transcription PCR data normalization. Anal Biochem 344: 141–143.
12. Ohl F, Jung M, Xu C, Stephan C, Rabien A, et al. (2005) Gene expression studies in prostate cancer tissue: which reference gene should be selected for normalization? J Mol Med 83: 1014–1024.
13. Wotschofsky Z, Meyer HA, Jung M, Fendler A, Wagner I, et al. (2011) Reference genes for the relative quantification of microRNAs in renal cell carcinomas and their metastases. Anal Biochem 417: 233–241.
14. Lee PD, Sladek R, Greenwood CM, Hudson TJ (2002) Control genes and variability: absence of ubiquitous reference transcripts in diverse mammalian expression studies. Genome Res 12: 292–297.
15. Kessler Y, Helfer-Hungerbuehler AK, Cattori V, Meli ML, Zellweger B, et al. (2009) Quantitative TaqMan real-time PCR assays for gene expression normalisation in feline tissues. BMC Mol Biol 10: 106.
16. Siegel R, Naishadham D, Jemal A (2012) Cancer statistics, 2012. CA Cancer J Clin 62: 10–29.
17. Baffa R, Fassan M, Volinia S, O'Hara B, Liu CG, et al. (2009) MicroRNA expression profiling of human metastatic cancers identifies cancer gene targets. J Pathol 219: 214–221.
18. Catto JW, Miah S, Owen HC, Bryant H, Myers K, et al. (2009) Distinct microRNA alterations characterize high- and low-grade bladder cancer. Cancer Res 69: 8472–8481.
19. Dyrskjot L, Ostenfeld MS, Bramsen JB, Silahtaroglu AN, Lamy P, et al. (2009) Genomic profiling of microRNAs in bladder cancer: miR-129 is associated with poor outcome and promotes cell death in vitro. Cancer Res 69: 4851–4860.
20. Friedman JM, Liang G, Liu CC, Wolff EM, Tsai YC, et al. (2009) The putative tumor suppressor microRNA-101 modulates the cancer epigenome by repressing the polycomb group protein EZH2. Cancer Res 69: 2623–2629.
21. Ichimi T, Enokida H, Okuno Y, Kunimoto R, Chiyomaru T, et al. (2009) Identification of novel microRNA targets based on microRNA signatures in bladder cancer. Int J Cancer 125: 345–352.
22. Lin T, Dong W, Huang J, Pan Q, Fan X, et al. (2009) MicroRNA-143 as a tumor suppressor for bladder cancer. J Urol 181: 1372–1380.
23. Hanke M, Hoefig K, Merz H, Feller AC, Kausch I, et al. (2010) A robust methodology to study urine microRNA as tumor marker: microRNA-126 and microRNA-182 are related to urinary bladder cancer. Urol Oncol 28: 655–661.
24. Neely LA, Rieger-Christ KM, Neto BS, Eroshkin A, Garver J, et al. (2010) A microRNA expression ratio defining the invasive phenotype in bladder tumors. Urol Oncol 28: 39–48.
25. Song T, Xia W, Shao N, Zhang X, Wang C, et al. (2010) Differential miRNA expression profiles in bladder urothelial carcinomas. Asian Pac J Cancer Prev 11: 905–911.
26. Han Y, Chen J, Zhao X, Liang C, Wang Y, et al. (2011) MicroRNA expression signatures of bladder cancer revealed by deep sequencing. PLoS One 6: e18286.
27. Cao Y, Yu SL, Wang Y, Guo GY, Ding Q, et al. (2011) MicroRNA-dependent regulation of PTEN after arsenic trioxide treatment in bladder cancer cell line T24. Tumour Biol 32: 179–188.
28. Yamada Y, Enokida H, Kojima S, Kawakami K, Chiyomaru T, et al. (2011) MiR-96 and miR-183 detection in urine serve as potential tumor markers of urothelial carcinoma: correlation with stage and grade, and comparison with urinary cytology. Cancer Sci 102: 522–529.
29. Villadsen SB, Bramsen JB, Ostenfeld MS, Wiklund ED, Fristrup N, et al. (2012) The miR-143/−145 cluster regulates plasminogen activator inhibitor-1 in bladder cancer. Br J Cancer 106: 366–374.
30. Ostenfeld MS, Bramsen JB, Lamy P, Villadsen SB, Fristrup N, et al. (2010) miR-145 induces caspase-dependent and -independent cell death in urothelial cancer cell lines with targeting of an expression signature present in Ta bladder tumors. Oncogene 29: 1073–1084.
31. Lin Y, Wu J, Chen H, Mao Y, Liu Y, et al. (2012) Cyclin-dependent kinase 4 is a novel target in microRNA-195-mediated cell cycle arrest in bladder cancer cells. FEBS Lett 586: 442–447.
32. Tatarano S, Chiyomaru T, Kawakami K, Enokida H, Yoshino H, et al. (2011) miR-218 on the genomic loss region of chromosome 4p15.31 functions as a tumor suppressor in bladder cancer. Int J Oncol 39: 13–21.
33. Wiklund ED, Bramsen JB, Hulf T, Dyrskjot L, Ramanathan R, et al. (2011) Coordinated epigenetic repression of the miR-200 family and miR-205 in invasive bladder cancer. Int J Cancer 128: 1327–1334.
34. Yoshino H, Chiyomaru T, Enokida H, Kawakami K, Tatarano S, et al. (2011) The tumour-suppressive function of miR-1 and miR-133a targeting TAGLN2 in bladder cancer. Br J Cancer 104: 808–818.
35. Hirata H, Hinoda Y, Ueno K, Shahryari V, Tabatabai ZL, et al. (2012) MicroRNA-1826 targets VEGFC, beta-catenin (CTNNB1) and MEK1 (MAP2K1) in human bladder cancer. Carcinogenesis 33: 41–48.
36. Wang G, Zhang H, He H, Tong W, Wang B, et al. (2010) Up-regulation of microRNA in bladder tumor tissue is not common. Int Urol Nephrol 42: 95–102.
37. Chang KH, Mestdagh P, Vandesompele J, Kerin MJ, Miller N (2010) MicroRNA expression profiling to identify and validate reference genes for relative quantification in colorectal cancer. BMC Cancer 10: 173.
38. Davoren PA, McNeill RE, Lowery AJ, Kerin MJ, Miller N (2008) Identification of suitable endogenous control genes for microRNA gene expression analysis in human breast cancer. BMC Mol Biol 9: 76.
39. Schaefer A, Jung M, Miller K, Lein M, Kristiansen G, et al. (2010) Suitable reference genes for relative quantification of miRNA expression in prostate cancer. Exp Mol Med 42: 749–758.
40. Shen Y, Li Y, Ye F, Wang F, Wan X, et al. (2011) Identification of miR-23a as a novel microRNA normalizer for relative quantification in human uterine cervical tissues. Exp Mol Med 43: 358–366.
41. van der Kwast TH, Bapat B (2009) Predicting favourable prognosis of urothelial carcinoma: gene expression and genome profiling. Curr Opin Urol 19: 516–521.
42. Schaefer A, Stephan C, Busch J, Yousef GM, Jung K (2010) Diagnostic, prognostic and therapeutic implications of microRNAs in urologic tumors. Nat Rev Urol 7: 286–297.

43. Wszolek MF, Rieger-Christ KM, Kenney PA, Gould JJ, Silva NB, et al. (2011) A MicroRNA expression profile defining the invasive bladder tumor phenotype. Urol Oncol 29: 794–801.

44. Adam L, Zhong M, Choi W, Qi W, Nicoloso M, et al. (2009) miR-200 expression regulates epithelial-to-mesenchymal transition in bladder cancer cells and reverses resistance to epidermal growth factor receptor therapy. Clin Cancer Res 15: 5060–5072.

45. Chiyomaru T, Enokida H, Tatarano S, Kawahara K, Uchida Y, et al. (2010) miR-145 and miR-133a function as tumour suppressors and directly regulate FSCN1 expression in bladder cancer. Br J Cancer 102: 883–891.

46. Huang L, Luo J, Cai Q, Pan Q, Zeng H, et al. (2011) MicroRNA-125b suppresses the development of bladder cancer by targeting E2F3. Int J Cancer 128: 1758–1769.

47. Fendler A, Stephan C, Yousef GM, Jung K (2011) MiRNAs as regulators of signal transduction in urological tumors. Clin Chem 57: 954–968.

48. Pfaffl MW, Tichopad A, Prgomet C, Neuvians TP (2004) Determination of stable housekeeping genes, differentially regulated target genes and sample integrity: BestKeeper–Excel-based tool using pair-wise correlations. Biotechnol Lett 26: 509–515.

49. Sobin LH, Wittekind C (2002) TNM classification of malignant tumours. New York: Wiley-Liss. 199 p.

50. Magi-Galluzzi C, Zhou M, Epstein JI (2007) Neoplasms of the urinary bladder. In: Zhou M, Magi-Galluzzi C, editors. Genitourinary pathology. Philadelphia: Churchill Livingstone Elsevier. 154–224.

51. Jung M, Mollenkopf HJ, Grimm C, Wagner I, Albrecht M, et al. (2009) MicroRNA profiling of clear cell renal cell cancer identifies a robust signature to define renal malignancy. J Cell Mol Med 13: 3918–3928.

52. Hellemans J, Mortier G, De PA, Speleman F, Vandesompele J (2007) qBase relative quantification framework and software for management and automated analysis of real-time quantitative PCR data. Genome Biol 8: R19.

53. Masotti A, Caputo V, Da SL, Pizzuti A, Dallapiccola B, et al. (2009) Quantification of small non-coding RNAs allows an accurate comparison of miRNA expression profiles. J Biomed Biotechnol 2009: 659028.

54. D'haene B, Mestdagh P, Hellemans J, Vandesompele J (2012) miRNA expression profiling: from reference genes to global mean normalization. Methods Mol Biol 822: 261–272.

55. Latham GJ (2010) Normalization of microRNA quantitative RT-PCR data in reduced scale experimental designs. Methods Mol Biol 667: 19–31.

56. Peltier HJ, Latham GJ (2008) Normalization of microRNA expression levels in quantitative RT-PCR assays: identification of suitable reference RNA targets in normal and cancerous human solid tissues. RNA 14: 844–852.

57. Jung M, Schaefer A, Steiner I, Kempkensteffen C, Stephan C, et al. (2010) Robust microRNA stability in degraded RNA preparations from human tissue and cell samples. Clin Chem 56: 998–1006.

58. Carlsson J, Helenius G, Karlsson M, Lubovac Z, Andren O, et al. (2010) Validation of suitable endogenous control genes for expression studies of miRNA in prostate cancer tissues. Cancer Genet Cytogenet 202: 71–75.

4

Detection of Bladder Cancer using Proteomic Profiling of Urine Sediments

Tadeusz Majewski[1], Philippe E. Spiess[2¤a], Jolanta Bondaruk[1], Peter Black[2¤b], Charlotte Clarke[3¤c], William Benedict[4], Colin P. Dinney[2], Herbert Barton Grossman[2], Kuang S. Tang[5], Bogdan Czerniak[1]*

1 Department of Pathology, The University of Texas MD Anderson Cancer Center, Houston, Texas, United States of America, 2 Department of Urology, The University of Texas MD Anderson Cancer Center, Houston, Texas, United States of America, 3 Ciphergen Biosystems, Inc., Fremont, California, United States of America, 4 Department of Genitourinary Medical Oncology, The University of Texas MD Anderson Cancer Center, Houston, Texas, United States of America, 5 Department of Biostatistics & Applied Math, The University of Texas MD Anderson Cancer Center, Houston, Texas, United States of America

Abstract

We used protein expression profiles to develop a classification rule for the detection and prognostic assessment of bladder cancer in voided urine samples. Using the Ciphergen PBS II ProteinChip Reader, we analyzed the protein profiles of 18 pairs of samples of bladder tumor and adjacent urothelium tissue, a training set of 85 voided urine samples (32 controls and 53 bladder cancer), and a blinded testing set of 68 voided urine samples (33 controls and 35 bladder cancer). Using t-tests, we identified 473 peaks showing significant differential expression across different categories of paired bladder tumor and adjacent urothelial samples compared to normal urothelium. Then the intensities of those 473 peaks were examined in a training set of voided urine samples. Using this approach, we identified 41 protein peaks that were differentially expressed in both sets of samples. The expression pattern of the 41 protein peaks was used to classify the voided urine samples as malignant or benign. This approach yielded a sensitivity and specificity of 59% and 90%, respectively, on the training set and 80% and 100%, respectively, on the testing set. The proteomic classification rule performed with similar accuracy in low- and high-grade bladder carcinomas. In addition, we used hierarchical clustering with all 473 protein peaks on 65 benign voided urine samples, 88 samples from patients with clinically evident bladder cancer, and 127 samples from patients with a history of bladder cancer to classify the samples into Cluster A or B. The tumors in Cluster B were characterized by clinically aggressive behavior with significantly shorter metastasis-free and disease-specific survival.

Editor: William C.S. Cho, Queen Elizabeth Hospital, Hong Kong

Funding: This work was supported by National Institute of Health Grants R01 CA 151489 (BC) and GU SPORE Grant P50 CA91846 (Project 1, BC). The funders had no role in study design, data collection and analysis, decision to publish, or preparation of the manuscript.

Competing Interests: CC was originally an employee of Ciphergen Biosystems, Inc., Fremont, California at the time of the initial study related to this project. Currently, she is working in the Office of the Vice President for Translational Research at The University of Texas M D Anderson Cancer Center.

* E-mail: bczernia@mdanderson.org

¤a Current address: Department of Genitourinary Oncology, H. Lee Moffitt Cancer Center & Research Institute, Tampa, Florida, United States of America
¤b Current address: Department of Urologic Sciences, University of British Columbia, and at Vancouver Prostate Centre, Vancouver, British Columbia, Canada
¤c Current address: Office of the Vice President for Translational Research, The University of Texas MD Anderson Cancer Center, Houston, Texas, United States of America

Introduction

Current pathogenetic concepts postulate that common neoplasms of the bladder arise in its epithelial lining (urothelium) via two distinct but somewhat overlapping pathways: the papillary and nonpapillary pathways. [1] Approximately 80% of the tumors that arise in the bladder are exophytic papillary lesions that originate from hyperplastic urothelial changes. They typically recur but usually do not invade the bladder wall or metastasize. The remaining 20% of bladder tumors are aggressive, nonpapillary carcinomas with a propensity for invading and metastasizing. Invasive bladder cancers typically occur in patients without a history of papillary tumors and originate from *in situ* preneoplastic lesions ranging from mild to moderate dysplasia (low-grade intraurothelial neoplasia, LGIN) to severe dysplasia and carcinoma *in situ* (high-grade intraurothelial neoplasia, HGIN). [2] The majority of aggressive high-grade non-papillary bladder carcinomas present at an advanced stage and necessitate chemotherapy and/or radical cystectomy to improve survival.

For studies of biomarkers, bladder carcinoma is an ideal disease model, because its development and progression can be monitored using noninvasive or minimally invasive techniques. [3] The mucosa of the bladder can be examined and biopsies can be obtained via an endoscopic procedure. In addition, the morphology of exfoliated urothelial cells and their constituents as well as secreted products can be scrutinized in urine at no risk to the patient.

Proteomic technologies that involve mass spectrometry coupled with ProteinChip Systems have been shown to facilitate the protein profiling of biological specimens. [4–6] The initial findings documenting the identification of serum and urine protein fingerprints for diagnosing several cancers [7–9] have been followed by reports raising concerns about problems with study design, reproducibility, calibration, and analytical procedures [10–13].

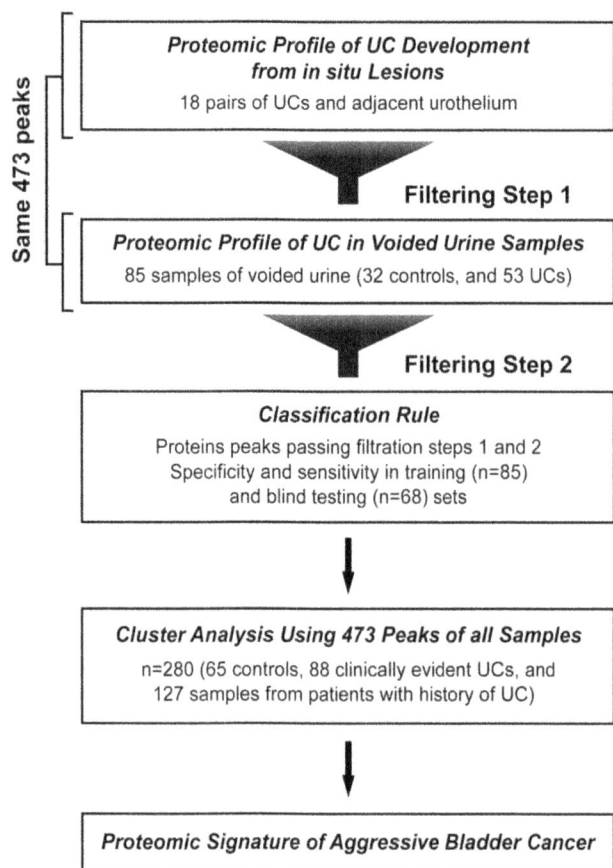

Figure 1. Analytical strategy used to develop classification rule for bladder cancer. The proteomic profile of bladder cancer development from *in situ* neoplasia was developed on a collection of proteomic spectra from paired samples of urothelial carcinoma (UC) and adjacent urothelium compared to normal urothelium. Using this approach, 473 protein peaks expressed in normal urothelium were identified. The same 473 were subsequently identified in the training set of voided urine samples from control subjects and patients with UC. The protein peaks first identified as abnormally expressed in tissue samples (filtering step 1) and then in the training set of voided urine samples (filtering step 2) were used to design a classification rule. The performance of the classification rule was assessed first in the training set and then in a blind testing set. Finally, a cluster analysis was performed using 473 protein peaks on all control and UC samples to identify the proteomic signature of aggressive bladder cancer.

This report outlines a strategy for protein profiling using surface-enhanced laser desorption and ionization time-of-flight (SELDI-TOF) mass spectroscopy to formulate a classification rule for detecting bladder cancer in voided urine samples and classifying clinically distinct classes of the disease.

Methods

Tumor and Urine Samples

All human tissues were collected wpith written informed consent under protocols approved by the M. D. Anderson Institutional Review Board and the samples were analyzed anonymously. We analyzed the protein expression profiles of 18 pairs of samples of bladder tumor and adjacent urothelium tissue, 88 voided urine samples from patients with clinically evident bladder cancer, and 127 voided urine samples from patients with a history of bladder cancer (HiUC) and no cystoscopic or pathologic evidence

(negative bladder biopsy and/or voided urine cytology) of bladder cancer at the time of urine collection. For paired samples of adjacent urothelium and bladder tumor tissue, we obtained baseline protein profiles from urothelial cell suspensions of 13 ureters with no evidence of urothelial neoplasia removed during nephrectomy for renal cell carcinoma. For urine samples, we obtained baseline protein profiles from 65 healthy individuals. The profiles were initially analyzed in paired samples of adjacent urothelium and bladder tumor tissue. They were then compared to the profiles identified in the initial 85 samples of urine (32 controls and 53 bladder cancer) referred to as the training set. Subsequently, the proteins that were significantly up- or down-regulated in both sets were used in a diagnostic algorithm first on the training set (n = 85) of urine samples and then on a blinded testing set (n = 68; 33 controls and 35 bladder cancer). Finally, the proteomic profiles of all samples (65 normal controls, 88 bladder cancers, and 127 HiUCs) were analyzed using unsupervised clustering.

The intraurothelial precursor conditions were classified on parallel sections from areas of adjacent mucosa as LGIN or HGIN. [2] The presence of normal, dysplastic, or malignant cells in scrapings from adjacent urothelium tissue was confirmed using microscopic evaluation of cytospin preparations. The tumors were classified according to the three-tiered World Health Organization histologic grading system and their growth patterns (papillary versus nonpapillary). [14] The depth of invasion was recorded according to the TNM (tumor–node–metastasis) staging system. [15] Stage T_1 (lamina propria invasion) has been divided into T_{1a} (no muscularis mucosae invasion) and T_{1b} (muscularis mucosae invasion), which has a significantly higher risk of progression. [16] The tumors were dichotomized into superficial (T_a-T_{1a}) and invasive (T_{1b} and higher) groups, as previously described. [17]

Cell suspensions from adjacent urothelium and bladder tumor tissue were prepared as described previously. [16] In brief, cystectomy samples of previously untreated urothelial carcinomas were used after obtaining informed consent from the patients. Each cystectomy sample was opened longitudinally along the anterior wall of the bladder and pinned down to a paraffin block. One representative section from the central area of grossly identified tumor was obtained for proteomic profiling. The presence of tumor in the tissue was confirmed via analysis of frozen sections. To minimize contamination with nontumor tissue, we dissected an area of tumor tissue from the frozen block. We prepared urothelial cell suspensions from adjacent urothelium tissue by scraping the mucosal surface. The purity of the samples was determined via cytologic examination of the cytospin preparations. Only the samples that yielded more than 90% microscopically intact normal, dysplastic, or malignant urothelial cells were used for protein analysis. For processing, the cells were transferred to conical tubes containing phosphate-buffered saline (PBS). The frozen tumor tissue was transferred to a similar conical tube containing PBS, which was mechanically agitated to release tumor cells. Before preparing cell lysates, we precleaned the cell suspensions via Ficoll Histopague-1077j (Sigma Diagnostics, Inc. St. Louis, MO, USA) gradient centrifugation. For storage, the cell pellets were resuspended in PBS containing 20% dimethyl sulfoxide and frozen in liquid nitrogen. Voided urine samples were treated in the same manner. [3]

Processing of the urine samples was completed within 1–4 hours of receipt. The volume of urine ranged from 10 to 50 ml. Urine samples were centrifuged at 2500 rpm for 10 minutes at room temperature. The cell pellet was resuspended in 2 ml Dulbecco's modified Eagle's medium (DMEM). The new conical tube (50 ml) was filled with 20 ml DMEM, and 5 ml Ficoll was placed in the

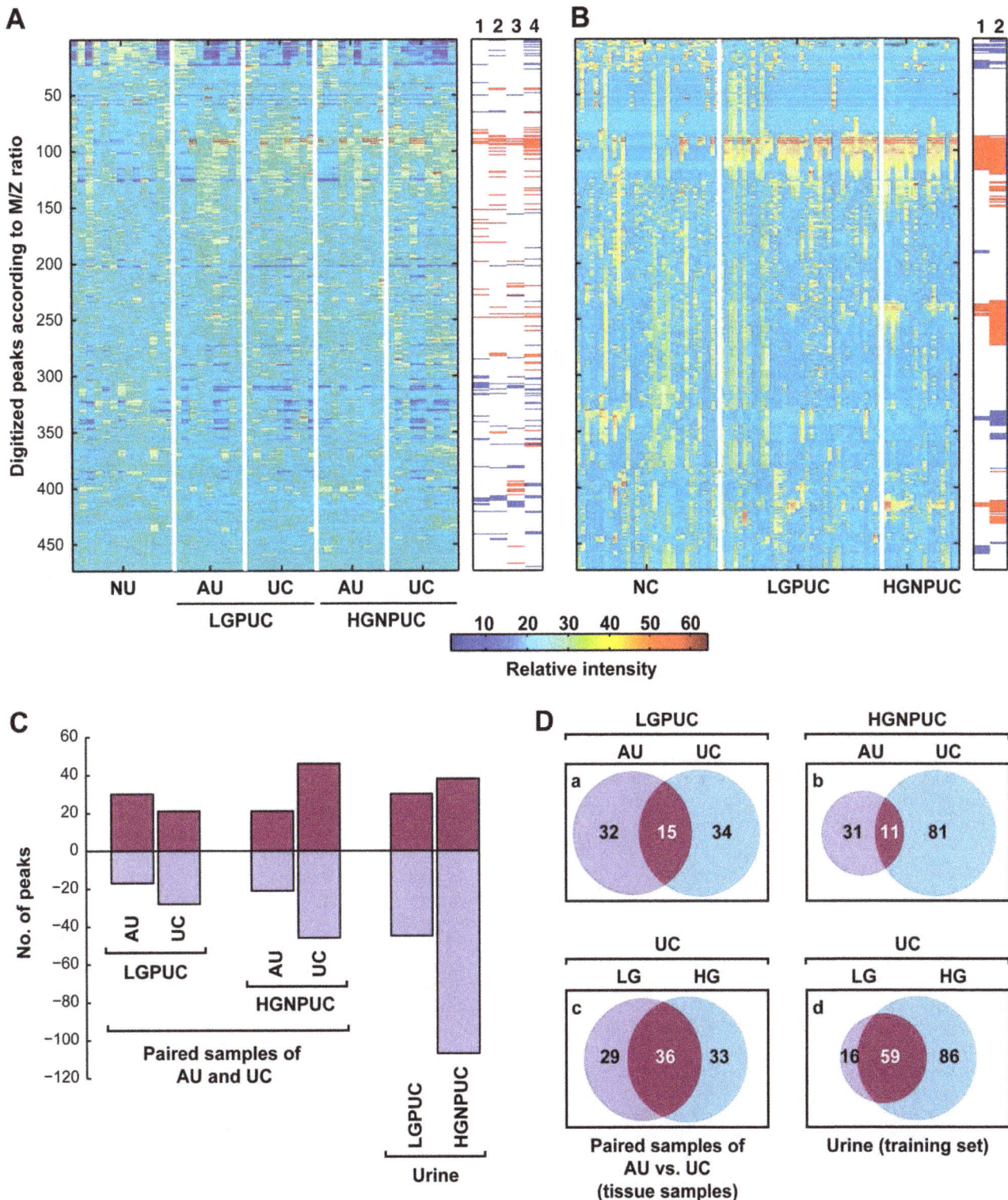

Figure 2. Proteomic profile of bladder cancer. (**A**) Digitalized proteomic profile of bladder cancer development from *in situ* neoplasia. Expression levels of protein peaks were analyzed on paired samples from adjacent urothelium (AU) and UCs compared to normal urothelium (NU). Each column represents UC or AU samples and each row corresponds to a digitalized protein peaks arranged according to *M/Z* ratios. Ratios of individual *M/Z* peak relative to NU are shown as a color saturation scale below the diagram. Samples corresponding to AU and UC are grouped according to their pathogenetic subsets representing low-grade (Grade 1–2) superficial papillary UC (LGPUC) and high grade (Grade 3) invasive UC (HGNPUC). The bar diagram on the right shows individual protein peaks with higher (red) and lower (blue) expression levels as compared to NU. Column 1: comparison between NU and AU LGPUC, 2: comparison between NU and LGPUC, 3: comparison between NU and AU HGNPUC, 4: comparison between NU and HGNPUC. (**B**) Proteomic profile of voided urine samples from control subjects (normal control, NC) and patients with UC dichotomized into LGPUC and HGNPUC categories. The bar diagram on the right shows individual protein peaks with higher (red) and lower (blue) expression levels as compared to NU. Column 1: comparison between NC and LGPUC; Column 2: comparison between NC and HGNPUC. (**C**) Number

of protein peaks with higher (maroon) and lower (purple) expression levels as compared to NU identified in paired tissue samples of AU and in voided urine samples of patients with UC compared to NC. (**D**) Proportion of proteins peaks with similar and dissimilar expression pattern.

bottom. The urinary cells were then transferred to the top of the solution. After centrifugation at 2500 rpm for 20 minutes at room temperature, the 10-ml upper layer was removed, and the interface (~8 ml) with urinary cells was transferred to a new conical tube (25 ml). The sample was centrifuged again at 2500 rpm for 10 minutes at 4°C. Finally the cells were collected, resuspended in 2 ml of DMEM with 10% dimethyl sulfoxide, and stored at −80°C for later use.

Preparation of Cell Lysates and Proteomic Analysis

Cell lysates were prepared as referenced in the Bio-Rad Web site. [18] Briefly, the samples were towed, centrifuged at 5000 g for 10 minutes, washed in PBS, and resuspended in a lysis buffer (10 mM Tris [pH = 9], 10 mM NaCl, 0.1% dodecyl mattoside). The protein lysates were prepared via sonication using a probe sonicator (Cole-Parmer Instrument Co., Chicago, IL, USA) set at 5 watts 10 times for 15 seconds with 45-second intervals of cooling on ice. Total protein content was measured in each sample using a Micro BCA protein assay reagent kit (Pierce, Rockford, IL, USA). Immobilized metal affinity IMAC3 capture chips (Ciphergen Biosystems, Fremont, CA, USA) were used for proteomic analysis. Chips activated by copper sulfate were briefly washed in deionized water and incubated with 100 mM sodium acetate (pH, 4.5) for 5 minutes to remove any excess Cu^{+2} and again washed with deionized water. The chips were briefly equilibrated with cell lysis buffer and incubated for 1 hour with protein lysates containing 1 µg of total protein in a volume of 3–8 µl of lysis buffer. Before reading, the chips were washed three times with lysis buffer, two times with deionized water, air-dried, and crystalized with 0.3 µl of sinapinic acid in 50% acetonitrile/1% trifluoroacetic acid. All preparatory steps were carried out at room temperature. The protein profiles were analyzed using a Ciphergen PBS II ProteinChip Reader (Ciphergen Biosystems Fremont, CA, USA). Before each series of measurements, the system was calibrated using an "all-in-1" standard from Ciphergen Biosystems, and the proteomic profile of a normal reference tissue, i.e., of normal urothelium tissue or of the urine sediment of normal individuals, was tested.

To assess the accuracy of the measurements, we performed several studies. [19] We evaluated the intensities of 26 peaks in 24 replicate spectra of the same sample from normal urothelium tissue to check reproducibility (**Figure S1**). Peak coefficients of variation (CVs) ranged from 13.7% to 63.1% of the mean. The median CV was 22.7%, and the interquartile range was from 19.4% to 27.7%. We also tested the sensitivity of the mass-to-charge ratio (M/Z) values to an amount of the total protein by varying loadings from 0.5 to 2 µg, and the M/Z readings varied by less than 1% (data not shown).

Analytical Procedures

All spectra were exported as *.xml files using Ciphergen software. The raw spectra were processed using MATLAB scripts developed in-house to (a) remove random noise, (b) subtract the low-frequency baseline, and (c) detect and quantify individual sample peaks. Denoising and baseline subtraction were performed using the wavelet thresholding approach. [20] After denoising, the spectra were normalized. Peak detection made use of the mean spectrum after denoising. [21] The data from all the spectra were summarized in a matrix of peak intensities, with each row corresponding to a specific M/Z value (a peak) and each column corresponding to a specific sample.

Classification accuracy was assessed via sensitivity and specificity and by positive and negative predictive values. The classification rule was also assessed using receiver operating characteristic (ROC) curves. The varying parameter in the ROC curve was the angle between the decision boundary line and the normal X axis: an angle of 0° led to all samples being classified as normal, and an angle of 90° led to all samples being classified as cancer. In addition, voided urine spectra were examined using unsupervised clustering to assess the degree of the associations between the two clusters and various clinicopathologic covariates, including follow-up.

Results

The analytical strategy used in our study to formulate a protein profile for detecting bladder cancer is summarized in **Figure 1**. To identify the optimal combination of protein peaks diagnostic of bladder cancer, we first analyzed a proteomic profile of its development from *in situ* neoplasia and compared it to the proteomic profile of voided urine sediment from bladder cancer patients. To identify the proteins that were abnormally expressed during early bladder cancer development, we analyzed the patterns of their expression in 18 paired samples of bladder tumor and adjacent urothelium tissue and compared them to their expression pattern in 13 samples of normal urothelium. We first selected peaks that were clearly identifiable in tissue samples and used t-tests to identify peaks that had significant differential expression across different categories of paired bladder tumor and adjacent urothelial samples. Using this approach, referred to as filtration step 1, we identified 473 protein peaks expressed in normal urothelium tissue and sets of up- and down-regulated proteins, which were somewhat overlapping but distinct, thereby signifying the development of bladder cancer from *in situ* neoplasia via papillary and nonpapillary pathways. Since voided urine sediments may contain a mixture of tumor and nontumor cells, including inflammatory, stromal, and peripheral blood cells as well as necrotic cells with degenerated proteins, we focused on the same 473 peaks identified in the tissue samples and examined their intensities in a training set of voided urine samples from 53 patients with clinically evident bladder cancer and 32 healthy individuals. In this phase, referred to as filtration step 2, we searched, again using t-tests, for peaks with significant differential expression between cancers and controls.

Examples of SELDI-TOF spectra from samples of normal urothelium tissue and paired samples of adjacent urothelium and tumor tissue as well as the results of filtration step 1 are shown in **Figure 2A**. The spectra from voided urine sediments of bladder cancer patients and normal controls and the results of filtration step 2 are shown in **Figure 2B**. The differences in the protein expression profiles of tumors identified in tissue and voided urine samples are summarized in **Figures 2C and D**. It is evident that HGINs or high-grade nonpapillary urothelial carcinomas (HGNPUC) have somewhat overlapping but distinct protein expression patterns that can be also identified in adjacent urothelium tissue. This finding implies that abnormal protein expression profiles can be identified in surface urothelium tissue before the development of clinically evident cancer. By comparing the patterns of abnormally expressed proteins in bladder tumors,

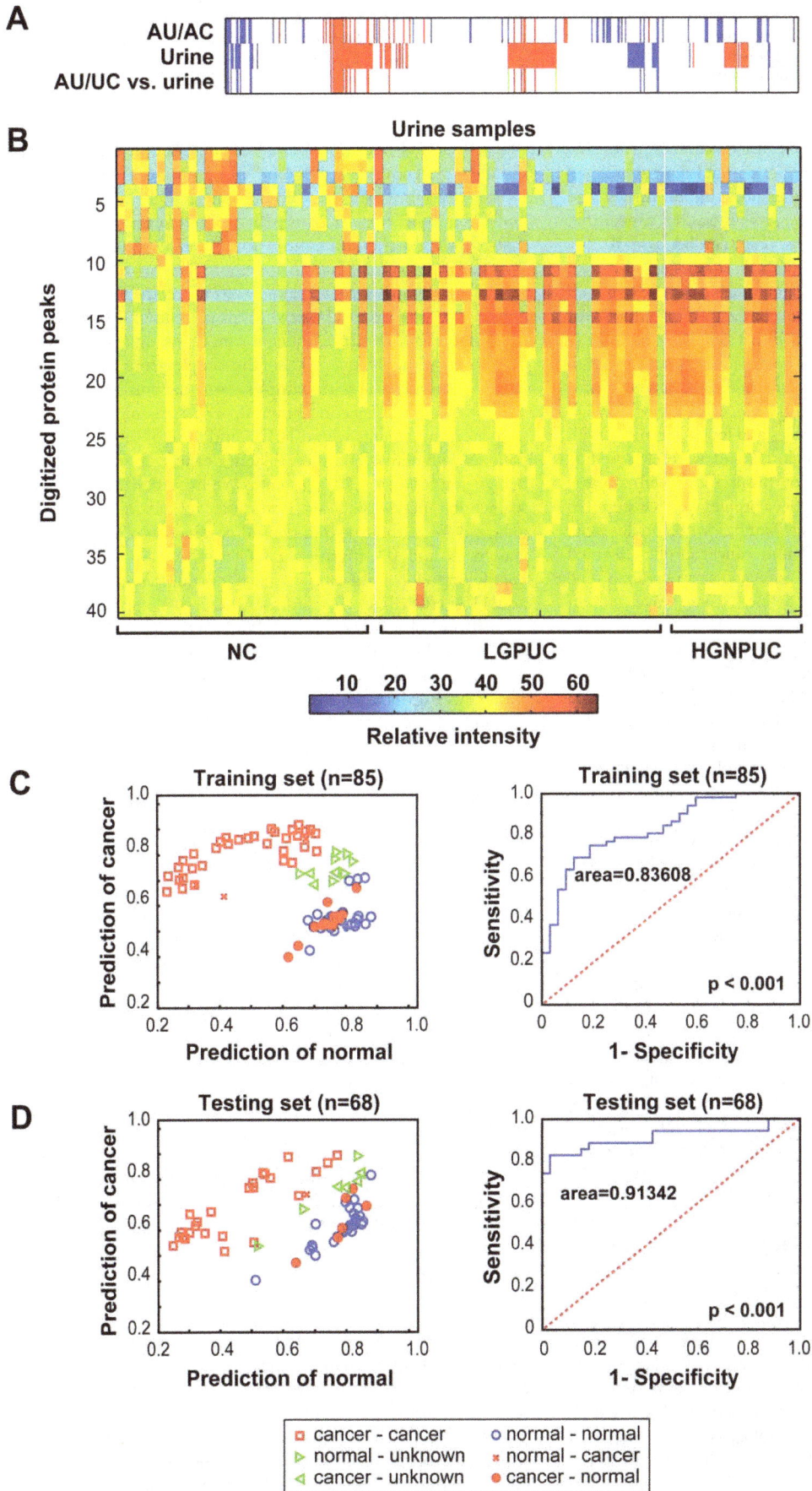

A

B

Urine samples

C

Training set (n=85)

Training set (n=85)

area=0.83608

p < 0.001

D

Testing set (n=68)

Testing set (n=68)

area=0.91342

p < 0.001

cancer - cancer   normal - normal
normal - unknown   normal - cancer
cancer - unknown   cancer - normal

Figure 3. Detection of bladder cancer by proteomic profiling using 41 protein peaks. (**A**) Up regulated (red) and down regulated (blue) protein peaks identified in AU and UC (upper row) and voided urine samples (mid row) and the protein peaks consistently found in both sets of samples (lower row). (**B**) Heat map for 41 protein peaks identified by filtering step 2. (See Figure 1) (**C**) Classification of individual samples (left panel) and ROC curve (right panel) in the training set. (**D**) Classification of individual samples (left panel) and ROC curve (right panel) in the testing set.

their adjacent urothelia, and voided urine samples from the training set, we identified a set of distinct up- and down-regulated proteins that were present in both bladder tumor tissues and voided urine sediment samples of patients with bladder cancer that was retained after both filtration steps. (**Figures 3A and B**).

Using only the peaks that passed both filtration steps, we used the matrix of 41 protein peak intensities to construct a classification rule for individual samples in the training and testing sets. (**Figure 3C**) The positions of individual samples in relation to the X (normal) and Y (cancer) axis were defined using a pair of numbers indicating their associations with both normal and cancer protein profiles. In this classification rule, samples with high associations with normal protein profiles and low associations with cancer profiles were clustered in region 1 and were classified as benign. In contrast, samples with low associations with normal profiles and high associations with cancer profiles were clustered in region 2 and were classified as cancer. Samples with equally weak or strong associations with normal and cancer profiles formed were clustered in region 3 and were designated as ambiguous. The boundaries of these clusters were defined using leave-one-out cross-validation.

Classification accuracy was initially assessed on the training set in terms of sensitivity of 0.59, specificity of 0.90, positive predictive value within the training set of 0.92, negative predictive value within the training set of 0.53, and ROC curve area of 0.84. (**Figure 3D**) Having defined the classification rule on the training set, we then validated its accuracy on the blinded testing set of 33 normal control samples and 35 bladder cancer samples, which yielded a sensitivity of 0.80, specificity of 1.0, positive predictive value on the testing set of 1.0, negative predictive value on the testing set of 0.83, and ROC curve area of 0.91. (**Figure 3D**) Cases that were deemed ambiguous were excluded when computing sensitivity, specificity, positive predictive value, and negative predictive value. All cases were retained for fitting ROC curves.

To assess how the classification rule based on the matrix of 41 protein peak intensities performed in different subsets of bladder cancer, we combined the training and testing sets and assessed its diagnostic accuracy for low-grade papillary urothelial carcinoma (LGPUC) and HGNPUC separately. Analysis of 65 benign control samples and 53 LGPUC samples yielded a sensitivity of 0.74, specificity of 0.95, positive predictive value of 0.91, negative predictive value of 0.84, and ROC curve area of 0.88. (**Figure 4A**) Similar analysis of 65 benign control samples and 35 HGNPUC samples yielded a sensitivity of 0.77, specificity of 0.95, positive predictive value of 0.90, negative predictive value of 0.88, and ROC curve area of 0.88. (**Figure 4B**) Analysis of the overall classification accuracy for the combined training and testing sets yielded a sensitivity of 0.75, specificity of 0.95, positive predictive value of 0.95, negative predictive value of 0.75, and ROC curve area of 0.88. (**Figures 4C and D**) Analysis of 39 samples from patients with bladder cancer for which the parallel data on the results of voided urine cytology were available indicated that classification based on the proteomic data correctly diagnosed 28 (72%) samples, whereas voided urine cytology correctly diagnosed 19 (49%) samples. (**Figure 4E**) Testing the difference between positive samples identified by proteomics and cytology using a z-test for proportions yielded a two-sided p value of 0.032.

Unsupervised clustering was carried out using Euclidean distance and complete linkage on all 65 normal control samples, 88 samples from patients with clinically evident bladder cancer, and 127 samples from patients with a HiUC. (**Figure 5**) Using the matrix of expression intensities for all 473 protein peaks, we classified the samples into two major groups. The first group (cluster A) consisted of a majority (97%) of the benign control samples. (**Figure 6A**) The second group (cluster B) consisted of 56% of the samples from patients with clinically evident bladder cancer. Interestingly, only 24% of the samples from patients with a HiUC co-segregated with samples from patients with clinically evident bladder cancer in cluster B. The remaining 76% of the samples from patients with a HiUC and 44% of the samples from patients with clinically evident bladder cancer co-segregated with benign control samples in cluster A. We hypothesized that this co-segregation may signify distinct classes of bladder cancer and analyzed the pathologic and clinical parameters of the samples in clusters A and B. (**Figure 6B**) Cluster A comprised predominantly normal control samples (62%) in addition to 27% LGPUC and 11% HGNPUC. In contrast, cluster B comprised only 4% normal control samples, 49% LGPUC, and 47% HGNPUC. The tumors in cluster B were characterized by significantly shorter metastasis-free and disease-specific survival than tumors from cluster A. (**Figures 6C and D**) Overall, the probability of dying of bladder cancer for patients in cluster B was approximately 12%, whereas the probability of dying for those in cluster A was less than 5%.

Although we did not perform the identification of the peaks used in a classification rule, we address their potential nature by focusing on the three most prominent peaks used in the analysis of our protein expression profiles. The cluster of three protein peaks with m/z values most likely corresponding to α-defensins was included in the classification rule. [22–24] The examples of SELDI-TOF spectra profiles between 3300 and 3600 m/z in representative urine samples of negative control, LGPUC and HGNPUC depicting the expression pattern of three peaks corresponding to α-defensins and the zoomed heat map in the training set are shown in **Figure 7A and B.** The expression pattern of the same proteins in the combined training and testing sets shows their overexpression in LGPUC and HGNPUC. (**Figure 7C**) The overexpression pattern of α-defensins is highly significant in both LGPUC and HGNPUC as compared to normal controls and even if taken out of context of the 41 anonymous protein peaks used in the classification rule, these proteins perform reasonably well as diagnostic markers (sensitivity 0.77 and specificity 0.84). (**Figure 7C**).

Discussion

The study design for proteomic profiling typically consists of a comparison of proteomic patterns of samples from patients with cancer and benign control samples using artificial intelligence algorithms such as genetic algorithms or tree analysis. [25–29] Such an approach identifies a limited number of anonymous protein peaks for discriminating cancer from benign tissue. When such peaks were identified by peptide sequencing, they represented, in general, the so-called acute phase proteins rather than tumor-specific products [28].

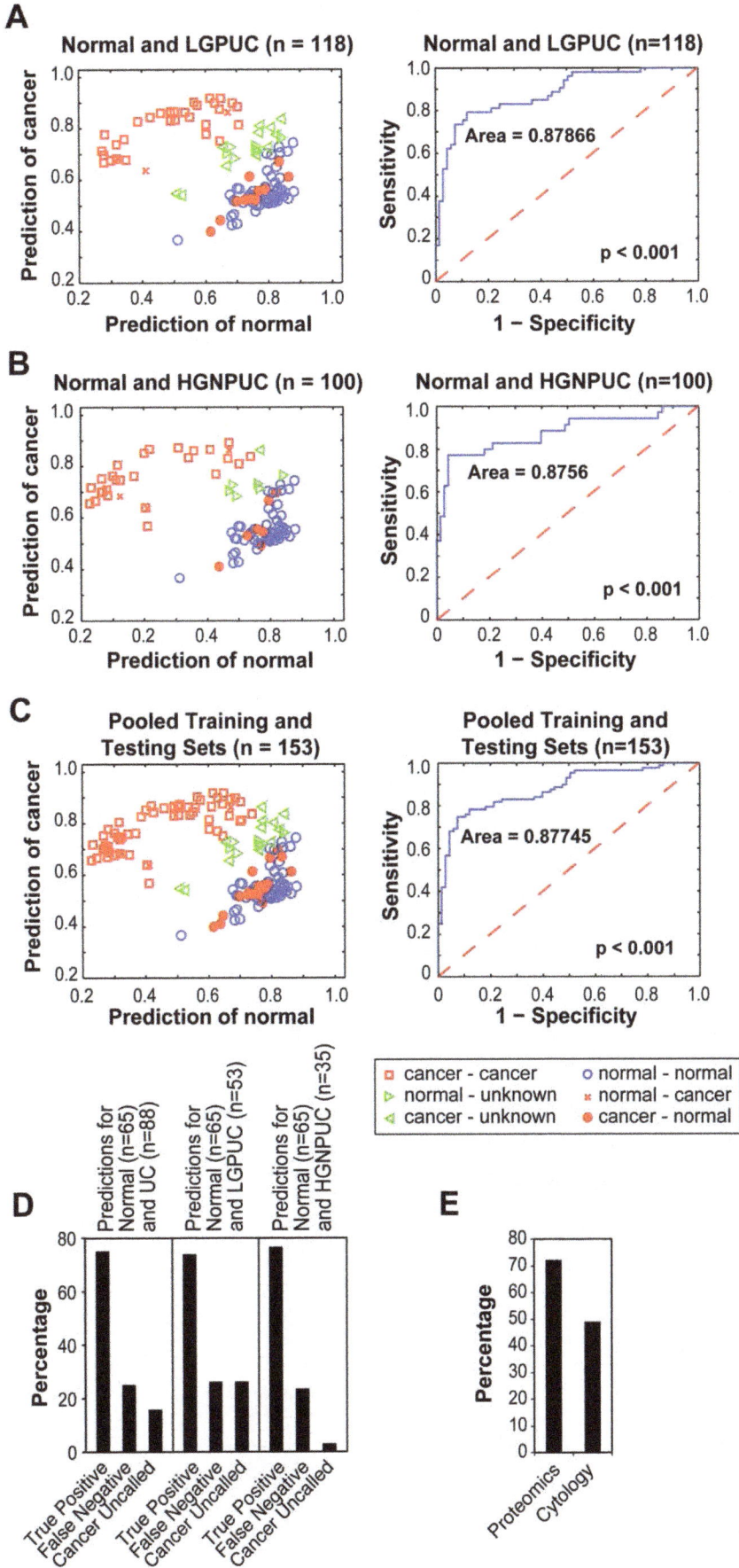

Figure 4. Detection of bladder cancer by proteomic profiling using 41 protein peaks in LGPUC and HGNPUC. (**A**) Classification of individual samples (left panel) and ROC curve (right panel) based on 65 benign control samples and 53 samples from patients with LGPUC. (**B**) Classificatin of individual samples (left panel) and ROC curve (right panel) based 65 benign control samples 35 samples from patients with HGNPUC. (**C**) Classification of individual samples (left panel) and ROC curve (right panel) based on 65 benign control samples and 88 samples from patients with UC.(combined training and testing sets) (**D**) Comparison of diagnostic accuracy of proteomics and cytology on 39 samples from patients with UC. (**E**) Classification of individual samples by proteomics based on the combined testing and training sets as well as for LGPUC and HGNPUC separately.

Several studies using proteomic profiling of voided urine for bladder cancer detection with SELDI platform were recently published. [30,31] These studies used various approaches to protein spectra analysis that range from the use of artificial intelligence algorithms combined with supervised clustering to individual peak and peak cluster identification as diagnostic discriminatory parameters. [30,31] As expected, the automatic clustering algorithm segregated controls from cancer samples with high sensitivity (80%) and specificity (>90%) in the training set but was associated with a dramatic drop of both sensitivity and specificity in the testing set to a range of approximately 50% and 60% respectively. [30] The combinatorial approach of individual biomarkers and biomarker clusters provided sensitivity of 87% and specificity of 66% but this study did not include separate training

and testing sets of samples. [31] Interestingly, the individual markers identified by this approach included the peaks corresponding to α-defensin family. Proteomic studies for diagnosis and prognosis of solid human malignancies including bladder cancer are based on serum or voided urine analysis and involve wide-range of technologies. The technologies used in biomarker design range from SELDI/MALDI-TOF MS through liquid chromatography or capillary electrophoresis mass spectroscopy and gel-based approaches to protein arrays. [32,33] More recent metabolic approaches combined several techniques such as high performance liquid chromatography (HPLC) with gas chromatography or mass spectroscopy (MS) for the analysis of human urine metabolites in search for diagnostic, prognostic, and therapy monitoring biomarkers. [34–36] These studies support the

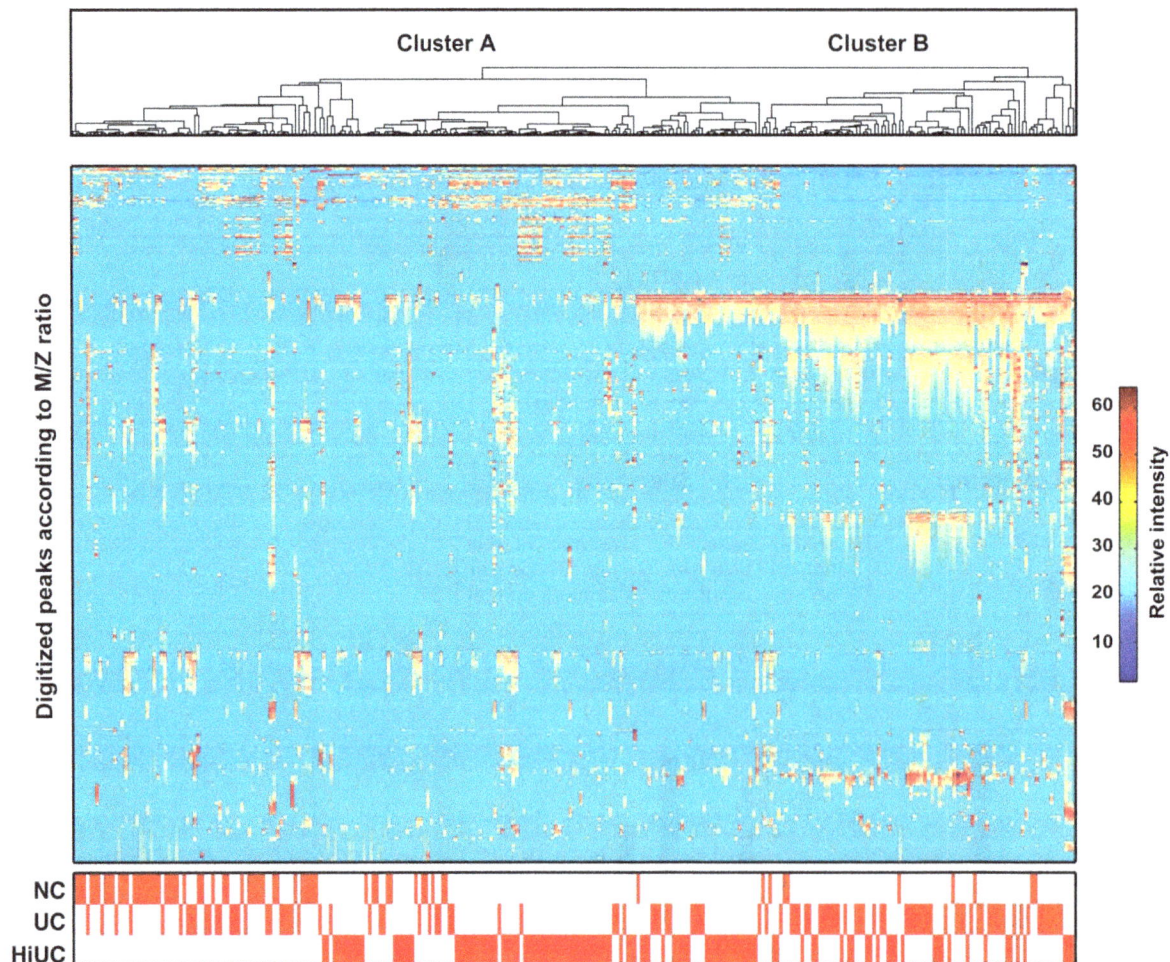

Figure 5. Unsupervised hierarchical clustering of voided urine samples (n = 280). The cohort included 65 normal controls (NC), 88 patients with clinically evident bladder cancer (UC) and 127 patients with a history of bladder cancer (HiUC). Clustering was performed using Euclidean distance and the matrix of expression intensities for 473 protein peaks. Each column represents a voided urine sample and each row corresponds to the digitalized protein peaks arranged according to M/Z ratios.

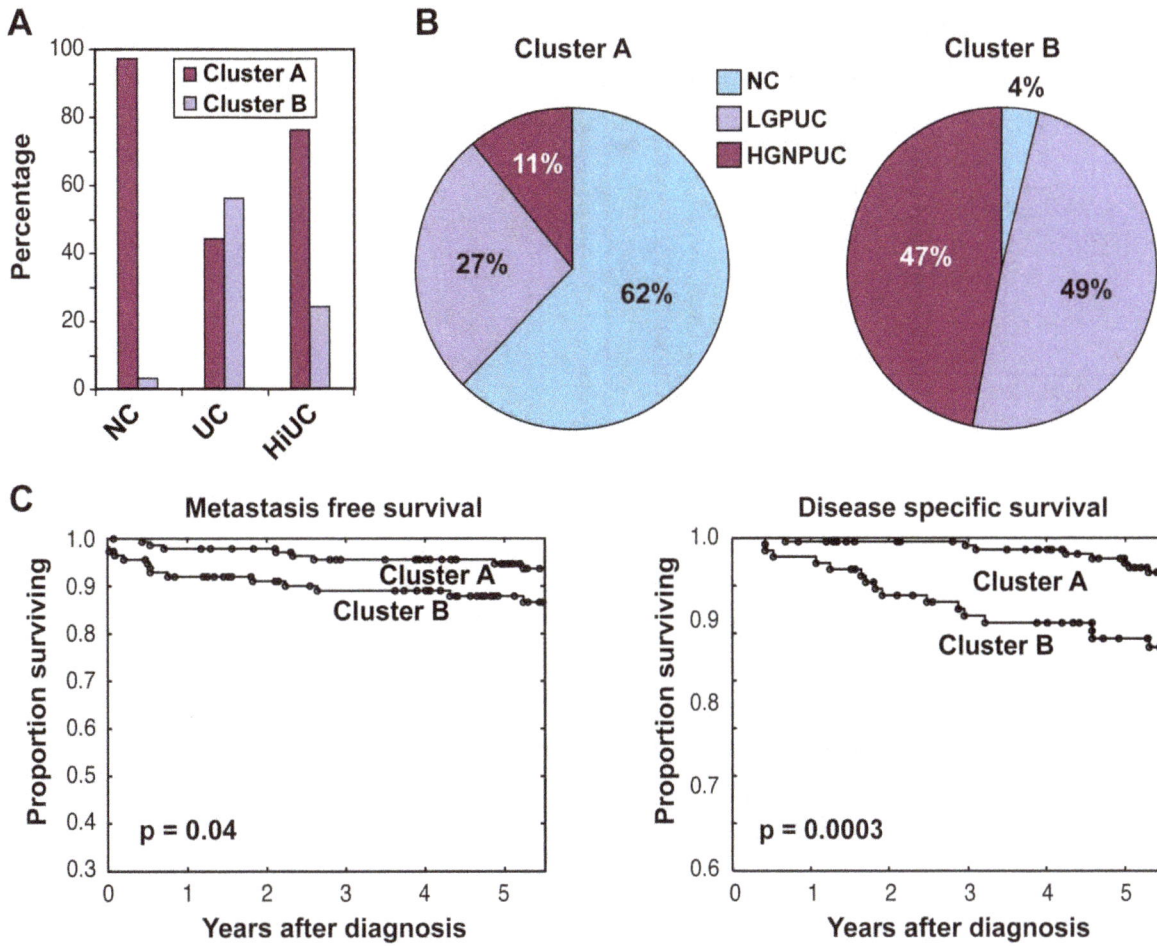

Figure 6. Distribution of various samples in clusters A and B. (A) Distribution of voided urine samples in cluster A and B of normal controls (NC), patients with clinically evident bladder cancer (UC) and patients with history of bladder cancer (HiUC). **(B)** Distribution of voided urine samples in Clusters A and B according to histologic grade and stage dichotomized into low grade invasive superficial papillary UC (LGPUC, pT_a – pT_{1a}) and high grade non-papillary UC (HGNPUC, T_{1b} and higher). **(C)** Kaplan – Mayer plots of metastasis and disease specific survival of patients with bladder cancer in Clusters A and B.

potential for proteomic profiling as a non-invasive tool for detecting and monitoring bladder cancer. Recent studies of the SELDI-TOF approach reported good reproducibility of peak intensities and stability of M/Z reading ratios among five participating laboratories when the same sample preparation protocol and analytical formula were used. [37] Our multi-laboratory reproducibility study revealed similar variability of peak intensities within the range of the median CV of approximately 20% and good stability of M/Z reading ratios, which varied by less than 1%. **(Figure S1)**.

The approach outlined in our study was designed after multiple attempts to identify protein fingerprints for diagnosing bladder cancer by comparing the protein profiles of voided urine from cancer patients with those of benign controls. In general, the attempts using artificial intelligence algorithms produced satisfactory results in the initial training set and failed in the second blind dataset, often performing no better than chance. The critical components of the successful strategy presented in this report were (1) the generation of proteomic profiles of bladder cancer development from *in situ* neoplasia, (2) the identification of the same 473 protein peaks in tissue and voided urine samples, and (3) the use of two filtration steps for identifying 41 protein peaks that were differentially expressed in cancer patients and controls that

could be identified in both tissue and voided urine. The matrix of these 41 protein intensities was used to define a classification rule, which detected cancer with a high degree of sensitivity and specificity in both training and blind testing sets. The proteomic classification rule performed with similar accuracy for LGPUC and HGNPUC. Moreover, the preliminary data indicated that proteomics may be more efficient in diagnosing bladder cancer than conventional voided urine cytology, but this finding must be verified in a larger independent sample set. The limited analysis of the diagnostic formula comprising 41 peaks and cytology on 39 samples indicate that the sensitivity of proteomics (72%) is significantly higher than voided urine cytology (49%). The recently published data comparing urine cytology and other biomarker tests, such as NMP22 and UroVysion FISH indicate high specificity (>90%) and low sensitivity (<30%) of cytology. [38] Although cytology is quite specific and sensitive for a high grade variant of urothelial carcinoma, it is considered to be inefficient for the detection of low grade urothelial tumors. [22,39–41] By comparing the performance of our proteomic diagnostic formula with cytology we show that proteomics may perform equally well in both high grade and low grade urothelial carcinomas. Therefore, combining proteomic profiling with other diagnostic

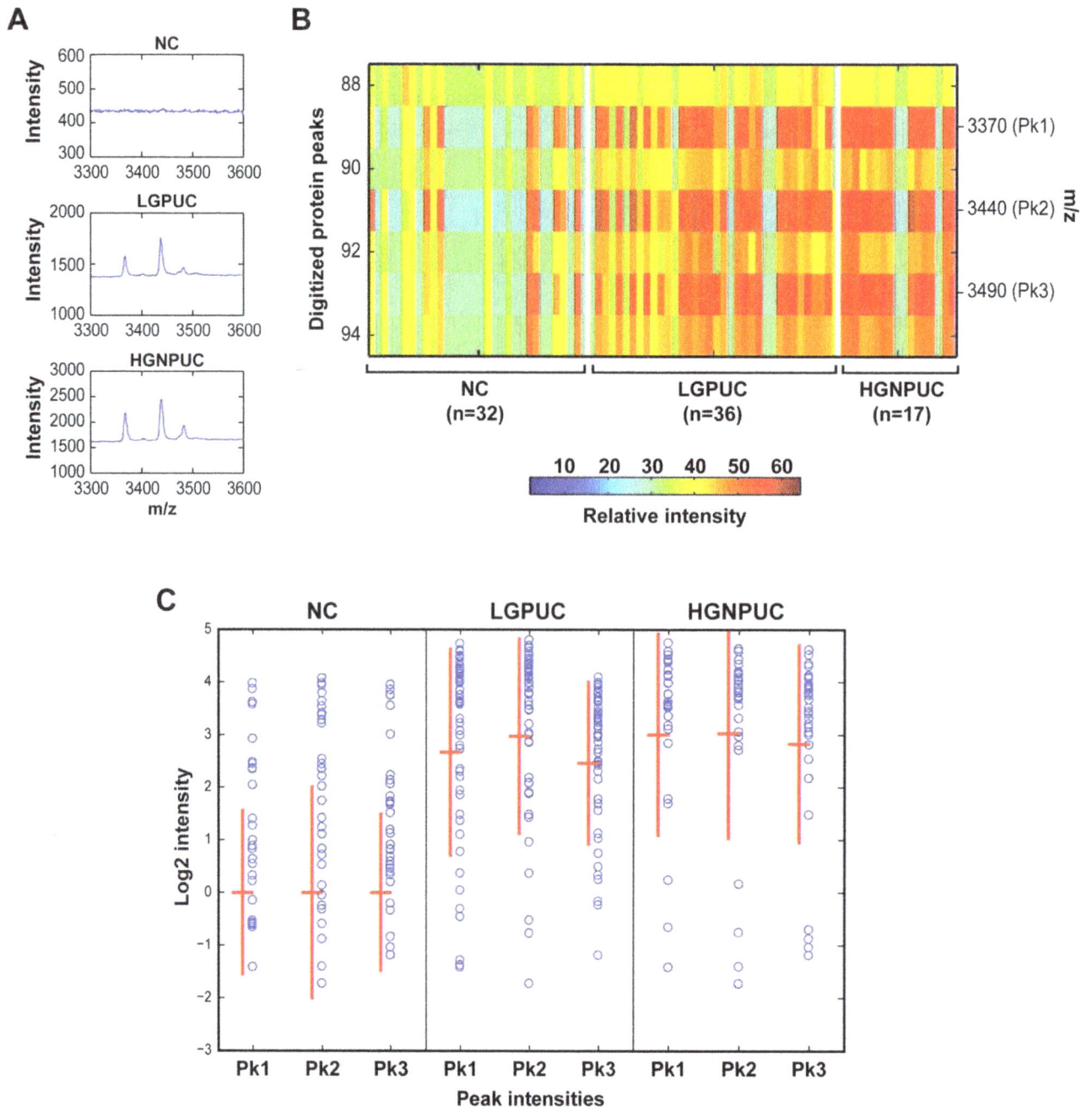

Figure 7. Expression patterns of selected protein peaks with molecular weights corresponding to α-defensins. (A) Protein profiles between 3300 and 3600 m/z of representative samples corresponding to NC, LGPUC and HGNPUC showing the expression pattern of three protein peaks with 3370, 3440 and 3490±10 m/z referred to as peaks 1–3 (pk 1–3) representing the cluster of α-defensins. **(B)** Zoomed heat map showing the expression pattern of α-defensin cluster in the training set. **(C)** The expression intensities of α-defensin cluster corresponding to pk 1–3 in pulled samples of testing and training sets of NC, LGPUC and HGNPUC. Crossed red lines and vertical bars represent mean and standard deviations. Two sample T-test was used to compare the log2-transformed peak intensities in cancer samples and controls for each respective peak ($p < 0.001$).

modalities including cytology may improve the detection of especially low grade urothelial tumors.

Unsupervised clustering using all 473 proteins identified clinically distinct subsets of bladder cancer corresponding to indolent and aggressive variants of the disease. In general, the proteomic profiles from voided urine sediments of patients with bladder cancer that clustered with benign controls were indicative of a better prognosis, with longer metastasis-free and disease-free

survival, than samples from patients with bladder cancer that formed a distinct cluster.

Our study of proteomic expression profiles concerns 473 anonymous protein peaks and 41 of them were used to construct a classification rule. The true nature of these peaks is unknown but as evidenced by prior studies the proteomic profiling of body fluids, including urine from cancer patients, typically do not identify oncogenic or tumor suppressor-like proteins. Most of the peaks in such profiles correspond to so-called acute phase proteins responsible for immune responses which are unlikely directly involved in tumor development. [42–46] The three most prominent proteins included in our analytic formula, as well as in the analysis of the global proteomic profiles, correspond by their molecular mass to such proteins and most likely represent α-defensins. [31,47–49] Defensins are involved in tissue specific regulation of inflammation but they were also documented as playing a role in tumor related cellular activities such as apoptosis and transcriptional regulation. [50] Their overexpression has been documented in several human malignancies including bladder cancer and was shown to be associated with tumor invasiveness. [23,32,49] Therefore, progressive deregulation of protein expression patterns in voided urine samples of patients with bladder cancer may be observed in aggressive variants of the disease. This may explain the relationship between global expression patterns of proteins in voided urine and clinical aggressiveness as identified by unsupervised clustering using the matrix of 473 protein peaks.

In summary, the analytical strategy described in this study facilitates the identification of protein expression peaks for diagnosis and prognosis of bladder cancer. The differences in protein expression profiles can be identified in voided urine samples of patients with bladder cancer compared to benign controls and in patients with low- versus high-grade bladder cancer and could be used as a noninvasive method for detecting and monitoring bladder cancer.

Acknowledgments

We would like to thank Stephanie Garza and Virginia Hurley for secretarial assistance and Kim-Anh T. Vu for computerized graphic design of figures.

Author Contributions

Conceived and designed the experiments: BC. Performed the experiments: TM CC. Analyzed the data: TM PES JB PB KST BC. Contributed reagents/materials/analysis tools: WB. Wrote the paper: TM BC. Provided clinical data: CPD HBG.

References

1. Dinney CP, McConkey DJ, Millikan RE, Wu X, Bar-Eli M, et al. (2004) Focus on bladder cancer. Cancer Cell 6: 111–116.
2. Spiess PE, Czerniak B (2006) Dual-track pathway of bladder carcinogenesis: practical implications. Arch Pathol Lab Med 130: 844–852.
3. Gazdar AF, Czerniak B (2001) Filling the void: urinary markers for bladder cancer risk and diagnosis. J Natl Cancer Inst 93: 413–415.
4. Rogers MA, Clarke P, Noble J, Munro NP, Paul A, et al. (2003) Proteomic profiling of urinary proteins in renal cancer by surface enhanced laser desorption ionization and neural-network analysis: identification of key issues affecting potential clinical utility. Cancer Res 63: 6971–6983.
5. Schaub S, Wilkins J, Weiler T, Sangster K, Rush D, et al. (2004) Urine protein profiling with surface-enhanced laser-desorption/ionization time-of-flight mass spectrometry. Kidney Int 65: 323–332.
6. Zhu W, Wang X, Ma Y, Rao M, Glimm J, et al. (2003) Detection of cancer-specific markers amid massive mass spectral data. Proc Natl Acad Sci U S A 100: 14666–14671.
7. Gaston KE, Grossman HB (2010) Proteomic assays for the detection of urothelial cancer. Methods Mol Biol 641: 303–323.
8. Petricoin EF, Ardekani AM, Hitt BA, Levine PJ, Fusaro VA, et al. (2002) Use of proteomic patterns in serum to identify ovarian cancer. Lancet 359: 572–577.
9. Petricoin EF, Liotta LA (2003) Clinical applications of proteomics. J Nutr 133: 2476S–2484S.
10. Baggerly KA, Edmonson SR, Morris JS, Coombes KR (2004) High-resolution serum proteomic patterns for ovarian cancer detection. Endocr Relat Cancer 11: 583–584; author reply 585–581.
11. Baggerly KA, Morris JS, Coombes KR (2004) Reproducibility of SELDI-TOF protein patterns in serum: comparing datasets from different experiments. Bioinformatics 20: 777–785.
12. Baggerly KA, Morris JS, Edmonson SR, Coombes KR (2005) Signal in noise: evaluating reported reproducibility of serum proteomic tests for ovarian cancer. J Natl Cancer Inst 97: 307–309.
13. Coombes KR, Morris JS, Hu J, Edmonson SR, Baggerly KA (2005) Serum proteomics profiling–a young technology begins to mature. Nat Biotechnol 23: 291–292.
14. FK M, IA S (1999) Histological typing of urinary bladder tumors. Histological Typing of urinary bladder tumors. New York Berlin: Springer.
15. Sobin OH, Wittekind C (1999) TNM classification of malignant tumors. International Union Against Cancer (UICC). New York: John Willey & Sons.
16. Kim JH, Tuziak T, Hu L, Wang Z, Bondaruk J, et al. (2005) Alterations in transcription clusters underlie development of bladder cancer along papillary and nonpapillary pathways. Laboratory Investigation 85: 532–549.
17. Sen S, Zhou H, Zhang RD, Yoon DS, Vakar-Lopez F, et al. (2002) Amplification/overexpression of a mitotic kinase gene in human bladder cancer. J Natl Cancer Inst 94: 1320–1329.
18. Thulasiraman V, McCutchen-Maloney SL, Motin VL, Garcia E (2001) Detection and identification of virulence factors in yersinia pestis using SELDI ProteinChip System. Biotechniques 30: 428–432.
19. Vorderwulbecke S, Cleverley S, Weinberger SR, Wiesner A (2005) Protein Quantification by the SELDI-TOF-MS-based ProteinChip System. Nature Methods 2: 393–395.
20. Coombes KR, Tsavachidis S, Morris JS, Baggerly KA, Hung MC, et al. (2005) Improved peak detection and quantification of mass spectrometry data acquired from surface-enhanced laser desorption and ionization by denoising spectra with the undecimated discrete wavelet transform. Proteomics 5: 4107–4117.
21. Morris JS, Coombes KR, Koomen J, Baggerly KA, Kobayashi R (2005) Feature extraction and quantification for mass spectrometry in biomedical applications using the mean spectrum. Bioinformatics 21: 1764–1775.
22. Zhang L, Yu W, He T, Yu J, Caffrey RE, et al. (2002) Contribution of human α-defensin 1, 2, and 3 to the anti-HIV-1 activity of CD8 antiviral factor. Science 298: 995–1000.
23. Holterman DA, Diaz JI, Blackmore PF, Davis JW, Shellhammer PF, et al. (2006) Overexpression of α-defensin is associated with bladder cancer invasiveness. Urologic Oncology: Seminary and Original Investigations. 24: 97–108.
24. Muller CA, Markovic-Lipkovski J, Klatt T, Gamper J, Schwarz G, et al. (2002) Human α-defensins HNPs-1, -2, and -3 in renal cell carcinoma: invludences on tumor cell proliferation. Am J Pathol 160: 1311–1324.
25. Abbod MF, Catto JWF, Chen M. Artificial Intelligence Techniques for the Prediction of Bladder Cancer Progression; 2005 April 27–29, 2005; Bruges, Belgium. 109–114.
26. Catto JW, Linkens DA, Abbod MF, Chen M, Burton JL, et al. (2003) Artificial intelligence in predicting bladder cancer outcome: a comparison of neuro-fuzzy modeling and artificial neural networks. Clin Cancer Res 9: 4172–4177.
27. Liu W, Guan M, Wu D (2005) Using tree analysis pattern and SELDI-TOF-MS to discriminate transitional cell carcinoma of the bladder cancer from noncancer patients. European Urology 47: 456–462.
28. Pisitkun T, Johnstone R, Knepper MA (2006) Discovery of urinary biomarkers. Mol Cell Proteomics 5: 1760–1771.
29. Qu Y, Adam BL, Yasui Y, Ward MD, Cazares LH, et al. (2002) Boosted decision tree analysis of surface-enhanced laser desorption/ionization mass spectral serum profiles discriminates prostate cancer from noncancer patients. Clin Chem 48: 1835–1843.
30. Mueller J, von Eggeling F, Driesch D, Schubert J, Melle C, et al. (2005) ProteinChip technology reveals distinctive protein expression profiles in the urine of bladder cancer patients. Eur Urol 47: 885–893; discussion 893–884.
31. Vlahou A, Schellhammer PF, Mendrinos S, Patel K, Kondylis FI, et al. (2001) Development of a novel proteomic approach for the detection of transitional cell carcinoma of the bladder in urine. Am J Pathol 158: 1491–1502.
32. Schwamborn K, Gaisa NT, Henkel C (2010). Tissue and serum proteomic profiling for diagnostic and prognostic bladder cancer biomarkers. Expert Rev Proteomics 7: 897–906.
33. Cho WC, Cheng CH (2007) Oncoproteomics 4: 401–410.
34. Pollard C, Nitz M, Baras A, Williams P, Moskaluk C, et al. (2009) Genoproteomic mining of urothelial cancer suggests γ-glutamyl hydrolase and diazepam-binding inhibitor as putative urinary markers of outcome after chemotherapy. Am J Pathol 175: 1824–1830.
35. Van QN, Veenstra TD, Issaq HJ (2011) Metabolic profiling for the detection of bladder cancer. Curr Urol Rep 12: 34–40.
36. Cho WS (2007) Contribution of oncoproteomics to cancer biomarker discovery. Mol Cancer 6: 1–13.
37. Diao L, Clarke CH, Coombes KR, Hamilton SR, Roth J, et al. (2011) Reproducibility of SELDI Spectra Across Time and Laboratories. Cancer Inform 10: 45–64.
38. Kehinde EO, Al-Mulla F, Kapila K, Anim JT (2011) Comparison of the sensitivity and specificty of urine cytology, urinary nuclear matrix protein-22 and

multitarget fluorescence in situ hybridization assay in the detection of bladder cancer. J Urol Nephrol 45: 113–121.

39. Sanchez-Carbayo M (2004) Recent advances in bladder cancer diagnostics. Clin Biochem 37: 562–571.

40. Goodison S, Rosser CJ, Urquidi V (2009). Urinary proteomic profiling for diagnostic bladder cancer biomarkers. Expert Rev Proteomics 6: 507–514.

41. Huang Z, Lin L, Gao Y, Chen Yongjing C, Yan X, et al. (2011) Bladder cancer determination via two urinary metabolites: a biomarker pattern approach. Mol Cell Proteomics 10: M111.007922, Epub 2011.

42. Lu M, Faull KF, Whitelegge JP, He J, Shen D, et al. (2007) Proteomics and mass spectrometry for cancer biomarker discovery. Biomarker Insights 2: 347–360.

43. Roesch-Ely M, Nees M, Karsai S, Ruess A, Bogumil R, et al. (2007) Proteomic analysis reveals successive aberrations in protein expression from healthy mucosa to invasive head and neck cancer. Oncogene 26: 54–64.

44. Khwaja FW, Nolen JDL, Mendrinos SE, Lewis MM, Olson JJ, et al. (2006) Proteomic analysis of cerebrospinal fluid discriminates maligant and nonmalignant disease of the central nervous system and identifies specific protein markers. Proteomics 6: 6277–6287.

45. Pan S, Chen R, Stevens T, Bronner MP, May D (2011) Proteomics portrait of archival lesions of chronic pancreatitis. Plos One 6: 1–12.

46. Conrad DH, Goyette J, Thomas PS (2007) Proteomics as a method for early detection of cancer: a review of proteomics, exhaled breath condensate, and lung cancer screening. J Gen Intern Med 23: 78–84.

47. Coffelt SB, Scandurro AB (2008) Tumors sound the alarmin(s). Cancer Res 68: 6482–6485.

48. Droin N, Hendra JB, Ducoroy P, Solary E (2009) Human defensins as cancer biomarkers and antitumour molecules. J Proteomics 72: 918–927.

49. Albrethsen J, Bogebo R, Gammeltoft S, Olsen J, Winther B, et al. (2005) Upregulated expression of human neutrophil peptides 1, 2 and 3 (HNP 1–3) in colon cancer serum and tumours: a biomarker study. BMC Cancer 5: 1–10.

50. Sun CQ, Arnold R, Fernandez-Golarz C, Parrish AB, Almekinder T, et al. (2006) Human β-defensin-1, a potential chromosome 8p tumor suppressor: control of transcription and induction of apoptosis in renal cell carcinoma. Cancer Res 66: 8542–8549.

5

Genistein Sensitizes Bladder Cancer Cells to HCPT Treatment In Vitro and In Vivo via ATM/NF-κB/IKK Pathway-Induced Apoptosis

Yong Wang[1ͻ], He Wang[1ͻ], Wei Zhang[1ͻ], Chen Shao[2], Peng Xu[3], Chang Hong Shi[4], Jian Guo Shi[5], Yu Mei Li[1], Qiang Fu[1], Wei Xue[1], Yong Hua Lei[1], Jing Yu Gao[1], Juan Ying Wang[1], Xiao Ping Gao[1], Jin Qing Li[6]*, Jian Lin Yuan[2]*, Yun Tao Zhang[2]*

1 Department of Urology, Tangdu Hospital, Fourth Military Medical University, Xi'an, Shaanxi, China, 2 Department of Urology, Xijing Hospital, Fourth Military Medical University, Xi'an, Shaanxi, China, 3 Department of Medical and Training Department, Tangdu Hospital, Fourth Military Medical University, Xi'an, Shaanxi, China, 4 Department of Experimental Animal, Fourth Military Medical University, Xi'an, Shaanxi, China, 5 Department of Cancer Research Institute, Fourth Military Medical University, Xi'an, Shaanxi, China, 6 Department of Plastic Surgery, Tangdu Hospital, Fourth Military Medical University, Xi'an, Shaanxi, China

Abstract

Bladder cancer is the most common malignant urological disease in China. Hydroxycamptothecin (HCPT) is a DNA topoisomerase I inhibitor, which has been utilized in chemotherapy for bladder cancer for nearly 40 years. Previous research has demonstrated that the isoflavone, genistein, can sensitize multiple cancer cell lines to HCPT treatment, such as prostate and cervical cancer. In this study, we investigated whether genistein could sensitize bladder cancer cell lines and bladder epithelial cell BDEC cells to HCPT treatment, and investigated the possible underlying molecular mechanisms. Genistein could significantly and dose-dependently sensitize multiple bladder cancer cell lines and BDEC cells to HCPT-induced apoptosis both in vitro and in vivo. Genistein and HCPT synergistically inhibited bladder cell growth and proliferation, and induced G2/M phase cell cycle arrest and apoptosis in TCCSUP bladder cancer cell and BDEC cell. Pretreatment with genistein sensitized BDEC and bladder cancer cell lines to HCPT-induced DNA damage by the synergistic activation of ataxia telangiectasia mutated (ATM) kinase. Genistein significantly attenuated the ability of HCPT to induce activation of the anti-apoptotic NF-κB pathway both in vitro and in vivo in a bladder cancer xenograft model, and thus counteracted the anti-apoptotic effect of the NF-κB pathway. This study indicates that genistein could act as a promising non-toxic agent to improve efficacy of HCPT bladder cancer chemotherapy.

Editor: Aamir Ahmad, Wayne State University School of Medicine, United States of America

Funding: This work was supported by grants from the National Natural Science Foundation of China (No. 30901498, No. 30100185, No. 81250036, No. 30973000, No. 30872583, No. 81072116) and the Natural Science Foundation of Shaan'xi Province, China (2009JQ4003). The funders had no role in study design, data collection and analysis, decision to publish, or preparation of the manuscript.

Competing Interests: The authors have declared that no competing interests exist.

* E-mail: jiangru@fmmu.edu.cn (YTZ); lijinqing@yahoo.cn (JQL); jianliny@fmmu.edu.cn (JLY)

ͻ These authors contributed equally to this work.

Introduction

Bladder cancer is one of the most common malignancies affecting the urinary system. A total of 44,690 males (29.8 per 100,000) and 16,730 females (11.2 per 100,000) were diagnosed in 2006, ranking bladder cancer as the fourth commonest male and ninth commonest female malignant disease in the United States [1]. In contrast, the incidence of bladder cancer in Asia is much lower. In 2009, Zhang et al. reported that although the rates rose between 1988 and 2002 (8.22 per 100,000 in 1988–1992, 9.45 per 100,000 in 1993–1997 and 9.68 per 100,000 in 1998–2002), the incidence of bladder cancer in China remains lower than the United States [2]. Similarly, in Eastern Asia, low incidences of bladder cancer have been reported in Korea (14.39 per 100,000), Japan and India (approximately 14 per 100,000) [3–5]. Additionally, the 5-year disease-specific survival rates of bladder cancer patients in Asia are higher than those in Western countries [6].

The chemotherapeutic agent, hydroxycamptothecin (HCPT), is primarily used for the treatment of bladder cancer. HCPT induces apoptosis in bladder cancer cells by forming a ternary complex with DNA and the DNA enzyme topoisomerase I via hydrogen bonds, thereby stabilizing the complex. The stable complex prevents DNA re-ligation and leads to the conversion of single-strand DNA breaks into double-strand breaks during the S-phase. At this point, the replication fork collides with DNA cleavage complexes, which induces apoptosis and cell cycle arrest [7].

Genistein, a well known isoflavone and natural botanical estrogen, has been shown to inhibit cancer cell growth, survival, metastasis and angiogenesis by increasing apoptotic cell death via the induction of several DNA-damaging stimuli [8–10]. Genistein has been shown to have an inhibitory effect on the growth of prostate cancer [11], cervical cancer [12], breast cancer [13], colon cancer [14] and renal cell carcinoma [15] cells. Genistein can also chemosensitize many malignant tumors to the effects of DNA toxic drugs. Previous reports have indicated that pretreatment with 10–30 µmol/l genistein can chemosensitize cervical, ovarian and normal fibroblast cells to treatment with HCPT by inducing a greater degree of growth inhibition and cell apoptosis [16]. However, whether genistein can enhance the chemotherapeutic effect of HCPT in bladder cells, and its molecular mechanism of action in this tissue type, remain unclear. Therefore, we explored whether genistein could chemosensitize bladder cancer cells to HCPT, and investigated the potential underlying mechanisms of this effect.

Materials and Methods

1. Cell lines

J82, SCaBER, and TCCSUP bladder cancer cell lines were purchased from the American Type Culture Collection (Manassas, VA, USA), BFTC905, HT1197, T24, TSGH-8301 bladder cancer cell lines were from the China Center for Type Culture Collection (CCTCC). The primary bladder epithelial cell line, BDEC, was from BioWhittaker (San Diego, CA, USA) and were maintained as exponentially growing cultures in DMEM supplemented with 10% fetal bovine serum, 100 U/ml penicillin and 100 µg/ml streptomycin. Genistein (Sigma, Shanghai, China) and HCPT (kindly provided by Sanofi, Shanghai, China) were dissolved in DMSO to prepare 10 mM stock solutions. For experiments, the cells were incubated for 3 days and then treated with or without 10 µM genistein and 1 µM HCPT for 24 h.

2. Cell growth inhibition by genistein and HCPT

Cells were seeded at a density of 5×10^3 cells/well and allowed to attach overnight. The culture medium was replaced with fresh media containing genistein at different concentrations for 24 h, and cells were then exposed to HCPT for an additional 72 h. For each single agent treatment, the cells were treated with genistein for 96 h and HCPT for 72 h. Cell growth was examined using the MTT assay.

3. Flow cytometry for apoptosis

Adherent cells were trypsinized, resuspended and treated as described previously [17]. Flow cytometry was performed using blue light argon-in laser (excitation wavelength, 488 nm; laser power, 200 mW) and red fluorescence from the PI that labels DNA was recorded. All tests for apoptosis were conducted in duplicate and the results shown are representative of at least three experiments.

4. Immunofluorescent staining for γ-H2AX and ATM

For γ-H2AX staining, cells were treated with different concentrations of HCPT and genistein, the media was removed at various time points and the cells were fixed in 1% paraformaldehyde for 10 min followed by 70% ethanol for 10 min. The cells were then incubated in 0.1% Triton X in phosphate buffered saline (PBS) for 10 min, permeabilized in 0.5% Triton in PBS for 10 min, washed three times in PBS and blocked with 5% bovine serum albumin (BSA) in PBS for 60 min. The cells were incubated with anti–γ-H2AX (1:2,000; Cell Signaling, Shanghai, China) or anti-ATM (1:300, Cell Signaling, Shanghai, China) in 5% BSA in PBS at 4°C overnight, washed four times in PBS, incubated in the dark with a FITC-labeled secondary antibody (1:2,000 for anti–γ-H2AX and 1:300 for anti-ATM) in 5% BSA for 1 h, washed 4 times in PBS, incubated in the dark with 1 µg/ml 4′,6-diamidino-2-phenylindole (DAPI; Invitrogen, Carlsbad, CA, USA) in PBS for 5 min, and mounted and coverslipped in Fluoromount G (Southern Biotech, Birmingham, AL, USA). The slides were examined on a Leica fluorescence

microscope (Wetzlar, Germany), images were captured using a Nikon fluorescence microscope (Nikon Eclipse E800) and imported into Nikon ACT-1 (Version 1.12) software. Images were combined into a publishing format using Adobe Photoshop CS2 software. For each treatment condition, the number of γ-H2AX or ATM foci was determined in at least 50 cells. All observations were validated by at least three independent experiments.

5. Western blotting

Bladder cancer cells were lysed in 400 µl 1% SDS lysis buffer (50 mM HEPES, pH 7.5, 100 mM NaCl, 10 mM EDTA, 4 mM NaPPi, 2 mM Na_3VO_4) for 5 min on ice to obtain total cell lysates. To collect nuclear protein, the monolayers were washed three times with ice-cold hypotonic lysis buffer (HLB, pH 7.5, 10 mM Tris, 10 mM KCl, 1 mM EDTA, 1 mM EGTA, 2 mM $MgCl_2$), and the cells were collected and transferred to a homogenizer (Wheaton Ltd, Millville, NJ, USA) in 500 µl HLB. The cells were swollen in HLB for 15 min, homogenized and the cell nuclei were collected by centrifugation and lysed in RIPA buffer. The pull-down assay was performed by the immunoprecipitation of 500 µg nuclear or cytosolic extract (precleared with Protein A/G beads) with primary antibody, and then 50–100 µg total or nuclear lysate was resolved on a 7.5–12.5% sodium dodecyl sulfate-polyacrylamide (SDS-PAGE) gel, electro-transferred to a Hybond ECL membrane (Amersham Pharmacia Biotech, Piscataway, NJ, USA), blocked in PBS containing 5% nonfat dried milk and 0.05% Tween-20, incubated with primary antibody overnight at 4°C, and then incubated with secondary antibodies for 1 h. The protein bands were visualized using the Phototope-HRP Western Detection System (Cell Signaling, Beverly, MA, USA) and Kodar film (Perkin Elmer, Waltham, MA, USA) and scanned and quantified using ImageJ (http://rsbweb.nih.gov/ij/). The anti-ATM, anti-phospho H2AX, anti-phospho ATM (Ser 1981), anti-IKK, anti-phospho IKK1/2, anti-β-actin, anti-GAPDH, anti-phospho-NEMO (NF-kappa-β essential modulator), anti-NBS1 (Nijimegen breakage syndrome 1) antibody, anti-caspase 3 and 9, anti-phospho PARP and anti-Oct1 antibodies were obtained from Cell Signaling.

6. siRNA transfection

Transfection of TCCSUP and BDEC cells with ATM siRNA (50 nmol/l; Invitrogen) was performed using Oligofectamine reagent (Invitrogen) according to the manufacturer's protocol.

7. In vivo tumor therapy studies

The experiment was approved by the Ethics Committee of the Fourth Military Medical University. Bladder cancer cells were premixed 1:1 with Matrigel (Becton Dickinson, Beijing, China) and subcutaneously inoculated (5×10^6 cells per site) into the flanks of 10-week-old female SCID nude mice (Department of Experimental Animals, the Fourth Military Medical University, Xi'an, Shaan'xi, China). Drug treatment started 22 days after tumor cell injection. Mice were randomly divided (5 mice/group) into five groups. The control group was compromised tumors that were treated with 0.01% DMSO. Mice were treated orally with food that contained genistein (1 g/kg) and/or the transperitoneal injection of 3 µg/ml HCPT. The percentage change in tumor size was calculated by comparisons with the baseline value at 22 days.

8. Electrophoretic mobility shift assay (EMSA)

Nuclear cell extracts were obtained as previously described, and 10 µg nuclear extract was incubated with purified ^{32}P-labeled NF-κB consensus double-stranded oligonucleotide and 0.25 mg/mL poly(dI-dC) in 5× binding buffer [18]. Samples were separated on 8% polyacrylamide gels, the gels were dried, exposed to X-ray film overnight at −80°C and developed using an All-Pro 100 Plus automated X-ray film processor (All-Pro Imaging Corporation, Hicksville, NY, USA).

9. Quantification and statistical methods

Groups were compared using the Student's t-test; P values ≤ 0.05 were considered statistically significant.

Results

1. Effects of HCPT and genistein on the viability of bladder cancer cells

Bladder cells were treated with genistein for 3 days, and cell viability was determined using the MTT assay. The treatment of a variety of bladder cancer cell lines and BDEC bladder cells with genistein resulted in the dose- and time-dependent inhibition of cell proliferation, which demonstrated that genistein reproducibly inhibits the growth of bladder cancer cells. However, a synergistic effect was observed when J82, T24, TSGH8301 and TCCSUP bladder cancer cells and BDEC bladder cells were treated with different concentrations of genistein and HCPT (Fig. 1A). MTT assays indicated that the synergistic effect of genistein and HCPT was concentration-dependent (Fig. 1B).

2. Synergistic cell cycle arrest by HCPT and genistein

Both HCPT (1 μm) and genistein (10 μm) for a 24-hour period showed a statistically significant ability to arrest the cell cycle (Fig. 1C). Compared with the vehicle, HCPT caused a cell cycle arrest in both the S phase (control: 57.6%, HCPT: 46.5%, genistein: 57.9%, HCPT+genistein: 31.1% for TCCSUP cells; control: 57.2%, HCPT: 43.1%, genistein: 53.6%, HCPT+genistein: 29.1% for BDEC cells) and the G2-M phase (control: 21.5%, HCPT: 30.6%, genistein: 22.1%, HCPT+genistein: 41.6% for TCCSUP cells; control: 21.7%, HCPT: 30.3%, genistein: 26.7%, HCPT+genistein: 36.3% for BDEC cells). Although genistein (10 μm) alone did not affect the cell cycle significantly compared with the controls, the addition of genistein to HCPT-treated (1 μm) cells significantly sensitized the cells to HCPT via inducing G2/M cell cycle arrest.

3. Synergistic induction of apoptosis by HCPT and genistein

Using FACS to quantify apoptosis, we observed that 10 μM genistein and 1 μM HCPT synergistically and dose-dependently induced apoptosis in bladder cancer cells (Fig. 1D). The induction of apoptosis was dose-dependent and directly correlated with an inhibition of cell growth (Fig. 1B, D).

4. NBS1-dependent ATM activation is induced by DNA damage

The results described in section 3.3 indicated that genistein may act synergistically with HCPT to induce apoptosis. As stated above, HCPT could induce cell apoptosis via inducing double strand breaks (DSB) in DNA. Therefore, we investigated whether this synergism of apoptosis is related to DSB. TCCSUP cells were treated with 1 μM HCPT and/or 10 μM genistein for 1 h, and the total protein from each group was extracted and underwent Western blotting for the chromosomal histone protein, γ-H2AX [19]. The Western blot demonstrated that HCPT and genistein could synergistically induce H2AX phosphorylation at 1 hour

after drug treatment, which indicated that these drugs could induce DSB. Furthermore, strong H2AX phosphorylation could still be seen in the co-treated group 24 h after treatment compared with the cells administered with single drugs only, which demonstrated a delayed DNA damage repair process (Fig. 2A). Additionally, 1 μM HCPT and 10 μM genistein synergistically activated the phosphorylation of ATM at Ser 794 in a dose-dependent manner (Fig. 2B). The spatial distribution of ATM and γ-H2AX after drug treatment was determined using a multiplexed immunofluorescence assay (Fig. 2C). Significantly more ATM and γ-H2AX nuclear foci were observed in TCCSUP cells treated with both HCPT and genistein for 30 min compared to the control, HCPT- and genistein-treated cells. Additionally, treatment with both these drugs significantly increased the co-localization of ATM and γ-H2AX in the cell nucleus. The ATM inhibitor, Ku55933, significantly decreased ATM foci formation, and thereby inhibited γ-H2AX/ATM co-localization in HCPT- and genistein-treated cells (Fig. 2C). An immunoprecipitation assay was performed to explore how ATM is phosphorylated after HCPT and genistein treatment. Treatment with both HCPT and genistein activated ATM and induced an interaction between ATM/H2AX and NBS1/H2AX in TCCSUP and BDEC cells. The NBS1 inhibitor, mirin, significantly attenuated HCPT- and/or genistein-induced ATM or NBS1 and H2AX binding in HCPT- and genistein-treated cells (Fig. 2D).

5. ATM inhibition downregulates NF-kB and induces apoptosis in HCPT- and genistein-treated cells

The levels of activated, phosphorylated ATM were investigated in TCCSUP cells. TCCSUP cells treated with 1 μM HCPT for 1 h exhibited a strong constitutive ATM phosphorylation, which could be inhibited by ATM siRNA or the small molecular specific ATM inhibitor, KU55933 (Fig. 3A). Immunoprecipitation assays indicated that ATM siRNA reduced ATM/NEMO binding in TCCSUP cells; however, HCPT and genistein could synergistically augment ATM/NEMO binding (Fig. 3B), which indicated that NEMO plays an important role in suppression of HCPT induced NF-κB activation. Additionally, the synergistic augmentation of ATM/NEMO binding in HCPT- and genistein-treated cells was accompanied by increased IκBα expression (Fig. 3C) and reduced IKK1/2 phosphorylation (Fig. 3D); in turn, these induced the increased cleavage of caspase 3, caspase 9 and PARP (Fig. 3E).

6. Genistein attenuated HCPT-induced NF-κB-activation and thus synergistically induced apoptosis in vivo

To verify the synergistic inhibitory effect on growth by genistein and HCPT in bladder cancer cells, we determined their effects in a xenograft model of SCID mice treated with the TCCSUP bladder cancer cell line. Genistein and HCPT exhibited a synergistic inhibitory effect on tumor growth in the xenograft (Fig. 4A). Furthermore, tumors treated with HCPT showed NF-κB activation, while genistein attenuated this activation (Fig. 4B). Decreased activation of the downstream molecules IKK1/2, increased phosphorylation of IκBα and increased cleavage of caspase 3, caspase 9 and PARP were observed in tumors treated with genistein and HCPT (Fig. 4C).

Discussion

Genistein is regarded to be a potentially ideal chemotherapy agent for bladder cancer, as it is natural, safe, with minimal side effects and relatively low costs [20]. Previous investigations have indicated that soybean isoflavone, which is present in large amounts of soybean products, may play an important role in the

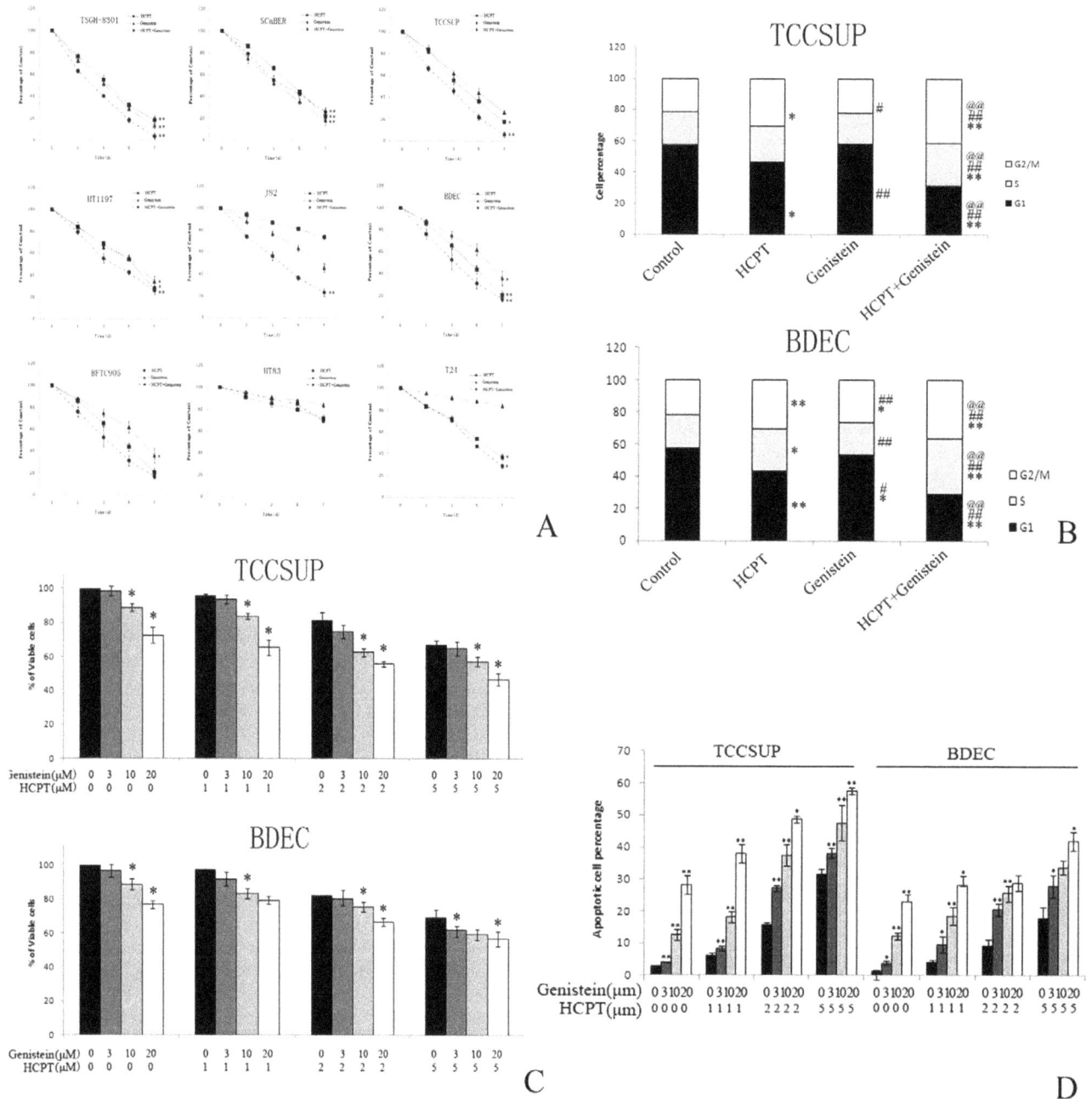

Figure 1. Genistein sensitizes bladder cancer cells to HCPT treatment. A. MTT assay of bladder cancer cell lines and BDEC cells treated with 10 μM genistein and/or 1 μM HCPT; results are expressed as percentage of control cells. **B.** MTT assay of TCCSUP and BDEC cells treated with different concentrations of HCPT and/or genistein for 48 h. **C.** Cell cycle distribution of TCCSUP or BDEC treated with 1 μM HCPT and/or 10 μM genistein for 24 h. **D.** Apoptosis measured by FACS in TCCSUP, and BDEC treated with 10 μM genistein and/or 1 μM HCPT. Values are mean ± SEM of three independent experiments; *$P<0.05$ and **$P<0.01$ compared with control group. #$P<0.05$ and ##$P<0.01$ compared with HCPT; @$P<0.05$ and @@$P<0.01$ compared with genistein.

inhibition of tumorigenesis [21]. It has also been shown to induce cell apoptosis via decreasing the expression of the 32 kDa caspase 3 precursor and increasing the levels of the cleaved active form of this caspase [22]. Zhou et al. reported that soybean isoflavones and soy phytochemical concentrates could inhibit the growth of murine and human bladder cell lines in vitro and in vivo in a dose-dependent manner [23]. Previous investigations revealed that the synergistic inhibitory effect of genistein and camptothecin in cervical cancer, ovarian carcinoma and mouse fibroblast cells

resulted from their inhibition of NF-κB translocation and the induction of G2/M cell cycle arrest and apoptosis [16].

Whether genistein could sensitize bladder cells to camptothecin treatment has not been studied previously. In this study, genistein and HCPT were found to inhibit the growth of multiple bladder cancer cell lines and the primary BDEC bladder epithelial cell line (Fig. 1A). Genistein and HCPT synergistically and dose-dependently inhibited cell survival (Fig. 1B), induced G2/M cell cycle arrest (Fig. 1C) and apoptosis (Fig. 1D) in the TCCSUP bladder

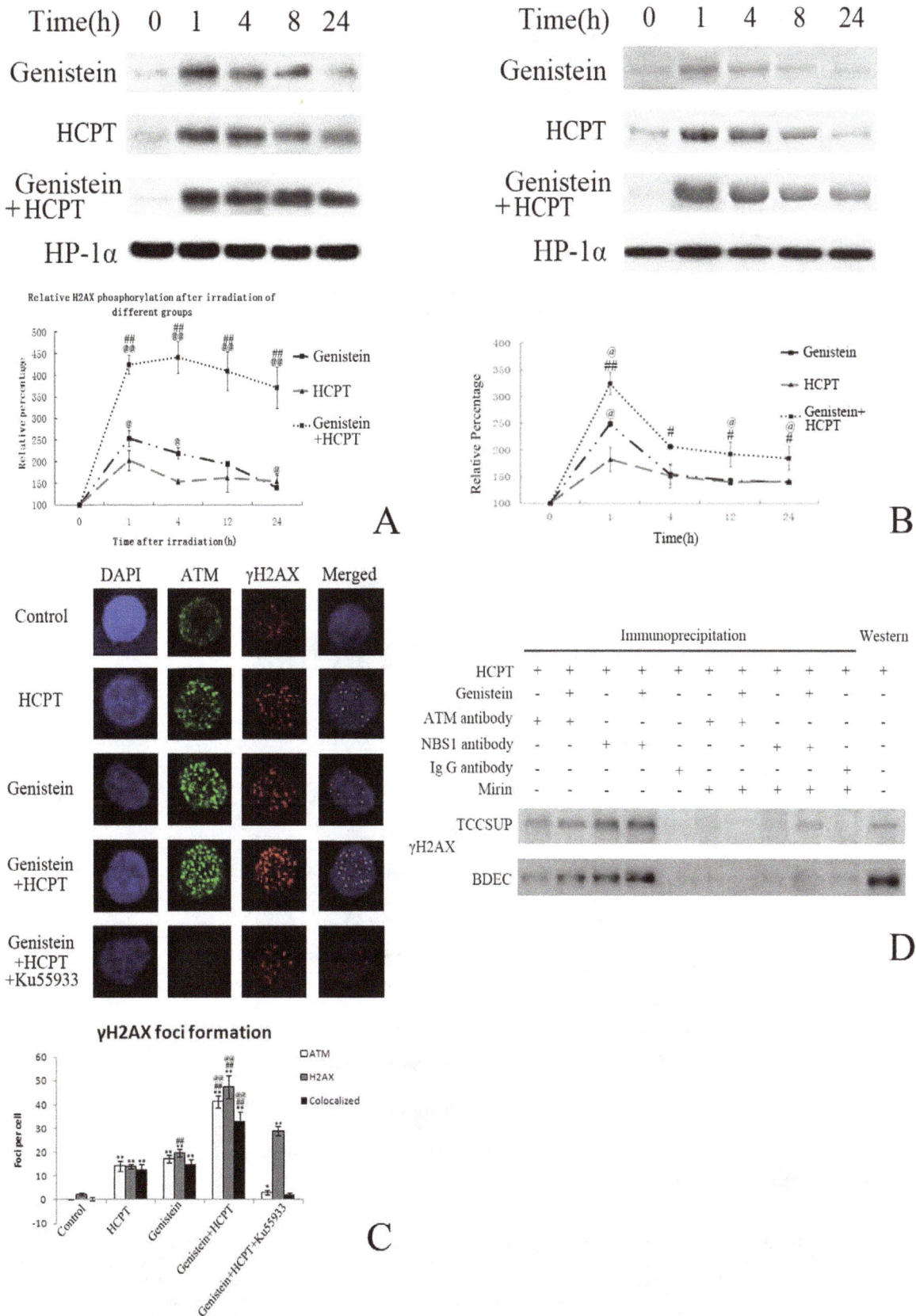

Figure 2. Genistein augments HCPT-induced cell DNA damage via the synergistic activation of nuclear ATM. A. Western blot and quantification of H2AX DNA damage repair after the pretreatment of 10 μM genistein and/or 10 μM HCPT. HP-1α was used as a loading control; results are expressed relative to the control group at 0 h. **B**. Western blot and quantification of ATM Ser 1981 phosphorylation after the pretreatment of TCCSUP cells with 10 μM genistein and/or 10 μM HCPT for 1 h. **C**. Representative images and quantification of ATM phosphorylation and H2AX

foci formation 30 min after treatment of TCCSUP cells with 1 μM HCPT and/or 10 μM genistein; discrete foci of ATM autophosphorylation appear at putative sites of double strand breaks. **D**. Identification of the NBS1-dependent ATM/H2AX interaction. TCCSUP cells and BDEC cells were treated with 1 μM HCPT and/or 10 μM genistein for 1 h with or without the NBS1 inhibitor, mirin, immunoprecipitated with anti-ATM or anti-NBS1 antibodies and immunocomplexes were detected by Western blotting. ATM foci increased linearly with dose after 1 h genistein and HCPT treatment. Values are mean ± SEM of three independent experiments; IP: immunoprecipitation, W: Western-blot. *$P<0.05$ and **$P<0.01$ compared with control group. #$P<0.05$ and ##$P<0.01$ compared with HCPT; @$P<0.05$ and @@$P<0.01$ compared with genistein.

cancer cell line and BDEC bladder epithelial cells. With regards to the underlying mechanism, the induction of dose-dependent synergistic DNA damage by genistein and HCPT and their inhibitory effect on the DNA damage repair process was observed for up to 24 h, compared with genistein or HCPT treatment alone (Fig. 2A). As previously reported, both HCPT [24] and genistein [25] could directly inhibit DNA topoisomerase I. We hypothesize that the induction of DNA damage by HCPT and genistein is due

to their inhibition on the DNA topoisomerase and thus their effects on the formation of the replication fork, which requires further investigation.

Then, we investigated the downstream signaling effects of genistein- and HCPT-induced DNA damage to determine how the synergistic induction of ATM phosphorylation is related to their pro-apoptotic effect. ATM kinase is a key regulator that is activated by DNA damage [26]. It has been reported to be closely

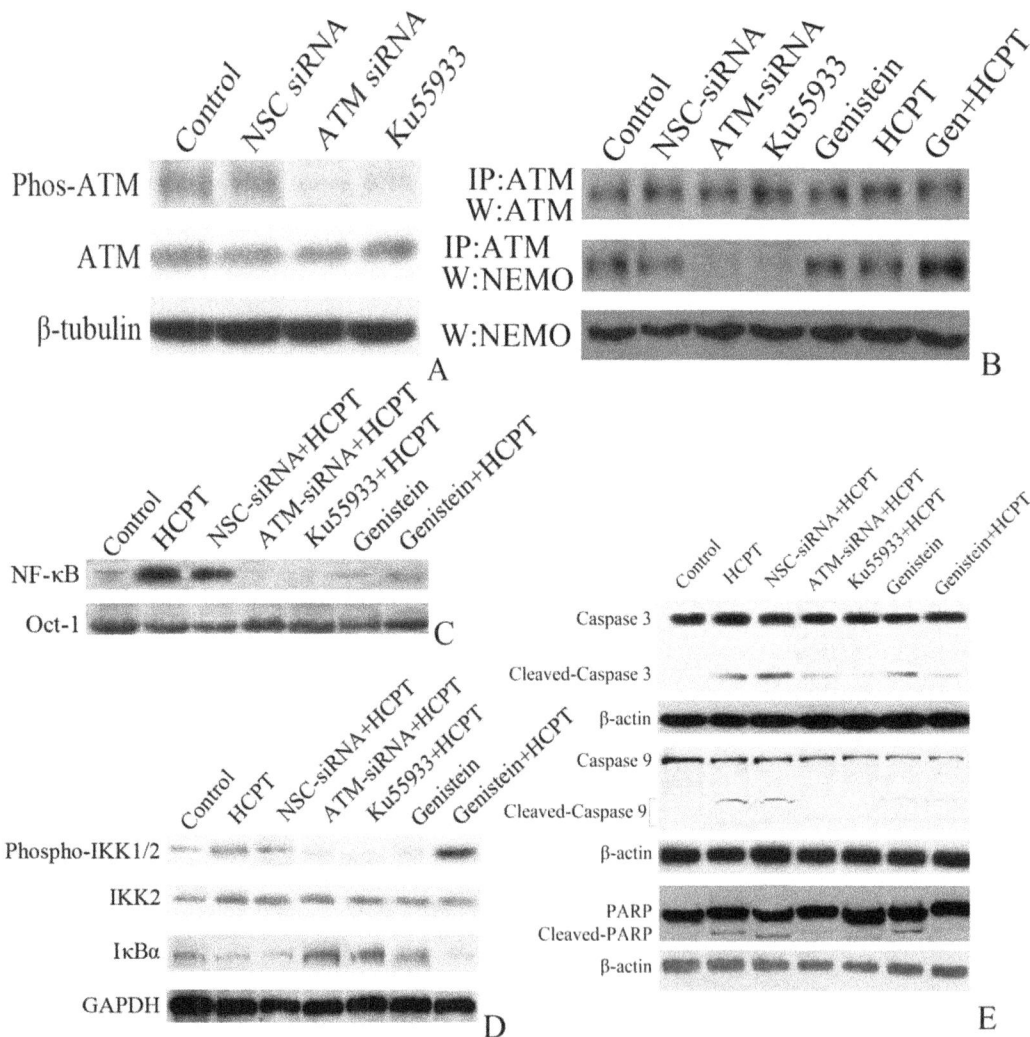

Figure 3. Genistein attenuates the activation of the ATM/NF-κB pathway by HCPT. A. Western blot of ATM phosphorylation in TCCSUP cells treated with 1 μM HCPT for 1 h transfected with non-silencing control (NSC) siRNA, ATM siRNA or treated with the ATM inhibitor, Ku55933 (10 μM,2 h). **B.** Immunoprecipitation and Western blot of ATM and NEMO in TCCSUP cells transfected with NSC siRNA or ATM siRNA, or treated with 10 μM Ku55933, 10 μM genistein and/or 1 μM HCPT. IP: immunoprecipitation, W: Western-blot. **C.** EMSA blot of NF-κB expression in TCCSUP cells treated with 10 μM genistein and/or 1 μM HCPT in the presence of NSC siRNA and ATM siRNA. **D.** Western blot of NF-κB, IKK2, IκBα expression and IKK1/2 phosphorylation in TCCSUP cells treated with 10 μM genistein and/or 1 μM HCPT in the presence of NSC siRNA and ATM siRNA, indicating that genistein and HCPT induce the phosphorylation of IKK1/2 and increase IκBα expression via ATM. **E.** Western blot of PARP, caspase 3 and caspase 9 cleavage in whole cell lysates prepared from TCCSUP cells treated with 10 μm genistein and/or 1 μM HCPT in the presence of ATM siRNA or Ku55933. All experiments were repeated three times, and similar results were obtained in each replicate.

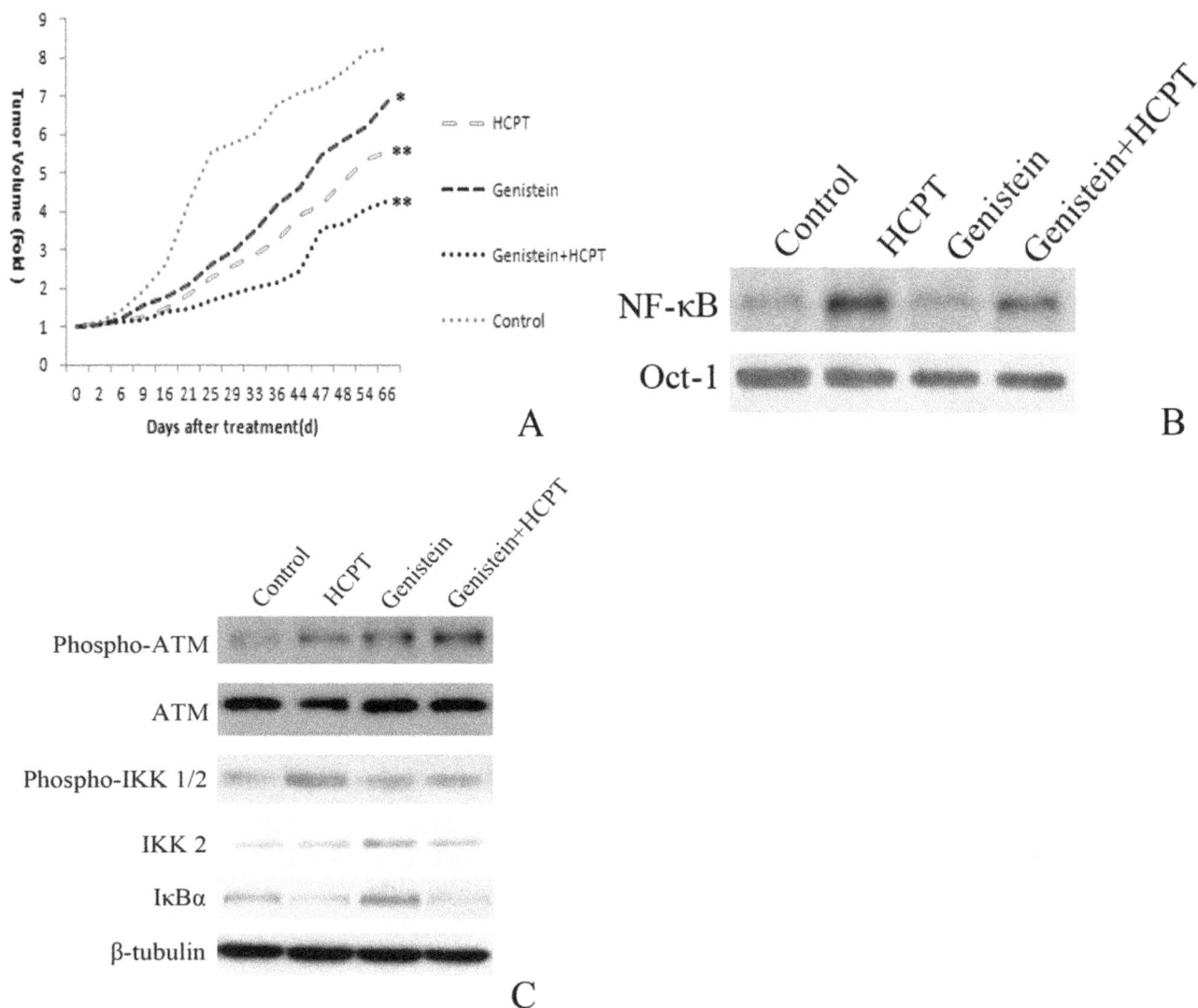

Figure 4. Genistein sensitizes TCCSUP tumors to HCPT in a SCID xenograft model. TCCSU bladder cancer cell tumors were allowed to establish for 22 days, then the animals were injected intratumorally with 10 μM genistein and/or 10 μM HCPT on day 0 and 7 of treatment. **A.** Growth curve of TCCSUP bladder cancer xenografts treated with genistein and/or HCPT; tumor volume is expressed relative to tumor size at the start of treatment. **B.** EMSA assay of NF-κB expression in xenograft tumor tissues from each group. **C.** Western blot analysis of phosphorylated IKK1/2, IKK2, IκBα expression in xenograft tumor tissues from each group.

correlated with cell apoptosis in multiple cancer cells. Zuco et al. reported that the camptothecin derivative, ST1968, can induce apoptosis via the activation of ATM [27]. Kawakami et al. reported that doxorubicin can induce apoptosis in A549 lung adenocarcinoma cells by ATM activation [28]. In this study, it was found that a combined treatment with genistein and HCPT synergistically induced ATM Ser 1981 phosphorylation (Fig. 2B) at sites of DNA damage. In cells treated with genistein and HCPT, the inhibition of ATM by its specific inhibitor, Ku55933, inhibited THE phosphorylation of ATM and H2AX, and thus inhibited their co-localization (Fig. 2C).

NBS1 has been proven to be the key element of the MRE11/ RAD50/NBS1 complex, which forms immediately after a DNA DSB forms to recruit related proteins to repair the damaged DNA sites [29]. ATM and NBS1 both bind to H2AX, a scaffold protein at sites of DNA damage. As previously described [30], we found that the ability of genistein and HCPT to synergistically induce DNA damage in bladder cancer cells via ATM activation was

dependent on NBS1, as the NBS1 inhibitor mirin specifically abrogated HCPT- and genistein-induced ATM/H2AX binding and NBS1/H2AX binding (Fig. 2D). These findings indicated that the synergistic DNA damaging effect of these two drugs was due to their inhibition of ATM, which is NBS1-dependent. The phosphorylation of ATM could activate NF-κB pathway via NEMO [31], which leads to the activation and expression of a variety of pro-proliferative and anti-apoptotic genes, thus protecting cancer cells from apoptosis. NEMO is thought to be a polyubiquitin binding subunit, which recruits IKK to linear or K63-linked polyubiquitin scaffolds that form as a consequence of receptor-initiated signaling events [32]. Therefore, after treatment with DNA toxic drugs, such as HCPT, DSB induced ATM activation, and the downstream NF-κB pathway is activated via NEMO (Fig. 3B). However, the NF-κB pathway has been shown to protect cells from cell apoptosis, which could in part attenuate the toxic effects of HCPT. In our research, genistein treatment could inactivate the NF-κB pathway in bladder cancer and epithelial cells. In summary, upon HCPT treatment, DNA damage may induce ATM phosphorylation, which activates the NF-κB pathway to protect cells from apoptosis. However, the multiple protease ability of genistein helps to abrogate HCPT-induced NF-κB activation [33]. The knockdown of ATM completely blocked the ability of HCPT and genistein to induce the activation of NEMO/IKK (Fig. 3D) and inhibited the cleavage of caspase 3, caspase 9 and PARP (Fig. 3E). This indicated that ATM plays a central role in HCPT- and genistein-induced apoptosis.

To confirm the synergistic effects of HCPT and genistein, we performed in vivo xenograft experiments. In xenografts of TCCSUP cells grown in SCID mice, combined treatment with HCTP and genistein synergistically inhibited tumor growth (Fig. 4A). This intracellular molecular event is in accordance with previously discovered findings in bladder cells. HCPT was shown to activate NF-κB, which was counteracted by genistein in SCID mice (Fig. 4B). Co-treatment with these two drugs synergistically activated ATM and inhibited IκBα (Fig. 4C).

This research indicates that the isoflavone, genistein, can significantly strengthen the effects of the bladder cancer chemotherapy agent, HCPT, both in vivo and in vivo. The synergistic pro-apoptotic effects of these two drugs induce more DSBs and delay the DNA damage repair process by activating the ATM/NBS1/NEMO/IKK pathway. However, some aspects of this mechanism remain to be elucidated. Firstly, it remains unknown as to whether the synergistic DSB inducing effect of HCPT and genistein occurs via interference with the replication fork and toposoimerase I. Secondly, it is still unclear how the DSB repair process is delayed, whether this is through the inhibition of homologous recombination, or the inhibition of non-homologous end joining. Thirdly, the role of the synergistic inhibition of NBS-1 activation by HCPT and genistein in the malformation of the MRN complex requires further exploration. In the end, genistein is a well-known botanic estrogen, and estrogen has been shown to be expressed in bladder transitional cell cancer, and it was negatively correlated with tumor grade [34]. Whether the estrogen effect of genistein is correlated with the synergistic growth inhibitory effect remain to be explored in the future.

In conclusion, this study demonstrates that genistein can sensitize bladder cancer cell lines to HCTP, leading to a synergistic dose-dependent inhibition of proliferation and an induction of cell cycle arrest and apoptosis. Genistein and HCTP induce double-

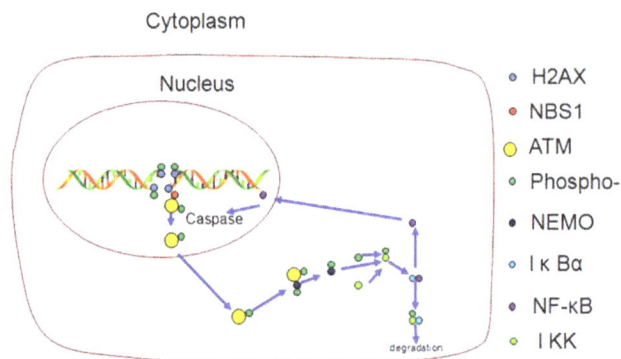

Figure 5. Schematic illustration of ATM activation and cytoplasmic translocation. ATM is phosphorylated at sites of double strand DNA breaks by NBS1 in the presence of H2AX phosphorylation. Activated ATM is transported to the cytoplasm, and activates NEMO, which phosphorylates IKK1/2. IKK1/2 activates and ubiquitinizes IκBα, leading to IκBα degradation. This stimulates the release and transport of NF-κB to the nucleus, where it binds to DNA, activates caspase cleavage and initiates apoptosis.

stranded DNA breaks, which leads to the synergistic activation of ATM, attenuates NEMO/NF-κB/IKK/caspase signal transduction, and thus induces apoptosis both in vitro and in vivo. Genistein could also counteract HCPT-induced NF-κB pathway activation, and thus attenuate the anti-apoptotic effect of the NF-κB pathway, as summarized in Fig. 5. These findings indicate that, although the underlying mechanisms require further exploration, the combined administration of HCTP and genistein might be a promising approach for the treatment of human bladder cancer.

Acknowledgments

We thank Dr. Claudia Buehnemann (University of Oxford, UK) for her excellent technical assistance.

Author Contributions

Provided the experimental lab and some funding: HW JLY YTZ. Conceived and designed the experiments: YW JQL. Performed the experiments: CS PX CHS JGS YML QF WX YHL JYW XPG. Analyzed the data: WZ. Contributed reagents/materials/analysis tools: JYG.

References

1. Jemal A, Siegel R, Ward E, Hao Y, Xu J, et al. (2006) Cancer statistics. CA Cancer J Clin 56: 106–130.

2. Zhang SW, Ma JH, Li M, Liu J, Shao MZ, et al. (2009) Incidence trends of bladder cancer in cities and counties in China. Chin J Urol 30: 673–676.

3. Cheon J, Kim CS, Lee ES, Hong SJ, Cho YH, et al. (2002) Survey of incidence of urological cancer in South Korea: a 15-year summary. Int J Urol 9: 445–454.

4. Kakehi Y, Hirao Y, Kim WJ, Ozono S, Masumori N, et al. (2010) Bladder Cancer Working Group report. Jpn J Clin Oncol Suppl 1:i57–64.

5. Manoharan N, Tyagi BB, Raina V (2010) Cancer incidences in rural Delhi–2004–05. Asian Pac J Cancer Prev 11:73–77.

6. Yee DS, Ishill NM, Lowrance WT, Herr HW, Elkin EB (2011) Ethnic Differences in Bladder Cancer Survival. Urology 78:544–549.

7. Morales R, Sriratana P, Zhang J, Cann IK (2011) Methanosarcina acetivorans C2A topoisomerase IIIα, an archaeal enzyme with promiscuity in divalent cation dependence.PLoS One 6(10):e26903.

8. Hilakivi-Clarke L, Onojafe I, Raygada M, Cho E, Skaar T, et al. (1999) Prepubertal exposure to zearalenone or genistein reduces mammary tumorigenesis. Br J Cancer 80:1682–1688.

9. Zhou JR, Mukherjee P, Gugger ET, Tanaka T, Blackburn GL, et al. (1998) Inhibition of murine bladder tumorigenesis by soy isoflavones via alterations in the cell cycle, apoptosis, and angiogenesis. Cancer Res 58:5231–5238.

10. Li C, Teng RH, Tsai YC, Ke HS, Huang JY, et al. (2005) H-Ras oncogene counteracts the growth-inhibitory effect of genistein in T24 bladder carcinoma cells. Br J Cancer 92:80–88.

11. Kumi-Diaka J, Merchant K, Haces A, Hormann V, Johnson M (2010) Genistein-selenium combination induces growth arrest in prostate cancer cells. J Med Food 13:842–50.

12. Kim SH, Kim SH, Kim YB, Jeon YT, Lee SC, et al. (2009) Genistein inhibits cell growth by modulating various mitogen-activated protein kinases and AKT in cervical cancer cells.Ann N Y Acad Sci 1171:495–500.

13. Ullah MF, Ahmad A, Zubair H, Khan HY, Wang Z, et al. (2011) Soy isoflavone genistein induces cell death in breast cancer cells through mobilization of endogenous copper ions and generation of reactive oxygen species.Mol Nutr Food Res 55:553–559.

14. Qi W, Weber CR, Wasland K, Savkovic SD (2011) Genistein inhibits proliferation of colon cancer cells by attenuating a negative effect of epidermal growth factor on tumor suppressor FOXO3 activity. BMC Cancer 11:219.

15. Wang Y, Zhang YT, Liu F, Zhang S, Wang W, et al. (2003) Effect of genistein on proliferation of renal cell carcinoma cell line GRC-1 and its correlation with p27. Chinese Journal of Cancer 22:1272–1275.

16. Papazisis KT, Kalemi TG, Zambouli D, Geromichalos GD, Lambropoulos AF, et al. (2006) Synergistic effects of protein tyrosine kinase inhibitor genistein with camptothecins against three cell lines in vitro. Cancer Lett 233:255–264.

17. Wang Y, Li JQ, Shao C, Shi CH, Liu F, et al. (2011) Androgen receptor coregulators NOCR1, TIF2, and ARA70 may account for the hydroxyflutamide insensitivity of prostate cancer cells. Ir J Med Sci 180:865–872.

18. Kobayashi J, Tauchi H, Chen B, Burma S, Tashiro S, et al. (2009) Histone H2AX participates the DNA damage-induced ATM activation through interaction with NBS1.Biochem Biophys Res Commun 380:752–757.

19. Fu S, Yang Y, Tirtha D, Yen Y, Zhou BS, et al. (2012) γ-H2AX Kinetics as a Novel Approach to High Content Screening for Small Molecule Radio-sensitizers.PLoS One 7(6):e38465.

20. Wang H, Li Q, Chen H (2012) Genistein Affects Histone Modifications on Dickkopf-Related Protein 1 (DKK1) Gene in SW480 Human Colon Cancer Cell Line.PLoS One 7(7):e40955.

21. Hilakivi-Clarke L, Cho E, Onojafe I, Raygada M, Clarke R (1999) Maternal exposure to genistein during pregnancy increases carcinogen-induced mammary tumorigenesis in female rat offspring. Oncol Rep 6:1089–1095.

22. Choi EJ, Lee BH (2004) Evidence for genistein mediated cytotoxicity and apoptosis in rat brain. Life Sci 75(4):499–509.

23. Zhou JR, Mukherjee P, Gugger ET, Tanaka T, Blackburn GL, et al. (1998) Inhibition of murine bladder tumorigenesis by soy isoflavones via alterations in the cell cycle, apoptosis, and angiogenesis. Cancer Res 58:5231–5238.

24. Tanizawa A, Fujimori A, Fujimori Y, Pommier Y (1994) Comparison of topoisomerase I inhibition, DNA damage, and cytotoxicity of camptothecin derivatives presently in clinical trials. J Natl Cancer Inst 86(11):836–42.

25. Okura A, Arakawa H, Oka H, Yoshinari T, Monden Y (1988) Effect of genistein on topoisomerase activity and on the growth of [Val 12]Ha-ras-transformed NIH 3T3 cells. Biochem Biophys Res Commun;157(1):183–9.

26. Lavin MF, Kozlov S, Gueven N, Peng C, Birrell G, et al. (2005) Atm and cellular response to DNA damage. Adv Exp Med Biol 570:457–476.

27. Zuco V, Benedetti V, Zunino F (2010) ATM- and ATR-mediated response to DNA damage induced by a novel camptothecin, ST1968. Cancer Lett 292:186–96.

28. Kawakami K, Nishida H, Tatewaki N, Nakajima Y, Konishi T, et al. (2011) Persimmon leaf extract inhibits the ATM activity during DNA damage response induced by Doxorubicin in A549 lung adenocarcinoma cells. Biosci Biotechnol Biochem 75:650–655.

29. Dheekollu J, Deng Z, Wiedmer A, Weitzman MD, Lieberman PM. (2007) A role for MRE11, NBS1, and recombination junctions in replication and stable maintenance of EBV episomes. PLoS One 2(12):e1257.

30. Perfettini JL, Nardacci R, Bourouba M, Subra F, Gros L, et al. (2008) Critical involvement of the ATM-dependent DNA damage response in the apoptotic demise of HIV-1-elicited syncytia.PLoS One 3(6):e2458.

31. Wu ZH, Miyamoto S (2008) Induction of a pro-apoptotic ATM-NF-kappaB pathway and its repression by ATR in response to replication stress.EMBO J 27(14):1963–73.

32. Adli M, Merkhofer E, Cogswell P, Baldwin AS (2010) IKKalpha and IKKbeta each function to regulate NF-kappaB activation in the TNF-induced/canonical pathway. PLoS One 5(2):e9428.

33. Davis JN, Kucuk O, Sarkar FH (1999) Genistein inhibits NF-kappa B activation in prostate cancer cells.Nutr Cancer 35(2):167–74.

34. Kontos S, Papatsoris A, Kominea A, Melachrinou M, Tanoglidi A, et al. (2011) Expression of ERβ and its co-regulators p300 and NCoR in human transitional cell bladder cancer. Urol Int87(2):151–8.

6

Downregulation of HIPK2 Increases Resistance of Bladder Cancer Cell to Cisplatin by Regulating Wip1

Jun Lin[1], Qiang Zhang[2], Yi Lu[1], Wenrui Xue[2], Yue Xu[2], Yichen Zhu[1], Xiaopeng Hu[2]*

1 Department of Urology, Beijing Friendship Hospital Affiliated to Capital Medical University, Beijing, P.R China, **2** Department of Urology, Beijing Chao-Yang Hospital Affiliated to Capital Medical University, Beijing, P.R China

Abstract

Cisplatin-based combination chemotherapy regimen is a reasonable alternative to cystectomy in advanced/metastatic bladder cancer, but acquisition of cisplatin resistance is common in patients with bladder cancer. Previous studies showed that loss of homeodomain-interacting protein kinase-2 (HIPK2) contributes to cell proliferation and tumorigenesis. However, the role of HIPK2 in regulating chemoresistance of cancer cell is not fully understood. In the present study, we found that HIPK2 mRNA and protein levels are significantly decreased in cisplatin-resistant bladder cancer cell *in vivo* and *in vitro*. Downregulation of HIPK2 increases the cell viability in a dose- and time-dependent manner during cisplatin treatment, whereas overexpression of HIPK2 reduces the cell viability. HIPK2 overexpression partially overcomes cisplatin resistance in RT4-CisR cell. Furthermore, we showed that Wip1 (wild-type p53-induced phosphatase 1) expression is upregulated in RT4-CisR cell compared with RT4 cell, and HIPK2 negatively regulates Wip1 expression in bladder cancer cell. HIPK2 and Wip1 expression is also negatively correlated after cisplatin-based combination chemotherapy *in vivo*. Finally, we demonstrated that overexpression of HIPK2 sensitizes chemoresistant bladder cancer cell to cisplatin by regulating Wip1 expression.

Conclusions: These data suggest that HIPK2/Wip1 signaling represents a novel pathway regulating chemoresistance, thus offering a new target for chemotherapy of bladder cancer.

Editor: Thomas G. Hofmann, German Cancer Research Center, Germany

Funding: The authors have no support or funding to report.

Competing Interests: The authors have declared that no competing interests exist.

* E-mail: xiaopenghu@sohu.com

Introduction

Human bladder cancer is the tenth most common malignancy in women, and the fourth most common in men [1,2]. Pathological studies indicate that bladder cancer comprises two major groups. The most common bladder cancer is urothelial carcinoma (UC) that usually recurs but rarely progress [3,4]. In addition, invasive bladder cancer is more aggressive, and one-half of patients with invasive bladder cancer develop distant metastasis [5,6]. Chemoradiation is a reasonable alternative to cystectomy in advanced/metastatic bladder cancer, but resistance to cancer chemotherapy is a common phenomenon especially in metastatic bladder cancer [7]. However, the advances in chemotherapy for the purpose of bladder cancer treatment have been limited because the underlying mechanisms causing chemoresistance are not known. Revealing the molecular mechanism of chemoresistance is indispensable for developing effective chemotherapeutic agents.

Homeodomain-interacting protein kinase-2 (HIPK2) is a serine/threonine kinase that as been shown to be involved in tumor suppressor [8,9,10]. HIPK2 is activated in response to various types of DNA-damaging agents, such as cisplatin, ultraviolet and roscovitine chemotherapeutic drugs [9]. HIPK2 phosphorylates p53 for specific activation of proapoptotic target genes, including p53AIP1, PIG3, Bax and Noxa and contributes to the regulation of p53-induced apoptosis [11,12,13]. Puca *et al* demonstrated that HIPK2 is an important regulator of p53 activity

in response to a chemotherapeutic drug [14]. HIPK2 is expressed differently in sensitive versus chemoresistant cells in response to different chemotherapeutic drugs (i.e., cisplatin and adriamycin). HIPK2 inhibition suppresses the adriamycin-induced apoptosis in chemoresistant cancer cells, whereas overexpression of HIPK2 triggers apoptosis in chemoresistant cells, associated with induction of p53Ser46-target gene AIP1 [14,15,16]. Lazzari *et al* showed that HIPK2 knockdown induces resistance to different anticancer drugs even by targetingΔNp63α in p53-null cells [17].

Wild-type p53-induced phosphatase 1 (Wip1) is a p53-inducible serine/threonine phosphatase that switches off DNA damage checkpoint responses by the dephosphorylation of certain proteins, such as p38 mitogen-activated protein kinase, p53, checkpoint kinase 1 and checkpoint kinase 2 [18,19]. Wip1 is targeted by HIPK2 for degradation [20]. Emerging data also indicate that Wip1 is overexpressed in various human tumors, and is associated with chemoresistance [19]. Wang *et al* showed that Wip1 knockdown increases DNA damage signaling and re-sensitizes oral squamous cell carcinoma (SCC) cells to cisplatin [21]. Using xenograft tumor models, they demonstrated that overexpression of Wip1 promotes tumorigenesis and its inhibition improves the tumor response to cisplatin [21]. Oppositely, Goloudina *et al* showed that Wip1 overexpression sensitizes colon cancer cells HCT116 (p53$^{-/-}$) to cisplatin in RUNX2-dependent transcriptional induction of the proapoptotic Bax protein [22]. However,

A

B

C

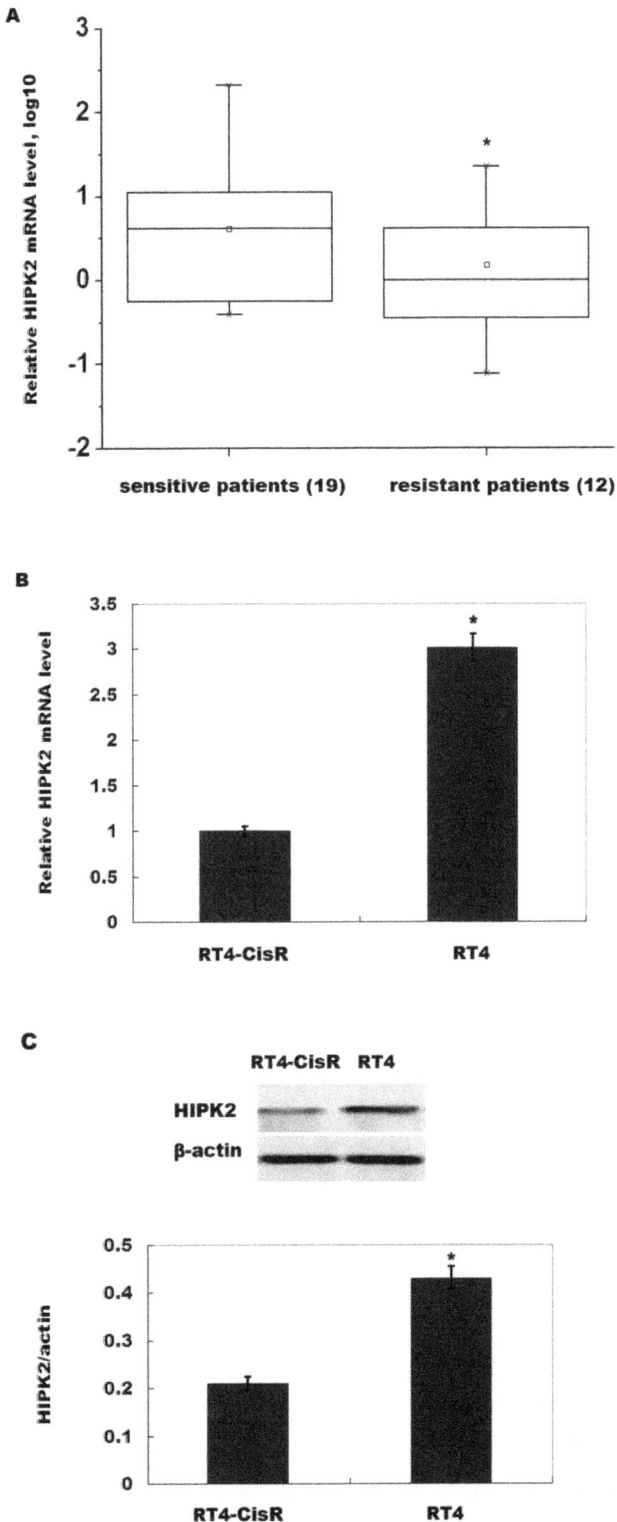

Figure 1. HIPK2 expression is decreased in chemo-resistant bladder cancer cell. (A) The analysis of the HIPK2 expression level was performed in blood samples with cisplatin-sensitive patients (n = 19) and cisplatin-resistant patients (n = 12). Total RNA was extracted and subjected to real-time RT-PCR to analyze the relative level of HIPK2 in each sample. Relative expression was calculated and normalized with respect to β-actin mRNA. All data were expressed as fold change relative to a tissue (control, expression = 1). The results were expressed as Log10 $(2^{-\Delta\Delta Ct})$. *$p<0.05$. (B) The cisplatin-resistant subline RT4-CisR was established by continuous exposure to increasing concentrations

of cisplatin over a time period of 12 months, and HIPK2 levels were analyzed by real-time PCR. Relative HIPK2 levels were calculated with respect to the control. *$p<0.05$. (C) Western blot analysis of HIPK2 protein level in RT4-CisR and RT4 cells (up). We also showed relative quantification of HIPK2 protein level (bottom, n = 3). *$p<0.05$.

the role of Wip1 in regulating cisplatin sensitivity of bladder cancer cell is not fully understood.

Based on these findings, we investigated whether HIPK2 regulates chemosensitivity by targeting Wip1 in bladder cancer cell. Here we found that upregulation of HIPK2 inhibits Wip1 expression, which sensitizes chemoresistant bladder cancer cell to cisplatin.

Materials and Methods

Cell lines and tissue samples

The protocols used in the study were approved by the Hospital's Protection of Human Subjects Committee. Blood specimens were acquired with written informed consent from the Beijing Friendship Hospital Affiliated to Capital University of Medical Sciences. A total of 31 unresectable/metastatic bladder cancer patients were included in the study, and all the patients received cisplatin-based combination chemotherapy between 12/2011 and 08/2013 (median age 62.3, range 51–80).

Human bladder cancer cell lines with wild type of p53 (RT4 and 253J) were obtained and maintained as recommended by American Type Culture Collection (ATCC, Manassas, VA). The cisplatin-resistant subline RT4-resistance (RT4-CisR) was established by continuous exposure to increasing concentrations of cisplatin over a time period of 12 months, as reported previously [23].

Real-time PCR

Total RNA was extracted from cells or tissues using Trizol reagent (Invitrogen, Carlsbad, CA), and reverse transcription (RT) reactions were performed according to the manufacturer's protocol. Real-time PCR was performed using a standard protocol from the SYBR Green PCR kit (Toyobo, Osaka, Japan). β-actin were used as references for mRNAs. ΔCt values were normalized to β-actin levels. The $2^{-\Delta\Delta Ct}$ method was used to determine the relative quantitation of gene expression levels. Each sample was analyzed in triplicate.

Western blot analysis

Western blot analysis to assess HIPK2, Wip1 and β-actin expression was performed as previously described [24]. HIPK2 (ab28507) and Wip1 (ab72000) primary antibodies were purchased from Abcam (Cambridge, MA, USA). The β-actin primary antibodies were purchased from Sigma (MO, USA).

Cell viability assay

Cells were plated and grown in 96-well plate in 0.1 ml Dulbecco's modified Eagle's medium containing 10% (v/v) fetal calf serum at 37°C for 24 h. Thereafter, the medium was changed and 0.1 ml fresh medium containing indicated drug was added and the cells were incubated for additional 48 h. The number of viable cells was determined by using the 3-(4,5-dimethylthiazol-2-yl)-2,5-diphenyltetrazolium bromide (MTT) assay as described [25].

RNAi and overexpression

RNAi was performed as described previously [26,27]. The siRNAs used in this study were mixtures of three siRNAs and were

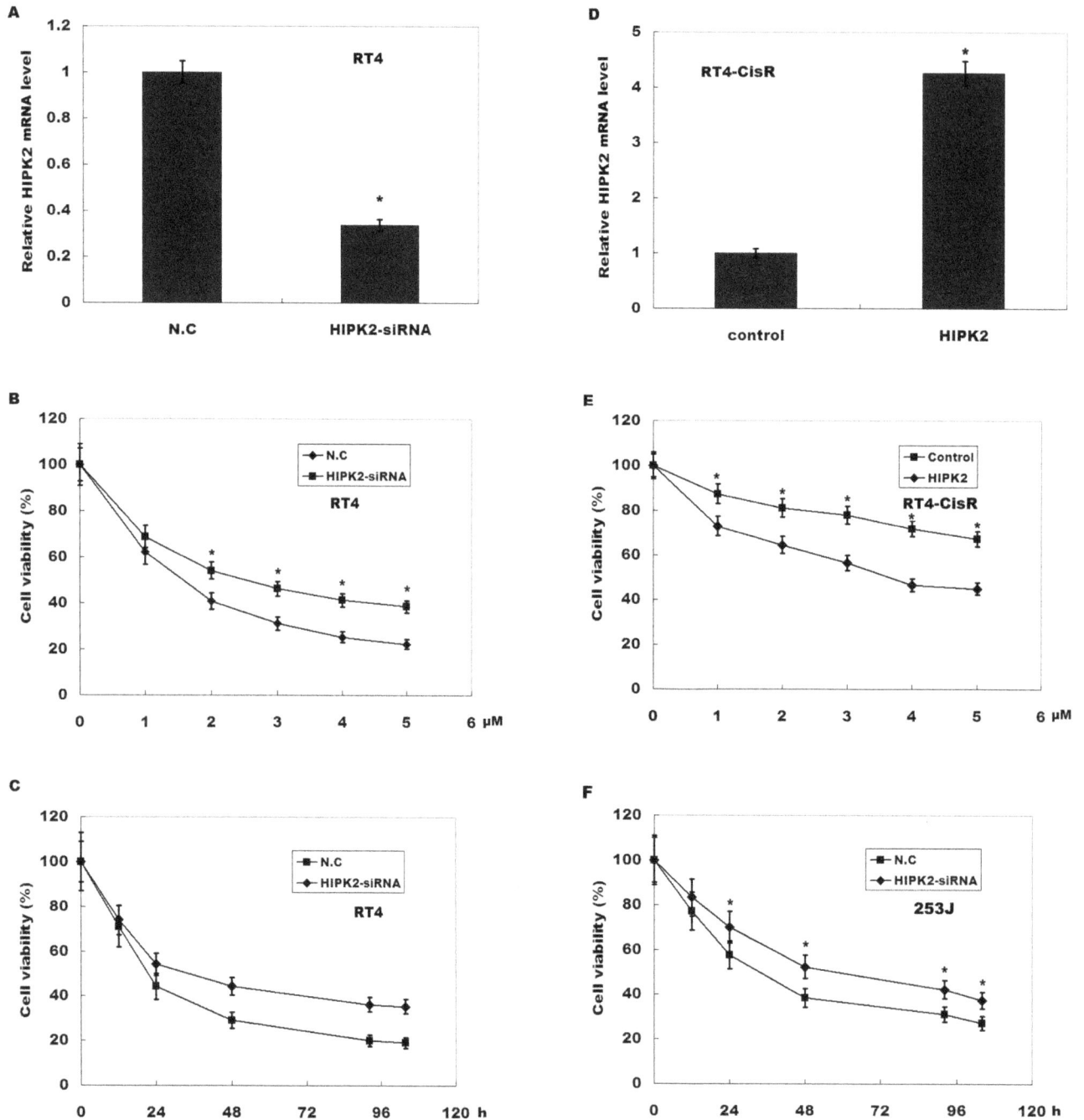

Figure 2. HIPK2 downregulation increases cell viability during cisplatin treatment in bladder cancer cell. (A) RT4 cells were transfected with HIPK2-siRNAs and HIPK2 expression level was assayed by real-time PCR. N.C = negative control (scrambled) siRNA. (B) RT4 cells were treated with HIPK2-siRNAs, and cell viability was assayed by using MTT following cisplatin treatment (1 to 6 μM). The results show data from six independent experiments, expressed as the mean ± SD. *$p < 0.05$. (C) RT4 cells were treated with HIPK2-siRNAs, and at the indicated time points, cell viability was assayed by using MTT following cisplatin treatment (6 μM). The results show data from six independent experiments, expressed as the mean ± SD. *$p < 0.05$. (D) RT4-CisR cells were transfected with pcDNA-HIPK2 and HIPK2 expression level was assayed by real-time PCR. (E) HIPK2 was overexpressed in RT4-CisR cells, and cell viability was assayed by using MTT following cisplatin treatment (1 to 6 μM). The results show data from six independent experiments, expressed as the mean ± SD. *$p < 0.05$. (F) 253J cells were treated with HIPK2-siRNAs, and cell viability was assayed by using MTT following cisplatin treatment (6 μM). *$p < 0.05$.

purchased from Genepharm (Shanghai, China). pcDNA-HIPK2 and pcDNA-Wip1 were constructed to overexpress HIPK2 or Wip1 by introducing a fragment containing the HIPK2 or Wip1 precursor into pcDNA plasmid.

Statistical analysis

All data are expressed as mean ± standard deviation (SD) from at least three separate experiments. The differences between groups were analyzed using Student's t test. Differences were deemed statistically significant at $p < 0.05$.

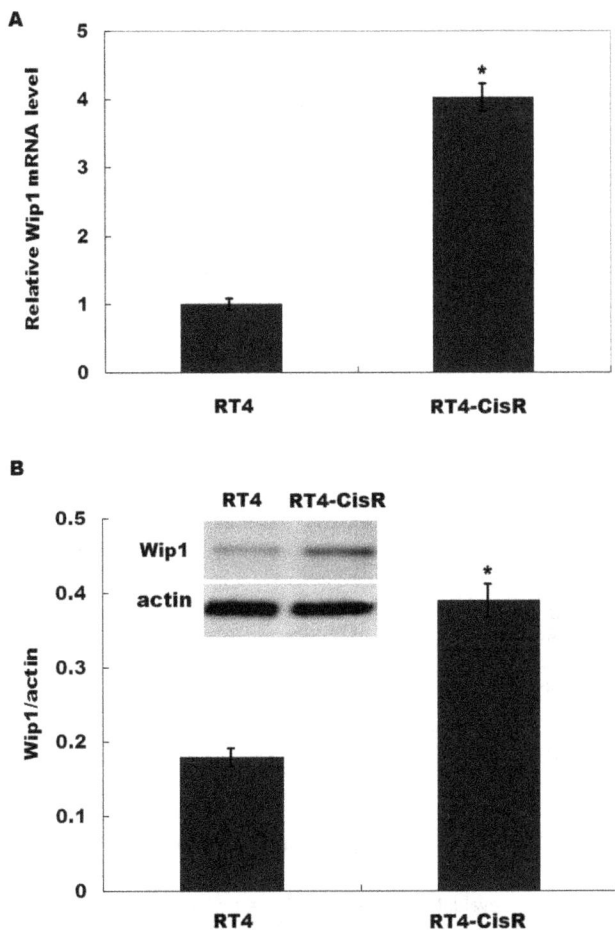

Figure 3. Wip1 expression is upregulated in RT4-CisR cell compared with RT4 cell. (A and B) Wip1 mRNA and protein expression levels were assayed in RT4 and RT4-CisR cells, respectively. *$p<0.05$.

Results

HIPK2 expression is decreased in chemo-resistant bladder cancer cell

Cisplatin is currently the most effective antitumor agent against advanced bladder cancer. However, resistance to cisplatin-based combination chemotherapy is a common phenomenon especially in metastatic bladder cancer. To clarify the molecular mechanisms underlying cisplatin resistance in bladder cancer, a total of 31 metastatic bladder cancer patients were included, and HIPK2 expression level was assayed after cisplatin-based combination chemotherapy. Figure 1A showed that HIPK2 expression in patients who are chemo-resistant is significantly decreased compared with chemo-sensitive patients. Then we established a cisplatin-resistant subline from the human bladder cancer cell line RT4 (RT4-CisR), and assayed the expression level of HIPK2. As shown in Figure 1B, HIPK2 mRNA levels were lower in RT4-CisR cells compared with RT4 cells. Similarly, HIPK2 protein levels were downregulated in RT4-CisR cells (Figure 1C). These data indicate that downregulation of HIPK2 may be related to cisplatin resistance of bladder cancer cells.

HIPK2 knockdown increases cell viability during cisplatin treatment in bladder cancer cell

To investigate the role of HIPK2 in cisplatin resistance, separate overexpression and ablation experiments were done using either pcDNA-HIPK2 or HIPK2 siRNA during cisplatin treatment and cell viability was assayed. Figure 2A showed that HIPK2 expression levels were decreased in RT4 cells treated with HIPK2-siRNA. Then RT4 cell were incubated with different concentrations of cisplatin (0, 1, 2, 3, 4, 5 and 6 μM) for 48 h. As shown in Figure 2B, HIPK2 inhibition markedly increases RT4 cell viability compared with negative control (N.C). Expectedly, knockdown of HIPK2 increases RT4 cell viability following cisplatin treatment in time-dependent manner (Figure 2C). In RT4-CisR cells, cisplatin treatment resulted in a modest inhibition of cell viability, whereas overexpression of HIPK2 re-sensitized RT4-CisR cells to cisplatin (Figure 2D and E). Similarly, HIPK2 expression was inhibited in 253J cells after HIPK2-siRNA treatment (Figure S1), and HIPK2 inhibition increases 253J cell viability in time-dependent manner (Figure 2F). These data suggest that HIPK2 increases cisplatin sensitivity of bladder cancer cells.

HIPK2 negatively regulates Wip1 expression

Previous studies showed that HIPK2 regulates tumor progression and drug resistance via several potential target genes, such as Bax, p53AIP1, Noxa, etc [14]. HIPK2 also plays a critical role in the initiation of double-strand break repair signaling by controlling Wip1 levels in response to ionizing radiation [20]. Recent studies indicate that Wip1 is overexpressed in various human tumors, and is associated with chemoresistance [19]. However, little is known about whether HIPK2 regulates cisplatin resistance by targeting Wip1. We first assayed the expression level of Wip1 in RT4 and RT4-CisR cells. Figure 3A and B showed that Wip1 mRNA and protein levels were significantly upregulated in RT4-CisR compared with RT4 cell. We then assayed whether HIPK2 negatively regulates Wip1 expression. HIPK2 knockdown increased Wip1 expression levels in bladder cancer cell lines (Figure 4A), whereas HIPK2 overexpression remarkably inhibited Wip1 mRNA level in bladder cancer cell lines (Figure 4B). Western blot analysis showed that HIPK2 knockdown increases Wip1 protein level (Figure 4C). *In vivo*, a significant negative correlation is also observed between the HIPK2 levels and the Wip1 levels in patients with bladder cancer after cisplatin-based combination chemotherapy ($r^2 = 0.1507$, $p = 0.0063$, Figure 4D). These data showed that downregulation of HIPK2 results in an increase of Wip1 expression.

HIPK2 overexpression sensitizes chemoresistant bladder cancer cell to cisplatin by regulating Wip1 expression

We next investigated the role of Wip1 in regulating cell viability during cisplatin treatment. Figure 5A showed that Wip1 overexpression increased cell viability in RT4 cells during cisplatin treatment. HIPK2 inhibits Wip1 expression and decreases cisplatin resistance, and a significant negative correlation is observed between the HIPK2 and the Wip1. We therefore speculated that the role of HIPK2 in regulating cisplatin resistance is mediated by Wip1. Figure 5B showed that HIPK2 inhibition markedly increases RT4 cell viability compared with N.C, whereas Wip1 inhibition in HIPK2-downregulating cells partly reduces cell viability. Similarly, Wip1 inhibition in HIPK2-downregulating cells partly reduces 253J cell viability (Figure 5C). More important, cell viability is decreased by HIPK2 overexpression, whereas Wip1 overexpression increased HIPK2-overexpressing cell viability

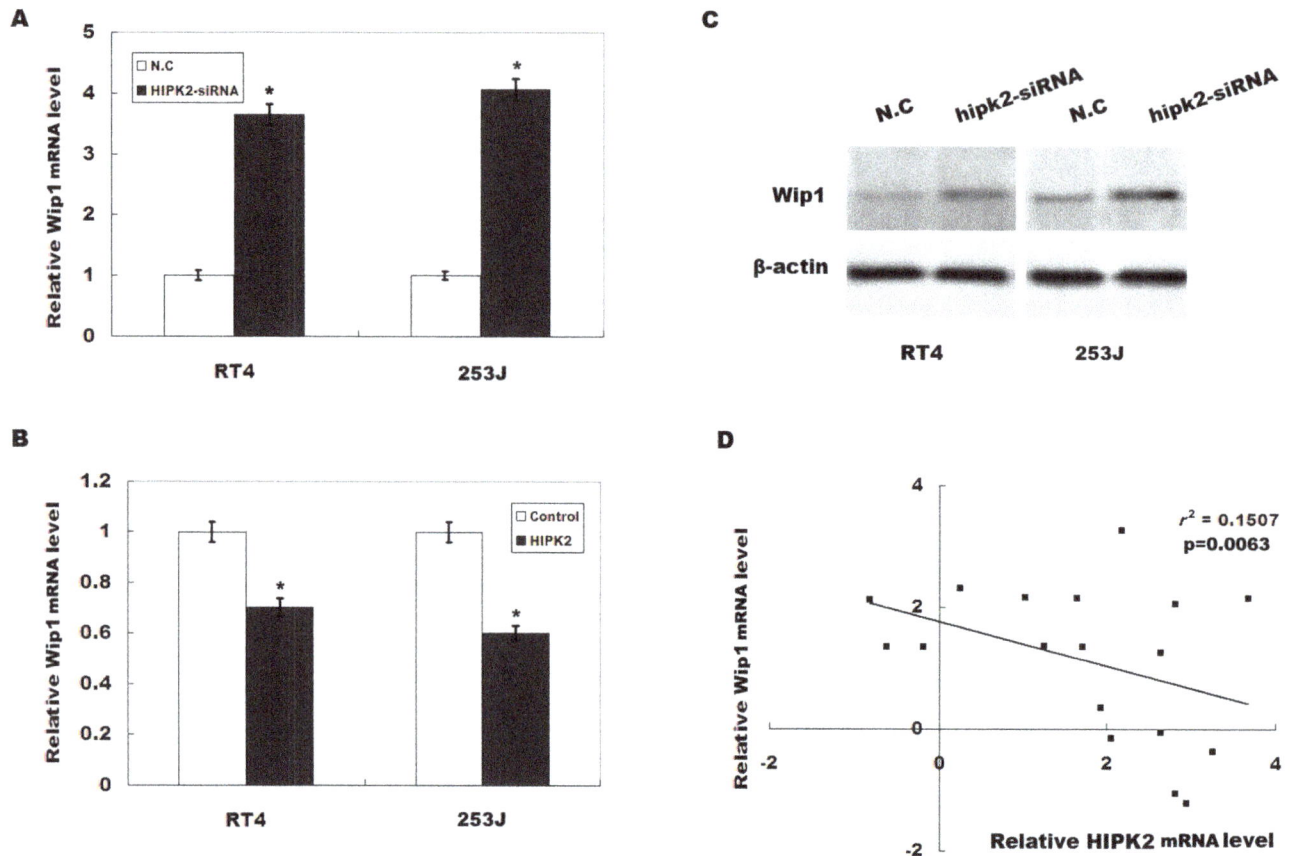

Figure 4. HIPK2 negatively regulates Wip1 expression. (A) Wip1 mRNA levels were evaluated by real-time PCR after HIPK2 inhibition in RT4 cells and 253J cells. *$p<0.05$. (B) Relative Wip1 mRNA level after HIPK2 overexpression in RT4 cells and 253J cells. *$p<0.05$. (C) Western blot analysis of Wip1 level after HIPK2 inhibition in RT4 and 253J cells. (D) Negative correlation between the HIPK2 levels and the Wip1 levels in 18 patients with bladder cancer after cisplatin-based combination chemotherapy ($r^2 = 0.1507$, $p = 0.0063$). Relative Wip1 or HIPK2 expression was calculated and normalized with respect to β-actin mRNA. All data were expressed as fold change relative to a tissue (control, expression = 1).

(Figure 5D). These data confirm that HIPK2 overexpression sensitizes chemoresistant bladder cancer cell to cisplatin by regulating Wip1 expression.

Discussion

Human bladder cancer is one of the most fatal cancers all over the world, and its incidence is increasing in many countries. Besides surgical treatments, systematic chemotherapy, play an important role in bladder cancer treatment especially for patients with advanced and metastatic bladder cancer [28,29]. However, despite a rapid shrinkage in tumor mass following chemotherapeutic cycles, the chemoresistance of cancer cells frequently results in the subsequent recurrence and metastasis of cancer [30,31]. Considering the poor prognosis for patients with bladder cancer, mainly because of late diagnosis and low response to chemotherapy, we attempted to identify predictive markers of therapeutic response and molecular targets to increase sensitivity to treatment.

Our studies provide a rationale for the potential use of HIPK2 transduction to sensitize chemoresistant bladder cancer cells to cisplatin. We showed that HIPK2 expression levels are significantly downregulated in cisplatin-resistant RT4 cell (RT4-CisR) compared with RT4 cell. Downregulation of HIPK2 increases the cisplatin resistance in a dose- and time-dependent manner in RT4 cell, whereas forced expression of HIPK2 reduces the cell viability during cisplatin treatment. Moreover, overexpression of HIPK2

partially overcomes cisplatin resistance in RT4-CisR cell. Previous studies showed that HIPK2 is activated in response to various types of DNA-damaging agents, such as cisplatin, ultraviolet and roscovitine chemotherapeutic drugs [14,32], and is an important regulator of p53 activity in response to a chemotherapeutic drug [11,14]. Overexpression of HIPK2 in p53 wild-type re-sensitizes chemoresistant ovarian cancer cells to chemotherapy by mediating p53 phosphorylation. However, the molecular mechanism of HIPK2 in regulating chemoresistance of cancer cell is not fully understood.

Wip1 is a p53-inducible serine/threonine phosphatase that switches off DNA damage checkpoint responses by the dephosphorylation of certain proteins involved in DNA repair and the cell cycle checkpoint [19]. The Wip1 gene is amplified in many tumor types [33]. Song et al showed that Wip1 interacts with and dephosphorylates BAX to suppress BAX-mediated apoptosis in response to γ-irradiation in prostate cancer cells [19]. Radiation-resistant LNCaP cells showed dramatic increases in Wip1 levels and impaired BAX movement to the mitochondria after c-irradiation, and these effects were reverted by a Wip1 inhibitor [19]. Wang et al showed that Wip1 is an effective drug target for enhanced cancer therapy [21]. Wip1 inhibition increases DNA damage signaling and resensitizes oral SCC cells to cisplatin. Wip1 upregulation promotes tumorigenesis and its inhbition improves the tumor response to cisplatin. Consistent with above results, we found that expression level of Wip1 is upregulated in RT4-CisR

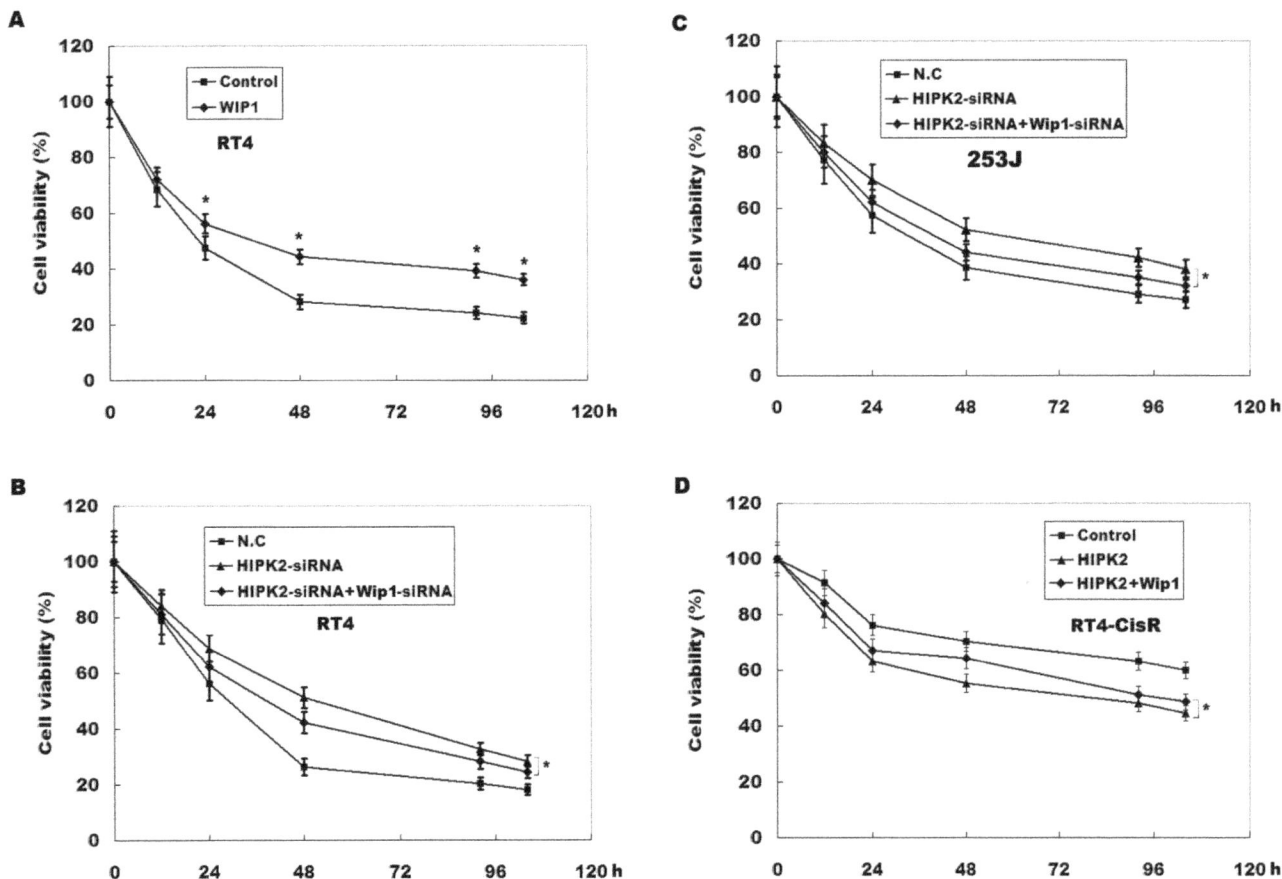

Figure 5. HIPK2 overexpression sensitizes chemoresistant bladder cancer cell to cisplatin by regulating Wip1 expression. (A) Wip1 was overexpressed in RT4 cells, and cell viability was assayed by using MTT following cisplatin treatment (6 μM). The results show data from six independent experiments, expressed as the mean ± SD. *$p < 0.05$. (B and C) RT4 and 253J cells were treated with HIPK2-siRNA or HIPK2-siRNA plus Wip1-siRNA, and at the indicated time points, cell viability was assayed by using MTT following cisplatin treatment (6 μM). (D) HIPK2 or HIPK2 plus Wip1 was overexpressed in RT4-CisR cells, and cell viability was assayed by using MTT following cisplatin treatment (6 μM). *$p < 0.05$.

cell compared with RT4 cell, and Wip1 overexpression increases cell viability during cisplatin treatment in RT4 cells. Importantly, we demonstrated that HIPK2 negatively regulates Wip1 expression in bladder cancer cell. HIPK2 and Wip1 expression is also negatively correlated after cisplatin-based combination chemotherapy *in vivo*. Forced expression of HIPK2 sensitizes chemoresistant bladder cancer cell to cisplatin by regulating Wip1 expression. **Conclusion**: These data demonstrated that HIPK2/Wip1 signaling represents a novel pathway regulating

chemoresistance. Thus, this study reveals that HIPK2/Wip1 is an effective drug target for enhanced cancer therapy.

Author Contributions

Conceived and designed the experiments: XH JL. Performed the experiments: JL QZ YL WX YX YZ. Analyzed the data: YZ XH. Contributed reagents/materials/analysis tools: YL WX YX. Wrote the paper: XH.

References

1. Cohen SM, Shirai T, Steineck G (2000) Epidemiology and etiology of premalignant and malignant urothelial changes. Scand J Urol Nephrol Suppl: 105–115.

2. Burger M, Catto JW, Dalbagni G, Grossman HB, Herr H, et al. (2013) Epidemiology and risk factors of urothelial bladder cancer. Eur Urol 63: 234–241.

3. Witjes JA, Comperat E, Cowan NC, De Santis M, Gakis G, et al. (2014) EAU Guidelines on Muscle-invasive and Metastatic Bladder Cancer: Summary of the 2013 Guidelines. Eur Urol 65: 778–792.

4. Kirkali Z, Chan T, Manoharan M, Algaba F, Busch C, et al. (2005) Bladder cancer: epidemiology, staging and grading, and diagnosis. Urology 66: 4–34.

5. Pollack A, Zagars GK, Cole CJ, Dinney CP, Swanson DA, et al. (1995) The relationship of local control to distant metastasis in muscle invasive bladder cancer. J Urol 154: 2059-2063; discussion 2063–2054.

6. Said N, Sanchez-Carbayo M, Smith SC, Theodorescu D (2012) RhoGDI2 suppresses lung metastasis in mice by reducing tumor versican expression and macrophage infiltration. J Clin Invest 122: 1503–1518.

7. Chang JS, Lara PN Jr, Pan CX (2012) Progress in personalizing chemotherapy for bladder cancer. Adv Urol 2012: 364919.

8. Wei G, Ku S, Ma GK, Saito S, Tang AA, et al. (2007) HIPK2 represses beta-catenin-mediated transcription, epidermal stem cell expansion, and skin tumorigenesis. Proc Natl Acad Sci U S A 104: 13040–13045.

9. D'Orazi G, Rinaldo C, Soddu S (2012) Updates on HIPK2: a resourceful oncosuppressor for clearing cancer. J Exp Clin Cancer Res 31: 63.

10. Hofmann TG, Glas C, Bitomsky N (2013) HIPK2: A tumour suppressor that controls DNA damage-induced cell fate and cytokinesis. Bioessays 35: 55–64.

11. Puca R, Nardinocchi L, Givol D, D'Orazi G (2010) Regulation of p53 activity by HIPK2: molecular mechanisms and therapeutical implications in human cancer cells. Oncogene 29: 4378–4387.

12. D'Orazi G, Cecchinelli B, Bruno T, Manni I, Higashimoto Y, et al. (2002) Homeodomain-interacting protein kinase-2 phosphorylates p53 at Ser 46 and mediates apoptosis. Nat Cell Biol 4: 11–19.

13. Winter M, Sombroek D, Dauth I, Moehlenbrink J, Scheuermann K, et al. (2008) Control of HIPK2 stability by ubiquitin ligase Siah-1 and checkpoint kinases ATM and ATR. Nat Cell Biol 10: 812–824.

14. Puca R, Nardinocchi L, Pistritto G, D'Orazi G (2008) Overexpression of HIPK2 circumvents the blockade of apoptosis in chemoresistant ovarian cancer cells. Gynecol Oncol 109: 403–410.

15. Hofmann TG, Moller A, Sirma H, Zentgraf H, Taya Y, et al. (2002) Regulation of p53 activity by its interaction with homeodomain-interacting protein kinase-2. Nat Cell Biol 4: 1–10.

16. Rinaldo C, Prodosmo A, Mancini F, Iacovelli S, Sacchi A, et al. (2007) MDM2-regulated degradation of HIPK2 prevents p53Ser46 phosphorylation and DNA damage-induced apoptosis. Mol Cell 25: 739–750.

17. Lazzari C, Prodosmo A, Siepi F, Rinaldo C, Galli F, et al. (2011) HIPK2 phosphorylates DeltaNp63alpha and promotes its degradation in response to DNA damage. Oncogene 30: 4802–4813.

18. Takekawa M, Adachi M, Nakahata A, Nakayama I, Itoh F, et al. (2000) p53-inducible wip1 phosphatase mediates a negative feedback regulation of p38 MAPK-p53 signaling in response to UV radiation. EMBO J 19: 6517–6526.

19. Song JY, Ryu SH, Cho YM, Kim YS, Lee BM, et al. (2013) Wip1 suppresses apoptotic cell death through direct dephosphorylation of BAX in response to gamma-radiation. Cell Death Dis 4: e744.

20. Choi DW, Na W, Kabir MH, Yi E, Kwon S, et al. (2013) WIP1, a homeostatic regulator of the DNA damage response, is targeted by HIPK2 for phosphorylation and degradation. Mol Cell 51: 374–385.

21. Wang L, Mosel AJ, Oakley GG, Peng A (2012) Deficient DNA damage signaling leads to chemoresistance to cisplatin in oral cancer. Mol Cancer Ther 11: 2401–2409.

22. Goloudina AR, Tanoue K, Hammann A, Fourmaux E, Le Guezennec X, et al. (2012) Wip1 promotes RUNX2-dependent apoptosis in p53-negative tumors and protects normal tissues during treatment with anticancer agents. Proc Natl Acad Sci U S A 109: E68–75.

23. Esaki T, Nakano S, Masumoto N, Fujishima H, Niho Y (1996) Schedule-dependent reversion of acquired cisplatin resistance by 5-fluorouracil in a newly established cisplatin-resistant HST-1 human squamous carcinoma cell line. Int J Cancer 65: 479–484.

24. Xu N, Shen C, Luo Y, Xia L, Xue F, et al. (2012) Upregulated miR-130a increases drug resistance by regulating RUNX3 and Wnt signaling in cisplatin-treated HCC cell. Biochem Biophys Res Commun 425: 468–472.

25. Wang F, Li X, Xie X, Zhao L, Chen W (2008) UCA1, a non-protein-coding RNA up-regulated in bladder carcinoma and embryo, influencing cell growth and promoting invasion. FEBS Lett 582: 1919–1927.

26. Yang C, Li X, Wang Y, Zhao L, Chen W (2012) Long non-coding RNA UCA1 regulated cell cycle distribution via CREB through PI3-K dependent pathway in bladder carcinoma cells. Gene 496: 8–16.

27. Yuan G, Regel I, Lian F, Friedrich T, Hitkova I, et al. (2013) WNT6 is a novel target gene of caveolin-1 promoting chemoresistance to epirubicin in human gastric cancer cells. Oncogene 32: 375–387.

28. Juffs HG, Moore MJ, Tannock IF (2002) The role of systemic chemotherapy in the management of muscle-invasive bladder cancer. Lancet Oncol 3: 738–747.

29. Gupta S, Mahipal A (2013) Role of systemic chemotherapy in urothelial urinary bladder cancer. Cancer Control 20: 200–210.

30. Kamat AM, Sethi G, Aggarwal BB (2007) Curcumin potentiates the apoptotic effects of chemotherapeutic agents and cytokines through down-regulation of nuclear factor-kappaB and nuclear factor-kappaB-regulated gene products in IFN-alpha-sensitive and IFN-alpha-resistant human bladder cancer cells. Mol Cancer Ther 6: 1022–1030.

31. Chung J, Kwak C, Jin RJ, Lee CH, Lee KH, et al. (2004) Enhanced chemosensitivity of bladder cancer cells to cisplatin by suppression of clusterin in vitro. Cancer Lett 203: 155–161.

32. Krieghoff-Henning E, Hofmann TG (2008) HIPK2 and cancer cell resistance to therapy. Future Oncol 4: 751–754.

33. Lu X, Nguyen TA, Moon SH, Darlington Y, Sommer M, et al. (2008) The type 2C phosphatase Wip1: an oncogenic regulator of tumor suppressor and DNA damage response pathways. Cancer Metastasis Rev 27: 123–135.

7

Expression Microarray Meta-Analysis Identifies Genes Associated with Ras/MAPK and Related Pathways in Progression of Muscle-Invasive Bladder Transition Cell Carcinoma

Jonathan A. Ewald[1,3], Tracy M. Downs[1,3], Jeremy P. Cetnar[2,3], William A. Ricke[1,3]*

1 Department of Urology, University of Wisconsin School of Medicine and Public Health, Madison, Wisconsin, United States of America, 2 Department of Medicine, Hematology/Oncology Unit, University of Wisconsin School of Medicine and Public Health, Madison, Wisconsin, United States of America, 3 University of Wisconsin Carbone Cancer Center, Madison, Wisconsin, United States of America

Abstract

The effective detection and management of muscle-invasive bladder Transition Cell Carcinoma (TCC) continues to be an urgent clinical challenge. While some differences of gene expression and function in papillary (Ta), superficial (T1) and muscle-invasive ($\geq$T2) bladder cancers have been investigated, the understanding of mechanisms involved in the progression of bladder tumors remains incomplete. Statistical methods of pathway-enrichment, cluster analysis and text-mining can extract and help interpret functional information about gene expression patterns in large sets of genomic data. The public availability of patient-derived expression microarray data allows open access and analysis of large amounts of clinical data. Using these resources, we investigated gene expression differences associated with tumor progression and muscle-invasive TCC. Gene expression was calculated relative to Ta tumors to assess progression-associated differences, revealing a network of genes related to Ras/MAPK and PI3K signaling pathways with increased expression. Further, we identified genes within this network that are similarly expressed in superficial Ta and T1 stages but altered in muscle-invasive T2 tumors, finding 7 genes (COL3A1, COL5A1, COL11A1, FN1, ErbB3, MAPK10 and CDC25C) whose expression patterns in muscle-invasive tumors are consistent in 5 to 7 independent outside microarray studies. Further, we found increased expression of the fibrillar collagen proteins COL3A1 and COL5A1 in muscle-invasive tumor samples and metastatic T24 cells. Our results suggest that increased expression of genes involved in mitogenic signaling may support the progression of muscle-invasive bladder tumors that generally lack activating mutations in these pathways, while expression changes of fibrillar collagens, fibronectin and specific signaling proteins are associated with muscle-invasive disease. These results identify potential biomarkers and targets for TCC treatments, and provide an integrated systems-level perspective of TCC pathobiology to inform future studies.

Editor: Natasha Kyprianou, University of Kentucky College of Medicine, United States of America

Funding: This work was supported by the National Institutes of Health [grant numbers: CA123199,DK093690, RC2ES018764 to WAR]. The funders had no role in study design, data collection and analysis, decision to publish, or preparation of the manuscript.

Competing Interests: The authors have declared that no competing interests exist.

* E-mail: rickew@urology.wisc.edu

Introduction

Bladder cancer is a disease receiving growing attention within the cancer biology community. Transition Cell Carcinoma (TCC) occurs as papillary tumors (Ta stage), superficial tumors (T1 stage), and muscle-invasive tumors of increasing severity (T2, T3 and T4 stage). Approximately 20% of primary bladder cancers are muscle-invasive at presentation and are associated with a poor prognosis, with 5 year survival estimates for muscle-invasive TCC approaching the low survival rates for advanced metastatic pancreatic cancers, small cell lung cancers, liver and bile-duct cancers, stomach and non-small cell lung carcinomas [1,2]. Although papillary and superficial tumors recur in 70% of patients after surgical removal, non-invasive tumors have a more favorable outcome than muscle-invasive tumors as only 10–20% of these recurrences progress to muscle-invasive disease [2]. The regulatory mechanisms that are altered and disrupted in muscle-invasive bladder cancer may represent a barrier to progression in superficial tumors, and are candidate targets for therapeutic intervention.

Accumulating evidence suggests that superficial and muscle-invasive tumors are pathobiologically distinct [3,4]. Superficial tumors frequently overexpress or express constitutively active mutants of HRAS and FGFR3 leading to hyperactivated Ras/ MAPK signaling activity [3,4]. Muscle-invasive tumors demonstrate disrupted activity of p53 and Rb and other tumor suppressors, overexpress EGFR and ErbB2, MMP2 and MMP9, and other pro-angiogenic factors, while having deleted cyclin-dependent kinase inhibitor genes CDKN2A (p16^{Ink4a}) and CDKN2B (p15^{Ink4b}) [4]. However, there is evidence that suggests that Ta tumors in some patients may progress and become muscle-invasive. In addition to observations that 10–20% of patients who initially have Ta tumors later develop muscle-invasive disease, tumors $\geq$T1 share common chromosomal deletions, gains and amplifications that are distinct from those found in Ta stage tumors, suggesting that accumulated chromosomal aberrations may be involved in the progression from papillary to muscle-invasive tumors [1,2]. Moreover, while activating mutations in *FGFR3*, *ras* isoforms, and *PI3K* are more common in papillary tumors, most high grade superficial tumors lack these mutations and are similar to invasive tumors, suggesting that these may be predisposed to progress to muscle-invasive disease [5]. At the same time, some tumor recurrences lose the activating mutations that are present in earlier tumors, which may also potentially drive progression [5]. In all, the relationship of superficial and muscle-invasive bladder cancer remains controversial and largely unresolved.

There are few effective systemic treatments for muscle-invasive bladder cancer, and an improved understanding of the molecular pathogenesis and progression of TCC is urgently needed. Analysis mRNA expression in different stages of bladder cancer could illustrate differences that exist which may promote progression from Ta and T1 tumors to higher stage recurrences, while similarities in expression patterns could clarify the relationship of tumor stages in progression of the disease. Insights into these molecular mechanisms of bladder tumor progression can provide targets for preventative and therapeutic interventions while providing biomarkers that reliably predict progression into muscle-invasive disease.

Microarray technology provides a powerful tool to measure mRNA expression across the entire genome of biological samples, allowing detailed analysis of large numbers of experimental and clinical samples in relatively little time. Typically in studies of various cancers, clinical samples are analyzed to identify genes expressed at relatively high or low amounts in common patterns that correlate with tumor stage and patient survival [6]. While this approach may be appropriate for identifying potentially useful diagnostic and prognostic biomarkers, it is often difficult to determine whether signature genes in advanced cancers are functionally relevant to tumor progression. Strategies to derive functional information from gene-expression datasets include expression clustering to identify genes with similar patterns of expression [7]and pathway enrichment programs including WebGestalt [8] that query Gene Ontology, Kyoto Encyclopedia of Genes and Genomes (KEGG), and other databases to identify processes in which gene expression changes are focused. Another strategy is to analyze the published literature using automated text-mining programs such as PubGene and Chilibot to identify functional associations between genes, phenotypes and diseases within publications indexed in PubMed [9–12]. Such resources have made computational informatic tools available to scientists who need to analyze and interpret microarray data, yet few studies have taken advantage of this information.

Studies of whole-genome expression using microarray technology require resources that may not be widely available to all researchers. Reliable microarray studies require large numbers of samples to provide for an adequate analysis and can be prohibitively expensive and time consuming. Access to human tissues required for relevant analyses is often not available to researchers outside of the medical field. The establishment of public microarray data archives, including the Gene Expression Omnibus (http://www.ncbi.nlm.nih.gov/geo/), has allowed free-access to a wealth of clinical and experimental data that can be analyzed and re-purposed by any investigator with the interest and the means to do so. The development of open-access analytical programs, including Oncomine (https://www.oncomine.org) [13] and Mayday [14], provide a means to investigate gene expression in data across multiple microarray studies. These advances allow

researchers to pursue genome-scale investigations in clinically-derived human tissues without the time, expense, and administrative efforts associated with generating primary genomic data.

Here, we use public data to identify genes that are associated with TCC tumor progression and muscle-invasive disease in male patients without metastases. We find that the differential expression of a network of genes related to the mitogenic Ras/MAPK and related signaling pathways are associated with progression beyond Ta stage. Additionally, we identified a subset of 7 genes within this network whose expression is associated with muscle-invasive TCC.

Materials and Methods

Microarray Dataset

The Gene Expression Omnibus (GEO) website (http://www.ncbi.nlm.nih.gov/geo/) was used to search publicly available datasets for recent studies of bladder cancers with at least 3 samples representing all tumor grades and performed using up-to-date whole-genome microarray chips. We chose a dataset (GEO# GSE 31684; accessed 2/29/2012) which was originally used to develop predictive models of bladder cancer outcome [15], as it fulfilled these requirements and provided detailed patient data. Data was further selected from male TCC patients without associated metastases, carcinoma *in situ* or sarcoma to reduce potential variation in data, resulting in a total of 36 patient datasets (Table 1).

Data selection, calculations and statistics

The meta-analysis of public data was performed according to PRISMA guidelines (Table S1, Table S2). Microarray expression data was organized, managed, and calculated using Microsoft Excel (Redmond, WA). The microarray expression data of all 36 sample datasets were expressed in $\log_2$ scale, and the average expression values were calculated for samples of each pathological tumor grade. To identify general expression changes associated with progression of TCC, the gene probe expression values of tumor stage T1, T2, T3 and T4 samples were individually normalized to Ta by subtracting their $\log_2$ averages. Gene probes were selected based on both an increase or decrease in expression by a factor of 2 ($\log_2 1/-1$) and statistical significance ($p<0.05$) in at least one tumor stage based on Student's t-test as a more stringent method of selection than either criterion alone. To identify expression changes associated with muscle-invasive disease, genes were selected that did not significantly change from Ta to T1 but are significantly different by a factor of 2 in T2 tumors in addition to significance based on Student's t-test. Further, the average expression values of selected gene probes in each tumor grade were compiled, and 3×3 matrix self-organizing map-based clustering analysis of relative gene expression across

Table 1. Tumor stage, sample size and age range of data selected from GSE 31684 dataset.

Tumor Stage	n =	Age Range
Ta	3	57–78
T1	7	57–74
T2	10	51–80
T3	9	66–84
T4	7	50–83

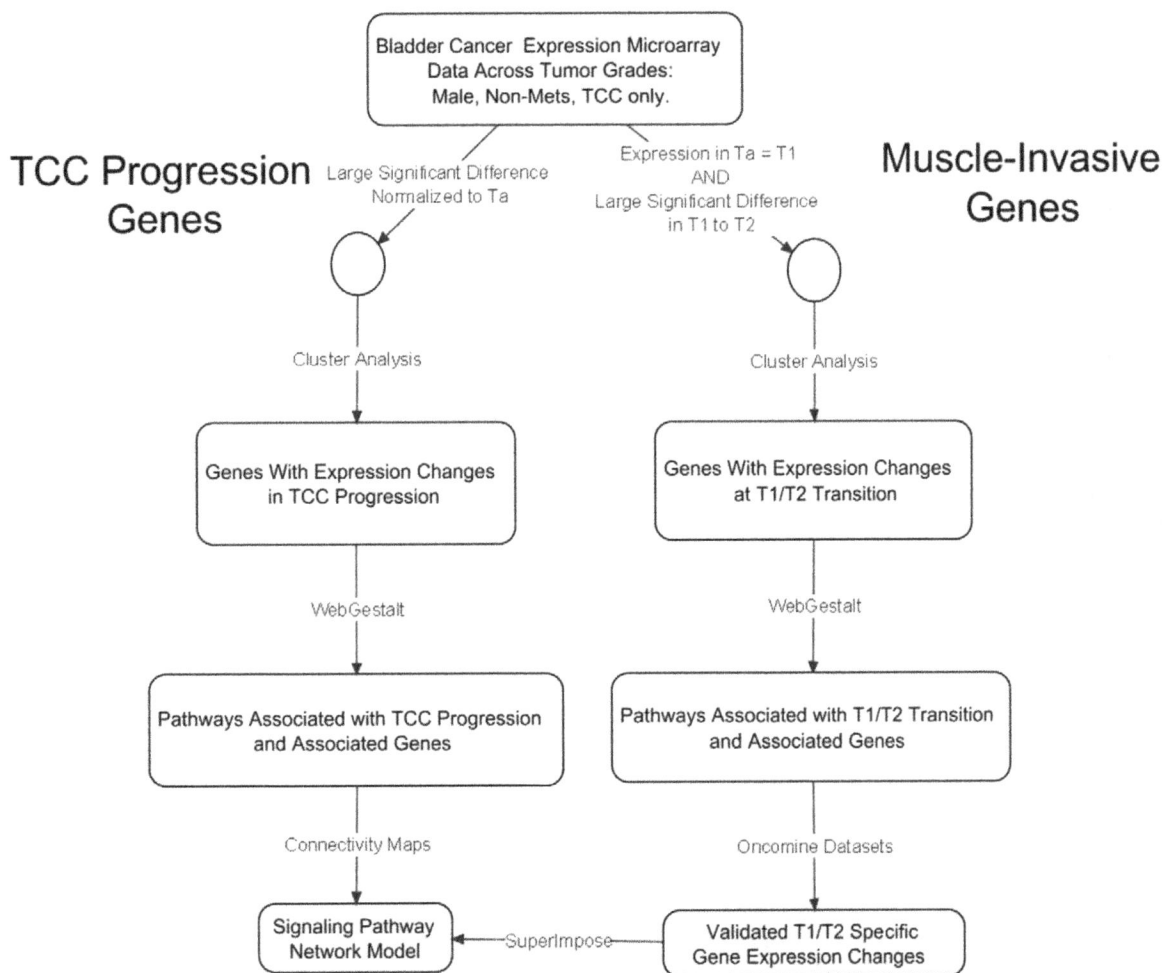

Figure 1. Flow diagram detailing the methods used to identify genes associated with TCC progression and muscle-invasive behavior from expression microarray data.

tumor stages was performed with 10,000 iterations using Mayday [14]. Clusters of gene probes with minimal expression changes, representing apparent false-positives, were arbitrarily omitted from subsequent analysis.

Statistical pathway enrichment analysis of differentially expressed genes

To perform pathway enrichment analysis on selected genes, gene probe IDs were annotated with Entrez gene symbols (Affymetrix Human Genome U133 Plus 2.0 [HG-U133_Plus_2]; GEO# GPL570) and analyzed using the WebGestalt website (http://bioinfo.vanderbilt.edu/webgestalt/) to identify defined KEGG pathways that are significantly over-represented in the dataset [8], using default settings and the Fisher's Exact test, selecting pathways where p<0.01. These results produced lists of the genes included in the enriched pathways, and provided a connectivity map of each pathway. A model network based on these pathways was generated using the Visual Understanding Environment (http://vue.tufts.edu/). Gene expression heatmaps were generated using Mayday (http://www-ps.informatik.uni-tuebingen.de/mayday/wp/) [14].

Statistical validation of muscle-invasive tumor gene signature using outside datasets

To determine whether muscle-invasive-specific expression changes identified in our initial dataset are typical across an expanded number of samples and studies, we obtained expression data for each gene compiled within the Oncomine database [13]. This included 8 datasets from 7 studies in which gene expression is measured in superficial and muscle-invasive bladder tumors [16–22]. The median expression of each gene in superficial and muscle-invasive tumors from each dataset was recorded and the averaged difference was calculated. A Mann-Whitney Rank-Sum test was performed to determine the significance of expression changes across datasets.

Bibliomic text-mining for functional gene association

To obtain published results that link functional interactions of genes and phenotypes, selected genes were analyzed using PubGene [10], while genes and keywords "bladder cancer", "metastasis", "angiogenesis", "invasive" were analyzed using Chilibot [11]. An association network based on co-occurrances and implied functional relationships determined by each program was constructed based on these results.

Table 2. KEGG pathway enrichment of genes differentially expressed in T1–T4 staged bladder tumors versus Ta-stage tumors.

KEGG Pathway	Number of Pathway Genes in Dataset	Enrichment Factor "R"	Fisher's Exact, Adjusted P-value
All Changes, Top 10			
Metabolic pathways	332	3.46	5.26E-93
Cell cycle*	68	6.11	2.46E-36
Spliceosome	68	6.11	2.46E-36
DNA replication	29	9.27	3.29E-23
Pyrimidine metabolism	47	5.52	1.05E-22
Ubiquitin mediated proteolysis	54	4.50	6.33E-21
Pathways in cancer*	86	3.00	2.50E-19
Focal adhesion*	63	3.61	1.30E-18
Huntington's disease	60	3.73	1.32E-18
Purine metabolism	52	3.96	1.75E-17
Selected Pathways			
MAPK signaling pathway*	60	2.57	6.88E-11
ErbB signaling pathway*	26	3.44	5.92E-08
Bladder cancer*	16	4.38	7.25E-07
Genes Up, Top 10			
Metabolic pathways	299	3.57	1.64E-85
Spliceosome	66	6.79	1.34E-37
Cell cycle*	62	6.38	2.13E-33
DNA replication	29	10.61	7.10E-25
Pyrimidine metabolism	46	6.18	3.64E-24
Ubiquitin mediated proteolysis	50	4.77	3.54E-20
Huntington's disease	58	4.13	7.22E-20
Purine metabolism	51	4.45	3.88E-19
Oocyte meiosis	42	4.85	1.95E-17
Alzheimer's disease	50	3.91	4.12E-16
Parkinson's disease	43	4.26	1.71E-15
Genes Down, Top 10			
Complement and coagulation cascades	11	14.12	1.22E-08
Pathways in cancer*	21	5.64	1.22E-08
Focal adhesion*	17	7.49	1.22E-08
MAPK signaling pathway*	17	5.60	4.00E-07
Small cell lung cancer	10	10.54	8.56E-07
Metabolic pathways	35	2.81	1.07E-06
p53 signaling pathway	9	11.55	1.31E-06
Tight junction	11	7.27	5.35E-06
NOD-like receptor signaling pathway	8	11.43	5.84E-06
Metabolism of xenobiotics by cytochrome P450	8	10.12	1.36E-05

(*)indicates KEGG pathways that involve mechanisms of signal transduction. P value represents the results of Fisher's Exact tests reported by WebGestalt.

Immunohistochemistry of Bladder Tumors

Samples (n = 5 each) of normal bladder and T1, T2 and T3 bladder tumors were purchased from Biomax.us (Rockville, MD). Samples were processed and stained by the TRIP Laboratory facility (Depatment of Pathology, University of Wisconsin School of Medince and Public Health) using standard immunostaining procedures. Antibodies to COL3A1 and COL5A1 were purchased from Santa Cruz Biotechnology (Santa Cruz, CA) and visualized using DAB and Warp Red stains. Nuclei were visualized using hematoxylin staining. Microscopy and image processing was performed as previously described [23].

Western Immunoblotting

T24 bladder cancer cells and E6-immortalized human urothelial cells (HUCs) were the kind gift of Dr. Dale Bjorling, University of Wisconsin. T24 cells were cultured in DMEM media +10% FBS, while HUCs were cultured in Ham's F12 media +10% FBS. Cells were cultured to 70% confluence, scraped from plates, collected, solubilized and processed, analyzed by western immu-

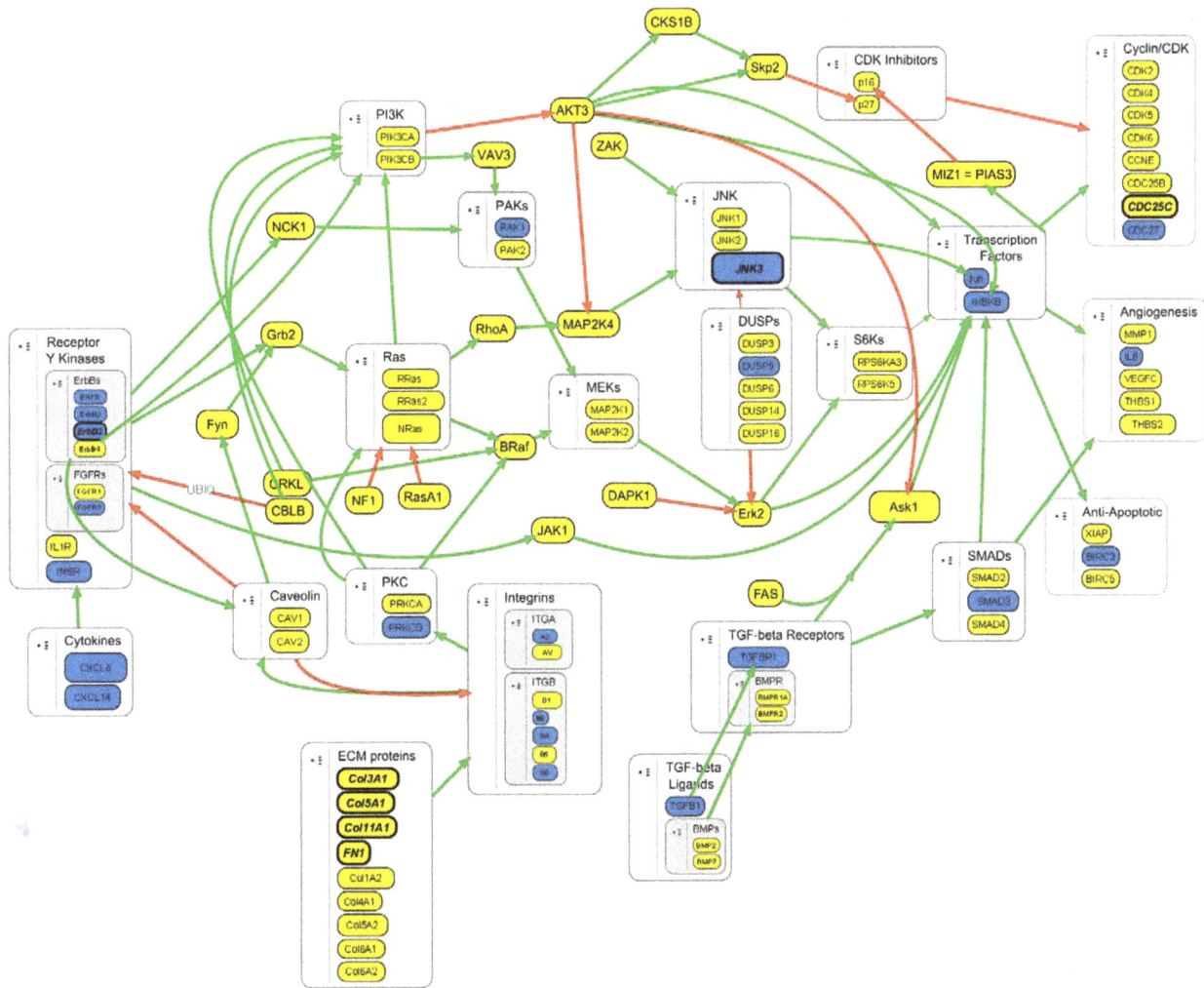

Figure 2. Altered expression in a network of Ras/MAPK associated signaling pathway genes in TCC progression. The stimulatory and inhibitory interactions of gene products differentially expressed in T1–T4 versus Ta tumors were mapped based on KEGG pathway maps. Node color denotes relative expression: Yellow = Increased expression in muscle-invasive tumors; Blue = Decreased expression in muscle-invasive tumors. Green and red arrows represent stimulatory and inhibitory interactions, respectively. The names of genes with supported associations with muscle-invasive tumors are highlighted in bold italics.

noblotting, and quantified using Image J, as previously described [23]. Antibodies to COL3A1 and COL5A1 are described above. Antibodies recognizing β-actin were used as a loading control.

Results

TCC progression is associated with differential expression of Ras/MAPK and related pathway genes

Our hypothesis was that gene expression differences exist between papillary/superficial and muscle-invasive bladder TCC tumors that define the regulation of tumor invasion, progression and metastasis. We developed an intuitive method, summarized in Figure 1, to select, analyze and interpret public microarray data using open access computational resources. We found a suitable dataset from the GEO database (GSE31684) containing expression data from 93 patient bladder tumors that were removed prior to any chemical treatment and used to identify gene expression signatures that predict outcome of high-risk bladder cancer [15]. To limit potential variation in sample expression data, sample data were selected from male patients with TCC of the bladder,

without metastatic tumors, CIS or sarcoma, producing 36 total datasets that represented at least three patients per stage for all stages of TCC tumors (Table 1).

First, we calculated expression differences between Ta and T1–T4 bladder tumors to identify changes broadly associated with bladder cancer progression beyond papillary tumor stages. Data were processed, averaged, normalized to the expression of Ta tumors, and selected based on a greater than 2-fold threshold difference in expression at any stage beyond Ta, and p<0.05 using Student's t-test. This produced a list of 8110 gene-associated probes. Expression data was retrieved for those selected probes and analyzed using the self-organizing map cluster analysis within Mayday [14] to arbitrarily remove probes that reflect little change in expression, selecting 5509 total probes.

As receptor tyrosine kinases, mitogenic signaling pathways and tumor suppressors are each involved in superficial and muscle-invasive bladder cancer, our aim was to identify changes in gene expression that could compliment the activities of these pathways. The list of selected probes was analyzed with WebGestalt [8] to identify defined pathways that are significantly represented in the

Table 3. KEGG pathway enrichment of genes differentially expressed in T2 versus Ta and T1 stage bladder tumors.

KEGG Pathway	Number of Pathway Genes in Dataset	Enrichment Factor "R"	Fisher's Exact, Adjusted P-value
All Changes, Top 10			
Focal adhesion*	14	8.4	1.44E-07
Tight junction	11	9.92	7.39E-07
Pancreatic cancer	8	13.43	4.23E-06
Androgen and estrogen metabolism	6	16.12	3.96E-05
Adherens junction	7	10.99	6.08E-05
ECM-receptor interaction	7	10.08	9.07E-05
Retinol metabolism	6	11.33	2.00E-04
MAPK signaling pathway*	11	4.94	2.00E-04
Ascorbate and aldarate metabolism	4	19.34	5.00E-04
Drug metabolism – other enzymes	5	11.85	5.00E-04
Selected Pathways			
Pathways in cancer*	10	3.6	1.90E-03
Cell cycle*	6	5.67	2.30E-03
Genes Up, Top 10			
Focal adhesion*	11	12.79	5.49E-08
ECM-receptor interaction	7	19.48	1.66E-06
Cell cycle*	5	9.13	2.10E-03
MAPK signaling pathway*	7	6.08	2.10E-03
Tight junction	5	8.72	2.50E-03
Regulation of actin cytoskeleton	6	6.49	2.70E-03
Progesterone-mediated oocyte maturation	4	10.87	2.90E-03
Valine, leucine and isoleucine degradation	3	15.93	4.60E-03
Sulfur metabolism	2	35.95	6.40E-03
Vascular smooth muscle contraction	4	8.13	6.60E-03
Genes Down, Top 10			
Retinol metabolism	6	12024	1.09E-05
Androgen and estrogen metabolism	5	27.68	1.63E-05
Adherens junction	6	19.41	1.63E-05
Drug metabolism – other enzymes	5	24.42	2.29E-05
Ascorbate and aldarate metabolism	4	39.86	2.73E-05
Pentose and glucuronate interconversions	4	36.91	3.14E-05
Pancreatic cancer	5	17.3	5.67E-05
Drug metabolism – cytochrome P450	5	17.3	5.67E-05
Metabolism of xenobiotics by cytochrome P450	5	17.79	5.67E-05

(*)indicates KEGG pathways that involve mechanisms of signal transduction. P value represents the results of Fisher's Exact tests reported by WebGestalt.

microarray data ($p < 0.05$). Whether the selected genes were analyzed as a single group or separated based on increased or decreased expression, many of the pathways reliably associated with these genes are related to cancer-related signal transduction and similar pathways (Table 2, Table S3). The ten best supported pathways associated with the entire set of genes include "Cell Cycle", "Pathways in Cancer", and "Focal Adhesion". Beyond these ten, "MAPK signaling", "ErbB signaling" and "Bladder Cancer" pathways were also well supported. Likewise, when this list was separated into separate lists of 4816 increasing and 693 decreasing genes, many similar cancer-related signal transduction pathways were found to be represented in these genes. While other pathways represented in the data could also be associated with

cancer progression and metastasis, such as "Metabolism" and "DNA Repair", the relationship of these pathways to current models of bladder progression is less direct. These results suggest that bladder cancer progression from Ta to T1+ stage tumors involves the increased expression of genes in mitogenic, cancer-associated pathways related to FGFR3 and ErbB family signaling.

KEGG pathways and other related ontologies and annotations are highly redundant, with individual genes associated with many multiple limited and interconnecting pathways. For this and other reasons, pathway enrichment analysis alone often does not adequately represent the global scope and relationships within the data. To better understand the relationships of these genes and how they may function in bladder cancer progression, we built an integrated pathway network model based on the KEGG maps of selected signaling pathways represented in the data (Table 2; Table S3). These results reveal that gene expression differences between Ta and T1 stage tumors largely occur within a signaling network related to Ras/MAPK signaling pathways, with increased expression of a majority of these genes (Figure 2).

Muscle-invasive TCC is associated with specific expression changes in ECM and signaling proteins

We further hypothesized that the expression of a subset of the genes within this signaling network model is specifically altered in muscle-invasive versus superficial tumors. Returning to the complete dataset, we selected genes that are expressed at similar levels within a 2 fold difference between Ta and T1 tumors, and are changed greater than 2 fold in T2 stage tumors with Student's t-test p<0.05 (Figure 1). After performing expression clustering analysis and arbitrarily removing clusters with minimal expression changes, as above, 496 total gene probes were selected for pathway enrichment analysis using WebGestalt. As before, these results show that the selected genes are associated with many signal transduction and cancer-related pathways that involve 23 of the selected genes (Table 3, Table S4, Figure 3). These genes were not focused in any single pathway, but instead were distributed across the network of pathways (Figure 2). Visualizing gene expression data relative to Ta tumors in a heatmap, the expression changes of selected genes are consistent in T2, T3 and T4 tumors (Figure 3). These results suggest that the differences of selected gene expression are distinct fundamental molecular characteristics of muscle-invasive tumors.

We then determined whether the relative expression of the selected genes could be observed in outside microarray datasets of superficial and muscle-invasive bladder tumors. Using Oncomine [24], we identified archived datasets containing expression data for each of the 23 selected candidate genes. The median gene expression of non-invasive and invasive tumors in each dataset was recorded, and the average change in expression of each gene was calculated across all datasets (Table 4). The Mann-Whitney Rank-Sum test was performed to determine the significance of the changes in median gene expression across datasets. These results show that expression of extracellular matrix genes COL3A1, COL5A1, COL11A1 and FN1 are significantly increased in muscle-invasive bladder tumors relative to Ta/T1 (p<0.05), while changes in CDC25C, MAPK10 and ErbB3 expression approached significance (p≤0.08) (Table 4). These final selected genes represent a sub-network of consistently-observed differences in gene expression of muscle-invasive and non-invasive bladder tumors that are associated with the activity of Ras/MAPK, PI3K and other signaling pathways (Figure 4).

While the consistent expression changes of the 7 selected genes are well supported by expression data from human clinical samples, the functional relationships of these genes were not immediate. With the expectation that functional relationships of selected genes would be reflected in the literature, we used the text-mining programs Chilibot and PubGeneto identify and visualize these relationships [10,11]. The results show that the genes can be placed in two functional groups of extracellular matrix proteins and signal transduction proteins (Figure 4). Outside genes that are functionally related to the selected genes showed little overlap between associated groups, suggesting that seven selected genes are critical nodes of regulation that coordinate the activities of outside gene pathway networks (Figure 4, and Data Not Shown). Further, the relationships of selected genes characteristics associated with advanced metastatic cancer were assessed using Chilibot. The CDC25C, ErbB3 and FN1 are previously

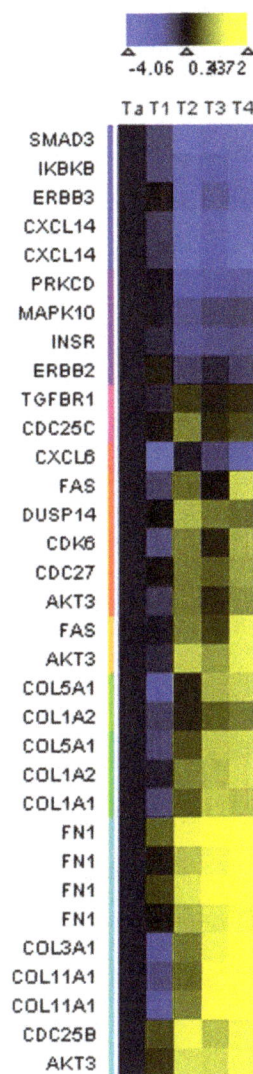

Figure 3. Expression heatmap of candidate muscle-invasive genes. Yellow and blue indicate increased and decreased expression in candidate muscle-invasive genes, respectively, relative to the average expression in Ta tumors.

associated with bladder cancer: The activity of CDC25C promotes proliferation and is a target for developing cancer therapies, including bladder cancer [25]; Decreased ErbB3 expression in bladder cancer is associated with poor prognosis [26]; and FN1 is a potential urine biomarker for bladder cancer [27]. All of the selected genes are associated with cancer and metastasis (Table 5). Interestingly, MAPK10 and FN1 were related to angiogenesis, COL5A1 and COL11A1 were associated only with invasion, while COL3A1, CDC25C and ErbB3 are associated with both. In all, the selected genes are associated with terms in published reports describe characteristics of muscle-invasive and metastatic tumors, and are relevant to mechanisms regulating the progression of advanced stage bladder cancer.

Increased COL3A1 and COL5A1 protein expression in muscle-invasive tumors and metastatic T24 cells

Because the expression changes of COL3A1 and COL5A1 are well supported statistically, the novelty of these genes' association with muscle-invasive bladder cancer, and the availability of

Table 4. Average normalized median expression of selected genes differentially expressed in non-invasive and muscle-invasive TCC in at least 3 datasets within the Oncomine Collection.

	Gene	Average Change in Median (Fold Increase vs Superficial)	St.Dev.	Mann-Whitney Rank-Sum p=	References
Validated	COL3A1	3.99	2.29	0.028	[16–21]
	COL5A1	5.07	1.74	0.047	[15–17,19,20]
	COL11A1	3.37	2.30	0.025	[15–17,19–21]
	FN1	5.45	2.25	0.028	[16,17,19–21]
	CDC25C	1.48	1.43	0.08	[15–17,19–21]
	MAPK10	0.55	1.70	0.08	[15–17,19–21]
	ERBB3	0.45	1.77	0.072	[16,17,19–21]
Rejected	AKT3	1.64	2.02	0.305	[15–17,19–21]
	DUSP14	1.53	1.26	0.105	[16,17,19–21]
	FAS	1.43	1.49	0.236	[15–17,19,21]
	COL1A1	3.72	2.52	0.101	[16–20]
	COL1A2	2.26	2.73	0.288	[16–20]
	CDC25B	1.53	1.54	0.189	[15–21]
	CDK6	1.53	1.36	0.189	[15–17,19–21]
	TGFBR1	1.24	1.41	0.443	[16,17,19,20]
	CDC27	1.17	1.42	0.222	[15–17,19–21]
	IKBKB	0.76	1.25	0.148	[15,16,19–21]
	ERBB2	0.71	1.65	0.417	[15–17,19–21]
	SMAD3	0.69	1.76	0.202	[15–19,21]
	PRKCD	0.58	1.65	0.202	[15–17,19,20]
	CXCL6	2.96	1.99	0.156	[15,16,19–21]
	CXCL14	1.02	1.35	0.5	[16,19,20]
	INSR	1.05	1.36	0.115	[15–17,19,21]

Genes selected based on significance ($p < 0.05$) or near-significance ($p < 0.10$) as determined by one-sided Mann-Whitney Rank-Sum tests. "References" contain the citations of the studies from which data analyzed by Oncomine were derived.

validated antibodies recognizing these proteins, we investigated whether their protein expression is increased in samples of muscle-invasive bladder tumors removed from patients. While the intensity and extent of staining results were variable, we found that COL3A1 and COL5A1 was detected in epithelial and stromal cells of T2 and T3 tumors, while little to no staining was detected in normal bladder tissue and T1 tumors (Figure 5A). Additionally, we found that T24 cells, which are metastatic in an *in vivo* xenograft model, show increased expression of these proteins compared to E6-immortalized HUCs derived from normal tissue (Figure 5B, Data Not Shown). These results validate the novel association of COL3A1 and COL5A1 expression with muscle-invasive bladder tumors.

Discussion

The outcome of bladder cancer treatment is largely dependent upon the pathobiology of individual bladder tumors [2]. Previous microarray-based gene expression studies of various stage bladder cancers have recognized the distinct behaviors and genetic nature of superficial and muscle-invasive tumors, suggesting the possibility that the two are discrete pathobiological entities [4]. However, no biomarkers have proven able to predict progression to muscle-invasive disease, and the physiological mechanisms that drive

bladder tumor progression and invasive behavior are not well understood.

We have analyzed a large collection of expression microarray-derived data to develop a functional picture of bladder cancer progression to muscle-invasive disease. We achieved this by using only publicly available microarray data and open-access computational resources. This avoids the need to generate custom tools to perform specific analyses to analyze large amounts of multi-dimensional data. Moreover, this strategy avoided the need to invest the time and resources to acquire appropriate clinical samples in large enough numbers to allow a meaningful analysis, as well as the time and resources to perform a large number of microarrays analyses. This is especially important given that a large amount of data already exists and is available to the biomedical research community. By re-purposing public data to address our specific interests, we have not only avoided significant expenses but we also help to increase the value drawn from existing data. This has resulted in a novel systems-level model of TCC progression and muscle-invasive disease that integrates gene expression data with functional information and relationships from previous experimental observations.

In the present study, we identified specific expression differences that occur with bladder cancer progression and muscle-invasive tumors. Our results show that progression from papillary Ta to more advanced stage tumors is associated with a general increase

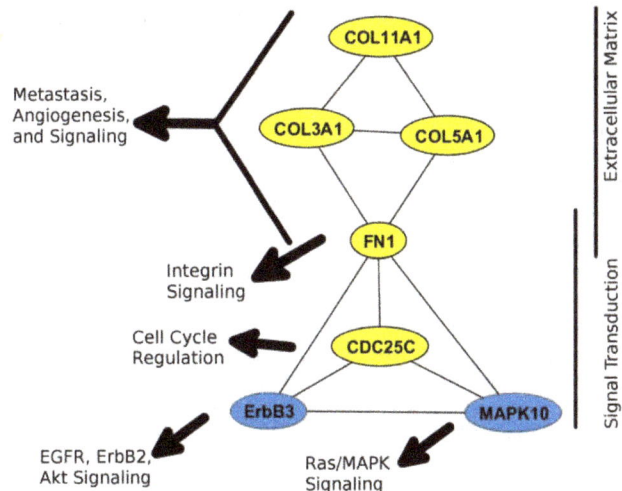

Figure 4. Bibliomic associations network in selected gene expression of muscle-invasive versus superficial tumors. Node color represents change in expression. Edges represent functional associations identified in the literature by text-mining programs PubGene and Chilibot. Selected genes separate into two functional groups of extracellular matrix and signal transduction genes. Black arrows represent generalized groups of outside genes with functional relationships to selected genes in the literature.

Table 5. Literature-based associations of selected genes and characteristics associated with advanced or metastatic cancers, identified using Chilibot [11].

Gene	Bladder Cancer	Cancer	Metastasis	Angio genesis	Invasion
COL11A1		*	*		*
COL5A1		*	*		*
COL3A1		*	*	*	*
CDC25C	*	*	*	*	*
ErbB3	*	*	*	*	*
MAPK10		*	*	*	
FN1	*	*	*	*	

*denotes identification of relationships between the terms and gene.

in expression of a network of genes involved in Ras/MAPK and associated signaling pathways (Figure 2). These pathways are closely associated with proliferation and are frequently disregulated in cancers, including bladder cancer. Interestingly, these pathways are downstream of the EGFR and ErbB2 family proteins whose expression and activity are related to bladder cancer progression, as well as ErbB3, FGFR3 and HRAS that are active in superficial tumors [4]. The increased expression of genes in

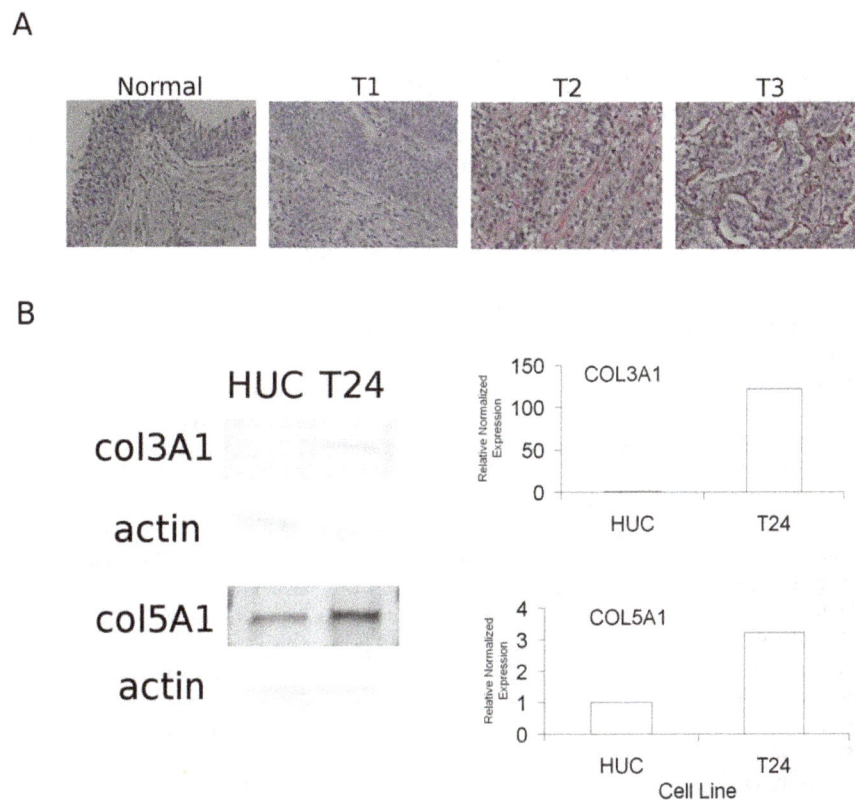

A

B

Figure 5. Elevated expression of COL3A1 and COL5A1 in muscle-invasive bladder tumors and metatstatic T24 cells. A. Immunohistochemistry of bladder tumors. DAB (brown) staining represents COL3A1 protein expression, while Warp Red staining represents COL5A1. Results are representative of five independent sample tissues per grade. B. Immunoblot analysis in immortalized non-cancer HUC cells and T24 bladder cancer cells. Expression of COL3A1 and COL5A1 was standardized to that of β-actin, and normalized to expression in HUC cells. These results are representative of 2 independent experiments.

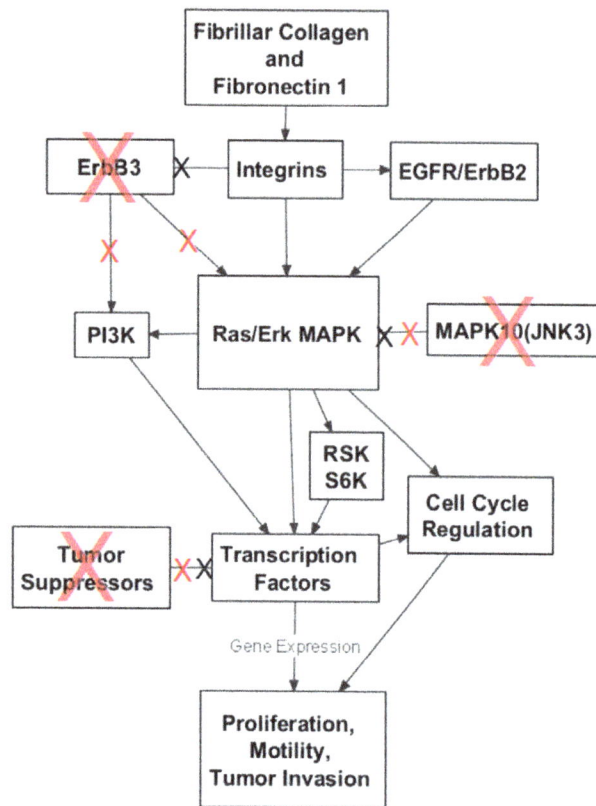

Figure 6. Model of muscle-invasive bladder cancer based on expression data and published observations. Arrows represent positive interactions. Black "X"s on arrows represent antagonistic interactions. Red "X"s represent disrupted or decreased activity.

hundreds of individual tumors, supporting the statistical validity of our observations.

The selected 7 genes can be separated into extracellular matrix proteins (COL3A1, COL5A1, COL11A1, FN1) and kinase signaling proteins (CDC25C, MAPK10, ErbB3). While the variation in expression data does not support the use of any of these genes as biomarkers individually (Data Not Shown), their expression may support a more specific means to identify muscle-invasive bladder tumors in the future. FN1 itself is a potential urine biomarker for bladder cancer detection [27]. While well supported, their functional relationships and relevance to muscle-invasive bladder cancer were not immediately apparent. To aid in our interpretation, the data were analyzed using text-mining programs that identify instances where gene names occur in potentially interactive contexts within abstracts and full texts of published reports in PubMed [10,11]. We found that these genes have been associated with cancer, bladder cancer, metastasis, angiogenesis, and invasion, suggesting that their involvement in cancer progression and/or muscle-invasive behaviors have been previously observed in various systems (Table 5).

The reported functions and interactions of the selected genes suggest a novel model of muscle-invasive disease in bladder cancer (Figure 6). COL3A1, COL5A1 and COL11A1 are fibrillar collagens, which act as "tracks" for metastatic invasion of breast tumors into secondary organs [28]. Formation of these fibrils is initiated by interactions between COL5A1 and COL11A1 proteins [29]. Tumor-secreted proteases diffuse along collagen fibrils and modify existing matrix to allow tumor cells a path of least-resistance along fibrils [30]. Collagens and FN1 are among many ligands for integrins, a class of surface receptor proteins that are functional heterodimers of 8 α and 18 β subunits that each bind specific ligands [31]. COL3A1 and COL5A1 are functionally related in connective tissue disorders [32], and expression of different collagens are associated with various cancers. FN1 "decorates" collagen fibrils and affects integrin binding specificity [31,33]. Integrin signaling stimulates RAS/MAPK signaling and modifies the activity of receptor tyrosine kinases, including EGFR/ErbB proteins, which are also upstream of Ras/MAPK [31,34]. Interestingly, FN1 has been reported to preferentially induce the activity of EGFR, ErbB2 and ErbB4 but not ErbB3 activity [34]. Our identification of decreased ErbB3 expression in muscle-invasive tumors is well supported by previous studies [26]. Formation of ErbB3/ErbB2 is kinetically preferred among ErbB family receptors, and ErbB3 is the only ErbB receptor that directly associates with and activates the PI3K signaling pathway [35]. In all, this evidence suggests a "class-switch" from ErbB3 to EGFR/ErbB2 mediated ErbB signaling, mediated in part by collagen and fibronectin-stimulated integrin signaling, is a key mechanism promoting muscle-invasion of bladder tumors. This may affect trafficking of active receptor proteins and impact the intensity and duration of downstream signaling [36], as well as alter the pathways that stimulate PI3K signaling.

Importantly, the effects of these gene expression differences in muscle-invasive tumors are likely augmented by increased expression of genes in mitogenic pathways that we find associated with general bladder cancer progression in the absence of activation mutations in RAS and PI3K pathways that are prevalent in superficial tumors. The ErbB and collagen-activated integrin proteins are upstream activators of Ras/MAPK signaling, which is associated with proliferative and tumorigenic activity and which our above expression data shows is generally increased in muscle-invasive bladder cancer (Figure 2). Changes in how Ras/MAPK and PI3K signaling are regulated by upstream receptors may fundamentally alter the nature of the responses to those

Ras/MAPK and PI3K pathways may be related to the disregulation of p53, Rb and other tumor suppressors in muscle-invasive bladder tumors [3,4]. The increased expression of components of this large pathway network may act to promote and enhance the effects of EGFR and ErbB2 activity, but the dependence of muscle-invasive tumors on the activities of these pathways in concert has not been investigated. Conversely, the relatively low expression of Ras/MAPK and PI3K pathways in superficial tumors may compensate for the elevated activity of ErbB3, FGFR3 and RAS isoforms, possibly a factor that limits the progression to muscle-invasive disease. These and other issues will be further addressed through the course of developing a systems-level understanding of bladder cancer progression.

We also used a similar approach to identify gene expression changes specifically associated with muscle-invasive tumors (Figure 2, Figure 3, Figure 4). We found that these initially selected genes occur sporadically across the initial network rather than focused on a particular pathway within the network, but the expression of these genes is consistent and distinct in superficial and muscle-invasive tumor samples (Figure 3). We then tested whether the expression differences of selected genes in our initial dataset were consistent with data from outside studies by using Oncomine to measure the median expression of each genes in 3 to 8 independent studies that include superficial and muscle-invasive bladder tumors, selecting a final set of 7 genes (Figure 4) [16–22]. Taking into account the number of samples within each study, these results ultimately represent the gene expression data of signaling pathways. The MAPK family protein MAPK10/JNK3 is generally involved in stress signaling and acts counter to Erk MAPK and PI3K signaling [37]. The decreased expression of antagonistic signaling proteins such as MAPK10 would further promote Ras/Erk MAPK signaling activity. Ultimately these activities modulate the expression and activities of proteins that affect proliferative, pro-metastatic and invasive behavior, including the CDC25C phosphatase which stimulates cyclin/CDK activity and mitosis. Metastasis and progression are further promoted by the disruption of tumor suppressors in muscle-invasive bladder cancer, including p53, Rb, myc and others that would act to limit proliferative and metastatic behavior [2–4]. As well as providing a basis for future systems-level studies of TCC, this model will inform efforts to identify and develop the therapeutic targets and predictive biomarkers that will guide the clinical treatment of muscle-invasive bladder cancer.

In summary, we have analyzed public expression microarray data of bladder tumors across stages, identifying the increased expression of the proliferative and pro-survival Ras/MAPK and PI3K pathways as a potential regulatory hallmark of tumor progression, while related genes, including fibrillar collagens are associated specifically with muscle-invasive bladder cancer. Translation of this information into clinical treatment may potentially improve the identification, treatment and outcome of bladder cancer in patients as well as in the treatment of other cancers.

Supporting Information

Table S1 Prefered Reporting Items for Systematic Reviews and Meta-Analyses (PRISMA) Guidelines Checklist.

Table S2 Prefered Reporting Items for Systematic Reviews and Meta-Analyses (PRISMA) Guidelines Checklist (Continued).

Table S3 Genes differentially expressed, both increased and decreased, in T1–T4 staged bladder tumors versus Ta-stage tumors and associated with KEGG pathways, including Top 10 pathways listed in Table 2. Pathways selected based on Fisher's Exact Scores ≤0.01.

Table S4 Genes differentially expressed, both increased and decreased, in Ta/T1-staged bladder tumors vs T2 tumors, and associated with KEGG pathways, including Top 10 pathways listen in Table 3. Pathways selected based on Fisher's Exact Scores ≤0.01.

Acknowledgments

The authors thank Glen Leverson Ph.D. and Chee Paul Lin of UW Department of Surgery for providing statistical analysis and support, and Sally A. Drew of The UW TRIP Lab for her expertise in immunohistochemistry. We thank Tihomir Miralem, Pamela Kreeger and Chad Vezina for their critical reviews and assistance in the writing of this manuscript.

Author Contributions

Conceived and designed the experiments: JAE TMD WAR. Performed the experiments: JAE WAR. Analyzed the data: JAE WAR TMD. Contributed reagents/materials/analysis tools: JAE. Wrote the paper: JAE TMD JPC WAR.

References

1. Howlander Nea (2012) SEER Cancer Statistics Review, 1975–2009 (Vintage 2009 Populations). Bethesda, MD, , USA: National Cancer Institute.
2. Knowles MA (2001) What we could do now: molecular pathology of bladder cancer. Mol Pathol 54: 215–221.
3. McConkey DJ, Lee S, Choi W, Tran M, Majewski T, et al. (2010) Molecular genetics of bladder cancer: Emerging mechanisms of tumor initiation and progression. Urol Oncol 28: 429–440.
4. Wu XR (2005) Urothelial tumorigenesis: a tale of divergent pathways. Nat Rev Cancer 5: 713–725.
5. Kompier LC, Lurkin I, van der Aa MN, van Rhijn BW, van der Kwast TH, et al. (2010) FGFR3, HRAS, KRAS, NRAS and PIK3CA mutations in bladder cancer and their potential as biomarkers for surveillance and therapy. PLoS One 5: e13821.
6. Simon R (2008) Microarray-based expression profiling and informatics. Curr Opin Biotechnol 19: 26–29.
7. Eisen MB, Spellman PT, Brown PO, Botstein D (1998) Cluster analysis and display of genome-wide expression patterns. Proc Natl Acad Sci U S A 95: 14863–14868.
8. Zhang B, Kirov S, Snoddy J (2005) WebGestalt: an integrated system for exploring gene sets in various biological contexts. Nucleic Acids Res 33: W741–748.
9. Ananiadou S, Pyysalo S, Tsujii J, Kell DB (2010) Event extraction for systems biology by text mining the literature. Trends Biotechnol 28: 381–390.
10. Jenssen TK, Laegreid A, Komorowski J, Hovig E (2001) A literature network of human genes for high-throughput analysis of gene expression. Nat Genet 28: 21–28.
11. Chen H, Sharp BM (2004) Content-rich biological network constructed by mining PubMed abstracts. BMC Bioinformatics 5: 147.
12. Faro A, Giordano D, Spampinato C (2012) Combining literature text mining with microarray data: advances for system biology modeling. Brief Bioinform 13: 61–82.
13. Rhodes DR, Kalyana-Sundaram S, Mahavisno V, Varambally R, Yu J, et al. (2007) Oncomine 3.0: genes, pathways, and networks in a collection of 18,000 cancer gene expression profiles. Neoplasia 9: 166–180.
14. Dietzsch J, Gehlenborg N, Nieselt K (2006) Mayday–a microarray data analysis workbench. Bioinformatics 22: 1010–1012.
15. Riester M, Taylor JM, Feifer A, Koppie T, Rosenberg JE, et al. (2012) Combination of a novel gene expression signature with a clinical nomogram improves the prediction of survival in high-risk bladder cancer. Clin Cancer Res 18: 1323–1333.
16. Blaveri E, Simko JP, Korkola JE, Brewer JL, Baehner F, et al. (2005) Bladder cancer outcome and subtype classification by gene expression. Clin Cancer Res 11: 4044–4055.
17. Dyrskjot L, Kruhoffer M, Thykjaer T, Marcussen N, Jensen JL, et al. (2004) Gene expression in the urinary bladder: a common carcinoma in situ gene expression signature exists disregarding histopathological classification. Cancer Res 64: 4040–4048.
18. Dyrskjot L, Thykjaer T, Kruhoffer M, Jensen JL, Marcussen N, et al. (2003) Identifying distinct classes of bladder carcinoma using microarrays. Nat Genet 33: 90–96.
19. Dyrskjot L, Zieger K, Real FX, Malats N, Carrato A, et al. (2007) Gene expression signatures predict outcome in non-muscle-invasive bladder carcinoma: a multicenter validation study. Clin Cancer Res 13: 3545–3551.
20. Modlich O, Prisack HB, Pitschke G, Ramp U, Ackermann R, et al. (2004) Identifying superficial, muscle-invasive, and metastasizing transitional cell carcinoma of the bladder: use of cDNA array analysis of gene expression profiles. Clin Cancer Res 10: 3410–3421.
21. Sanchez-Carbayo M, Socci ND, Lozano J, Saint F, Cordon-Cardo C (2006) Defining molecular profiles of poor outcome in patients with invasive bladder cancer using oligonucleotide microarrays. J Clin Oncol 24: 778–789.
22. Stransky N, Vallot C, Reyal F, Bernard-Pierrot I, de Medina SG, et al. (2006) Regional copy number-independent deregulation of transcription in cancer. Nat Genet 38: 1386–1396.
23. Ewald JA, Jarrard DF (2012) Decreased skp2 expression is necessary but not sufficient for therapy-induced senescence in prostate cancer. Transl Oncol 5: 278–287.
24. Rhodes DR, Yu J, Shanker K, Deshpande N, Varambally R, et al. (2004) ONCOMINE: a cancer microarray database and integrated data-mining platform. Neoplasia 6: 1–6.
25. Aressy B, Ducommun B (2008) Cell cycle control by the CDC25 phosphatases. Anticancer Agents Med Chem 8: 818–824.
26. Memon AA, Sorensen BS, Meldgaard P, Fokdal L, Thykjaer T, et al. (2006) The relation between survival and expression of HER1 and HER2 depends on the expression of HER3 and HER4: a study in bladder cancer patients. Br J Cancer 94: 1703–1709.
27. Eissa S, Zohny SF, Zekri AR, El-Zayat TM, Maher AM (2010) Diagnostic value of fibronectin and mutant p53 in the urine of patients with bladder cancer:

impact on clinicopathological features and disease recurrence. Med Oncol 27: 1286–1294.

28. Gritsenko PG, Ilina O, Friedl P (2012) Interstitial guidance of cancer invasion. J Pathol 226: 185–199.

29. Wenstrup RJ, Smith SM, Florer JB, Zhang G, Beason DP, et al. (2011) Regulation of collagen fibril nucleation and initial fibril assembly involves coordinate interactions with collagens V and XI in developing tendon. J Biol Chem 286: 20455–20465.

30. Collier IE, Legant W, Marmer B, Lubman O, Saffarian S, et al. (2011) Diffusion of MMPs on the surface of collagen fibrils: the mobile cell surface-collagen substratum interface. PLoS One 6: e24029.

31. Juliano RL, Reddig P, Alahari S, Edin M, Howe A, et al. (2004) Integrin regulation of cell signalling and motility. Biochem Soc Trans 32: 443–446.

32. Zoppi N, Gardella R, De Paepe A, Barlati S, Colombi M (2004) Human fibroblasts with mutations in COL5A1 and COL3A1 genes do not organize collagens and fibronectin in the extracellular matrix, down-regulate alpha2beta1 integrin, and recruit alphavbeta3 Instead of alpha5beta1 integrin. J Biol Chem 279: 18157–18168.

33. Exposito JY, Valcourt U, Cluzel C, Lethias C (2011) The fibrillar collagen family. Int J Mol Sci 11: 407–426.

34. Cabodi S, Moro L, Bergatto E, Boeri Erba E, Di Stefano P, et al. (2004) Integrin regulation of epidermal growth factor (EGF) receptor and of EGF-dependent responses. Biochem Soc Trans 32: 438–442.

35. Citri A, Yarden Y (2006) EGF-ERBB signalling: towards the systems level. Nat Rev Mol Cell Biol 7: 505–516.

36. Resat H, Ewald JA, Dixon DA, Wiley HS (2003) An integrated model of epidermal growth factor receptor trafficking and signal transduction. Biophys J 85: 730–743.

37. Turjanski AG, Vaque JP, Gutkind JS (2007) MAP kinases and the control of nuclear events. Oncogene 26: 3240–3253.

8

Cyclooxygenase-2 Expression in Bladder Cancer and Patient Prognosis: Results from a Large Clinical Cohort and Meta-Analysis

Maciej J. Czachorowski[1], **André F. S. Amaral**[1], **Santiago Montes-Moreno**[2], **Josep Lloreta**[3,4,5], **Alfredo Carrato**[6,7], **Adonina Tardón**[8], **Manuel M. Morente**[9], **Manolis Kogevinas**[10], **Francisco X. Real**[5,11], **Núria Malats**[1]*, for the SBC/EPICURO investigators[¶]

1 Genetic and Molecular Epidemiology Group, Spanish National Cancer Research Centre (CNIO), Madrid, Spain, 2 Servicio de Anatomía Patológica, Hospital Universitario Marqués de Valdecilla, Santander, Spain, 3 Institut Municipal d'Investigació Mèdica – Hospital del Mar, Barcelona, Spain, 4 Departament de Patologia, Hospital del Mar – Parc de Salut Mar, Barcelona, Spain, 5 Departament de Ciències Experimentals i de la Salut, Universitat Pompeu Fabra, Barcelona, Spain, 6 Hospital General Universitario de Elche, Elche, Spain, 7 Hospital Ramon y Cajal, Madrid, Spain, 8 Universidad de Oviedo, Oviedo, Spain, 9 Tumor Bank Unit, Spanish National Cancer Research Centre (CNIO), Madrid, Spain, 10 Centre de Recerca en Epidemiologia Ambiental (CREAL), Barcelona, Spain, 11 Epithelial Carcinogenesis Group, Spanish National Cancer Research Centre (CNIO), Madrid, Spain

Abstract

Aberrant overexpression of cyclooxygenase-2 (COX2) is observed in urothelial carcinoma of the bladder (UCB). Studies evaluating COX2 as a prognostic marker in UCB report contradictory results. We determined the prognostic potential of COX2 expression in UCB and quantitatively summarize the results with those of the literature through a meta-analysis. Newly diagnosed UCB patients recruited between 1998–2001 in 18 Spanish hospitals were prospectively included in the study and followed-up (median, 70.7 months). Diagnostic slides were reviewed and uniformly classified by expert pathologists. Clinical data was retrieved from hospital charts. Tissue microarrays containing non-muscle invasive (n = 557) and muscle invasive (n = 216) tumours were analyzed by immunohistochemistry using quantitative image analysis. Expression was evaluated in Cox regression models to assess the risk of recurrence, progression and disease-specific mortality. Meta-hazard ratios were estimated using our results and those from 11 additional evaluable studies. COX2 expression was observed in 38% (211/557) of non-muscle invasive and 63% (137/216) of muscle invasive tumors. Expression was associated with advanced pathological stage and grade (p<0.0001). In the univariable analyses, COX2 expression - as a categorical variable - was not associated with any of the outcomes analyzed. As a continuous variable, a weak association with recurrence in non-muscle invasive tumors was observed (p-value = 0.048). In the multivariable analyses, COX2 expression did not independently predict any of the considered outcomes. The meta-analysis confirmed these results. We did not find evidence that COX2 expression is an independent prognostic marker of recurrence, progression or survival in patients with UCB.

Editor: Xiaolin Zi, University of California Irvine, United States of America

Funding: The work was partially supported by the Fondo de Investigaciones Sanitarias, Instituto de Salud Carlos III, Ministry of Science and Innovation, Spain (G03/174, 00/0745, PI051436, PI061614 and G03/174); Red Temática de Investigación Cooperativa en Cáncer- RD06/0020-RTICC; Consolider ONCOBIO; EU-FP6-STREP-37739-DRoP-ToP; EU-FP7-HEALTH-F2-2008-201663-UROMOL; EU-FP7-HEALTH-F2-2008-201333-DECanBio; USA-NIH-RO1-CA089715; and a PhD fellowship awarded to MJC from the "la Caixa" foundation, Spain, and a postdoctoral fellowship awarded to AFSA from the Fundación Científica de la AECC. The funders had no role in study design, data collection and analysis, decision to publish, or preparation of the manuscript.

Competing Interests: The authors have declared that no competing interests exist.

* E-mail: nmalats@cnio.es

¶ Membership of the Spanish Bladder Cancer (SBC)/EPICURO Study investigators is provided in the Acknowledgments.

Introduction

Urothelial carcinoma of the bladder (UCB) is the most common bladder cancer type in developed nations [1]. UCB predominantly manifests (70–80% of patients) as a non-muscle invasive tumor (NMIBC: pTa-pT1) characterized by an overall good prognosis following transurethral resection in patients with low-grade tumors (pTaG1/2), and intravesical chemotherapy and/or Bacillus Calmette Guerin (BCG) instillation in patients with high-grade tumors (pTaG3 or pT1G2/3) [2]. Approximately 70% of NMIBC patients suffer a recurrence following treatment and a further 15% progress, developing new tumors exhibiting muscle invasion (MIBC: pT2-pT4); the risk of progression being higher among patients with high-grade tumors [2]. Due to a high rate of recurrence and the need for close follow-up over a patient's lifetime, UCB remains one of the most expensive tumors to treat on a per patient basis [3]. A lower proportion (20–30%) of UCB patients are diagnosed with muscle invasive tumors (MIBC; pT2-pT4) characterized by poor prognosis: 50% of these patients die from their cancer [2]. Genomic profiling and gene expression analyses indicate a strong correlation between these pathologic classifications and the underlying molecular architecture of UCB [4].

Growing evidence indicates that chronic inflammation may increase the risk of UCB [5]. Studies investigating the prolonged use of cyclooxygenase-2 (COX2) inhibiting non-steroidal anti-inflammatory drugs (NSAIDs) have reported a decrease in UCB risk [6,7]. COX2 is a prostaglandin endoperoxide synthetase that catalyzes the production of prostanoids upon induction by proinflammatory cytokines, growth factors, tumor promoters and other external stimuli [8]. COX2 activation mediates cellular processes also implicated in carcinogenesis such as angiogenesis, cell survival/proliferation and apoptosis [9]. Moreover, studies have shown that bladder tissue from patients with cystitis or UCB exhibits elevated COX2 levels in contrast to benign bladder tissue [10,11].

While numerous groups have investigated the prognostic potential of COX2 expression in UCB [12–31], there is no clear consensus on its utility. The objective of this study was to assess whether COX2 protein expression in UCB cells is associated with prognosis using a large and standardized cohort of newly diagnosed bladder cancer patients. A meta-analysis was also done to summarize these results together with those from other studies published on the topic.

Materials and Methods

Study Population

A total of 773 newly diagnosed UCB cases aged 22–80 years (mean $\pm$ SD $= 66 \pm 10$ yrs) with a median follow-up of 70.7 months (range 0.7–117.7 months) and available tumor tissue were used in the current analysis. All cases were recruited between 1998 and 2001 from 18 hospitals in five regions of Spain as part of the Spanish Bladder Cancer (SBC)/EPIdemiology of Cancer of the UROthelium (EPICURO) study, a hospital-based case-control study described previously [32]. A pathologist review panel uniformly classified the T stage and grade (G) of each tumor biopsy according to the criteria of the TNM classification and the WHO-ISUP [33], using the three grade redefinition provided by the WHO [34,35]. All bladder tumor samples used in the study were collected prior to the administration of any intravesical or systemic therapy. Clinical information related to diagnostic procedures, tumor characteristics and treatment was collected from medical records, and a computerized questionnaire was used for the collection of sociodemographic data. NMIBCs were removed by transurethral resection and patients received intravesical chemo- or immunotherapy (i.e. BCG) as appropriate. The majority of patients presenting with MIBCs were treated by radical cystectomy; in cases where surgery was not possible, radiotherapy or systemic chemotherapy were administered. Follow-up information was collected annually from hospital records and through direct telephone interviews by trained monitors using structured questionnaires. Among NMIBCs, recurrence was defined as the appearance of a new NMIBC following a previous negative follow-up cystoscopy, and progression, as the development of a MIBC. In patients initially presenting with MIBCs, any tumor reappearance after treatment was considered progression, regardless of whether the tumor relapse was local or distal. Tumour-specific survival was assessed only for patients with MIBCs. Informed written consent was obtained from study participants in accordance with the Ethics Committees of each participating hospital.

Immunohistochemistry

Tissue blocks of formalin-fixed, paraffin-embedded primary bladder tumors were used to construct tissue microarrays (TMA) containing tumor cores of 0.6-mm in diameter represented in duplicate and selected from the most representative regions of the tumor on which T and G were based. After deparaffinisation and heat-induced antigen retrieval, all slides were stained simultaneously at the Histology and Immunohistochemistry Core Unit of the CNIO using the PT LINK system as per manufacturer's instructions (Dako Inc., Glostrup, Denmark). Briefly, tissue sections were incubated with anti-COX2 rabbit monoclonal antibody (ThermoFisher Scientific, Fremont, CA, USA; #RM-9121-R7; pre-diluted, ready-to-use) at room temperature, followed by visualization using the EnVision Flex Visualization system (Dako Inc., Glostrup, Denmark) and exposure to diaminobenzedine. Tissues were then counterstained with haematoxylin, dehydrated and mounted. A section of colon tissue was used as a positive control.

Evaluation of COX2 Immunostaining

COX2 expression was quantified using the Ariol SL-50 (version 3.1.2, Applied Imaging Corp., San Jose, CA, USA) high-throughput slide imaging scanner. All cores were imaged and processed using a light microscope and the accompanying TMA Multistain Imaging software. The program was trained by a pathologist (SM) to maximize the inclusion of positively stained tumor epithelium while minimizing stromal material, as described previously [36]. COX2 expression score was calculated as the product of the mean intensity of staining (by defining the background and saturation limits of the antibody and imaging sensor, respectively) and the proportion of cellular antibody-positive area divided by total cellular area. Values from replicate cores were averaged to provide a final expression score for each patient. Furthermore, one randomly selected TMA (representing 10% of all cores) was analyzed by direct visual microscopic inspection by an independent pathologist (MMM) to enable comparison with the automated scoring approach. The pathologist-derived score was calculated as the product of COX2 staining intensity (1 = weak, 2 = intermediate, 3 = strong) and a quartile of the percentage of epithelial tumor cells stained (0–4; with 0 representing 0% staining), providing a final categorical score in the range of 0–12. There was a high and significant correlation between the machine and pathologist derived scores (Spearman rho $= 0.85$; 95%CI $= 0.79$–0.90; p-value<0.00001). COX2 expression was analyzed as both a continuous variable and categorical variables partitioned at the median and extreme tertiles. Additionally, expression was examined as a categorical variable dichotomized at a threshold (0.340 arbitrary units [au]) above which COX2 expression was considered to be *positive*. This expression threshold was derived by comparing the pathologist's (MMM) binary assignment of positive expression (i.e. score of 0 vs. score ≥ 1, as described above) to the machine-derived continuous score using receiver operating characteristic (ROC) curve analysis (area under the curve $= 0.95$; 86% sensitivity and 92% specificity) [37].

Meta-analysis

The meta-analysis included COX2 expression results from our own series (using the ROC-derived categorical expression variable) and relevant studies published before 1 January 2012 identified by searching PubMed and ISI Web of Knowledge. The search string used was: (cox2 OR cox-2 OR cyclooxygenase-2 OR "cyclooxygenase 2" OR ptgs2) AND (prognos* OR survival OR mortality OR recurrence OR relapse OR progression) AND ("bladder cancer"). Studies were considered eligible if: (i) they reported the effect measure (as HRs, survival curves or log-rank p-values) of COX2 protein expression on recurrence, progression or disease-specific survival; (ii) COX2 was assessed in primary tumors exhibiting homogeneity in tumor histology (≥75% UCB), and subphenotype (≥75% NMIBC *or* MIBC); (iii) they were written in English or Spanish (Table S1). Reviews, abstracts, non-clinical studies, and duplicate publications were excluded. HRs and 95%CIs were directly extracted from the publications whenever available. For those reporting only the log-rank p-value or the Kaplan–Meier survival curves, the HRs and 95%CIs were independently calculated by two of the co-authors (MJC, AFSA) using the spreadsheet prepared by Sydes and Tierney with any discrepancies resolved by discussion [38]. In a few indicated cases, authors were directly contacted for clarification or provision of data not shown in the published manuscripts (Table S1). The level of heterogeneity among studies was calculated by means of the I^2 statistic [39], and publication bias was assessed by analyzing funnel plots and Egger's asymmetry test [40].

Statistical Analysis

Associations between demographic and clinico-pathological parameters and COX2 expression were assessed using Fisher's exact test. In NMIBCs, expression was also assessed distinctly in low-grade/risk (pTaG1/G2) and high-grade/risk (pTa/pT2G3) tumors, based on our previous evidence suggesting differential prognostic, genetic and molecular profiles between these subgroups [41,42]. Recurrence-free, progression-free, and overall disease-specific survival curves were generated using the Kaplan-Meier method, with statistical significance assessed using the log-rank test. Time to each endpoint was calculated from date of primary treatment to the date of event, date of last follow-up, or date of patient's death. Individuals who did not present any event until the end of the study, those lost to follow-up, or those who died from other causes were censored either at the time of last medical visit or at death. Time to recurrence and progression were defined by applying the "mid-time" between the date of the previous disease-free visit and that when a new event was diagnosed. Survival time was measured as the time from initial treatment to death resulting from cancer. Univariable and multivariable Cox-proportional hazards analysis was used to calculate hazard ratios (HR) and 95% confidence intervals (CI). Schoenfeld residual analysis did not suggest any departure from the proportional hazards assumption in multivariable models.

All statistical analyses were done using STATA (version 10.1 SE, StataCorp, College Station, TX, USA). Statistical tests were two-sided and p-values less than 0.05 were considered significant. The REMARK [43] guidelines for prognostic studies as well as the PRISMA [44] guidelines for systematic reviews and meta-analyses were adhered to in the preparation of the manuscript.

Results

Patients and COX2 Expression in Bladder Cancer TMAs

COX2 expression was assessed in 557 patients with NMIBCs and 216 individuals with MIBCs. Median COX2 expression was 0.121 au (range 0–42.590; interquartile range 1.382) in NMIBCs, and 0.760 au (0–30.806; 3.600) in MIBCs (p-value = 4×10^{-12}). Representative COX2 immunostaining patterns in UCBs are shown in Figure S1. Of patients with NMIBCs, 41% (230/557) were treated only by transurethral resection, with the remainder (56%) receiving endovesical BCG immunotherapy and/or chemotherapy following transurethral resection, or other treatment (3%; Table 1). Nearly half (46%) of patients with MIBCs were treated by cystectomy, with the remainder receiving systemic chemotherapy, radiotherapy, superficial or other treatment, or some combination thereof (Table 2).

Table 1. Distribution of characteristics of patients with NMIBCs by COX2 expression.

Patient characteristics	Total, N	COX2 expression* negative, n	COX2 expression* positive, n	P value[†]
	557	346	211	
Area				0,506
Barcelona	98	68	30	
Valles	105	66	39	
Elche	51	32	19	
Tenerife	122	71	51	
Asturias	181	109	72	
Age (yrs.)				0,385
≤60	140	81	59	
>60 and ≤70	210	130	80	
>70	207	135	72	
Gender				0,891
Men	494	306	188	
Women	63	40	23	
Tumor Invasion				<0,0001
Ta	477	277	200	
T1	80	69	11	
Grade				<0,0001
GI	200	131	69	
GII	219	95	124	
GIII	138	120	18	
Low/High Grade				<0,0001
Low (TaG1/TaG2)	408	221	187	
High (TaG3/T1G2/T1G3)	149	125	24	
Number of tumors				0,106
1	348	209	139	
>1	178	120	58	
missing	31	17	14	
Tumour Size				0,564
≤3 cm	294	188	106	
>3 cm	111	67	44	
missing	152	91	61	
Number of Recurrences				0,409
none	366	232	134	
at least 1	191	114	77	
Treatment[‡]				0,393
TUR	230	133	97	
TUR+BCG	158	105	53	
TUR+Chem.	132	83	49	
TUR+BCG+Chem.	19	14	5	
Other	18	11	7	

*COX2 expression score dichotomised at the threshold of positivitiy (0,340 au).
[†]Fisher's exact test comparing distribution of COX-2 negative versus positive patients; missing values excluded from analysis where applicable.
[‡]TUR: transurethral resection; BCG: Bacillus Calmette-Guerin instillation; Chem.: chemotherapy via endovesical instillation.

Table 2. Distribution of characteristics of patients with MIBCs by COX2 expression.

| Patient Characteristics | Total, N | COX2 expression* | | P value† |
		negative, N	positive, N	
	216	79	137	
Area				0,207
Barcelona	39	16	23	
Valles	36	9	27	
Elche	15	9	6	
Tenerife	39	14	25	
Asturias	87	31	56	
Gender				0,816
Men	194	72	122	
Women	22	7	15	
Age (yrs.)				0,426
≤60	45	14	31	
>60 and ≤70	84	35	49	
>70	87	30	57	
Tumor invasion				0,896
T2	114	42	72	
T3	55	21	34	
T4	47	16	31	
Grade				0,326
GII	19	9	10	
GIII	197	70	127	
Metastases				0,296
M0	168	57	111	
M1	29	13	16	
Mx	19	9	10	
Lymphatic invasion				0,862
N0	141	50	91	
N1, N3	49	16	33	
Nx	26	13	13	
Number of tumors				0,008
1	146	63	83	
>1	54	12	42	
missing	16	4	12	
Tumour size				0,572
≤3 cm	53	19	34	
>3 cm	66	28	38	
missing	97	32	65	
Treatment‡				0,417
Cystectomy	67	19	48	
Cystectomy+Chem.	32	15	17	
Chem. only	23	9	14	
RT +/− Chem.	19	7	12	
Superficial Treatment	13	3	10	
Others	61	25	36	
missing	1	1	0	

*COX2 expression score dichotomised at the threshold of positivity (0,340 au).
†Fisher's exact test comparing distribution of patients with negative or positive COX-2 expression; missing, Nx and Mx values excluded from analysis where applicable.
‡Chem.: Systemic chemotherapy; RT: Radiation therapy.

COX2 Expression and Clinicopathological Features

Two-hundred eleven (38%) NMIBCs and 137 (58%) MIBCs expressed COX2 (Tables 1 and 2, respectively), with positive expression defined as a score equal to or greater than the ROC-derived threshold of 0.340 au. Patient and tumor characteristics in the analyzed sample did not differ significantly from the initial SBC/EPICURO study population with the exception of geographic region and tumor size in NMIBC patients (data not shown). The distribution of COX2 positivity was assessed according to established bladder cancer prognosticators including tumor invasion and grade, tumor multiplicity, tumor size and treatment, among others. Demographic factors like age, gender and region were not associated with COX2 expression, nor was the type of primary treatment received by patients (Tables 1 and 2). In NMIBCs, COX2 expression was significantly associated only with T and G; being more prominent in low-grade/risk pTaG1/2 tumors than in high-grade/risk pTa/pT1G3 tumors (p-value<0.0001; Table 1). Further assessment of COX2 distribution in relevant molecular subtypes of UCB [4], revealed a greater proportion of pTaG2 than pTaG1 tumors positively expressing COX2 in low-grade NMIBCs (p<0.0001, subtype 1; Figure S2). COX2 expression did not differ among high-grade/risk NMIBCs (p = 0.075), but a greater proportion of MIBCs positively expressed COX2 than did all high-grade/risk NMIBCs combined (p<0.0001, subtype 2; Figure S2). Only tumor multiplicity was associated with positive COX2 expression in MIBC patients (p-value = 0.008; Table 2).

COX2 Expression and Prognosis in Bladder Cancer Patients

We analyzed the association of COX2 expression with tumor recurrence and progression in patients with NMIBCs and with progression and disease-specific survival in patients with MIBCs (Table 3; Figure 1). When considered as a continuous variable in the univariable analysis, COX2 expression was marginally associated with an increased risk of recurrence in NMIBCs (HR = 1.02, 95%CI = 1.00–1.04, p-value = 0.048; Table 3). However, this association disappeared upon multivariable analysis when adjusting for region, gender, tumor stage and grade, multiplicity, tumor size, and treatment. Moreover, COX2 expression was not significantly associated with recurrence in NMIBCs when considered as a categorical variable, neither in the univariable nor multivariable analyses (Figure 1A; Figure S3AC; Table 3). Lastly, no significant association between COX2 expression and progression or survival was observed in patients with NMIBCs or MIBCs, regardless of whether expression was considered as a continuous or categorical variable in non-adjusted or adjusted analyses (Figure 1B–D; Figure S3B, 3D–H; Table 3).

Meta-analysis of COX2 Expression and Bladder Cancer Prognosis

Twenty publications on COX2 expression and bladder cancer prognosis were identified through the literature review (Table S1) [12–31]. Three of them lacked prognostic data, two overlapped with other larger studies and four included patient cohorts that did not meet the eligibility criteria outlined earlier, leaving 11 evaluable publications [12–14,19,21–25,28,29] plus the current study for the meta-analysis (Figure S4). Studies were classified by the tumor subtype(s) they reported on (i.e. NMIBC or MIBC), and whether adjustment for covariates was considered for each prognostic endpoint examined (i.e. univariable or multivariable; Figures 2 and 3). Of the four meta-analyses conducted with univariable data, only the metaHR of the association between

COX2 expression and recurrence in NMIBCs showed marginal significance (metaHR = 1.35, 95%CI = 1.00–1.83; Figure 2). This result was not affected by study heterogeneity (I^2 p-value = 0.13) but exhibited significant publication bias, as evidenced by Egger's test (p-value = 0.019). The remaining meta-analyses considering univariable data suggested increased, albeit non-significant, risks of tumor progression in patients with NMIBCs (metaHR = 2.07, 95%CI = 0.76–5.64) and MIBCs (metaHR = 1.45, 95%CI = 0.77–2.74), and death in patients with MIBCs (metaHR = 1.13, 95%CI = 0.8–1.59; Figure 2). Notably, the summary effect for progression in NMIBCs and that observed for survival in MIBCs were both significantly affected by study heterogeneity (I^2 p-values: 0.006 and 0.004, respectively), with the former also significantly influenced by publication bias (Egger's test p-value = 0.001).

Due to a paucity of published prognostic studies performing multivariable analysis on patients with NMIBCs, we could only address the multivariable meta-association with progression and survival in patients with MIBCs (Figure 3). A small, non-significant increased summary risk of progression (metaHR = 1.12, 95%CI = 0.53–2.35; Figure 3) was observed in COX2 expressing MIBCs that was unaffected by study heterogeneity (I^2 p-value = 0.139). Similarly, a null summary effect was observed for survival (metaHR = 0.97, 95%CI = 0.69–1.36; Figure 3). This effect was influenced neither by study heterogeneity (I^2 p-value = 0.114) nor by publication bias (Egger's test p-value = 0.108).

Discussion

Despite many published studies, contradictory findings prevail on COX2 expression as an independent prognostic marker in patients with UCB. The current study suggests that COX2 expression is not an independent marker associated with recurrence, progression or survival in patients with UCB.

Using the largest cohort of patients with NMIBCs evaluated for COX2 expression to date, we observed that 38% of these tumors expressed the protein. Other groups have reported frequencies ranging from 53–88%; however, these studies used different COX2 antibodies and expression evaluation techniques and had smaller sample sizes [16,28,29,45,46]. In accordance with reported results [11,18,45] we observed significantly higher COX2 expression in MIBCs (58%) than in NMIBCs. This frequency is similar to that observed in other large, histologically homogeneous studies [21,28], while groups using heterogeneous cohorts of squamous and transitional cell carcinomas report frequencies different from our own [12,29]. Collectively, these findings reiterate the importance of homogeneity, or stratification, in tumor marker studies.

The association between COX2 and clinico-pathological characteristics remains a contentious issue in the literature. The majority of studies report an association between COX2 overexpression and advanced tumor invasion and grade, but use heterogeneous populations of NMIBCs *and* MIBCs in their assessments [21,25,26,28,47]. Given the known disparity in COX2 expression between NMIBCs and MIBCs, an association of this type would be expected in a mixed tumor population. After pooling NMIBCs and MIBCs in our study we also observe a strong significant association between COX2 overexpression and advanced tumor invasion (p>0.0001) and grade (p>0.0001). Notably, several groups report no association between COX2 expression and T and G [14,29,45]; especially those working strictly with homogeneous cohorts of MIBCs [12,23]. Similarly, in our study, COX2 expression did not differ significantly among pT2, pT3 and pT4 tumors (p = 0.896). Interestingly, we observed

Table 3. Analysis of COX2 expression in NMIBCs and MIBCs; univariable and multivariable analyses.

Score Categorization*	Univariate COX-regression					Multivariate COX-regression[†]				
	Patients, n	Events, n	HR	(95% CI)	P value[‡]	Patients, n	Failures, n	HR	(95% CI)	P value[‡]
Non-muscle invasive tumors										
Recurrence [§]										
Continuous	556	191	1,02	1,00–1,04	0,048	401	141	1,02	1,00–1,04	0,140
Negative vs. Positive	556	191	1,08	0,81–1,44	0,612	401	141	1,11	0,78–1,59	0,555
Median	556	191	1,08	0,82–1,44	0,583	401	141	1,17	0,82–1,67	0,390
Extreme tertiles	370	127	1,06	0,89–1,27	0,483	268	94	1,08	0,86–1,37	0,510
Progression										
Continuous	557	48	0,92	0,84–1,01	0,094	526	43	0,96	0,87–1,05	0,350
Negative vs. Positive	557	48	0,72	0,39–1,33	0,302	526	43	1,38	0,61–3,11	0,434
Median	557	48	0,67	0,38–1,20	0,181	526	43	1,11	0,53–2,33	0,780
Extreme tertiles	371	33	0,71	0,49–1,01	0,059	351	29	0,92	0,54–1,56	0,750
Muscle invasive tumors										
Progression										
Continuous	216	131	0,99	0,96–1,03	0,617	189	110	0,99	0,96–1,03	0,750
Negative vs. Positive	216	131	0,94	0,66–1,34	0,734	189	110	0,85	0,56–1,29	0,448
Median	216	131	0,97	0,69–1,37	0,869	189	110	0,89	0,60–1,32	0,560
Extreme tertiles	144	85	0,92	0,75–1,14	0,464	128	75	0,90	0,70–1,15	0,410
Disease specific survival										
Continuous	216	110	1,00	0,97–1,04	0,908	187	89	1,01	0,97–1,05	0,730
Negative vs. Positive	216	110	0,91	0,61–1,34	0,627	187	89	0,77	0,48–1,23	0,267
Median	216	110	0,94	0,64–1,36	0,726	187	89	0,78	0,50–1,23	0,290
Extreme tertiles	144	68	0,90	0,71–1,15	0,407	126	57	0,78	0,58–1,04	0,090

*Expression cut-points used for categorical variables: "Neg. vs. Pos." - NMIBC/MIBC: 0.340; "Median" - NMIBC: 0.121, MIBC: 0.760; "Extreme tertiles" - NMIBC: (<0.0239, >0.586), MIBC: (<0.270, >2.149).
[†]Multivariate models adjusted for established bladder cancer prognostic factors as follows: NMIBC Recurrence adjusted by region, gender, tumour stage and grade, # tumours, size of tumours, and treatment; NMIBC Progression adjusted by region, # recurrences, age, tumour stage and grade, # tumours, and treatment; MIBC Progression adjusted by region, tumour stage, treatment, and presence of nodes; MIBC Survival adjusted by region, tumour stage, treatment, presence of nodes, and metastases.
[‡]Cox proportional hazards analysis.
[§]One patient excluded due to incomplete follow-up record.

lower COX2 positivity in pT1 and high-grade/risk NMIBCs, than in pTa and low-grade/risk NMIBCs tumors. This result may seem counterintuitive if grade progression is considered a linear trait and COX2 expression is deemed to increase linearly with T and G. However, there is strong evidence indicating that UCB exists as two molecularly distinct subtypes, with high-grade/risk NMIBCs having a molecular signature more similar to MIBCs than to low-grade/risk NMIBCs [4,42]. In this respect, we observed that COX2 positivity increased significantly with increasing T and G within each molecular tumor subtype (Figure S2). Shirahama et al. [26] reported a COX2 distribution similar to ours, observing 8% positivity in pT1 tumors and 50% in MIBCs when using whole section staining and a 5% expression threshold. Collectively, these results reiterate the disparity in COX2 expression between NMIBCs and MIBCs first reported by Komhoff et al. [47], and highlight the importance of considering expression within the proper molecular context.

To minimize the effects resulting from selecting an arbitrary expression threshold, we investigated COX2 protein expression as a continuous variable and three categorical variables. Only when considered as a continuous variable in the univariable analysis was COX2 expression found to be associated with a slight increase in the risk of recurrence. The meta-analysis,

consisting of five other univariable studies, reiterated this association and showed a 35% increased risk of recurrence in patients with COX2 expressing NMIBCs. However, both effect estimates exhibit only marginal significance, suggesting that the observed associations may be due to chance. Moreover, the association observed in the univariable analysis did not hold after adjustment for conventional prognostic factors of recurrence in the multivariable analysis. Lastly, the summary effect observed in the meta-analysis may have been skewed by two small studies which selected only high risk NMIBCs (T1G3 [19] and Cis [24]). When a sensitivity analysis was performed removing these two studies from the meta-analysis, the association between recurrence and COX2 expression was no longer maintained (metaHR = 1.14, 95%CI = 0.94–1.38). The observed disparity between effect estimates of progression in the present study and the meta-analysis could also be attributed to the inclusion of these two studies. Upon their exclusion, the summary HR showed no association with progression (metaHR = 0.98, 95%CI = 0.47–2.03). These results do not support a role for COX2 expression in NMIBCs as an independent prognostic marker of recurrence or progression.

Several groups have investigated the ability of COX2 expression to predict outcome in patients with MIBCs. Despite wide inter-

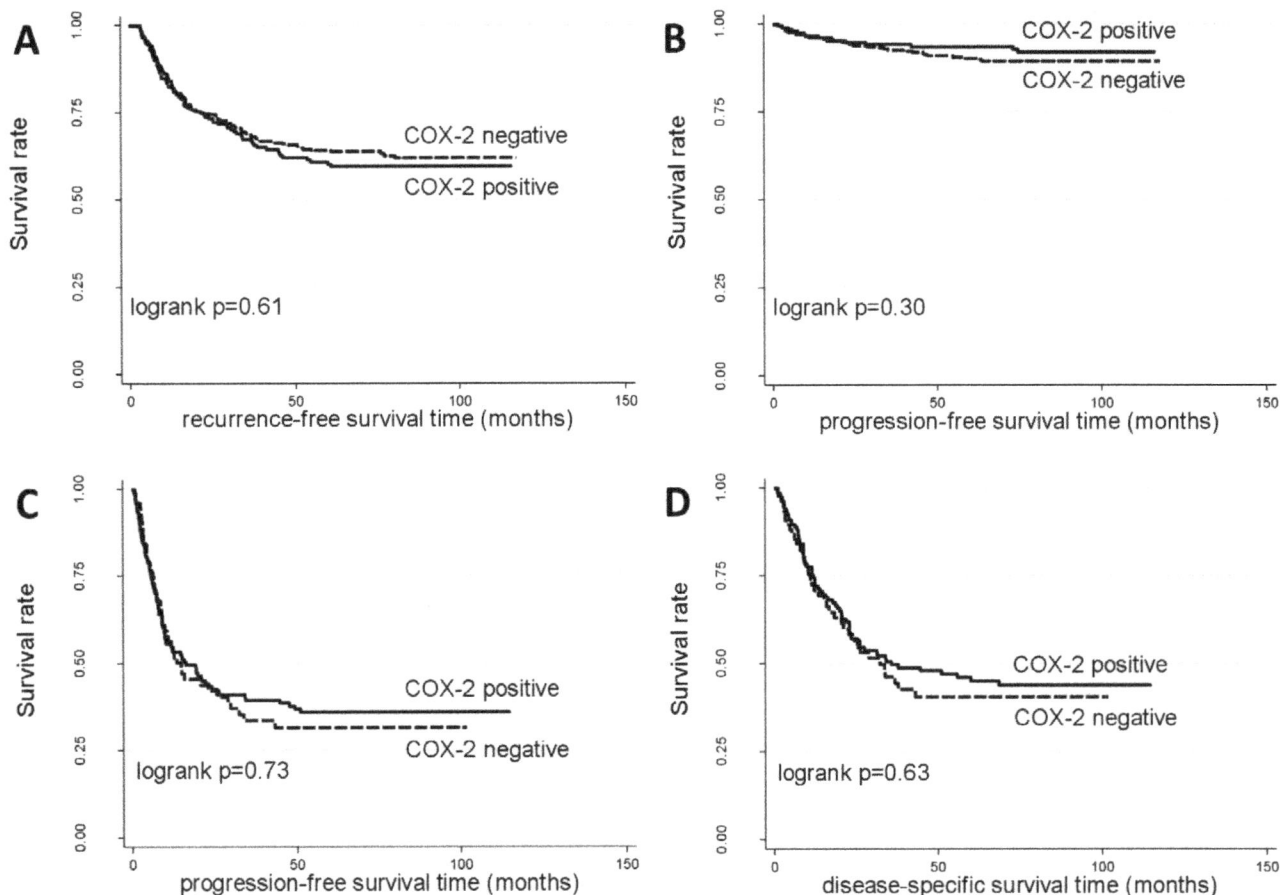

Figure 1. Kaplan-Meier survival curves corresponding to failures in superficial (A, B) and invasive (C, D) tumors for specified prognostic endpoints. Dashed curves: patients with tumors positive for COX2 protein staining; solid curves: patients with tumors negative for COX2 protein staining. Significance values from two-sided logrank test.

study variation in methodology, antibodies used, sample size, and adjustment parameters in the case of multivariable analyses, the majority of these studies did not identify any significant association between COX2 expression and progression or survival, consistent with our findings [13,14,23,28,29]. Shariat and Margulis and their colleagues observed a negative association between high COX2 expression and tumor progression and mortality [21,25]. However, both studies relied on heterogeneous sample populations which included a small proportion of patients with NMIBCs; potentially accounting for the observed associations given the disparity in COX2 expression between superficial and advanced bladder tumors [45]. In another study, Wulfing et al. reported that high COX2 expression was an independent predictor of poor overall survival in a subgroup of 62 patients with MIBC treated with cisplatin-based chemotherapy [29]. We did not identify any meaningful interaction between COX2 expression and treatment (data not shown), and were unable to replicate their findings in a smaller subset of 39 patients treated with cisplatin (HR = 1.47, 95%CI = 0.48–4.51, p-value = 0.497). Aziz et al. reported a 36% survival advantage associated with increased COX2 levels in a cohort of 266 patients with MIBCs (221 with UCB) that was independent of lymph node status and neo/adjuvant chemotherapy [12]. While we also observed improved survival among patients with COX2 overexpressing MIBCs, this association did not reach significance, consistent with other univariable [23,28] and multivariable [26] analyses.

Our study had a large sample size, included only incident cases and relied on extensive and accurately acquired follow-up information spanning ten years. Additionally, we used automated scoring of immunostained TMAs, a strategy providing a reproducible assessment of expression that correlated highly with the independent evaluation of a subset of samples by an independent pathologist. COX2 staining was done in one laboratory to avoid heterogeneity in immunohistochemical staining and scoring, and evaluated as a continuous variable in the prognostic analyses to avoid potential bias related to selection of an expression threshold. Moreover, the sample population provides an accurate representation of bladder cancer in the general population as no inclusion criteria were applied in the recruitment process which included a good mix of referral centers and county hospitals. Lastly, the recommendations of the REMARK and PRISMA studies were followed in all of the reported analyses.

Despite these considerations and attempts to accurately quantify COX2 expression only in epithelial cells, the pathologist-trained automated imaging system may have incorporated some immunostained stromal material found on the tissue core, thereby increasing type I error. To reduce potential error we averaged the expression scores from duplicate cores and also explored a method investigated by Henriksen et al. [48] in which the higher score was used (data not shown). Both methods produced similar material associations between COX2 expression and clinico-pathological parameters or HRs. Moreover, adjusted analyses for progression

COX-2 and bladder cancer prognosis
Univariate analysis

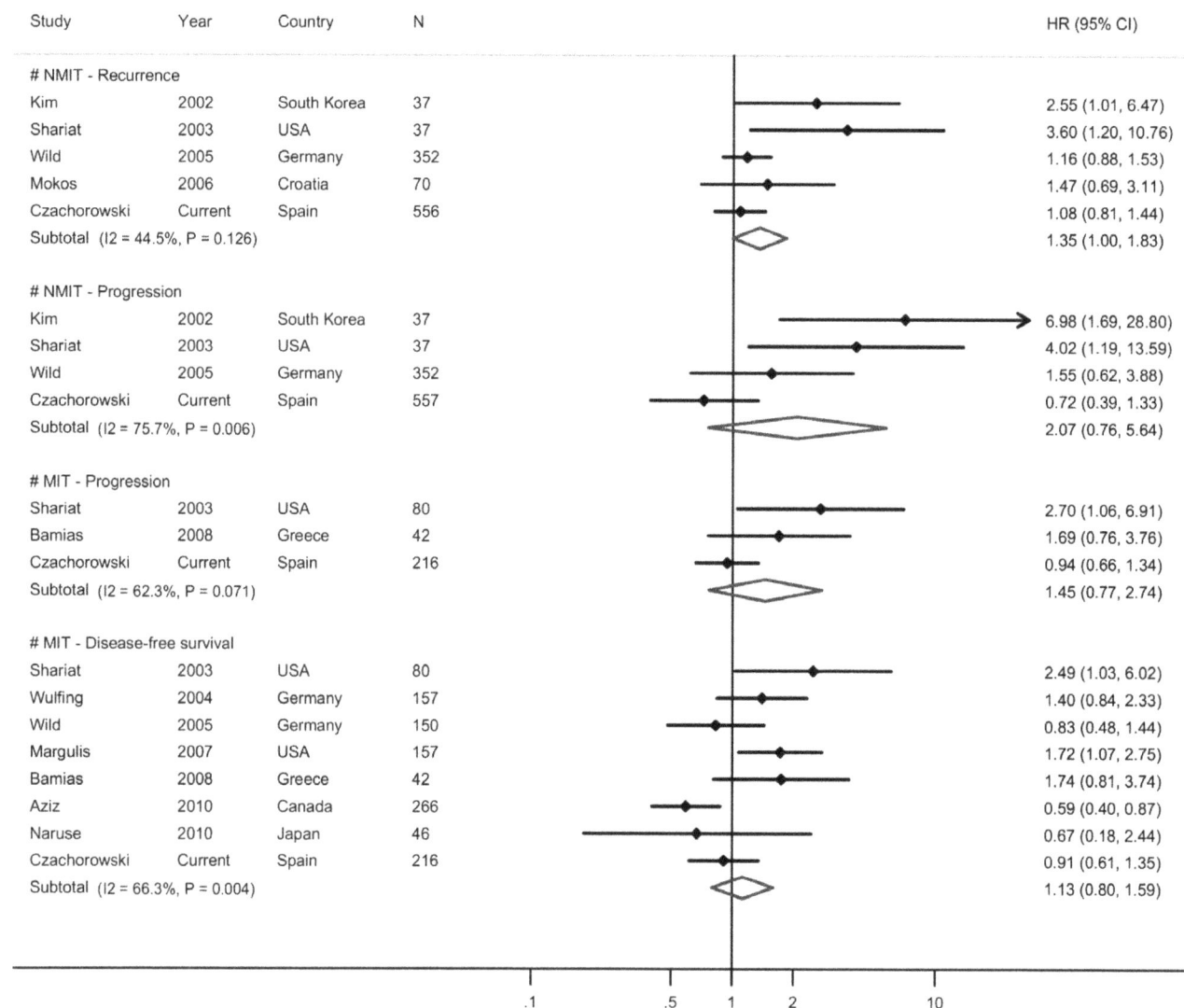

Figure 2. Forest plots from selected univariable studies indicating the risk of reaching the indicated prognostic endpoints in non-muscle invasive (NMIBC; two upper panels), and muscle invasive (MIBC; two lower panels) UCBs in the presence of urothelial COX2 expression.

in NMIBCs should be interpreted cautiously given the low number of events in relation to covariates. Also, different patient management practices across recruitment hospitals could increase sample heterogeneity, necessitating the inclusion of both recruitment area and treatment regimen in our multivariable analyses.

The results presented herein focus on COX2 expression levels measured in tumor epithelial cells – only one aspect of the complex interplay between the tumor and the host immune/inflammatory response [49]. The prognostic potential of COX2 (if any) may only be revealed when considered together with other tumoral markers. When investigating several potential prognostic parameters in UCB, Hilmy et al. concluded that systemic factors of the inflammatory response such as levels of C-reactive protein were superior to tumor-based factors such as grade, COX2 expression

or T-lymphocytic infiltration [18]. Moreover, in models of cervical cancer, Ferrandina et al. observed that while COX2 expression was mutually exclusive in the tumor and stromal inflammatory cells, high expression in both cell types could be used as an independent marker of poor survival [50]. Future studies investigating the prognostic value of COX2 expression in UCB should take into consideration the multi-factorial and multi-dimensional context of the inflammatory response during carcinogenesis.

The current study is the largest to investigate COX2 expression as an independent marker of outcome in a prospective cohort of UCB patients. These findings, supported by a meta-analysis that included our own data and that from other relevant studies, do not

COX-2 and bladder cancer prognosis
Multivariate analysis

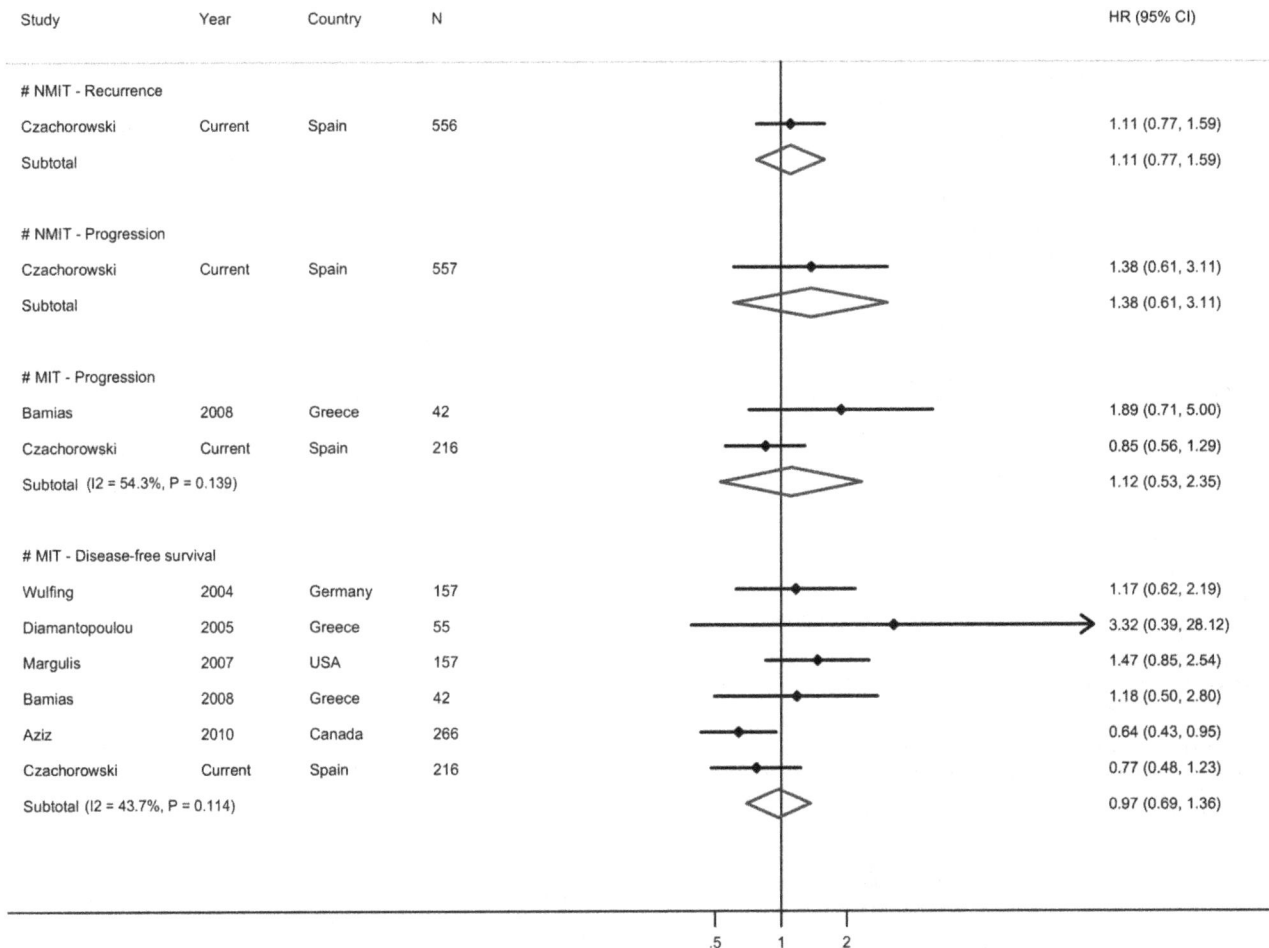

Study	Year	Country	N		HR (95% CI)
# NMIT - Recurrence					
Czachorowski	Current	Spain	556		1.11 (0.77, 1.59)
Subtotal					1.11 (0.77, 1.59)
# NMIT - Progression					
Czachorowski	Current	Spain	557		1.38 (0.61, 3.11)
Subtotal					1.38 (0.61, 3.11)
# MIT - Progression					
Bamias	2008	Greece	42		1.89 (0.71, 5.00)
Czachorowski	Current	Spain	216		0.85 (0.56, 1.29)
Subtotal (I2 = 54.3%, P = 0.139)					1.12 (0.53, 2.35)
# MIT - Disease-free survival					
Wulfing	2004	Germany	157		1.17 (0.62, 2.19)
Diamantopoulou	2005	Greece	55		3.32 (0.39, 28.12)
Margulis	2007	USA	157		1.47 (0.85, 2.54)
Bamias	2008	Greece	42		1.18 (0.50, 2.80)
Aziz	2010	Canada	266		0.64 (0.43, 0.95)
Czachorowski	Current	Spain	216		0.77 (0.48, 1.23)
Subtotal (I2 = 43.7%, P = 0.114)					0.97 (0.69, 1.36)

.5   1   2

Figure 3. Forest plots from selected multivariable studies indicating the risk of reaching the indicated prognostic endpoints in non-muscle invasive (NMIBC; two upper panels), and muscle invasive (MIBC; two lower panels) UCBs in the presence of urothelial COX2 expression.

support COX2 tumor cell expression being an independent prognosticator of UCB.

Supporting Information

Figure S1 Immunohistochemical staining of COX2 in primary UCBs on TMAs. Expression was scored as a product of the percentage of epithelial area stained and the staining intensity using automated imaging analysis. A score of <0.340 au was considered negative for COX2 expression, while a score of ≥0.340 was considered positive. Representative sections of a pTaG1 UCB lacking COX2 expression (**A and D**) and a pT2G3 UCB expressing COX2 (**B and E**) are shown. Normal colon tissue was used as a positive control (**C and F**). Upper panels show sections under 100x magnification (**A-C**); lower panels show sections under 200x magnification (**D–F**).

Figure S2 Distribution of positive COX2 expression in urothelial carcionomas of the bladder classified by their molecular and pathological stage-grade subtypes. Positive COX2 expression assessed as described in Figure S1. Statistical significance assessed using Fisher's exact test with a 0.05 significance level. pT1G2 tumors excluded due to low sample size in the current study (n = 11), and a reported tendency to overlap both molecular subtypes.

Figure S3 Kaplan-Meier survival curves corresponding to failures in superficial (A, B, C, D) and invasive (E, F, G, H) tumors for specified prognostic endpoints and quantiles of COX2 expression. Dashed curves: patients with tumors expressing COX2 at lower specified quantiles; solid curves: patients with tumors expressing COX2 at upper specified quantiles. Significance values from two-sided logrank test.

Figure S4 Flow diagram of study selection and inclusion in meta-analysis.

Table S1 Main characteristics of eligible studies used in meta-analysis.

Acknowledgments

The authors acknowledge the corresponding authors of the studies indicated in Table S1 for providing additional data used in the meta-analysis; members of MJC's thesis committee for scientific and methodological comments to the work; the Histology and Immunohistochemistry Core Unit at the CNIO for help with immunohistochemical staining of TMAs; and the patients, technicians, field workers and coordinators who made the study possible.

Spanish Bladder Cancer/EPICURO Study investigators
Institut Municipal d'Investigació Mèdica, Universitat Pompeu Fabra, Barcelona – Coordinating Center (M. Kogevinas, N. Malats, F.X. Real, M. Sala, G. Castaño, M. Torà, D. Puente, C. Villanueva, C. Murta-Nascimento, J. Fortuny, E. López, S. Hernández, R. Jaramillo, G. Vellalta, L. Palencia, F. Fernández, A. Amorós, A. Alfaro, G. Carretero); Hospital del Mar, Universitat Autònoma de Barcelona, Barcelona (J. Lloreta, S. Serrano, L. Ferrer, A. Gelabert, J. Carles, O. Bielsa, K. Villadiego); Hospital Germans Trias i Pujol, Badalona, Barcelona (L. Cecchini, J.M. Saladié, L. Ibarz); Hospital de Sant Boi, Sant Boi de Llobregat, Barcelona (M. Céspedes); Consorci Hospitalari Parc Taulí, Sabadell (C. Serra, D. García, J. Pujadas, R. Hernando, A. Cabezuelo, C. Abad, A. Prera, J.

Prat); Centre Hospitalari i Cardiològic, Manresa, Barcelona (M. Domènech, J. Badal, J. Malet); Hospital Universitario de Canarias, La Laguna, Tenerife (R. García-Closas, J. Rodríguez de Vera, A.I. Martín); Hospital Universitario Nuestra Señora de la Candelaria, Tenerife (J. Taño, F. Cáceres); Hospital General Universitario de Elche, Universidad Miguel Hernández, Elche, Alicante (A. Carrato, F. García-López, M. Ull, A. Teruel, E. Andrada, A. Bustos, A. Castillejo, J.L. Soto); Universidad de Oviedo, Oviedo, Asturias (A. Tardón); Hospital San Agustín, Avilés, Asturias (J.L. Guate, J.M. Lanzas, J. Velasco); Hospital Central Covadonga, Oviedo, Asturias (J.M. Fernández, J.J. Rodríguez, A. Herrero), Hospital Central General, Oviedo, Asturias (R. Abascal, C. Manzano, T. Miralles); Hospital de Cabueñes, Gijón, Asturias (M. Rivas, M. Arguelles); Hospital de Jove, Gijón, Asturias (M. Díaz, J. Sánchez, O. González); Hospital de Cruz Roja, Gijón, Asturias (A. Mateos, V. Frade); Hospital Alvarez-Buylla (Mieres, Asturias): P. Muntañola, C. Pravia; Hospital Jarrio, Coaña, Asturias (A.M. Huescar, F. Huergo); Hospital Carmen y Severo Ochoa, Cangas, Asturias (J. Mosquera).

Author Contributions

Conceived and designed the experiments: NM FXR MK JL AC AT. Performed the experiments: MJC NM FXR MK JL AC AT SMM MMM. Analyzed the data: MJC AFSA. Contributed reagents/materials/analysis tools: NM FXR MK AC AT. Wrote the paper: MJC AFSA NM. Revised the manuscript: SMM MMM.

References

1. Jemal A, Bray F, Center MM, Ferlay J, Ward E, et al. (2011) Global cancer statistics. CA Cancer J Clin 61: 69–90.
2. Wu XR (2005) Urothelial tumorigenesis: a tale of divergent pathways. Nat Rev Cancer 5: 713–725.
3. Botteman MF, Pashos CL, Redaelli A, Laskin B, Hauser R (2003) The health economics of bladder cancer: a comprehensive review of the published literature. Pharmacoeconomics 21: 1315–1330.
4. Lindgren D, Frigyesi A, Gudjonsson S, Sjodahl G, Hallden C, et al. (2010) Combined gene expression and genomic profiling define two intrinsic molecular subtypes of urothelial carcinoma and gene signatures for molecular grading and outcome. Cancer Res 70: 3463–3472.
5. Michaud DS (2007) Chronic inflammation and bladder cancer. Urol Oncol 25: 260–268.
6. Fortuny J, Kogevinas M, Garcia-Closas M, Real FX, Tardon A, et al. (2006) Use of analgesics and nonsteroidal anti-inflammatory drugs, genetic predisposition, and bladder cancer risk in Spain. Cancer Epidemiol Biomarkers Prev 15: 1696–1702.
7. Daugherty SE, Pfeiffer RM, Sigurdson AJ, Hayes RB, Leitzmann M, et al. (2011) Nonsteroidal antiinflammatory drugs and bladder cancer: a pooled analysis. Am J Epidemiol 173: 721–730.
8. Harris RE (2007) Cyclooxygenase-2 (cox-2) and the inflammogenesis of cancer. Subcell Biochem 42: 93–126.
9. Greenhough A, Smartt HJ, Moore AE, Roberts HR, Williams AC, et al. (2009) The COX-2/PGE2 pathway: key roles in the hallmarks of cancer and adaptation to the tumour microenvironment. Carcinogenesis 30: 377–386.
10. Wheeler MA, Hausladen DA, Yoon JH, Weiss RM (2002) Prostaglandin E2 production and cyclooxygenase-2 induction in human urinary tract infections and bladder cancer. J Urol 168: 1568–1573.
11. Shirahama T (2000) Cyclooxygenase-2 expression is up-regulated in transitional cell carcinoma and its preneoplastic lesions in the human urinary bladder. Clin Cancer Res 6: 2424–2430.
12. Aziz A, Lessard A, Moore K, Hovington H, Latulippe E, et al. (2010) Improved cancer specific-survival in patients with carcinoma invading bladder muscle expressing cyclo-oxygenase-2. BJU Int 108: 531–537.
13. Bamias A, Kyriakou F, Chorti M, Kavantzas N, Noni A, et al. (2008) Microvessel density (MVD) and cyclooxygenase-2 (COX-2)/beta-catenin interaction are associated with relapse in patients with transitional carcinoma receiving adjuvant chemotherapy with paclitaxel/carboplatin: a hellenic cooperative oncology group (HECOG) study. Anticancer Res 28: 2479–2486.
14. Diamantopoulou K, Lazaris A, Mylona E, Zervas A, Stravodimos K, et al. (2005) Cyclooxygenase-2 protein expression in relation to apoptotic potential and its prognostic significance in bladder urothelial carcinoma. Anticancer Res 25: 4543–4549.
15. Eltze E, Wulfing C, Von Struensee D, Piechota H, Buerger H, et al. (2005) Cox-2 and Her2/neu co-expression in invasive bladder cancer. Int J Oncol 26: 1525–1531.
16. Friedrich MG, Toma MI, Petri S, Huland H (2003) Cyclooxygenase-2 promotes angiogenesis in pTa/T1 urothelial bladder carcinoma but does not predict recurrence. BJU Int 92: 389–392.

17. Gudjonsson S, Bendahl PO, Chebil G, Hoglund M, Lindgren D, et al. (2011) Can tissue microarray-based analysis of protein expression predict recurrence of stage Ta bladder cancer? Scand J Urol Nephrol 45: 270–277.
18. Hilmy M, Campbell R, Bartlett JM, McNicol AM, Underwood MA, et al. (2006) The relationship between the systemic inflammatory response, tumour proliferative activity, T-lymphocytic infiltration and COX-2 expression and survival in patients with transitional cell carcinoma of the urinary bladder. Br J Cancer 95: 1234–1238.
19. Kim SI, Kwon SM, Kim YS, Hong SJ (2002) Association of cyclooxygenase-2 expression with prognosis of stage T1 grade 3 bladder cancer. Urology 60: 816–821.
20. Liedberg F, Anderson H, Chebil G, Gudjonsson S, Hoglund M, et al. (2008) Tissue microarray based analysis of prognostic markers in invasive bladder cancer: much effort to no avail? Urol Oncol 26: 17–24.
21. Margulis V, Shariat SF, Ashfaq R, Thompson M, Sagalowsky AI, et al. (2007) Expression of cyclooxygenase-2 in normal urothelium, and superficial and advanced transitional cell carcinoma of bladder. J Urol 177: 1163–1168.
22. Mokos I, Jakic-Razumovic J, Marekovic Z, Pasini J (2006) Association of cyclooxygenase-2 immunoreactivity with tumor recurrence and disease progression in superficial urothelial bladder cancer. Tumori 92: 124–129.
23. Naruse K, Yamada Y, Nakamura K, Aoki S, Taki T, et al. (2010) Potential of molecular targeted therapy of HER-2 and Cox-2 for invasive transitional cell carcinoma of the urinary bladder. Oncol Rep 23: 1577–1583.
24. Shariat SF, Kim JH, Ayala GE, Kho K, Wheeler TM, et al. (2003) Cyclooxygenase-2 is highly expressed in carcinoma in situ and T1 transitional cell carcinoma of the bladder. J Urol 169: 938–942.
25. Shariat SF, Matsumoto K, Kim J, Ayala GE, Zhou JH, et al. (2003) Correlation of cyclooxygenase-2 expression with molecular markers, pathological features and clinical outcome of transitional cell carcinoma of the bladder. J Urol 170: 985–989.
26. Shirahama T, Arima J, Akiba S, Sakakura C (2001) Relation between cyclooxygenase-2 expression and tumor invasiveness and patient survival in transitional cell carcinoma of the urinary bladder. Cancer 92: 188–193.
27. Tiguert R, Lessard A, So A, Fradet Y (2002) Prognostic markers in muscle invasive bladder cancer. World J Urol 20: 190–195.
28. Wild PJ, Kunz-Schughart LA, Stoehr R, Burger M, Blaszyk H, et al. (2005) High-throughput tissue microarray analysis of COX2 expression in urinary bladder cancer. Int J Oncol 27: 385–391.
29. Wulfing C, Eltze E, von Struensee D, Wulfing P, Hertle L, et al. (2004) Cyclooxygenase-2 expression in bladder cancer: correlation with poor outcome after chemotherapy. Eur Urol 45: 46–52.
30. Yoshimura R, Sano H, Mitsuhashi M, Kohno M, Chargui J, et al. (2001) Expression of cyclooxygenase-2 in patients with bladder carcinoma. J Urol 165: 1468–1472.
31. Youssef RF, Shariat SF, Kapur P, Kabbani W, Mosbah A, et al. (2011) Prognostic Value of Cyclooxygenase-2 Expression in Squamous Cell Carcinoma of the Bladder. J Urol 185: 6.
32. Garcia-Closas M, Malats N, Silverman D, Dosemeci M, Kogevinas M, et al. (2005) NAT2 slow acetylation, GSTM1 null genotype, and risk of bladder cancer: results from the Spanish Bladder Cancer Study and meta-analyses. Lancet 366: 649–659.

33. Epstein JI, Amin MB, Reuter VR, Mostofi FK (1998) The World Health Organization/International Society of Urological Pathology consensus classification of urothelial (transitional cell) neoplasms of the urinary bladder. Bladder Consensus Conference Committee. Am J Surg Pathol 22: 1435–1448.

34. Mostofi F, Davis C, Sesterhen I (1999) Histological typing of urinary bladder tumours. World Health Organization international classification of histological tumours. Berlin: Springer Verlag.

35. Eble JN, Sauter G, Epstein JI, Sesterhen I (2004) Pathology and genetics of tumours of the urinary system and male genital organs. WHO classification of tumours. Lyon, France IARC Press.

36. Wahlin BE, Aggarwal M, Montes-Moreno S, Gonzalez LF, Roncador G, et al. (2010) A unifying microenvironment model in follicular lymphoma: outcome is predicted by programmed death-1–positive, regulatory, cytotoxic, and helper T cells and macrophages. Clin Cancer Res 16: 637–650.

37. Metz CE (1978) Basic principles of ROC analysis. Semin Nucl Med 8: 283–298.

38. Tierney JF, Stewart LA, Ghersi D, Burdett S, Sydes MR (2007) Practical methods for incorporating summary time-to-event data into meta-analysis. Trials 8: 16.

39. Higgins JP, Thompson SG (2002) Quantifying heterogeneity in a meta-analysis. Stat Med 21: 1539–1558.

40. Egger M, Davey Smith G, Schneider M, Minder C (1997) Bias in meta-analysis detected by a simple, graphical test. BMJ 315: 629–634.

41. Hernandez S, Lopez-Knowles E, Lloreta J, Kogevinas M, Amoros A, et al. (2006) Prospective study of FGFR3 mutations as a prognostic factor in nonmuscle invasive urothelial bladder carcinomas. J Clin Oncol 24: 3664–3671.

42. Lopez-Knowles E, Hernandez S, Kogevinas M, Lloreta J, Amoros A, et al. (2006) The p53 pathway and outcome among patients with T1G3 bladder tumors. Clin Cancer Res 12: 6029–6036.

43. McShane LM, Altman DG, Sauerbrei W, Taube SE, Gion M, et al. (2005) REporting recommendations for tumour MARKer prognostic studies (REMARK). Br J Cancer 93: 387–391.

44. Moher D, Liberati A, Tetzlaff J, Altman DG, The PG (2009) Preferred reporting items for systematic reviews and meta-analyses: the PRISMA Statement. Open Med 3: e123–e130.

45. Ristimaki A, Nieminen O, Saukkonen K, Hotakainen K, Nordling S, et al. (2001) Expression of cyclooxygenase-2 in human transitional cell carcinoma of the urinary bladder. Am J Pathol 158: 849–853.

46. Mohammed SI, Knapp DW, Bostwick DG, Foster RS, Khan KN, et al. (1999) Expression of cyclooxygenase-2 (COX-2) in human invasive transitional cell carcinoma (TCC) of the urinary bladder. Cancer Res 59: 5647–5650.

47. Komhoff M, Guan Y, Shappell HW, Davis L, Jack G, et al. (2000) Enhanced expression of cyclooxygenase-2 in high grade human transitional cell bladder carcinomas. Am J Pathol 157: 29–35.

48. Henriksen KL, Rasmussen BB, Lykkesfeldt AE, Moller S, Ejlertsen B, et al. (2007) Semi-quantitative scoring of potentially predictive markers for endocrine treatment of breast cancer: a comparison between whole sections and tissue microarrays. J Clin Pathol 60: 397–404.

49. Mantovani A, Allavena P, Sica A, Balkwill F (2008) Cancer-related inflammation. Nature 454: 436–444.

50. Ferrandina G, Lauriola L, Zannoni GF, Distefano MG, Legge F, et al. (2002) Expression of cyclooxygenase-2 (COX-2) in tumour and stroma compartments in cervical cancer: clinical implications. Br J Cancer 87: 1145–1152.

9

A Novel Mechanism of PPAR Gamma Induction via EGFR Signalling Constitutes Rational for Combination Therapy in Bladder Cancer

Jose Joao Mansure, Roland Nassim, Simone Chevalier, Konrad Szymanski, Joice Rocha, Saad Aldousari, Wassim Kassouf*

McGill Urologic Oncology Research, Division of Urology, McGill University Health Center, Montreal, Quebec, Canada

Abstract

Background: Two signalling molecules that are attractive for targeted therapy are the epidermal growth factor receptor (EGFR) and the peroxisome proliferator-activated receptor gamma (PPARγ). We investigated possible crosstalk between these 2 pathways, particularly in light of the recent evidence implicating PPARγ for anticancer therapy.

Principal Findings: As evaluated by MTT assays, gefitinib (EGFR inhibitor) and DIM-C (PPARγ agonist) inhibited growth of 9 bladder cancer cell lines in a dose-dependent manner but with variable sensitivity. In addition, combination of gefitinib and DIM-C demonstrated maximal inhibition of cell proliferation compared to each drug alone. These findings were confirmed *in vivo*, where combination therapy maximally inhibited tumor growth in contrast to each treatment alone when compared to control (p<0.04). Induction of PPARγ expression along with nuclear accumulation was observed in response to increasing concentrations of gefitinib via activation of the transcription factor CCAT/enhancer-binding protein-β (CEBP-β). In these cell lines, DIM-C significantly sensitized bladder cancer cell lines that were resistant to EGFR inhibition in a schedule-specific manner.

Conclusion: These results suggest that PPARγ agonist DIM-C can be an excellent alternative to bladder tumors resistant to EGFR inhibition and combination efficacy might be achieved in a schedule-specific manner.

Editor: Aamir Ahmad, Wayne State University School of Medicine, United States of America

Funding: This study was supported by the Cancer Research Society. (http://www.src-crs.ca/en-CA) W. Kassouf is a recipient of a clinical research scholar award from the FRSQ. (http://www.frsq.gouv.qc.ca/en/index.shtml). The funders had no role in study design, data collection and analysis, decision to publish, or preparation of the manuscript.

Competing Interests: The authors have declared that no competing interests exist.

* E-mail: wassim.kassouf@muhc.mcgill.ca

Introduction

Almost all patients with metastatic bladder cancer succumb to disease, with median survival of 18 months even with the best available chemotherapeutic regimens. As understanding of biology of urothelial carcinoma (UC) improves, novel approaches need to be studied. Two signalling molecules that are attractive for targeted therapy are the epidermal growth factor receptor (EGFR) and the peroxisome proliferator-activated receptor γ (PPARγ). Inhibition of EGFR function is extremely attractive among the wide array of biological targets implicated in urothelial carcinoma (UC) progression. Although mechanism by which EGFR regulates tumor biology in bladder cancer is not clearly defined, it has been demonstrated that EGFR signalling regulates cell survival, proliferation, differentiation, and invasion [1]. Moreover, EGFR is implicated in tumor-induced angiogenesis and metastasis [2]. However, clinical trials with EGFR inhibitors in head and neck, lung, and colon cancer demonstrated that only a minority of patients seemed to benefit from this approach. In context of Non Small Cancer Lung Cells (NSCLC), it was shown that clinical responses were linked to activating mutations within EGFR

tyrosine kinase domain, suggesting that better understanding of biological effects of EGFR inhibitors on cancer will help identify tumors that will respond to therapy [3,4]. Although none of 17 human UC cell lines nor any of 75 primary tumors evaluated at M. D. Anderson Cancer Center contained activating EGFR kinase domain mutations [5], EGFR inhibitors blocked cell cycle progression in 6/17 UC cell lines. We have shown that high EGFR expression is associated with an aggressive phenotype [6] and that modulation of GSK-3β might be a predictor of response to EGFR inhibitors in bladder cancer [7]. We do believe that EGFR remains a strong signalling axis in progression of bladder cancer where its inhibition may benefit selected patients.

Another receptor of interest is PPARγ, a ligand-activated receptor and a member of the nuclear receptor superfamily of transcription factors [8,9]. Importantly, PPARγ plays an important role in carcinogenesis. PPARγ is highly expressed in tumor samples from different sites, including bladder cancer (reviewed in reference [10]). PPARγ is an interesting target for cancer therapy not only because of its elevated expression in tumors, but also because PPARγ activation results in decreased cell proliferation, decreased G_0/G_1 to S phase progression, increased terminal differentiation, and apoptosis [11,12,13]. Further, PPARγ agonists are potent angiogenesis inhibitors *in vitro* and *in vivo*, in part due to downregulation of VEGF [14,15]. Recently, a new class of PPARγ agonists, 1,1-bis(3′-indolyl)-1-(*p*-substitutedphenyl)methanes (PPARγ-active DIM-Cs), has been developed and shown to be significantly more potent than the previous generation of drugs. We published the first report on significant antitumorigenic activity of PPARγ-active DIM-Cs in UC cells *in vitro* and *in vivo* [16]. Use of potent PPARγ-active DIM-Cs was attractive and warrants further evaluation in treatment of UC.

A prior study has shown that PPARγ agonists increase gefitinib's antitumor activity, possibly mediated through induction of PTEN expression *in vitro* [17]. Additionally, curcumin was shown to induce PPARγ expression and inhibit proliferation in hepatic stellate cells [18]. Others have shown that curcumin can also inhibit EGFR activation and these findings further corroborate the potential crosstalk between the two signaling axes of interest.

The aim of this study is to investigate crosstalk between these two signalling axes as they share some common downstream signalling effectors and evaluate whether combination of PPARγ agonist and an EGFR inhibitor may overcome resistance to EGFR therapy in bladder cancer.

Materials and Methods

Cell Culture

The UC cell line 253J B-V was generated from the 253J human UC cell line as previously described [19] and was kindly provided by Dr Colin P.N. Dinney from M.D. Anderson Cancer Center, Houston, Texas. The UM-UC series of urothelial carcinoma cell lines used in this study were genotypically characterised and provided by the Specimen Core of the Genitourinary Specialized Programs of Research Excellence in bladder cancer at M. D. Anderson Cancer Center [20].

Drugs

Gefitinib (Iressa ZD1839) was supplied by AstraZeneca, London, United Kingdom) and the orally available PPARγ-active DIM-C was generously provided by Dr. S. Safe, Houston, TX as dry powder.

Cell Proliferation Assay

Bladder cancer cells were treated with different concentrations of gefitinib (0.001 μM to 100 μM) and DIM-C (0.01 μM to 10 μM) in EMEM's supplemented with 10% FBS for 48 hs Cell proliferation was evaluated using MTT assays (Sigma-Aldrich, Canada). The GI50 value was defined as the mean concentration of drug that generated 50% of growth inhibition.

Western Blot Analysis

Cells were harvested at ~75% to 80% confluence in lysis buffer (RIPA) and a cocktail of phosphatase and protease inhibitors (Roche Diagnostics, Germany). Proteins were subjected to SDS-PAGE, transferred onto nitrocellulose membranes (Bio-Rad, Hercules, CA) by semidry electroblotting. Primary monoclonal antibodies [EGF Receptor (15F8), tubulin and b-actin (Cell Signaling Technology, New England, MA)] and PPARγ (sc-7273, Santa Cruz Biotechnology, California, US) were applied to detect bands of interest. Additionally, the following rabbit antibodies from cell signaling were used : Akt; phospho-Akt (Ser473); GSK-3β; phospho-GSK-3β (Ser9); p21 Waf1/Cip1; p44–42 MAPK (Erk1/2); phosphor-p44/42 MAPK (Erk1/2). Anti-rabbit and anti-mouse immunoglobulins (IgGs) coupled to

HRP/horseradish were used as secondary antibodies according to the primary antibody.

Immunofluorescence

Cells cultured in eight-well plastic chambers were washed on ice with cold PBS containing protease inhibitors (Roche Diagnostics, Germany) and fixed with 3.7% paraformaldehyde. Cells were incubated with different concentrations of gefitinib (0, 2, 4 and 8 μM) for 24 hs and then incubated with mouse monoclonal PPARγ primary antibody (1:50) overnight. Immunofluorescence was revealed using anti-mouse antibodies coupled to FITC (Alexa Fluor 488) or rhodamine (CY3; Invitrogen). 4,6-Diamidino-2-phenylindole (DAPI) was used to stain the nuclei. Photomicrographs were taken with an inverted Olympus IX-81 microscope equipped with a CoolSnap HQ digital camera and the ImagePro+ software (version 5.0.1; Media Cybernetics).

RNA Isolation and Real Time PCR

Total RNA was extracted from cells using Trizol reagent (Invitrogen, Carlsbad, CA), according to the protocol provided by the manufacturer. The synthesis of cDNA was performed using the Quantitec Reverse Transcription Kit (Qiagen, Mississauga, ON). For RT-PCR amplification, validated primers from Qiagen (Hs_CEBPB_2_SG QuantiTect Primer Assay QT00998494) were used. No genomic DNA contamination or pseudogenes were detected by PCR without the reverse transcription step in the total RNA used. β actin was used as an internal control. The reactions started at 95°C for 10 min, followed by 40 cycles of 95°C for 10 s, 60°C for 20 s. Melting peaks of PCR products were determined by heat-denaturation over a 35°C temperature gradient at 0.2°C/s from 60 to 95°C. The cycle numbers crossing an arbitrary threshold (Ct) were determined using MyIQ system software, version 1.0.410 (BioRad, CA, U.S.A.). Fold change in target mRNA relative to β actin was calculated as follow: Fold change $= 2^{-\Delta\Delta Ct}$ where $\Delta\Delta Ct = (Ct_{target} - Ct\ \beta\ actin)_{time\ X} - (Ct_{target} - Ct\ \beta\ actin)_{time\ 0}$ Time X is time point after 3 hs gefitinib. Time 0 represents the experiment starting time (no drug added).

Bladder Tumor Xenografts

Female nude mice (purchased from Charles Rivers, Wilmington, MA) were injected subcutaneously with the KU-7 cells (10^6 cells per injection). Animals of each series (10 mice per group) were randomised and assigned to treatment and a placebo arms. DIM-C was given 60 mg/kg 3 times per week and gefitinib was given 2 mg/day, 5 times per week. All drugs and placebo were given by oral gavage. Treatment was continued for 4 weeks and subsequently tumors were harvested and weighted. Tumors were snap-frozen in liquid nitrogen for further analysis.

This study was carried out following the Standard Operating Procedures for Care and Use of Laboratory Animals of the McGill University Animal Care Committee. The protocol was approved by the Facility Animal Care Committee of the Research McGill University Health Center (Permit Number: 5428). All surgery was performed under sodium pentobarbital anesthesia, and all efforts were made to minimize suffering.

Immunohistochemistry

Serial sections of tumor xenografts from mice treated with placebo and combination treatment (gefitinib plus DIM-C) were incubated overnight at 4°C, with primary specific antibodies against PPARγ (sc-7273 mouse monoclonal IgG₁ antibody 1:1000 dilution, Santa Cruz, CA, USA), p21 (12D1 rabbit antibody 1:100 dilution, cell signaling, MA, USA). Goat polyclonal anti-rabbit

A

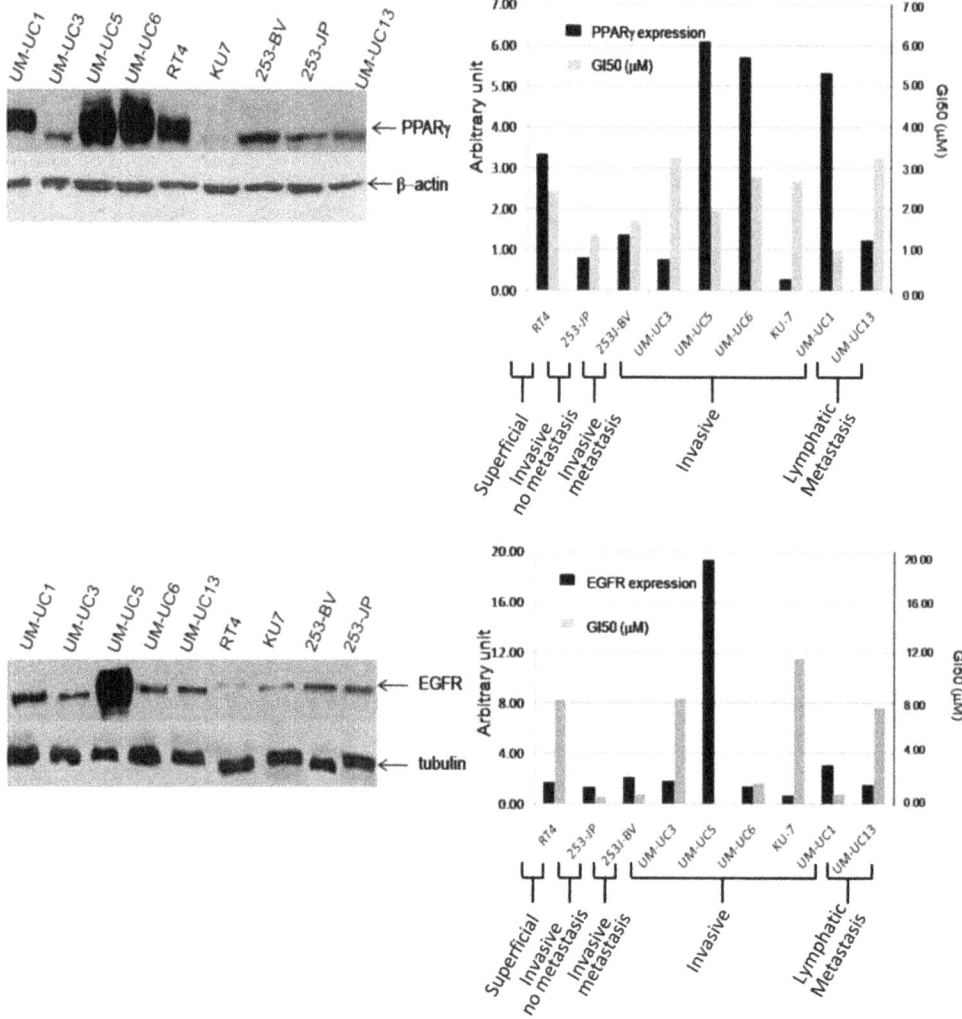

B

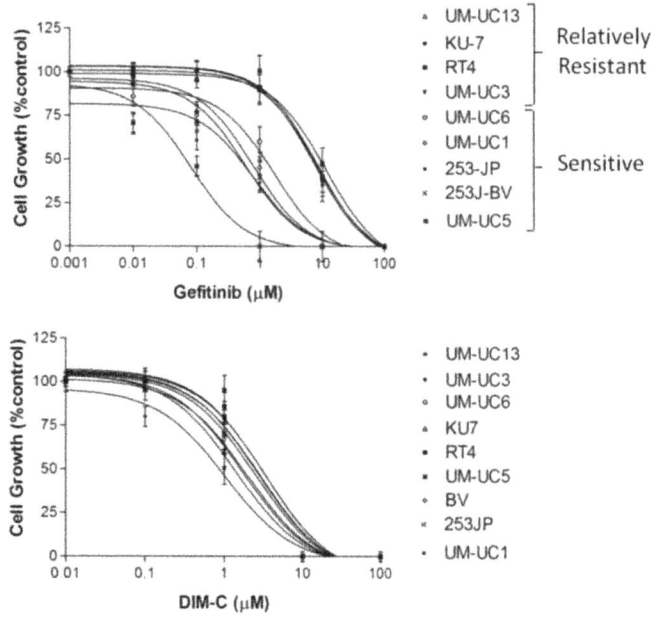

Figure 1. Baseline expression of PPARγ and EGFR. (A) Expression of PPARγ and EGFR relative to endogenous levels of β-actin and tubulin, respectively, and represented in units among 9 bladder cancer cell lines reflecting different stages of the disease (from Superficial to Invasive & no Metastasis, Invasive and Lymphatic Metastasis). (B) Dose-response of bladder cancer cell lines to PPARγ agonist (DIM-C) and EGFR inhibitor (gefitinib). The GI50 value was defined as the mean concentration of drug that generates 50% of growth inhibition as compared to controls.

IgG secondary antibody, conjugated with HRP was added and incubated for 1 h at room temperature. Color development was performed with DAB substrate (Sigma Aldrich, Canada), according to manufacturer's instructions. Immunostaining was evaluated in a semiquantitative method based on the average of five foci on percentage of viable cells showing positive expression. Specimens were scored based on the intensity of antibody nuclear and cytoplasmic staining in each slide. Values were compared using unpaired Student's t test.

Microarray Analysis

Bladder tumors xenografts, were sectored stained by hematoxilin and eosin and the tumors were mapped for further isolation. Total RNA was extracted as previously described. RNA was quantified using a NanoDrop-ND1000 spectrophotometer (Thermo Fisher Scientific, Wilmington, DE) and quality was monitored with the Agilent 2100 Bioanalyzer (Agilent Technologies, Genome Quebec Innovation Center, CA). Microarray analyses were performed at McGill University and Genome Quebec Innovation Center, using Illumina BeadArray™ technology. The HumanHT-12 Expression BeadChip™ was used and contained more than 22,000 probes from the NCBI RefSeq database, which provides higher throughput processing of 12 samples per chip. There is a coverage of >99.99% of all bead types on any given HumanHT-12. TotalPrep RNA Amplification kit from Ambion was used to perform one round of amplification from 50–500 ng of total RNA. The cDNA synthesis and *in vitro* transcription amplification were followed by hybridization. The BeadChips were imaged using Illumina's BeadArray or iScan reader. Statistical analysis and visualization of data from microarray experiments was performed using the software package

FlexArray version 1.6 developed and provided by Genome Quebec. Functional and signalling pathway analyses were assessed using Ingenuity Pathway Analysis (IPA) software.

Statistical Analysis

All data were analyzed using the STATA version 10.0 software. Results from *in vivo* were compared using repeated measure ANOVA and Fischer's exact test. $P < 0.05$ was considered to be statistically significant.

Results

Baseline Expression of PPARγ and EGFR in a Panel of Urothelial Carcinoma Cell Lines

We have previously reported that inhibition of EGFR signalling axis and activation of PPARγ axis are both effective in significantly inhibiting proliferation of human carcinoma cells through different pathways, in part converging to PI3K/Akt, cyclin D1, and cyclin-dependent kinase inhibitors [7,16]. In our previous work, we have shown significant expression of the HER family members across various UC cell lines [7]. To further investigate for interaction between the two signalling axes, we first screened to characterize the levels of EGFR and PPARγ expression across a panel of 9 UC cell lines. As revealed in Figure 1 A, all the cell lines tested expressed various levels of EGFR and PPARγ. We did not demonstrate a correlation between baseline levels of expression and stage of disease of which the 9 cell lines were derived from (from superficial to invasive to metastatic). We have also determined the dose response of among the urothelial carcinoma cell lines (UM-UC1, UM-UC3, UM-UC5, UM-UC6, UM-UC13, RT4, 253JP, 253J-BV, KU7) to different concentrations of EGFR

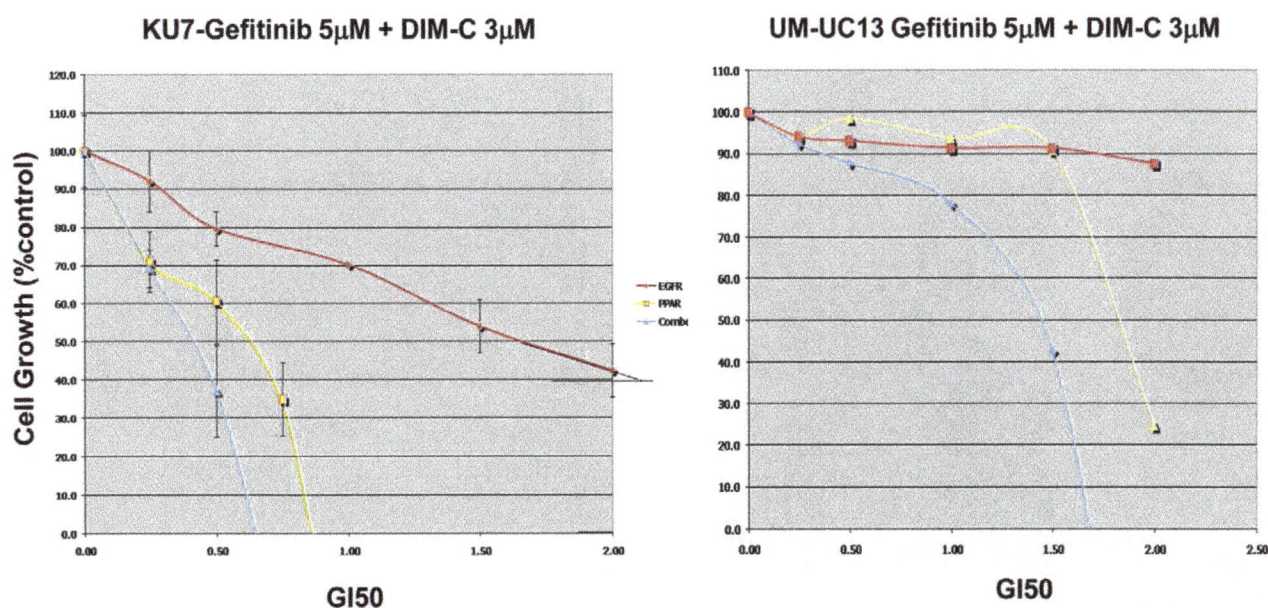

Figure 2. Antiproliferative effects of combined therapy. Growth was monitored by MTT assays. Cells were treated with gefitinib 5 μM and DIM-C 3 μM and compared to each drug alone. Red: gefitinib; Yellow: DIM-C; Blue: gefitinib+DIM-C.

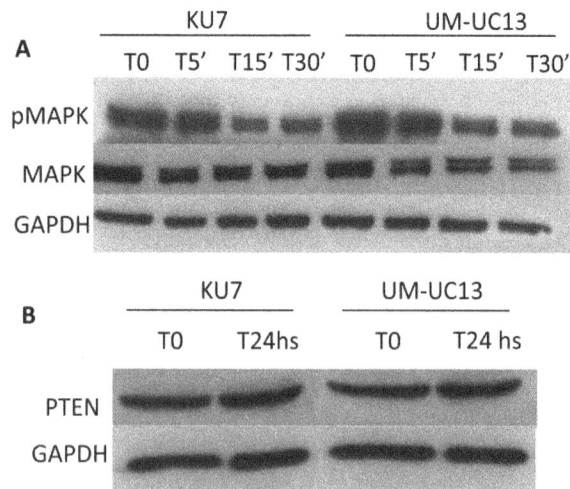

Figure 3. Effect of combination therapy on EGFR downstream signaling. (A) Phosphorylation pattern of p42/44 MAPK (Erk1/2) in cells treated with gefitinib 5 µM and DIM-C 3 µM for 5, 15 and 30 minutes. T0 is the untreated control. Whole-cell lysates were immunoblotted with phosho-p42/44 MAPK and p42/44 MAP. GAPDH was used as loading control on the Western blotting. (B) Comparison of PTEN expression in cell lines treated with gefitinib 5 µM and DIM-C 3 µM for 24 hs. T0 is the untreated control.

sensitive cell line to gefitinib, is different from the rest of the cell lines as it contains EGFR gene amplification.

Effects of Combined EGFR Inhibitors and PPARγ Agonists Therapy

We investigated the antiproliferative effects of combined therapy, gefitinib and DIM-C, compared to each drug alone on bladder cancer cell growth *in vitro*. Growth and cell proliferation were monitored by MTT assays and conducted on two relatively EGFR-resistant cell lines (KU7 and UM-UC13). Cells were treated for 72 hs and used a fixed-ratio of different fractions of GI50 (0.25, 0.5, 1.0 and 2.0) of each drug alone according to median effect method. Maximal inhibition of cell proliferation was demonstrated in the combined treatment compared to either drug alone (Figure 2). DIM-C rendered the resistant cells sensitive to EGFR inhibition.

Effect of Combination on the EGFR Downstream Signaling and PTEN Expression

Binding of EGFR to its ligand leads to activation of various signals, including the Ras/Raf/mitogen-activated protein kinase pathway (MAPK) [21]. Therefore, we investigated the effect of combination in the phosphorylation status of p42/44 MAPK (Erk1/2). As seen in Figure 3A, a significant time course deactivation of the Erk pathway was observed, compared to control, among cells treated with gefitinib 5 µM and DIM-C 3 µM. Additionally, as previously mentioned, expression of PTEN increases in non-small cell lung cancer (NSCLC) treated with the PPARγ agonists, rosiglitazone [17]. Therefore, we also investigated the effect of combination treatment in PTEN expression. As shown in Figure 3B, no difference in PTEN expression was observed, as compared to control, when cells were treated with combined gefitinib and DIM-C for 24 hs.

inhibitor (gefitinib) and PPARγ agonist (DIM-C) after 72 hs of treatment (Figure 1 B). We were able to stratify several UC cell lines ranging from highly sensitive to relatively resistant to EGFR inhibition, while no significant changes were observed to justify a stratification in response to DIM-C. Of note, UC5, the most

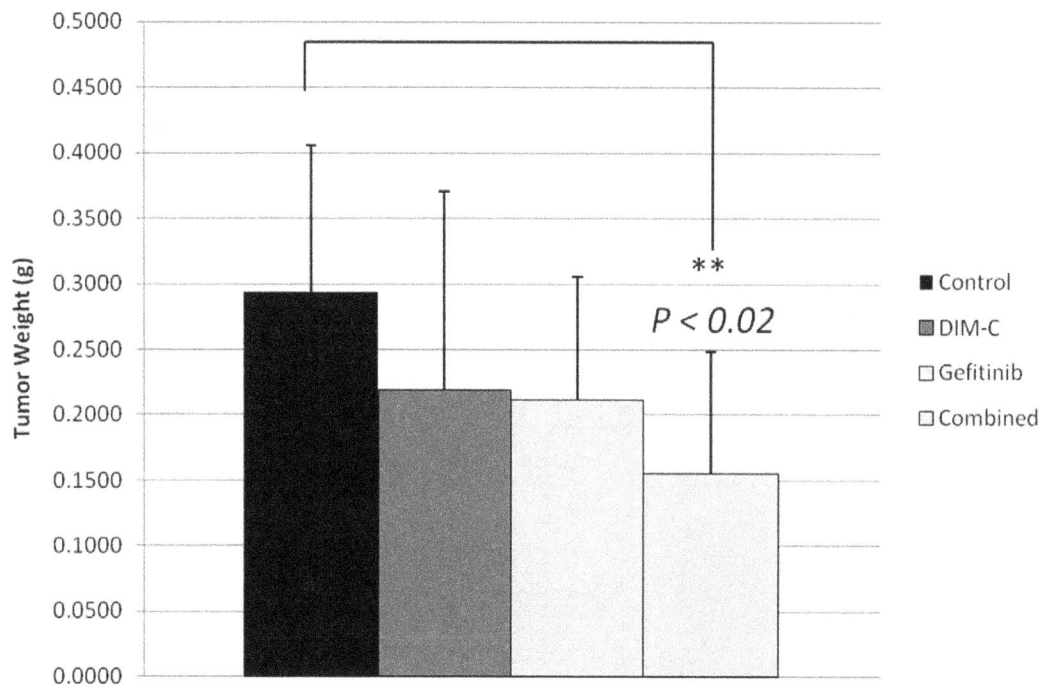

Figure 4. Effects of combination therapy *in vivo*. Bladder tumor growth of combination treatment arm compared to control arm (P<0.02). Ten mice per group were treated with placebo; DIM-C was given 60 mg/Kg 3 times per week; Gefitinib was given 2 mg/day, 5 times per week. All drugs were administrated by oral gavage. Treatment was continued for 4 weeks.

A

B

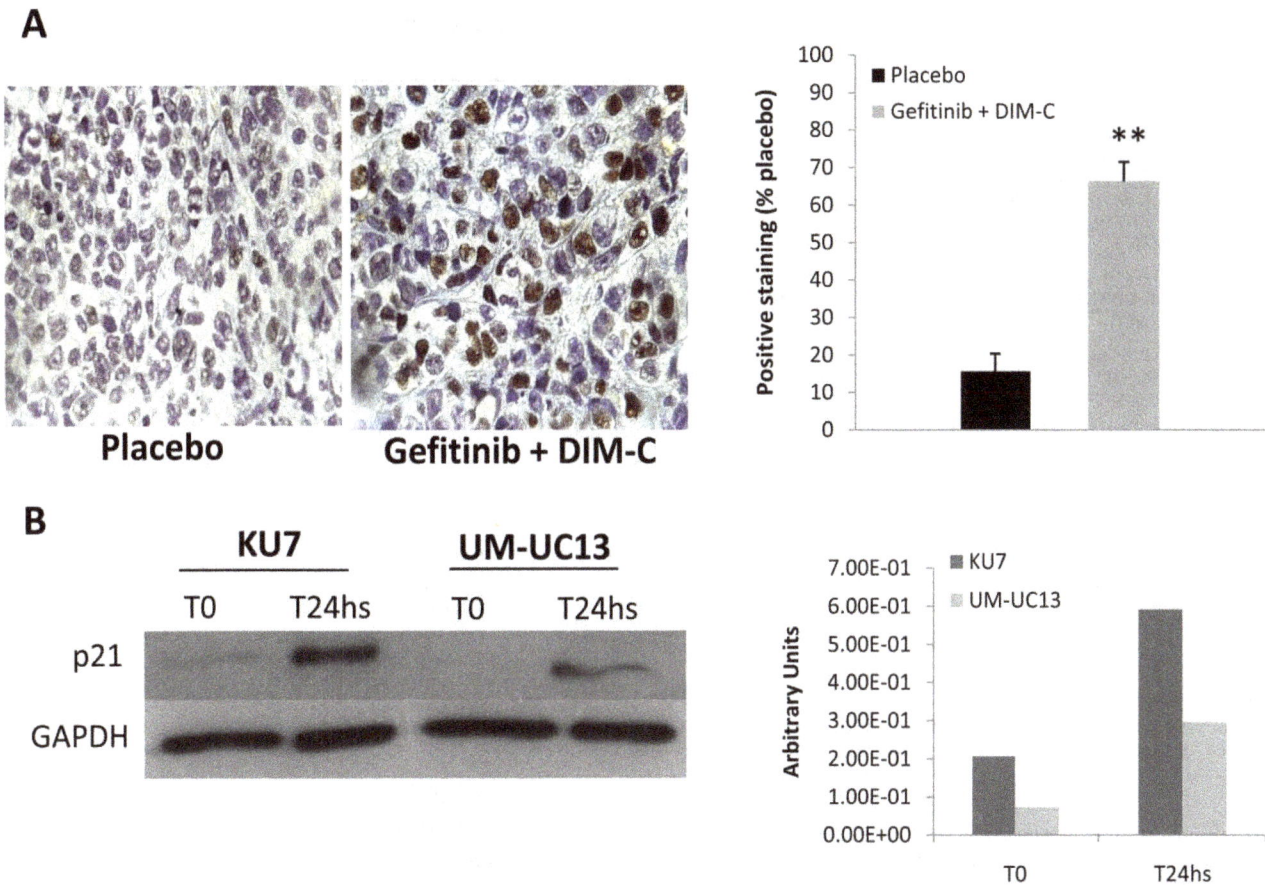

Figure 5. Effects of combination therapy on p21 expression *in vivo* **and** *in vitro*. (A) Immunohistochemistry (IHC) staining for p21 in tumor xenograft tissues. Mice were treated with placebo or combination therapy (Gefitinib 2 mg/day, 5 times per week and DIM-C 60 mg/Kg, 3 times per week). Graphic on the right side represents quantification of positive staining cells. (B) In vitro expression of p21 in Western blot of lysate cells treated with gefitinib 5 μM and DIM-C 3 μM for 24 hs. Graphic on the right side, represents quantification of p21 expression related to GAPDH.

Effects of Treatment on Bladder Tumor Growth in vivo

To evaluate whether these findings can be translated *in vivo*, nude mice were inoculated subcutaneously with relatively resistant bladder cancer cells (KU-7 cells). The mice were treated with targeted agents via oral gavage (PPARγ-active DIM-Cs given 60 mg/kg 3 times per week, gefitinib given 2 mg/day 5 times per week, or both) for 4 weeks. As shown in Figure 4, tumor weights were markedly reduced in combined group in contrast to each drug alone when compared to control (*p*<0.02). These findings suggest combined treatment has a better antitumor activity. Furthermore, gene expression profiling analysis of the bladder tumor xenografts, showed that several genes involved in cell cycle, cell death, cellular growth and proliferation were differently expressed in the combined treatment group as compared to the control group. (Table 1). Remarkably, cyclin-dependent Kinase inhibitor (CDKN1A or p21), which functions as a regulator of cell cycle progression at G1, was significantly upregulated (Fold change 2.6, *p* value <0.02) and this was validated by immuno-histochemistry showing higher percentage of p21 positive cells in the combined arm *in vivo* (66% vs 15%, p<0.001) (Figure 5A) as well as *in vitro* (Figure 5B). Interestingly, it has been reported that PPARγ plays an important role mediating the differentiation-dependent cascade expression of cyclin-dependent kinase inhibitors, thereby providing a molecular mechanism coupling growth arrest and adipocyte differentiation [22].

EGFR Inhibition Induces Gene Expression of PPARγ in a Dose-dependent Manner

We evaluated the effect of gefitinib on members of the PPARγ signalling axes. Two resistant cells (KU-7 and UM-UC13) were treated with different concentrations of EGFR inhibitor for 24 hs. PPARγ expression was determined by western blotting analyses as previously described. As shown in Figure 6A, a dramatic induction of PPARγ expression was observed in both cell lines, in a dose dependent manner, followed EGFR inhibition. Interestingly, a nuclear accumulation of PPARγ was also observed following its upregulation, which is in fact the active form of the receptor. (Figure 6B). These findings were confirmed *in vivo*, as seen in Figure 7, that shows PPARγ expression is higher among the xenograft tumors treated with gefitinib as compared to the placebo group. Of note, a nuclear staining was also observed, suggesting a nuclear translocation of PPARγ following induction of its expression.

Schedule-specific Efficacy of Combination Therapy

If cells are sensitized to EGFR inhibition via induction of PPARγ expression, then one would expect that efficacy of combination therapy may also be significantly affected and improved by sequence of administration of gefitinib and DIM-C. In fact, we observed marked effect on proliferation among three relatively resistant and one sensitive cell lines to gefitinib (KU-7,

Table 1. Analysis of molecular pathways and functions of the differentially expressed mRNAs of combined treatment compared to control group in bladder tumor xenografts.

Molecules in Network	P - Value	Top Functions
AXIN2, BACH2 **CDKN1A**, DUSP6, DYRK1B, FOXO4, HAS2, MED16, MMP9, NCOR2, P38 MAPK, PDGF BB, PLTP, SCGB1A1, STK39, SYNE1, TNFSF11, VTN, XAF1	10E-38	Cell Cycle, Tumor Morphology, Cell Morphology
ALDH3A1, AMT, APOF, BDP1, CCDC11, CDK18, **CDKN1A**, Cyclin D1/cdk4, NEURL2, NKAP, POMT1, STX17, TAPBPL, VEZT	10E-23	Cell Death, Genetic Disorder,
ARMCX3, CAMTA2, CDC42EP1, FKBP2, HNRNPM, HSPBP1, HTR1E KCNAB1, PIP4K2B, SRGAP2, TUSC3, WDR17, ZFP91	10E-23	Cell Cycle, Tumor Morphology, Cellular Assembly and Organization
DLX2, DLX3, EXOC1, FANCD2, HAS2, HAUS6, HEATR3, IL1RAPL1, MDN1, MYC, OSBPL1A, PROCKLE1, PXMP4	10E-22	Gene Expression, Cancer and Immunological Disease
ARPC3, CFB, CFP, COL12A1, DDAH2, KCNK6, KCTD7, KLHL4, PILRA, PTPRB, SLC14A1, SMPDL3B	10E-17	Cell Signaling, and Inflammatory Response
MYCN	10E-2	Cancer, Cell Cycle, Cell-To-Cell Signaling and Interaction

IPA analysis was performed in order to identify the molecular pathways and functions of the differentially expressed mRNAs of combined treatment compared to control group in bladder tumor xenografts. Most significantly enriched groups relating to molecular and cellular functions are shown. The networks were generated on the basis of the published literature and ranked by the P-value calculated by Fisher's exact Test.

UM-UC3; UM-UM13) when cells were pre-treated with gefitinib for 24 hs to allow for induction of PPARγ expression compared to when the cells were simultaneous exposure to gefitinib and DIM-C (Figure 8). These findings strongly suggest PPARγ agonist could significantly sensitize UC cell lines, particularly those that were resistant to EGFR inhibition, in a schedule-specific manner and provide an excellent potential for combination therapy.

C/EBPβ Expression After Gefitinib Induced-PPARγ Expression

Considerable evidence indicates that CCAAT/enhancer-binding protein beta (C/EBPβ) acts as a transcriptional activator for PPARγ genes [23,24]. This belief is supported by the fact that the proximal of its promoters possess C/EBP regulatory elements that are essential for transactivation of PPARγ promoter-reporter transgenes. Here we report compelling evidence that sequential induction of PPARγ expression by EGFR inhibition is mediated by C/EBPβ (Figure 9). When cells were pre-treated with gefitinib at the same concentrations used to induce expression of PPARγ, an increase in C/EBPβ was also observed suggesting gefitinib induced-PPARγ expression may be mediated by C/EBPβ.

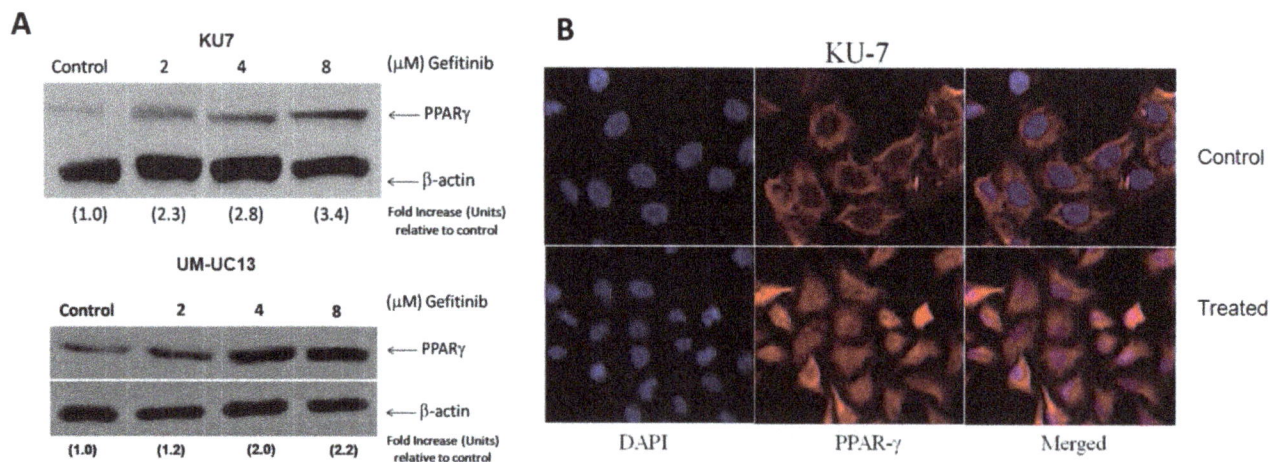

Figure 6. Induction of PPARγ expression in response to different concentrations of gefitinib. (A) Fold increase relative to control was determined after normalization with β-actin as external loading control. (B) Upregulation and nuclear accumulation of PPARγ following treatment with gefitinib (24 hs).

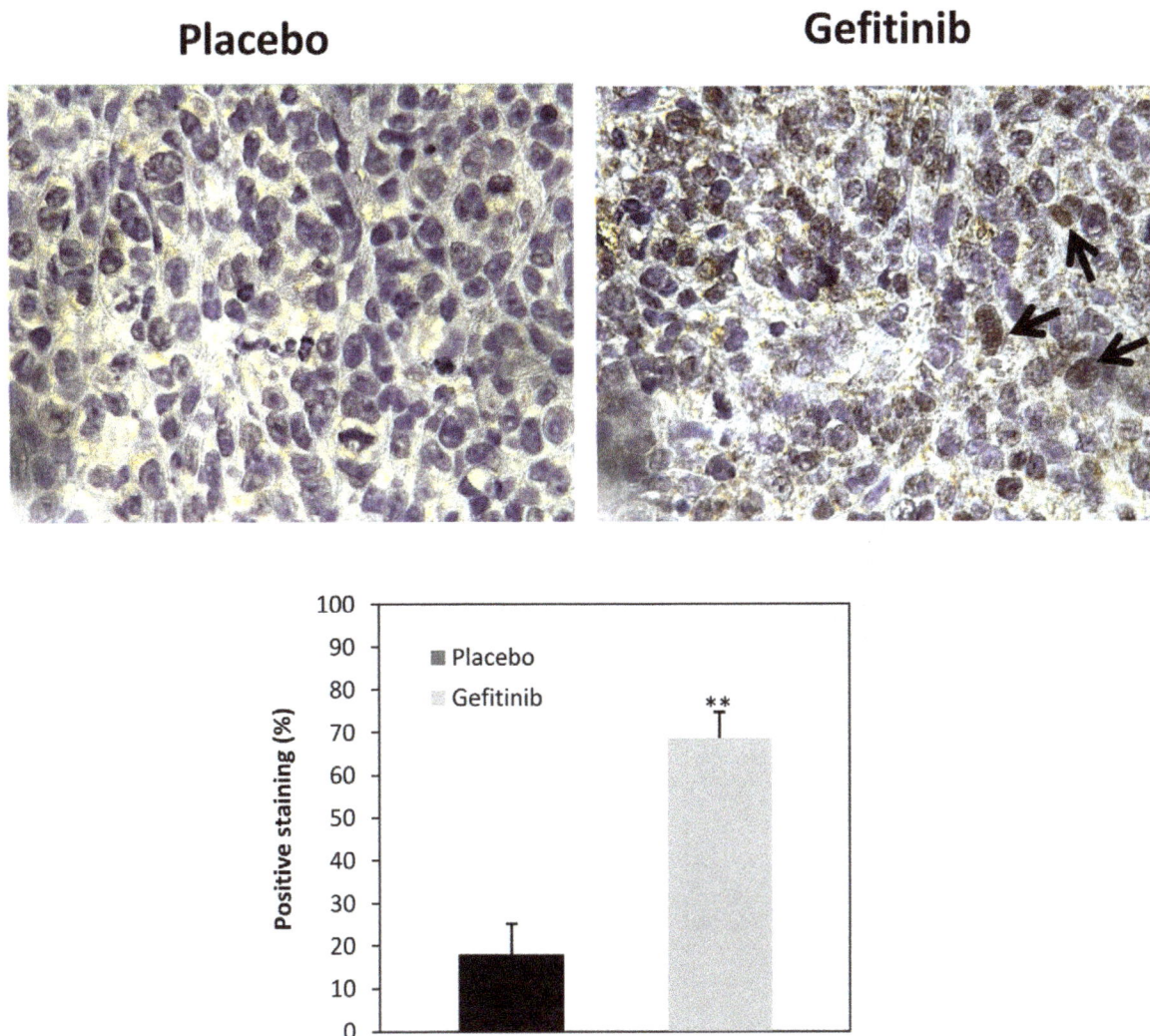

Figure 7. Immunohistochemistry (IHC) staining for PPARγ in tumor xenograft tissues Mice were treated with placebo or gefitinib (Gefitinib 2 mg/day, 5 times per week). Graphic on the lower level represents quantification of positive staining cells. Black arrows indicate nuclear staining.

Discussion

Results from a large body of preclinical studies and clinical trials suggest that targeting EGFR represents a significant contribution to cancer therapy. However, the issue of constitutive resistance in a large number of patients and the development of acquired resistance in the responders remains an unexplored subject of investigation. Cancer cell resistance to EGFR antagonists could be due to several reasons, such as genetic alterations, which enable them to have an intrinsic resistance to anticancer drugs. In addition, several different molecular changes important in EGFR dependent or -independent cellular signalling pathways could be responsible for the development of resistance to these inhibitors. For instance, we have previously shown uncoupling of EGFR with mitogenic pathways can cause resistance to EGFR antagonists [7]. Currently, combined therapy has become a breakthrough in treating cancer. In a range of tumor entities, such approach has produced impressive results. Combination therapy of PPARγ agonists and other agents has been shown to be more effective than using either agent alone. [25,26]. In bladder cancer cells *in vitro* and in bladder tumor *in vivo*, we demonstrated that PPARγ

active DIM-Cs showed significant anti-tumorigenic activity and were more potent inhibitors of bladder cancer growth when compared with rosiglitazone, the currently used synthetic PPARγ agonist [16]. Taken together, combined targeting of both EGFR and PPARγ axes can reveal promising molecules to target in bladder cancer. However, our results have shown that human urothelial cancer cell lines display marked heterogeneity towards sensitivity to EGFR inhibitors. Of high interest, the levels of expression of EGFR and PPARγ varied significantly among the different cell lines but did not correlate with stage of disease (range from superficial papillary to invasive to metastatic tumors). Furthermore, this correlation was not perfect as well to sensitivity either to EGFR inhibitor or PPARγ agonist with exception of UM-UC5 that shows high levels of EGFR expression and display high sensitivity to EGFR inhibitor. These findings corroborate results from other groups that have reported, in a panel of 17 human bladder cancer cell lines, that despite the strong correlation among gefitinib-responsiveness, EGFR surface expression and p27Kip1 protein expression in the most responsive lines, gefitinib-responsiveness was not as tightly linked to surface EGFR expression within the panel of cell lines as a whole [27]. These

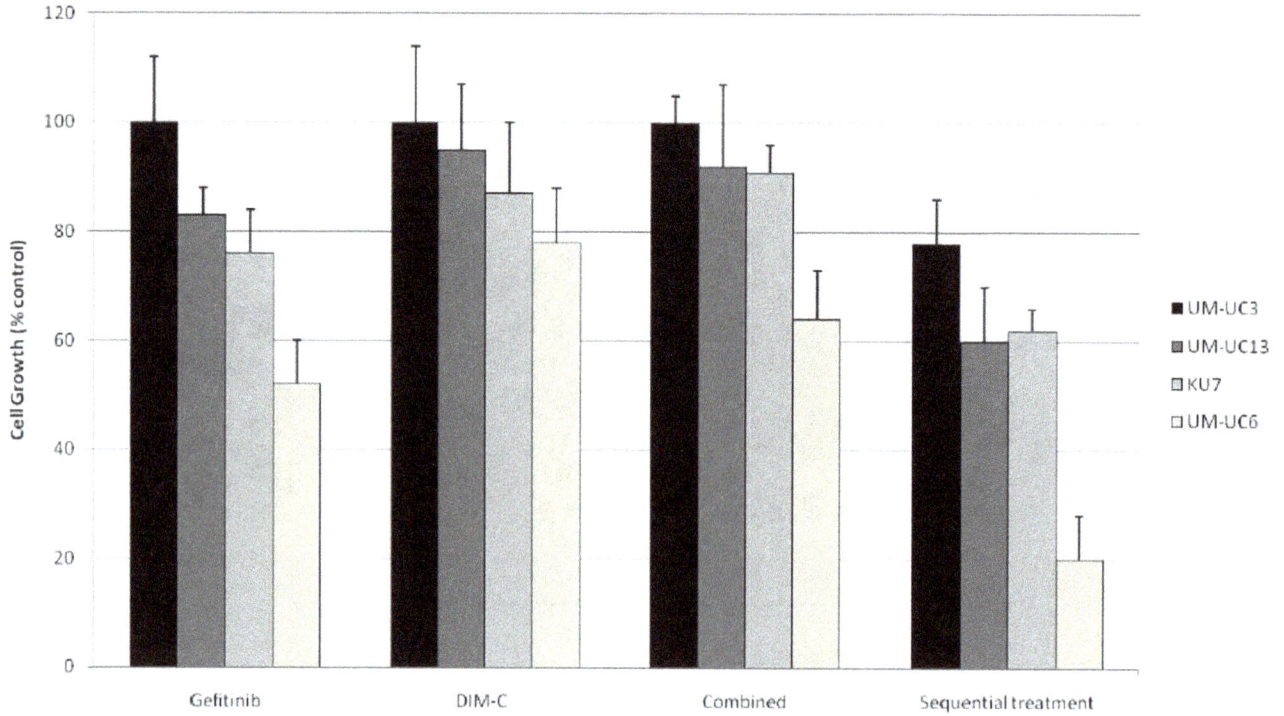

Figure 8. Schedule-specific efficacy of combination therapy. Three relatively resistant cell lines to gefitinib (UM-UC3, UM-UC13, and KU-7) and one sensitive (UM-UC6). Growth (MTT assays) after 48 hs treatment. Gefitinib: 2 µM. DIM-C: 2 µM.

results are remarkable but remain unclear whether baseline expression could predict EGFR dependent growth in bladder cancer. Conversely, when two resistant cell lines (KU-7 and UM-UC13) were treated with fixed-ratio of different fractions of GI50 of each drug alone (gefitinib or DIM-C), combination therapy potentially exerts additive inhibition of UC cell proliferation. These results provided further insight into the potential of combined therapy to overcome resistance to either drug alone, particularly to EGFR inhibitor. Indeed, our *in vivo* findings, showed positively the effects of combined EGFR inhibitors and PPARγ agonists on the growth of human urothelial tumors. In fact, xenografts nude mice with the relatively resistant bladder cancer cells (KU-7 cells) showed a markedly reduced tumor weight in combined group, in contrast to each treatment alone when compared to control. These findings indicate that even relatively resistant cells, *in vitro*, demonstrated sensitivity *in vivo* in the

combined treatment, suggesting PPARγ agonist could potentially be used to sensitize bladder cancer cell lines that were resistant to EGFR inhibition.

Recently, curcumin was shown to induce PPARγ expression in hepatic stellate cells and inhibit cell proliferation potentially *via* inhibiting EGFR activation [28]. In this study, Zhou et al, reported that interruption of the PDGF and EGF signalling pathways by curcumin, stimulates gene expression of PPARγ in activated Hepatic Stellate Cells (HSC), leading to the reduction in cell growth, including induction of cell arrest and apoptosis. Similarly, we observed an induction of PPARγ expression upon inhibition of EGFR in resistant KU-7 and UM-UC13 cells. This was an attractive result, since induction of PPARγ expression was observed in a dose dependent manner, and was followed by a nuclear accumulation of PPARγ, which is, in fact, the functional form of the receptor. Our novel observation reflects that efficacy of

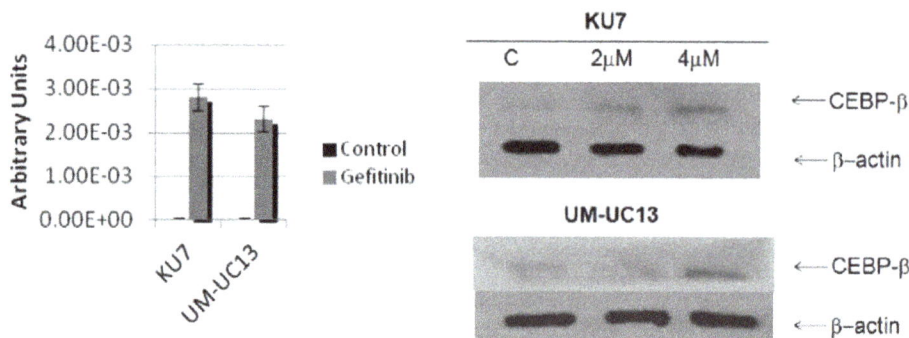

Figure 9. mRNA expression of CEBPβ after treatment with gefitinib. (A) RT-PCR of cells treated with gefitinib (B) Western blot of CEBPβ expression in KU-7 and UM-UC-13 cell lines in response to different concentrations of gefitinib.

combination therapy may also be significantly affected and improved by sequenced administration of gefitinib and PPARγ agonist. In reality, PPARγ agonist markedly sensitized bladder cancer cell lines, particularly those that were resistant to EGFR inhibition, in a schedule-specific manner, suggesting it can be an excellent alternative when cells are resistant to the aforementioned monotherapies. The mechanism of induction of PPARγ gene expression by gefitinib is still not clear. During adipogenesis, considerable evidences indicate that CEBP/β act as a transcriptional activator of PPARγ genes [23]. This belief is supported by the fact that proximal promoters of PPARγ posses C/EBP regulatory elements essential for its transactivation. Moreover, it has been shown that CEBP/β is expressed at early stage subsequently to treatment with differentiation inducers [29] followed by expression of PPARγ. Indeed, our findings shows EGFR inhibition induced CEBP/β expression and interestingly, its upregulation was also observed at early stage after gefitinib treatment, a process very similar to activation of adipogenic genes during differentiation, and which precedes induction of PPARγ

gene expression. However, future studies are needed in order to determine the direct role of C/EBPβ in the induction of PPARγ expression mediated by gefitinib. When interpreting our results, it is important to recognize the limitations of preclinical studies. Additionally, long-term use of PPARγ agonist such as pioglitazone has been associated with risk of bladder cancer while short-term use has shown no association [30,31]. Therefore, despite our promising findings show PPARγ agonists are more effective in combination therapy and particularly render bladder tumor sensitive to EGFR inhibition, a better understanding of the mechanism of activated PPARγ and EGFR inhibition is needed to evaluate the benefits from such therapy in future clinical applications.

Author Contributions

Conceived and designed the experiments: JJM SC WK. Performed the experiments: JJM RN KS SA JR. Analyzed the data: JJM SC WK. Wrote the paper: JJM SC WK.

References

1. Ciardiello F (2000) Epidermal growth factor receptor tyrosine kinase inhibitors as anticancer agents. Drugs 60 Suppl 1: 25–32; discussion 41–22.
2. Mendelsohn J, Dinney CP (2001) The Willet F. Whitmore, Jr., Lectureship: blockade of epidermal growth factor receptors as anticancer therapy. J Urol 165: 1152–1157.
3. Paez JG, Janne PA, Lee JC, Tracy S, Greulich H, et al. (2004) EGFR mutations in lung cancer: correlation with clinical response to gefitinib therapy. Science 304: 1497–1500.
4. Lynch TJ, Bell DW, Sordella R, Gurubhagavatula S, Okimoto RA, et al. (2004) Activating mutations in the epidermal growth factor receptor underlying responsiveness of non-small-cell lung cancer to gefitinib. N Engl J Med 350: 2129–2139.
5. Blehm KN, Spiess PE, Bondaruk JE, Dujka ME, Villares GJ, et al. (2006) Mutations within the kinase domain and truncations of the epidermal growth factor receptor are rare events in bladder cancer: implications for therapy. Clin Cancer Res 12: 4671–4677.
6. Kassouf W, Black PC, Tuziak T, Bondaruk J, Lee S, et al. (2008) Distinctive expression pattern of ErbB family receptors signifies an aggressive variant of bladder cancer. J Urol 179: 353–358.
7. Kassouf W, Dinney CP, Brown G, McConkey DJ, Diehl AJ, et al. (2005) Uncoupling between epidermal growth factor receptor and downstream signals defines resistance to the antiproliferative effect of Gefitinib in bladder cancer cells. Cancer Res 65: 10524–10535.
8. Fajas L, Auboeuf D, Raspe E, Schoonjans K, Lefebvre AM, et al. (1997) The organization, promoter analysis, and expression of the human PPARgamma gene. J Biol Chem 272: 18779–18789.
9. Motomura W, Okumura T, Takahashi N, Obara T, Kohgo Y (2000) Activation of peroxisome proliferator-activated receptor gamma by troglitazone inhibits cell growth through the increase of p27KiP1 in human. Pancreatic carcinoma cells. Cancer Res 60: 5558–5564.
10. Mansure JJ, Nassim R, Kassouf W (2009) Peroxisome proliferator-activated receptor gamma in bladder cancer: a promising therapeutic target. Cancer Biol Ther 8: 6–15.
11. Guan YF, Zhang YH, Breyer RM, Davis L, Breyer MD (1999) Expression of peroxisome proliferator-activated receptor gamma (PPARgamma) in human transitional bladder cancer and its role in inducing cell death. Neoplasia 1: 330–339.
12. Suzuki T, Nakagawa T, Endo H, Mitsudomi T, Masuda A, et al. (2003) The sensitivity of lung cancer cell lines to the EGFR-selective tyrosine kinase inhibitor ZD1839 ('Iressa') is not related to the expression of EGFR or HER-2 or to K-ras gene status. Lung Cancer 42: 35–41.
13. Burgermeister E, Tencer L, Liscovitch M (2003) Peroxisome proliferator-activated receptor-gamma upregulates caveolin-1 and caveolin-2 expression in human carcinoma cells. Oncogene 22: 3888–3900.
14. Xin X, Yang S, Kowalski J, Gerritsen ME (1999) Peroxisome proliferator-activated receptor gamma ligands are potent inhibitors of angiogenesis in vitro and in vivo. J Biol Chem 274: 9116–9121.
15. Bishop-Bailey D, Hla T (1999) Endothelial cell apoptosis induced by the peroxisome proliferator-activated receptor (PPAR) ligand 15-deoxy-Delta12, 14-prostaglandin J2. J Biol Chem 274: 17042–17048.
16. Kassouf W, Chintharlapalli S, Abdelrahim M, Nelkin G, Safe S, et al. (2006) Inhibition of bladder tumor growth by 1,1-bis(3'-indolyl)-1-(p-substitutedphenyl)methanes: a new class of peroxisome proliferator-activated receptor gamma agonists. Cancer Res 66: 412–418.
17. Lee SY, Hur GY, Jung KH, Jung HC, Kim JH, et al. (2006) PPAR-gamma agonist increase gefitinib's antitumor activity through PTEN expression. Lung Cancer 51: 297–301.
18. Zhou Y, Zheng S, Lin J, Zhang QJ, Chen A (2007) The interruption of the PDGF and EGF signaling pathways by curcumin stimulates gene expression of PPARgamma in rat activated hepatic stellate cell in vitro. Lab Invest 87: 488–498.
19. Dinney CP, Fishbeck R, Singh RK, Eve B, Pathak S, et al. (1995) Isolation and characterization of metastatic variants from human transitional cell carcinoma passaged by orthotopic implantation in athymic nude mice. J Urol 154: 1532–1538.
20. Sabichi A, Keyhani A, Tanaka N, Delacerda J, Lee IL, et al. (2006) Characterization of a panel of cell lines derived from urothelial neoplasms: genetic alterations, growth in vivo and the relationship of adenoviral mediated gene transfer to coxsackie adenovirus receptor expression. J Urol 175: 1133–1137.
21. Ono M, Kuwano M (2006) Molecular mechanisms of epidermal growth factor receptor (EGFR) activation and response to gefitinib and other EGFR-targeting drugs. Clin Cancer Res 12: 7242–7251.
22. Morrison RF, Farmer SR (1999) Role of PPARgamma in regulating a cascade expression of cyclin-dependent kinase inhibitors, p18(INK4c) and p21(Waf1/Cip1), during adipogenesis. J Biol Chem 274: 17088–17097.
23. Zhu Y, Qi C, Korenberg JR, Chen XN, Noya D, et al. (1995) Structural organization of mouse peroxisome proliferator-activated receptor gamma (mPPAR gamma) gene: alternative promoter use and different splicing yield two mPPAR gamma isoforms. Proc Natl Acad Sci U S A 92: 7921–7925.
24. Pettaway CA, Pisters LL, Dinney CP, Jularbal F, Swanson DA, et al. (1995) Sentinel lymph node dissection for penile carcinoma: the M. D. Anderson Cancer Center experience. J Urol 154: 1999–2003.
25. Emmans VC, Rodway HA, Hunt AN, Lillycrop KA (2004) Regulation of cellular processes by PPARgamma ligands in neuroblastoma cells is modulated by the level of retinoblastoma protein expression. Biochem Soc Trans 32: 840–842.
26. Hau P, Kunz-Schughart L, Bogdahn U, Baumgart U, Hirschmann B, et al. (2007) Low-dose chemotherapy in combination with COX-2 inhibitors and PPAR-gamma agonists in recurrent high-grade gliomas - a phase II study. Oncology 73: 21–25.
27. Shrader M, Pino MS, Brown G, Black P, Adam L, et al. (2007) Molecular correlates of gefitinib responsiveness in human bladder cancer cells. Mol Cancer Ther 6: 277–285.
28. Lin J, Chen A (2008) Activation of peroxisome proliferator-activated receptor-gamma by curcumin blocks the signaling pathways for PDGF and EGF in hepatic stellate cells. Lab Invest 88: 529–540.
29. Tang QQ, Lane MD (1999) Activation and centromeric localization of CCAAT/enhancer-binding proteins during the mitotic clonal expansion of adipocyte differentiation. Genes Dev 13: 2231–2241.
30. Lewis JD, Ferrara A, Peng T, Hedderson M, Bilker WB, et al. (2011) Risk of bladder cancer among diabetic patients treated with pioglitazone: interim report of a longitudinal cohort study. Diabetes Care 34: 916–922.
31. Dormandy J, Bhattacharya M, van Troostenburg de Bruyn AR (2009) Safety and tolerability of pioglitazone in high-risk patients with type 2 diabetes: an overview of data from PROactive. Drug Saf 32: 187–202.

10

A MicroRNA-7 Binding Site Polymorphism in HOXB5 Leads to Differential Gene Expression in Bladder Cancer

Junhua Luo[1], Qingqing Cai[2], Wei Wang[3], Hui Huang[4], Hong Zeng[5], Wang He[1], Weixi Deng[6], Hao Yu[1], Eddie Chan[7], Chi-fai NG[7], Jian Huang[1]*, Tianxin Lin[1,6]*

1 Department of Urology, Sun Yat-sen Memorial Hospital, Sun Yat-sen University, Guangzhou, China, 2 Department of Internal Medicine, Cancer Center, Sun Yat-sen University, Guangzhou, China, 3 Department of Urology, Guangzhou General Hospital of Guangzhou Military Command (Guangzhou Liuhuaqiao Hospital), Guangzhou, China, 4 Department of Cardiology, Sun Yat-sen Memorial Hospital, Sun Yat-sen University, Guangzhou, China, 5 Department of Pathology, Sun Yat-sen Memorial Hospital, Sun Yat-sen University, Guangzhou, China, 6 Lin Bai-xin Research Center, Sun Yat-sen Memorial Hospital, Sun Yat-sen University, Guangzhou, China, 7 Division of Urology, Department of Surgery, The Chinese University of Hong Kong, Hong Kong, China

Abstract

Purpose: To investigate the biological function of HOXB5 in human bladder cancer and explore whether the HOXB5 3'-UTR SNP (1010A/G), which is located within the microRNA-7 binding site, was correlated with clinical features of bladder cancer.

Methods: Expression of HOXB5 in 35 human bladder cancer tissues and 8 cell lines were examined using real-time PCR and immunohistochemistry. Next, we explored the biological function of HOXB5 *in vitro* using cell proliferation, migration and colony formation assays. Using bioinformatics, a SNP (1010A/G) was found located within the microRNA-7 binding site in the 3'-UTR of HOXB5. Real-time PCR was used to test HOXB5 expression affected by different alleles. Finally, multivariate logistic regression analysis was used to determine the relationship between SNP (1010A/G) frequency and clinical features in 391 cases.

Results: HOXB5 was frequently over-expressed both in bladder cancer tissues and cell lines. Inhibition of HOXB5 suppressed the oncogenic function of cancer cells. Next, we demonstrated that a SNP (1010A/G), located within the microRNA-7 binding site in the 3'-UTR of HOXB5, could affect HOXB5 expression in bladder cancer mainly by differential binding activity of microRNA-7 and SNP-related mRNA stability. Finally, we also showed the frequency of 1010G genotype was higher in cancer group compared to normal controls and correlated with the risk of high grade and high stage.

Conclusion: HOXB5 is overexpressed in bladder cancer. A miRNA-binding SNP (1010A/G) located within 3'-UTR of HOXB5 is associated with gene expression and may be a promising prognostic factor for bladder cancer.

Editor: Lorenzo Chiariotti, Università di Napoli Federico II, ITALY

Funding: This work was supported by the National Natural Science Foundation of China (81071688, 30972983, 81172431, 91029742), Guangdong province Natural Scientific Foundation (07117366, 6104605), Yat-sen Scholarship for Young Scientists (For Tianxin Lin), Clinical Key Project of Public Health Ministry (for Jian Huang), and the Program for New Century Excellent Talents in University (NCET-10-0852, for Tianxin Lin). The funders had no role in study design, data collection and analysis, decision to publish, or preparation of the manuscript.

Competing Interests: The authors have declared that no competing interests exist.

* E-mail: tianxinl@sina.com (TL); yehjn@yahoo.com.cn (JH)

Introduction

Urinary bladder cancer is the most common urological tumor in China [1]; however, the mechanisms of bladder cancer tumorigenesis have not been well illustrated. Data show that most of the bladder cancers are induced by carcinogens that damage the DNA. The sensitivity of the transitional epithelium's microenvironment may be another important factor during tumorigenesis [2]. Oncogenes and tumor suppressors have also been reported to play important roles in bladder cancer [3]. Recently, genetic changes including SNPs, deletions, insertions, and changes of DNA copy number have been found to be involved in bladder carcinogenesis.

A homeobox (HOX) is a sequence of about 180 nucleotides within genes that code for a protein domain called homeodomain. Studies showed that HOX genes constitute as much as 0.1–0.2% of the whole vertebrate genome [4]. HOX genes are highly conserved across vast evolutionary distances and encode nuclear proteins that act as transcription factors (TF) during normal organ development [5]. In recent years, the HOX gene family has also been associated with human diseases especially cancers. For instance, loss of HOXA5 in breast cancer [6], overexpression of HOXA10 in acute myeloid leukemia (AML) [7], gene mutations of HOXD4 in renal and colon cancer [8] and overexpression of HOXC4 in human bladder cancer [9] have been reported. HOXB5 (NM_002147.3), located on human chromosome 17, is a member of the HOX gene family that is involved in normal lung and gut development in mouse and human [10]. HOXB5 has been reported to be related to human diseases including AML [11], congenital cystic adenomatoid malformation (CCAM) [12] and bronchopulmonary sequestration (BPS) [13]. Also, the HOXB5 gene was found to be highly expressed in ovarian cancer and was considered to be an important potential targets in the treatment of ovarian cancer [14]. The biological function of HOXB5 in urological carcinomas have not been reported. In a pilot study, we found that HOXB5 was frequently over-expressed in human bladder cancer tissues and cell lines, suggesting that it may be a candidate oncogene in bladder cancer.

In the past ten years, the involvement of microRNAs (miRNAs) in human cancers has been widely studied. MiRNAs repress the expression of the target mRNA by binding to the 3' untranslated region (3'-UTR) of the mRNA. In human bladder cancer, miRNAs had been shown to be important factors during tumorigenesis. In a previous study, we reported that miRNA-143 and miRNA-125b acted as tumor suppressors in human bladder cancer [15,16]. In another study it was reported that miR-7 was down-regulated in bladder cancer and may suppress tumor growth by inhibiting growth factor receptor expression and by impairing the anti-apoptotic Akt pathway [17].

Single-nucleotide polymorphisms (SNPs), the most common form of genetic variations in the human genome, contribute to different human phenotypes. SNPs have been associated with many human diseases, especially cancers. In recent years, SNPs located within the miRNA-binding site of a miRNA target (also called miRNA-binding SNP) have been found to be important during tumorigenesis. In a previous study, our group suggested that SNP (1805C/T) in the miR-181a binding site of the Mel-18 gene was related to some clinical features of prostate cancer [18]. In a pilot study, we found a possible miRNA-binding SNP (1010A/G) in the 3'-UTR of the HOXB5 gene using the NCBI SNP database (http://www.ncbi.nlm.nih.gov/snp/) and miRbase (http://www.mirbase.org/).

In this study, we showed that the HOXB5 gene was over-expressed and acted as an oncogene in human bladder cancer. We also found a SNP (1010 A/G) in the 3'-UTR of the HOXB5 gene which is within the miRNA-7 binding site. We have shown that this SNP could affect the expression of HOXB5 mainly by interfering with the function of miRNA-7 and SNP-related mRNA stability; Furthermore, the frequency of 1010G genotype was higher in cancer group compared to normal controls, and was found to be correlated with the risk of high grade and high stage. To our knowledge, this is the first study of the involvement of polymorphisms in the miRNA binding site of HOXB5 in human bladder cancer.

Materials and Methods

Patients and Tissues

391 bladder cancer patients were enrolled in our study. This study was approved by the Institute Research Ethics, Sun Yat-sen University, China. Informed consent was written and obtained from all the subjects in our study. All the patients had primary bladder cancers; no previous treatment had been conducted before the operation. The cancer samples were obtained from patients who underwent resection of bladder cancer. The samples were collected between 2007 and 2010 at the Department of Urology, Sun Yat-sen Memorial Hospital, Sun Yat-sen University, Guangzhou, China and Department of Urology, Southwest Hospital, Chongqing, China. All bladder specimens were immediately snap frozen in liquid nitrogen and stored at $-80°C$. Histology of the tissues was independently evaluated by two pathologists, and the clinical stage of bladder cancer was determined using the 2002 tumor-node-metastasis (TNM) classification system.

Cell Lines and Cell Culture

Cell lines used in our study were obtained from American Tissue Type Culture Collection (ATCC, Manassas, VA, USA); they include T24, 5637, TCCSUP, HT-1376, UM-UC-3, J82, RT4, EJ and the SV40-transformed kidney cell line 293T. The cells were cultured in a humidified air atmosphere of 5% CO_2 at 37°C, and all media were supplemented with 10% fetal bovine serum (Hyclone, Logan, UT, USA). T24 was cultured in McCoy's 5a medium (modified); 5637 was cultured in RPMI 1640 medium; J82, UM-UC-3, TCCSUP and HT-1376 were cultured in Eagle's minimum essential medium (EMEM) (Hyclone); and RT4, EJ and SV40-transformed kidney cell line 293T were cultured in Dulbecco's modified Eagle's medium (DMEM) (Hyclone).

RNA Extraction and Quantitative Real-time PCR

Total RNA was extracted from the patients' bladder samples or cell lines using TRIzol reagent (Invitrogen, Carlsbad, California, USA) according to the manufacturer's protocol. Quantitative real-time PCR (qPCR) was done using the SYBR green assay (TaKaRa Biotechnology, Dalian, China) on a Roche LightCycler 480 machine (Roche Applied Science, Mannheim, Germany). qPCR was performed as followed: an initial predenaturation step for 30 seconds at 95°C, followed by amplification of 40 cycles at 95°C for 5 seconds and at 60°C for 20 seconds, melting curve analysis was performed at the end. All reactions were done in a 20 μL reaction volume in triplicate. The expression level of HOXB5 was evaluated using the comparative Ct method. GAPDH was used as an internal control. The primers used for HOXB5 were: sense, 5'-TGAAGCACAGGGTTATAACGACCA-3', antisense, 5'-GCAGCGGGATCCCTGTAAGA-3'; and for GAPDH the primers were: sense, 5'- GAAGGTGAAGGTCGGAGTC-3', antisense, 5'- GAAGATGGTGATGGGATTTC-3'.

Immunohistochemistry

Paraffin-embedded, formalin-fixed tissues were cut into 5-μm section, placed on a polylysine-coated slide, deparaffinized in xylene, rehydrated using graded ethanol, quenched for endogenous peroxidase activity in 0.3% hydrogen peroxide and processed for antigen retrieval by microwave heating in 10 mM citrate buffer (pH 6.0). Sections were incubated at 4°C overnight with HOXB5 rabbit polyclonal antibody (1:100, AbCam, Cambridge, MA, USA). Immunostaining was performed using the ChemMate[TM] DAKO EnVision[TM] Detection Kit (DakoCytomation, Glostrup, Denmark), which resulted in a brown precipitate at the antigen site. Subsequently, sections were counterstained with hematoxylin (Zymed Laboratories, South San Francisco, CA, USA) and mounted in nonaqueous mounting medium. The primary antibody was omitted for the negative controls.

Western Blot

Protein was extracted from bladder cancer tissues and cell lines as described [19]. Briefly, 30 μg of protein from each sample was separated by electrophoresis in a sodium dodecyl sulfate poly-acrylamide gel before being transferred to polyvinylidene fluoride membranes (Millipore, Billerica, MA, USA) for 2 hours. Then the membranes were blocked for 1 hour at room temperature using 5% bovine serum albumin (BSA), and incubated in TBST (Tris buffered saline with 0.05% tween) containing rabbit polyclonal IgG2a anti-HOXB5 (1:1000, AbCam) or GAPDH (1:1000, Cell Signaling Technology, Beverly, MA, USA) overnight at 4°C. The membranes were incubated with peroxidase-conjugated goat anti-rabbit immunoglobulin (1:5000, Cell

Signaling Technology) as secondary antibody and then visualized using a commercial ECL kit (Pierce, Rockford, IL, USA).

Cell Transfection with si-HOXB5 and miRNA-7

siRNAs designed to HOXB5 and miRNA-7 mimics were transfected into the bladder cancer cells T24, 5637 and TCCSUP using Lipofectamine-RNAiMAX (Invitrogen). The sequences used for si-HOXB5 were, sense: 5′-GGAUGGACCUCAGCGU-CAATT-3′, antisense: 5′-UUGACGCUGAGGUCCAUCCTT-3′; for miR-7 mimics, sense: 5′-CAACAAAUCACAGUCUGC-CAUA-3′, antisense: 5′-UAUGGCAGACUGUGAUUUGUUG-3′; and for the negative control, sense: 5′-UUCUCCGAACGU-GUCACGUTT-3′, antisense: 5′-ACGUGACACGUUCGGA-GAATT-3′. All the RNA oligoribonucleotides were purchased from Genepharma (Shanghai, China). One day before transfection, 2×10^5 cells were seeded onto a six-well plate. The next day, when the cells reached 70–80% confluence, they were transfected with RNA at a final concentration of 100 nM according to Lipofectamine-RNAiMAX's protocol. The transfection efficiency measured by qPCR, was 70% for T24, 72% for 5637 and 75% for TCCSUP (data not shown).

Cell Proliferation Assay

Human bladder cancer cell lines T24, 5637 and TCCSUP were plated onto 6-well plates and incubated at 37°C in a 5% CO2 incubator one day before transfection. After transfection with siRNAs (100 nM) or a negative control for 24 hours, the cells were collected and plated onto 96-well plates for cell viability evaluation using a CCK8 assay (Cell Counting Kit-8) (Dojindo Laboratories, Japan) according to the protocol [20].

In vitro Cell Migration Assay

After the bladder cancer cell lines T24, 5637 and TCCSUP were transfected with si-HOXB5 (100 nM) or nonspecific control (NC) siRNA for 24 hours, the cells were harvested and suspended in 100 μL serum-free medium and then plated (1×10^4 cells) in the upper compartment of Transwell plates (Corning, NY, USA). The Transwell inserts were then placed into the lower compartment of a 24-well plate containing 600 μL of the medium with 20% FBS as the chemo-attractant. After a 24 hour incubation period, the cells remaining on the top surface of the membrane were removed and the cells on the lower surface were fixed in 100% methanol for 30 minutes, followed by staining with 0.1% crystal violet solution for 30 minutes. Cells that stained purple were defined as positive and the images were captured using a microscope (10×) (Olympus, Center Valley, PA, USA).

Colony Formation Assay

After transfection with si-HOXB5 (100 nM) or NC siRNA for 24 hours, the human bladder cancer cells T24, 5637 and TCCSUP were collected and placed onto a fresh six-well plate (500 cells for T24, and 1,000 cells for 5637 and TCCSUP). The cells were cultured for about 2 weeks to form colonies. Colonies were fixed with 100% methanol and stained with 0.1% crystal violet in 20% methanol for 15 min. Colony-forming efficiency was calculated as colonies/plated cells ×100%.

Bioinformatics

The NCBI SNP database (http://www.ncbi.nlm.nih.gov/snp/) was used to find SNPs located within the 3′-UTR of the HOXB5 gene. Four publicly available algorithms, PicTar (http://pictar.mdc-berlin.de/), TargetScan (http://www.targetscan.org/), mi-Randa (http://www.microrna.org/) and DIANA microT (http://diana.pcbi.upenn.edu/) were used to predict which of the human miRNAs in miRbase (http://www.mirbase.org/) may bind to the 3′-UTR of HOXB5. The miRNAs that were predicted by at least 2 of the algorithms to bind were accepted as candidates for further study. The mRNA secondary structure prediction tool MFOLD (http://mfold.rna.albany.edu/) was used to predict the secondary structure of the HOXB5 mRNA. Small minimal free energy (MFE) indicates high stability of the predicted mRNA secondary structure.

Luciferase Reporter Assay

We construct luciferase reporter plasmids with the HOXB5 3′-UTR fragment that contained the putative binding sites for the candidate miRNA and subcloned them into the psiCHECK-2 Vector (Promega, Madison, WI, USA) to produce the psi-CHECK-2-3′-UTR-WT plasmid. The mutant HOXB5 3′-UTR was generated using the fusion PCR method and then it also subcloned into the psiCHECK-2 Vector to produce the psiCHECK-2-3′-UTR-MUT plasmid. DNA sequencing analysis was used to confirm the sequence of the constructed plasmids.

For the luciferase reporter assay, HEK-293T cells (2×10^4) were placed onto a 24-well plate one day before transfection. The next day 0.5 μg of either the psiCHECK-2-3′-UTR-WT or the psiCHECK-2-3′-UTR-MUT, and either the miRNA or the negative control were cotransfected into the HEK-293T cells using Lipofectamine2000 (Invitrogen). Assays were performed 48 hours after transfection using the Dual-Luciferase Reporter Assay System (Promega). Luciferase activity was detected using the GloMax-Multi Detection System (Promega). The Renilla luciferase signals were normalized to the internal firefly luciferase transfection control. Transfections were done in triplicate in independent experiments.

DNA Extraction and HOXB5 Genotyping Analysis

Total DNA was extracted from the patients' bladder cancer samples and cell lines using QIAamp reagent (QIAGEN, Germantown, MD, USA) according to the manufacturer's protocol. HOXB5 genotyping was performed using a DNA sequencing assay. A 334 bp DNA fragment containing the SNP in the 3′-UTR of HOXB5 gene was amplified from genomic DNA. The PCR primers used were, forward 5′-GCGCATGAAGTGGAA-GAAGG-3′, reverse 5′-TTGGGACAAGCAGAAGGGAG-3′. The amplified DNA fragment was sequenced using GENESCAN software (Applied Biosystems, Foster City, CA, USA).

Measurement of the Expression of HOXB5 mRNA

The HOXB5 mRNA level was measured in 3 bladder cancer cell lines (5637, J82 and RT4) and 13 bladder cancer tissues. Region-specific Taqman probes were designed to detect the SNP in the 3′-UTR of the HOXB5 mRNA. The cDNA from the cell lines and cancer tissues were subjected to qPCR and the fluorescence (VIC for 1010A, FAM for 1010G) was measured using LightCycler 480 Probes Master (Roche Applied Science, Mannheim, Germany).

Genomic DNA was also extracted from cell lines and cancer tissues as mentioned. As an internal control, qPCR was performed to determine the genomic DNA levels of HOXB5 using the same region-specific Taqman probes.

HOXB5 mRNA Half-life

qPCR was also used to measure the half-life of the HOXB5 mRNA. 1×10^6 T24 and TCCSUP bladder cancer cells were

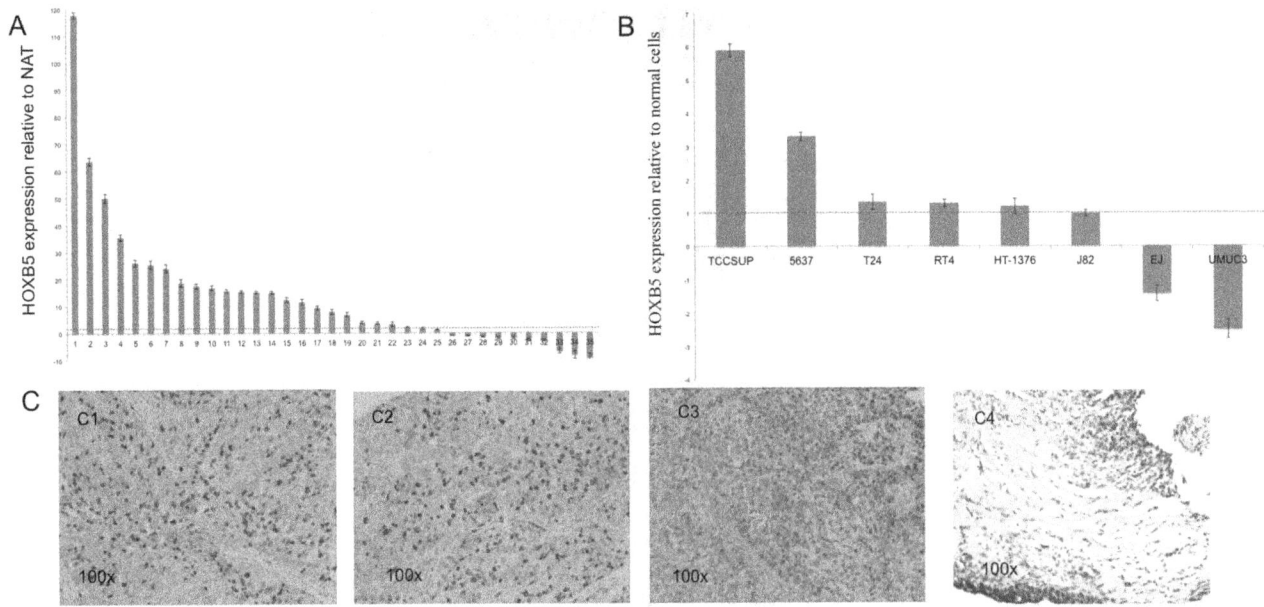

Figure 1. HOXB5 is over-expressed in human bladder tumors. A. Expression of HOXB5 in 35 bladder cancer tissues relative to normal adjacent tissues (NAT). Columns above the X-axis indicate overexpression of HOXB5; those below the X-axis indicate down-expression of HOXB5 relative to NAT. B. Expression of HOXB5 in eight bladder cancer cell lines relative to normal bladder cells. Columns above the X-axis indicate overexpression of HOXB5; those below the X-axis indicate down-expression of HOXB5 relative to normal cells. Fold changes >1 was considered to be positive. C. HOXB5 expression in primary transitional cell bladder cancer tissues detected by immunohistochemistry. C1 and C2, Bladder cancer tissues, G2 grade. C3, Bladder cancer tissue, G3 grade. C4, Normal bladder tissue. All images are ×100. Staining: brown, HOXB5.

plated onto a 10-cm dish one day before actinomycin D (5 µg/ml), which inhibits genetic transcription, was added to the cells. After treated with actinomycin D, the cells were lysed using TRIzol at different time points, 0 h, 4 h, 8 h, 12 h, 24 h and

48 h. Total RNA was extracted and the HOXB5 mRNA level was quantified by qPCR using the Taqman assay as previously described above.

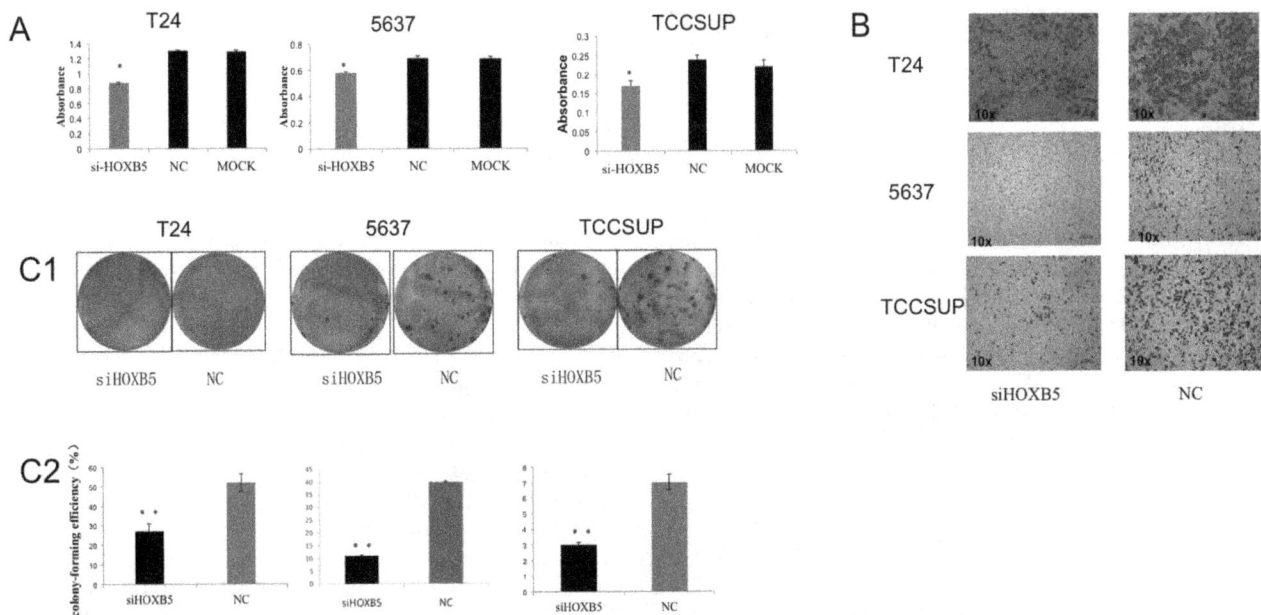

Figure 2. si-HOXB5 inhibited the biological function of bladder cancer cells *in vitro.* A. Proliferation of bladder cancer cell lines T24, 5637 and TCCSUP. A CCK8 assay was used to examine cell growth of bladder cancer cells. B. Migration of bladder cancer cell lines. Left column, si-HOXB5 transfected group; right column, NC siRNA transfected group. All images are ×10. Staining: purple, migration cells. C. Colony formation (C1) and colony-forming efficiency (C2) of bladder cancer cells after transfection with si-HOXB5 or NC siRNA. Colony-forming efficiency = colonies/plated cells ×100%. *p<0.05, **p<0.01. NC, nonspecific control. MOCK, Lipofectamine only.

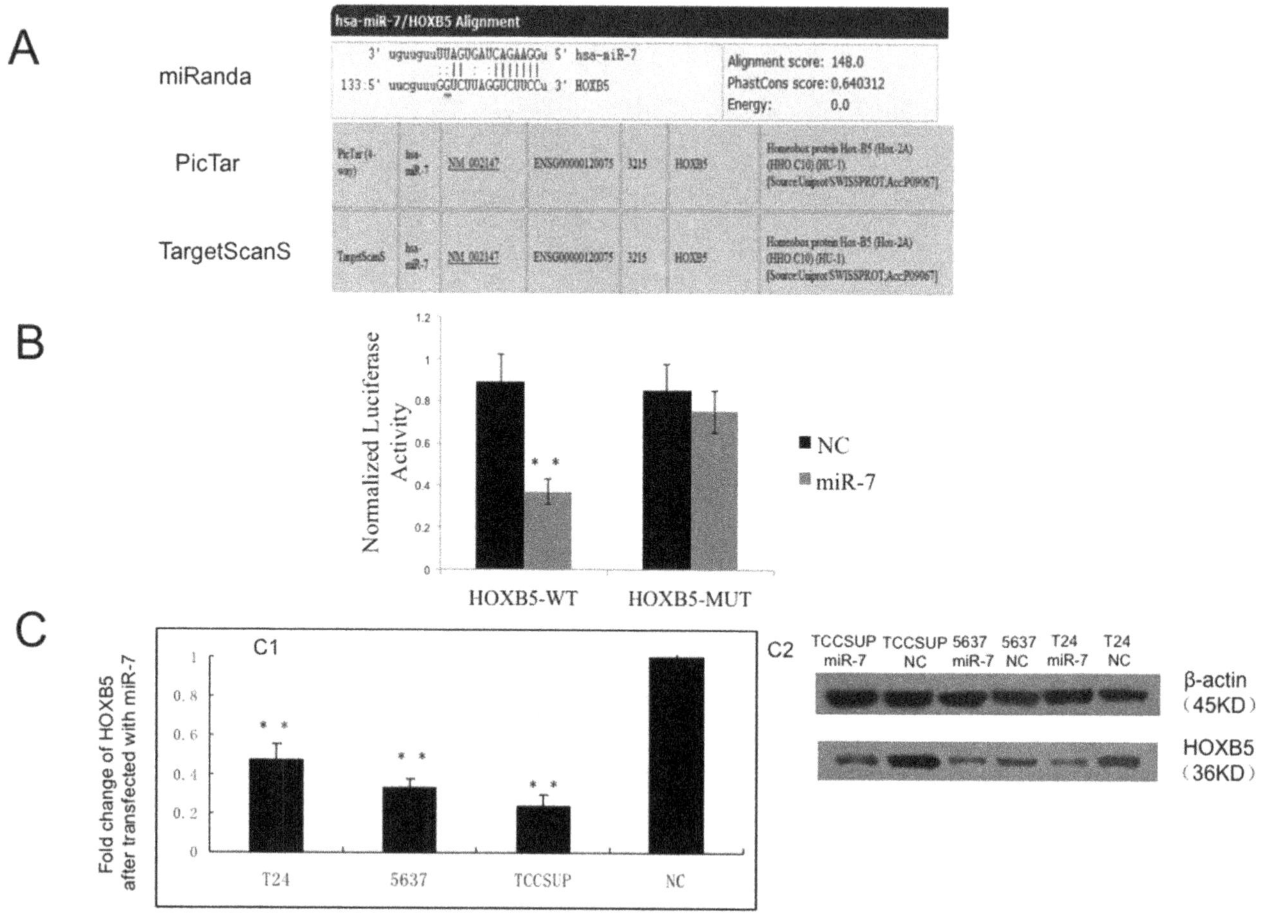

Figure 3. HOXB5 is a target of miR-7. A. HOXB5 was predicted as a direct target of miR-7 by miRanda, PicTar and TargetScan. B. Luciferase analysis in HEK-293T cells. WT, wild type. MUT, mutant type. C. Effect of miR-7 overexpression on the expression levels of endogenous HOXB5 in T24, 5637 and TCCSUP cells. Endogenous HOXB5 mRNA and protein levels were assayed by qPCR (C1) and Western blot (C2) respectively. β-actin, internal control. **p<0.01, compared with NC transfectants. NC, nonspecific control.

Statistic

All data are expressed as the mean ± SEM from at least three separate experiments. The differences between groups were analyzed using Student's t test when only two groups were compared, or, by one-way analysis of variance (ANOVA) when more than two groups were compared. The age-adjusted odds ratio (aOR) and 95% confidence interval (CI) for the relationship between the HOXB5 3'-UTR genotype frequencies and clinical or histological features were determined by multivariate logistic regression analysis using SPSS 17.0 with age considered as a factor. All statistical tests were two-sided. Differences were considered statistically significant at p<0.05.

Results

HOXB5 was Over-expressed in Human Bladder Cancer Tissues and Cell Lines

RNA was extracted from 35 bladder cancer patients and 8 bladder cancer cell lines and the expression of HOXB5 was measured using qPCR. As shown in Figure 1A, of 35 samples, 23 (~70%) exhibited higher expression of HOXB5 compared with normal adjacent tissue (NAT). The expression of HOXB5 was also higher in 6 of 8 bladder cancer cell lines (TCCSUP, 5637, T24, RT4, HT-1376, and J82) than in normal bladder cells (Figure 1B).

Immunohistochemical studies using the HOXB5-specific antibody confirmed that the expression of HOXB5 is higher in bladder cancer tissues than normal bladder tissues (Figure 1C). However, there was no correlation between the expression of HOXB5 and the tumor grade or stage (data not shown). These results suggested that the overexpression of HOXB5 may be common in some bladder cancer tissues and in cell lines.

HOXB5 Promotes Cell Proliferation and Migration of Bladder Cancer Cells

We found that HOXB5 was over-expressed in bladder cancer tissues and in cell lines, indicating that HOXB5 may act as an oncogene. To investigate the oncogenic function of HOXB5, we transfected si-HOXB5 and NC siRNA into T24, 5637 and TCCSUP cells. 48 hours after transfection, a CCK8 assay showed that cell growth was significantly decreased in si-HOXB5 transfected groups compared with the NC group or mock group (Lipofectamine only) (Figure 2A, p<0.05). We also found that the migration ability of si-HOXB5 transfected cells was significantly inhibited compared with the NC group or mock group (Figure 2B). These results indicated that HOXB5 may promote cell proliferation and the migration of bladder cancer cells, consistent with a role of an oncogene.

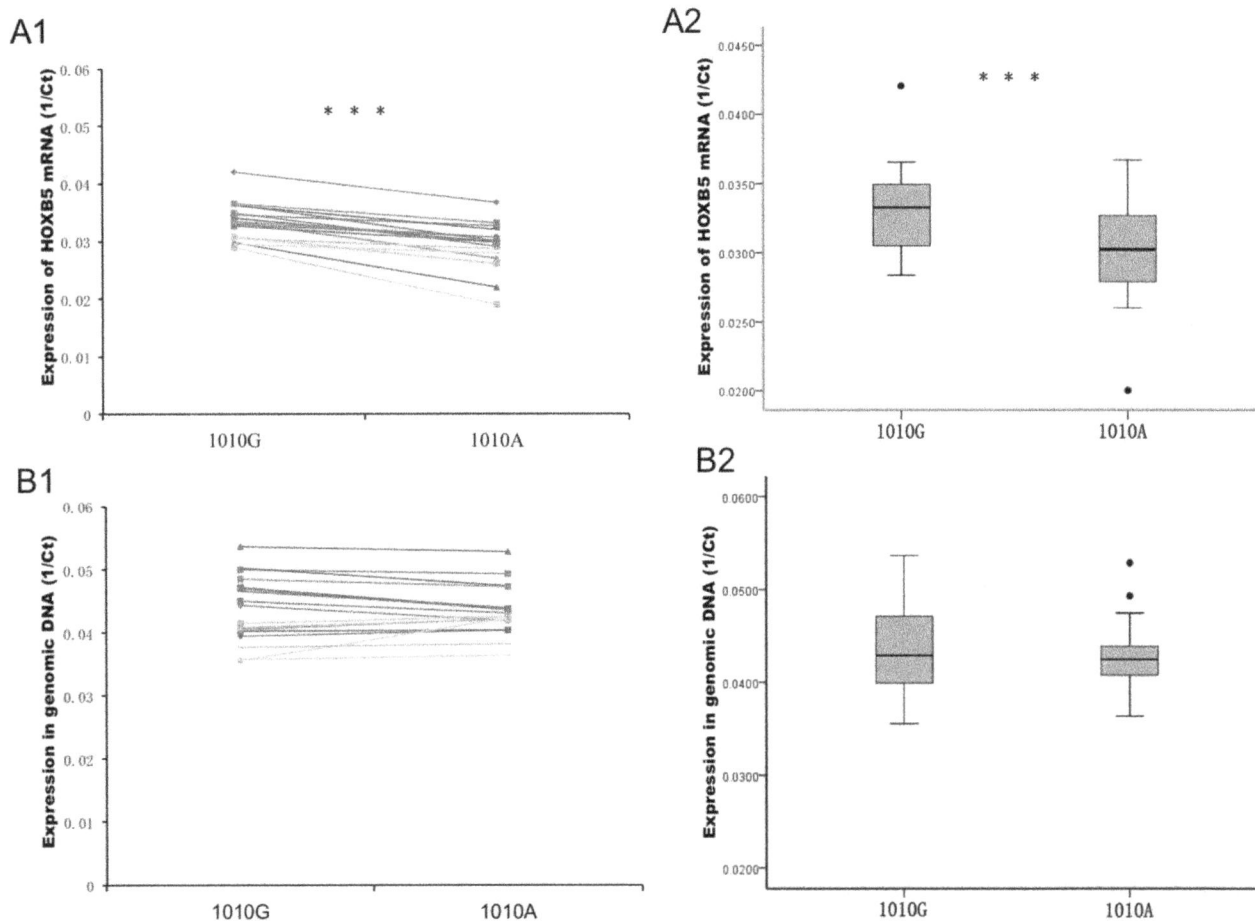

Figure 4. Expression of HOXB5 mRNA for each allele in heterozygous bladder cancer tissues and cell lines. A1. Expression of mRNA for each allele in the heterozygous GA genotype cell lines (5637, RT4 and J82) and tissues (13 cases). A2. Expression of mRNA (Mean) for each allele in heterozygous GA genotype cell lines and tissues. Y-axis, expression of HOXB5 mRNA. Ct: cycle threshold, calculated from Realtime-PCR machine. B1. Expression of the heterozygous genomic DNA as an internal control. B2. Expression of the heterozygous genomic DNA (Mean) as an internal control. Y-axis, expression in genomic DNA. ***p<0.001.

si-HOXB5 Suppresses Clonogenicity *in vitro*

To further explore the potential role of HOXB5 in tumorigenesis, we investigated the effect of HOXB5 on colony formation of cancer cells *in vitro*. Three bladder cancer cell lines (T24, 5637 and TCCSUP) were transfected with an si-HOXB5 or NC duplex, and allowed to grow at very low density (500 cells for T24, 1,000 cells for 5637 and TCCSUP) for about 14 days. Notably, si-HOXB5 inhibited, both in size and number, the ability of bladder cancer cells to form colonies (Figure 2 C1). Further, the si-HOXB5 transfected cells showed lower colony-forming efficiency than the NC-transfected cells (Figure 2 C2, p<0.01). These data further supported the oncogenic effect of HOXB5 in bladder cancer cells.

SNP-1010A/G is Located within miRNA-7 Binding Site in HOXB5 3'-UTR

We found SNP rs9299 (1010 A/G) is located within the 3'-UTR of the HOXB5 gene using the NCBI SNP database. HOXB5 was also predicted to be one of the target genes of miRNA-7 according to 3 of the different systemic bioinformatics software that we used, and the SNP (1010 A/G) was located within the miRNA-7 binding site (Figure 3A).

To validate HOXB5 as a bona fide target of miR-7, a human HOXB5 3'-UTR fragment containing either the wild-type or mutant miR-7-binding sequence was subcloned downstream of the Renilla luciferase reporter gene as described in the Materials and Methods section. The relative luciferase activity of the reporter containing the wild-type HOXB5 3'-UTR was significantly suppressed when miR-7 was co-transfected (p<0.01). In contrast, the luciferase activity of the reporter containing the mutant miR-7-binding site was almost unaffected (p>0.05) (Figure 3B).

To further explore the regulation of HOXB5 expression by miR-7, we transfected miR-7 mimics and NC into the cell lines T24, 5637 and TCCSUP. After 48 hours, we examined the HOXB5 mRNA and protein levels using qPCR and western blot. We found that the HOXB5 mRNA and protein levels were downregulated in the miR-7 transfected groups compared with the NC groups (Figure 3 C1 & C2).

These results indicated that miR-7 may regulate HOXB5 expression at both the post-transcription and mRNA levels.

SNP 1010A/G affects HOXB5 Expression

To investigate the affect of SNP 1010A/G on the expression of HOXB5, we examined the mRNA levels of HOXB5 for the 1010A and 1010G alleles in the heterozygous GA genotype bladder cancer tissues (13 cases) and cell lines (5637, RT4 and J82), using the Taqman assay as described above. We found that

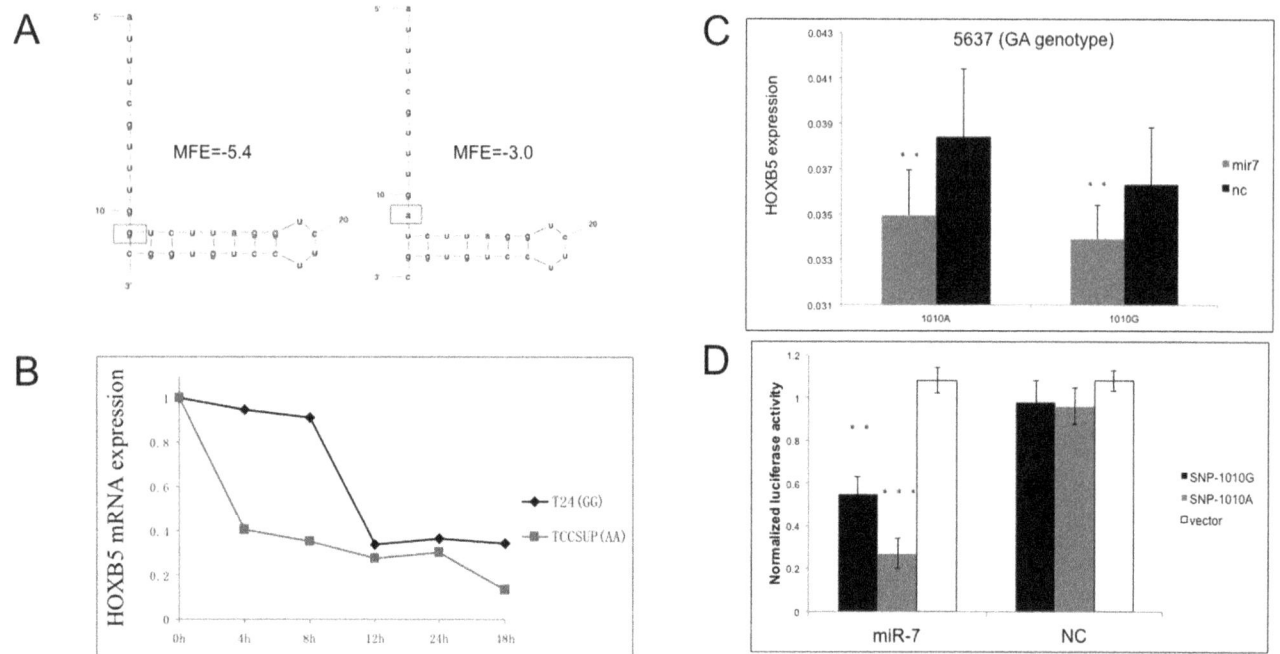

Figure 5. Different alleles affect HOXB5 mRNA stability and the activity of miR-7 binding. A. Secondary structures of HOXB5 mRNA predicted by MFOLD. Minimal free energy (MFE) may reflect mRNA stability. B. Half-life of HOXB5 mRNA in T24 (GG genotype) and TCCSUP (AA genotype) cells. The half-life for the mRNA with the G allele was about 11 hours, and about 3.7 hours with the A allele. C. HOXB5 expression level after transfection with miR-7 relative to NC in 5637 cells (GA genotype). Both A and G alleles of the mRNA transfected with miR-7 exhibited down-regulation relative to the NC group. The level of HOXB5 mRNA with the A allele decreased more than mRNA with the G allele. D. Luciferase analysis in HEK-293T cells of miR-7 activity. Vector, psiCHECK-2 Vector. *p<0.05, **p<0.01, ***p<0.001.

the expression of the HOXB5 mRNA with the 1010G allele was significantly higher than the mRNA with the 1010A allele in both cancer tissues and cell lines (Figure 4A1 and A2). However, the expression ratio of 1010G to 1010A in the genomic DNA from these heterozygous cancer tissues and cell lines were similar (Figure 4B1 and B2). These results showed that the 1010A/G SNP in the HOXB5 3'-UTR affected the expression of HOXB5 mRNA.

The Different Alleles Affect mRNA Stability and HOXB5 Expression Levels

To predict possible mechanisms how the 1010A/G SNP results in differential HOXB5 expression levels, we used the mRNA secondary structure prediction tool MFOLD to predict

the secondary structure of the mRNAs with the A and G alleles. We found that the predicted minimal free energy (MFE) of the secondary structure of the mRNA with the G allele was lower than that of the mRNA with the A allele (−5.4 vs −3.0). This result indicated that the structure of the mRNA with the G allele may be more stable than that for the mRNA with the A allele (Figure 5A).

To further explore which allele (A or G) conferred more stability, we measured the mRNA half-life because it has been shown that the steady state of mRNA is closely related to the mRNA half-life [21]. We examined the half-life of HOXB5 mRNA in the homozygous T24 and TCCSUP bladder cancer cells (GG for T24 and AA for TCCSUP) after treatment with actinomycin D, using qPCR. The results showed that the half-life

Table 1. Genotype frequencies of the HOXB5 polymorphism in bladder cancer subgroups (G1 and G2–G3 groups).

HOXB5 1010A/G genotype	G1	G2–G3	aOR[a] (95%CI[b])	p
	N[c] (%)	N (%)		
AA	51 (37.8%)	32 (12.5%)	Ref	
AG	68 (50.4%)	163 (63.7%)	3.82 (2.26–6.48)	0.001
GG	16 (11.9%)	61 (23.8%)	6.07 (2.99–12.31)	0.001
AG+GG (against AA)	84 (62.2%)	224 (87.5%)	4.25 (2.58–7.07)	<0.001
AG+AA (against GG)	119 (88.1%)	195 (76.2%)	0.40 (0.22–0.73)	0.003

[a]age-adjusted odds ratio,
[b]95% confidence interval,
[c]Numbers of people.

Table 2. Genotype frequencies of the HOXB5 polymorphism in bladder cancer subgroups (Non-muscle invasive and Muscle-invasive groups).

HOXB5 1010A/G genotype	Non-muscle invasive	Muscle-invasive	aOR[a] (95%CI[b])	p
	N[c] (%)	N (%)		
AA	59 (26.8%)	24 (14%)	Ref	
AG	119 (54.1%)	112 (65.5%)	2.31 (1.35–3.47)	0.002
GG	42 (19.1%)	35 (20.5%)	2.05 (1.06–3.94)	0.031
AG+GG (against AA)	161 (73.2%)	147 (85.9%)	2.25 (1.33–3.79)	0.003
AG+AA (against GG)	178 (80.9%)	136 (79.5%)	0.91 (0.56–1.51)	0.917

[a]age-adjusted odds ratio,
[b]95% confidence interval,
[c]Numbers of people.

of HOXB5 mRNA in the cells with the GG genotype was 3.5 fold (11 h) than the mRNA half-life (3.4 h) in the cells with the AA genotype (Figure 5B), indicating that the mRNA with the G allele was more stable than the mRNA with the A allele. This different stability on the two mRNAs may be the possible mechanism that explains the different effect of the SNP on HOXB5 expression.

The Binding Activity of miR-7 for Different Alleles of mRNA affects HOXB5 Expression Level

We transfected miR-7 to a bladder cancer cell line (5637) with the heterozygous GA genotype for 48 hours and measured the HOXB5 mRNA level using the Taqman assay. We observed that the overexpression of miR-7 could significantly inhibit the expression level of HOXB5 mRNA compared with the NC group? Interestingly, the expression level of the HOXB5 mRNA with the A allele decreased much more than the level of the mRNA with the G allele (Figure 5C), indicating that the binding of miR-7 to the HOXB5 mRNA with the A allele was greater than the mRNA with the G allele.

To validate our hypothesis, we carried out a luciferase assay. The relative luciferase activity was suppressed much more in the reporter containing the 1010A transfected with miR-7 than that containing the 1010G allele (Figure 5D). These results showed that the binding activity of miR-7 with either the 1010A or 1010G allele may be another important mechanism involved in the different HOXB5 expression levels affected by the SNP.

The Association between the 1010A/G HOXB5 Genotype Frequency and Bladder Cancer

Next, we examined the association between 1010A/G HOXB5 genotype frequency and the clinical features of bladder cancer. DNA was extracted from 391 patients with bladder cancer that was confirmed by pathologists, and from 391 normal controls, and the SNP (1010A/G) genotypes for each sample were analyzed. We found that G allele (AG+GG) genotypes were associated with the risk of high grade (Grade 2 and 3, aOR = 4.25, p<0.001, Table 1) and high stage (T2–T4, muscle invasive type, aOR = 2.25, p = 0.003, Table 2) cancers as against low grade (Grade1) and low stage (T1, non-muscle invasive type) cancers. We also showed that the frequency of G genotypes (AG+GG) was higher in bladder cancer group compared with the normal controls (aOR = 1.48, p = 0.017) (Table 3).

Discussion

The HOX gene family has recently been identified as one of the main factors in the normal development of the human organs. The HOXB5 gene, which was found to be involved in lung and gut development, was reported to be an important factor in human disease, including cancers [14]. Here, we showed that the HOXB5 gene was frequently over-expressed in human bladder cancer tissues and in cancer cell lines. In vitro experiments showed that HOXB5 may act as an oncogene in human bladder cancer. We found a SNP (1010 A/G) in the 3′-UTR of the HOXB5 gene, which was also within a miRNA-7 binding site. We observed that this SNP could affect the expression of the HOXB5 gene.

Table 3. Genotype frequencies of the HOXB5 polymorphism in controls and bladder cancer groups.

HOXB5 1010A/G genotype	Controls	Bladder cancer	aOR[a] (95%CI[b])	p
	N[c] (%)	N (%)		
AA	113 (28.6%)	83 (21.2%)	Ref	
AG	195 (50.4%)	231 (59.1%)	1.58 (1.12–2.22)	0.009
GG	83 (21%)	77 (19.7%)	1.263 (0.83–1.92)	0.276
AG+GG (against AA)	278 (71.4%)	308 (78.8%)	1.487 (1.07–2.06)	0.017
AG+AA (against GG)	308 (79%)	314 (80.3%)	0.922 (0.65–1.31)	0.646

[a]age-adjusted odds ratio,
[b]95% confidence interval,
[c]Numbers of people.

Accordingly, we proposed that miR-7 binding activity and mRNA stability which can be affected by SNP may be involved in the differential expression of HOXB5. Finally, the frequency of 1010G genotype was higher in bladder cancer group compared to normal controls, and was related to the risk of high grade and high stage bladder cancers.

Homeobox genes code for transcription factors that are primarily involved in embryonic development. Several homeobox gene families, including HOX, EMX, PAX, MSX and many isolated divergent homeobox genes have been identified. The HOX gene family is the one that has most often been found to play a role in regulating network structure organization [22]. Over 10 years ago, the HOX genes were found to control embryonic organ-specific patterning. During embryogenesis, these genes were shown to code for transcription factors that regulate the expression of subordinate genes [23]. The HOX gene family was also found to be involved in human tumorigenesis [6,7,8,9]. Among HOX gene family, HOXB5 gene has been found to play a role in the patterning of airway branches during mouse lung morphogenesis in Volpe et al's study [10]. Later, they found HOXB5 gene was also related to human lung morphogenesis and may play a role in controlling airway patterning [19]. The HOXB5 gene was found to related with vasculogenesis by its interaction with vascular endothelial growth factor receptor-2 (VEGFR-2) and angiopoietin-2 (Ang2) [24,25], indicating that HOXB5 may be involved in tumorigenesis. Until now, the biological function of HOXB5 in human bladder cancer has not been reported. In the present study, we found that HOXB5 was over-expressed in human bladder cancer and our *in vitro* experiment showed that HOXB5 may act as an oncogene in bladder cancer.

In recent years, genome-wide association studies (GWAS) have given us a deeper insight into the mechanisms related to genomic changes in various cancers. Chang *et al.* identified several susceptibility loci in human bladder cancer, including rs9642880 (nearest gene: MYC), rs710521 (nearest gene: TP63), and rs2294008 (nearest gene: PSCA) among others [26].

The involvement of miRNAs in human cancer has been discovered recently. In a previous study, we reported that miRNA-143 and miRNA-125b act as tumor suppressors in human bladder cancer by binding to the oncogenes RAS and E2F3 respectively [15,16]. 3'-UTR polymorphisms in certain genes have been reported to related with human disease, including hereditary thrombophilia [27], urolithiasis [28], and increased sensitivity to 5-fluorouracil chemotherapy [29]. SNPs in miRNA-binding sites have recently been discovered. Yu et al. conducted a genome-wide analysis of SNPs located in the miRNA-binding sites of the 3'-UTR of various human genes associated with human cancers. They found 1,265 SNPs that were located within the miRNA-binding sites, and suggested that these SNPs may affect expression of the miRNA binding target [30]. Mishra et al. showed that SNP 829C/T located within the miRNA-24 binding site of the 3'-UTR of the DHFR gene led to overexpression of its target gene and resulted in resistance to methotrexate [21]. In a previous study from our group, we reported that the Mel-18 gene functioned as a tumor suppressor in prostate cancer, and a SNP (1805A/G) in the miRNA-181a binding site

correlated with Mel-18 expression and clinical features in prostate cancer [18].

Until now, no SNPs in miRNA-binding sites have been reported in human bladder cancer. MiR-7 was shown to be down-regulated in human glioblastoma and bladder cancer and a further study showed that miR-7 may suppress tumor growth in human bladder cancer by inhibiting growth factor receptor expression and by impairing the antiapoptotic Akt-pathway [17]. Bioinformatics analyses predicted a miR-7-binding SNP (1010A/G) within the 3'-UTR of the HOXB5 gene. Here, we reported a SNP (1010A/G) that was located within the miR-7 binding site of the 3'-UTR of the HOXB5 gene, and found that the different SNP (A or G) genotype could affect HOXB5 mRNA expression. Many 3'-UTR polymorphisms had been shown related with altered gene expression, but the possible mechanisms were not fully understood [21]. We propose that the SNP (1010A/G) may affect the expression of HOXB5 in bladder cancer by differential mRNA stability and binding activity of miR-7. Furthermore, multivariate logistic regression analysis showed that genotypes with the G allele (GG and AG) were associated with the risk of high grade (Grade 2 and 3, aOR = 4.25, p<0.001) and high stage (T2–T4, muscle invasive type, aOR = 2.25, p = 0.003) cancers. We also showed that compared with normal controls, the genotypes with the G allele were associated with the risk of bladder cancer (aOR = 1.48, p = 0.017). These results suggested that the SNP located within the miR-7 binding sites may affect HOXB5 expression, which in turn may affect bladder tumorigenesis. In addition, this SNP may have the potential to become a prognostic factor for bladder cancer.

miRNA binding site polymorphisms have only recently been investigated. These polymorphisms may not only affect gene expression, but could also have a relationship with clinical features of cancer or even with the prognosis of cancer. In future studies, we intend to source many more bladder cancer cases and use them to carry out a longer-term study to discover whether or not this SNP (rs9299) could be a good prognostic and prognosis factor for bladder cancer.

In summary, in this study we showed for the first time that the HOXB5 gene may act as an oncogene in human bladder cancer. We found that a SNP (1010A/G) within the miR-7 binding site of HOXB5 3'-UTR affects HOXB5 expression and this SNP may be correlated with bladder tumorigenesis and the risk of high grade and high stage human bladder cancers. These results suggested a possible mechanism for the effects of the miRNA binding site polymorphism during bladder tumorigenesis and revealed a possible prognostic and prognosis factor for bladder cancer.

Acknowledgments

The authors thank Zhiping Chen (Department of Urology, Southwest Hospital, Chongqing, China) for giving us cancer samples.

Author Contributions

Conceived and designed the experiments: TL JH. Performed the experiments: JL QC HZ. Analyzed the data: JL WW EC CN. Contributed reagents/materials/analysis tools: WD WH HY HH. Wrote the paper: JL TL. Proof read and approved of final version: TL.

References

1. Yu S, Zan MF, Xia M (2004) General description of urothelial tumors of the bladder. In: Wu JP. Urology. Jinan: Shan Dong Science and Technology. pp. 959–81.

2. Messing EM (2007) Urothelial tumors of the bladder. In: Wein AJ, Kavoussi LR, Novick AC, Partin AW, Peters CA. In: Campbell-Walsh Urology: WB Saunders Co. pp. 2407–46.

3. Feber A, Clark J, Goodwin G, Dodson AR, Smith PH, et al. (2004) Amplification and overexpression of E2F3 in human bladder cancer. Oncogene 23: 1627–30.

4. Stein S, Fritsch R, Lemaire L, Kessel M (1996) Checklist: vertebrate homeobox genes. Mech Dev 55: 91–108.

5. Gehring WJ, Hiromi Y (1986) Homeotic genes and the homeobox. Annu Rev Genet 20: 147–73.

6. Raman V, Martensen SA, Reisman D, Evron E, Odenwald WF, et al. (2000) Compromised HOXA5 function can limit p53 expression in human breast tumours. Nature 405: 974–78.

7. Drabkin HA, Parsy C, Ferguson K, Guilhot F, Lacotte L, et al. (2002) Quantitative HOX expression in chromosomally defined subsets of acute myelogenous leukemia. Leukemia 16: 186–95.

8. Cillo C, Barba P, Freschi G, Bucciarelli G, Magli MC, et al. (1992) Hox gene expression in normal and neoplastic human kidney. Int. J. Cancer 51: 892–7.

9. Cantile M, Cindolo L, Napodano G, Altieri V, Cillo C (2003) Hyperexpression of locus C genes in the HOX network is strongly associated in vivo with human bladder transitional cell carcinomas. Oncogene 22: 6462–8.

10. Volpe MV, Martin A, Vosatka RJ, Mazzoni CL, Nielsen HC (1997) Hoxb-5 expression in the developing mouse lung suggests a role in branching morphogenesis and epithelial cell fate. Histochem Cell Biol 108: 495–504.

11. Giampaolo A, Sterpetti P, Bulgarini D, Samoggia P, Pelosi E, et al. (1994) Key functional role and lineage-specific expression of selected HOXB genes in purified hematopoietic progenitor differentiation. Blood 84: 3637–47.

12. Wang X, Wolgemuth DJ, Baxi LV (2011) Overexpression of HOXB5, Cyclin D1 and PCNA in Congenital Cystic Adenomatoid Malformation. Fetal Diagn Ther 29: 315–20.

13. Volpe MV, Chung E, Ulm JP, Gilchrist BF, Ralston S, et al. (2009) Aberrant cell adhesion molecule expression in human bronchopulmonary sequestration and congenital cystic adenomatoid malformation. Am J Physiol Lung Cell Mol Physiol 297: L143–52.

14. Morgan R, Plowright L, Harrington KJ, Michael A, Pandha HS (2010) Targeting HOX and PBX transcription factors in ovarian cancer. BMC Cancer 10: 89.

15. Lin T, Dong W, Huang J, Pan Q, Fan X, et al. (2009) MicroRNA-143 as a tumor suppressor for bladder cancer. J Urol 181: 1372–80.

16. Huang L, Luo J, Cai Q, Pan Q, Zeng H, et al. (2011) MicroRNA-125b suppresses the development of bladder cancer by targeting E2F3. Int J Cancer 128: 1758–69.

17. Veerla S, Lindgren D, Kvist A, Frigyesi A, Staaf J, et al. (2009) MiRNA expression in urothelial carcinomas: Important roles of miR-10a, miR-222, miR-125b, miR-7 and miR-452 for tumor stage and metastasis, and frequent homozygous losses of miR-31, Int. J. Cancer 124: 2236–42.

18. Wang W, Yuasa T, Tsuchiya N, Ma Z, Maita S, et al. (2009) The novel tumor-suppressor Mel-18 in prostate cancer: its functional polymorphism, expression and clinical significance. Int J Cancer 125: 2836–43.

19. Volpe MV, Pham L, Lessin M, Ralston SJ, Bhan I, et al. (2003) Expression of Hoxb-5 During Human Lung Development and in Congenital Lung Malformations. Birth Defects Research 67: 550–6.

20. Hamamoto R, Furukawa Y, Morita M, Iimura Y, Silva FP, et al. (2004) SMYD3 encodes a histone methyltransferase involved in the proliferation of cancer cells. Nat Cell Biol 6: 731–40.

21. Mishra PJ, Humeniuk R, Mishra PJ, Longo-Sorbello GS, Banerjee D, et al. (2007) A miR-24 microRNA binding-site polymorphism in dihydrofolate reductase gene leads to methotrexate resistance. Proc Natl Acad Sci U S A 104: 13513–8.

22. Cillo C, Cantile M, Faiella A, Boncinelli E (2001) Homeobox Genes in Normal and Malignant Cells. Journal of Cellular Physiology 188: 161–9.

23. Krumlauf R (1994) Hox genes in vertebrate development. Cell 78: 191–201.

24. Wu Y, Moser M, Bautch VL, Patterson C (2003) HoxB5 is an upstream transcriptional switch for differentiation of the vascular endothelium from precursor cells. Mol Cell Biol 23: 5680–91.

25. Winnik S, Klinkert M, Kurz H, Zoeller C, Heinke J, et al. (2009) HoxB5 induces endothelial sprouting in vitro and modifies intussusceptive angiogenesis in vivo involving angiopoietin-2. Cardiovasc Res 83: 558–65.

26. Wu X, Hildebrandt MA, Chang DW (2009) Genome-wide association studies of bladder cancer risk: a field synopsis of progress and potential applications. Cancer Metastasis Rev 28: 269–80.

27. Gehring NH, Frede U, Neu-Yilik G, Hundsdoerfer P, Vetter B, et al. (2001) Increased efficiency of mRNA 3' end formation: a new genetic mechanism contributing to hereditary thrombophilia. Nat Genet 28: 389–92.

28. Tsai FJ, Lin CC, Lu HF, Chen HY, Chen WC (2002) Urokinase gene 3'-UTR T/C polymorphism is associated with urolithiasis. Urology 59: 458–61.

29. Lu JW, Gao CM, Wu JZ, Cao HX, Tajima K, et al. (2006) Polymorphism in the 3'-untranslated region of the thymidylate synthase gene and sensitivity of stomach cancer to fluoropyrimidine-based chemotherapy. J Hum Genet 51: 155–60.

30. Yu Z, Li Z, Jolicoeur N, Zhang L, Fortin Y, et al. (2007) Aberrant allele frequencies of the SNPs located in microRNA target sites are potentially associated with human cancers. Nucleic Acids Res 35: 4535–41.

11

Atomic Force Microscopy Reveals a Role for Endothelial Cell ICAM-1 Expression in Bladder Cancer Cell Adherence

Valérie M. Laurent[1,2]*, Alain Duperray[3,4,5], Vinoth Sundar Rajan[3,4,5], Claude Verdier[1,2]

1 Univ. Grenoble Alpes, LIPHY, F-38000, Grenoble, France, **2** CNRS, LIPHY, F-38000, Grenoble, France, **3** INSERM, IAB, F-38000, Grenoble, France, **4** Univ. Grenoble Alpes, IAB, F-38000, Grenoble, France, **5** CHU de Grenoble, IAB, F-38000, Grenoble, France

Abstract

Cancer metastasis is a complex process involving cell-cell interactions mediated by cell adhesive molecules. In this study we determine the adhesion strength between an endothelial cell monolayer and tumor cells of different metastatic potentials using Atomic Force Microscopy. We show that the rupture forces of receptor-ligand bonds increase with retraction speed and range between 20 and 70 pN. It is shown that the most invasive cell lines (T24, J82) form the strongest bonds with endothelial cells. Using ICAM-1 coated substrates and a monoclonal antibody specific for ICAM-1, we demonstrate that ICAM-1 serves as a key receptor on endothelial cells and that its interactions with ligands expressed by tumor cells are correlated with the rupture forces obtained with the most invasive cancer cells (T24, J82). For the less invasive cancer cells (RT112), endothelial ICAM-1 does not seem to play any role in the adhesion process. Moreover, a detailed analysis of the distribution of rupture forces suggests that ICAM-1 interacts preferentially with one ligand on T24 cancer cells and with two ligands on J82 cancer cells. Possible counter receptors for these interactions are CD43 and MUC1, two known ligands for ICAM-1 which are expressed by these cancer cells.

Editor: Andrew Pelling, University of Ottawa, Canada

Funding: The sources of funding that have supported the work are Nanosciences Foundation, ANR Transmig, La Ligue contre le cancer, LabeX Tec21. The funders had no role in study design, data collection and analysis, decision to publish, or preparation of the manuscript.

Competing Interests: The authors have declared that no competing interests exist.

* E-mail: valerie.laurent@ujf-grenoble.fr

Introduction

Adhesive interactions of cancer cells with the endothelium are key events in the metastasis process (i.e. the dispersion of cancer cells from one organ to other parts of the body) [1,2]. During the formation and growth of tumors, cancer cells manage to escape from primary tumors and penetrate the blood flow, thus can travel over long distances. At distant sites within the human body, cancer cells interact with the endothelium, adhere and eventually extravasate, i.e. migrate through the endothelial barrier. Leukocytes and cancer cells use similar mechanisms for interacting with endothelial cells (ECs), but while the phenomena of adhesion and migration of leukocytes through the endothelium has been particularly studied during inflammation, few results are available regarding the role of the key molecules involved in the adhesion and transmigration of cancer cells [1,3,4,5].

Similarly to leukocyte recruitment, tethering and rolling of tumor cells (TCs) on the endothelium have been demonstrated for some cancer cells and are mediated by selectins. After this initial interaction, firm adhesion takes place, mediated by several cell adhesion molecules belonging to the integrin family [6] as well as the Intercellular Adhesion Molecule-1 (ICAM-1) and Vascular Cell Adhesion Molecule-1 (VCAM-1) from the immunoglobulin family, leading to tumor invasion [7,8]. VCAM-1 is expressed by the endothelium after stimulation, and interacts with the $\alpha4\beta1$ integrin, while ICAM-1 is expressed by ECs, leukocytes and some TCs, and can be upregulated by inflammatory cytokines. ICAM-1 is involved in leukocyte adhesion to the endothelium through its interactions with LFA-1 and Mac-1 leukocyte integrins ($\beta2$ integrin). TCs lack $\beta2$ integrins, but neutrophils can act as a bridge between TCs and ECs, with LFA-1 on leukocytes binding to ICAM-1 expressed on both endothelial and TCs [5]. In addition, ICAM-1 is a receptor for other molecules, such as CD43 [9] and MUC1 [10], which are expressed by some TCs.

Cancer progression is associated with alterations in the expression of some adhesive molecules. Some works investigated the relationship between the N-cadherin expression and the progression of tumor malignancy [11,12]. An increase of cancer cell invasiveness is combined with switching of E-cadherin by N-cadherin and an increase in the expression of some integrin subunits [13]. From a quantitative point of view, the comparison of adhesive properties in non-malignant and malignant epithelial bladder cells have shown that an enhanced N-cadherin level in T24 malignant cells was accompanied by changes in unbinding properties of individual N-cadherin molecules [14]. In addition, the ICAM-1 expression has been associated with a more aggressive tumour phenotype [15,16]. Nevertheless, the ligands involved in the firm adhesion of TC are not yet as clearly defined as for leukocytes, and the quantification of such adhesive interactions between ECs and cancer cells has not been investigated so far.

Quantitative information on the cell adhesive forces can be obtained using different force spectroscopy techniques: the biomembrane force probe [17], optical tweezers [18] and the atomic force microscope (AFM) [19]. All these techniques operating under an optical microscope allow to visualise the cells and simultaneously measure adhesion forces from a few pN to a few hundreds pN or more. In this work, we choose to use the single-cell force spectroscopy mode of the AFM to study cell-cell interactions involved in the adhesion of TCs on ECs. In contrast with other methods of adhesion strength, this technique allows to carry out measurements in a configuration close to the *in vivo* situation. A cancer cell is attached to a soft cantilever and put in contact with an EC-monolayer and the force signal is monitored thanks to the AFM cantilever deflection [19,20]. The signal also allows detecting events such as possible breakups of receptor-ligand bonds as well as the global adhesion strength at the cell level.

Determination of cell-cell interactions was carried out for different cantilever retraction speeds to study how rupture force (involved in cell-cell adhesive bonds) is modified. We investigated the relationship between the measured receptor-ligand bonds and the corresponding metastatic potential of human bladder cancer cells, in order to determine the adhesive signature of such cancer cells. Finally, we show that the ICAM-1 receptor on the ECs acts as a key mediator for the adhesive interaction with the most invasive cancer cells. Our findings indicate that the more invasive bladder cancer cells interact thanks to one or two types of ICAM-1 ligands: CD43 and MUC1 are good candidates, as demonstrated by flow cytometry experiments. This knowledge about such interactions is essential for the understanding of cancer cell adhesion to the endothelium, a mechanism leading to invasion and metastasis.

Materials and Methods

Cells and cell culture

Three bladder cell lines were used in this study: RT112, T24 and J82 (ATCC, Rockville, MD). These cell lines represent progression from well to poorly differentiated phenotypes and arise from superficial to invasive epithelial human bladder cancer. RT112 cancer cells are moderately differentiated and are characterized by a cytological grade 2 (or differentiation) [21]. T24 and J82 cancer cells are poorly differentiated and characterized by a cytological grade 3. To distinguish cancer cells from HUVECs, cancer cells were transfected with a plasmid expressing GFP (Green Fluorescent Protein – pEGFP). Human Vascular Umbilical Endothelial Cells (HUVECs) were purchased from Promocell (Heidelberg, Germany). Cancer cells were grown at 37°C in a humidified 5% CO_2 atmosphere, in RPMI 1640 medium supplemented with 10% fetal calf serum, 100 UI/mL penicillin and 100 μg/mL streptomycin (complete RPMI medium). ECs were maintained in Promocell culture medium. The ECs were plated in complete culture medium on glass coverslips coated with collagen I (BD Biosciences, Le pont de Claix, France) and left 3 days to spread in order to achieve confluence. For AFM experiments, the culture medium was supplemented with HEPES (20 mM, pH 7.4).

Atomic Force Microscopy

We used a Nanowizard II AFM (JPK Instruments, Berlin, Germany) mounted on a Zeiss microscope (Carl Zeiss, Jena, Germany). This configuration allows to carry out AFM measurements and simultaneously observe the cells using phase contrast or fluorescence modes. This AFM is also equipped with the 'CellHesion' module (JPK Instruments, Berlin, Germany). This module enables a long-range vertical displacement of the stage up to 100 μm which makes force spectroscopy measurements possible including cell-cell interactions. In parallel, a vertical piezo-translator (PIFOC, Physik Instrumente, Karlsruhe, Germany) is mounted on the microscope objective to move the objective

concurrently with the microscope stage and focus on cells while carrying out AFM measurements. All the measurements were carried out at 37°C using the Petri Dish Heater (JPK Instruments, Berlin, Germany).

Cantilever coating

Soft cantilevers were V-shaped ones without tips (MLCT-O, Bruker, France). They were calibrated using the thermal fluctuations analysis method [22] and exhibit a spring constant close to 0.01 N/m. To enable the adhesion of cancer cells to the cantilever, the latter was functionalized using biotin-conA (Interchim, Montluçon, France) [23]. After rinsing with PBS, cantilevers were incubated overnight at 37°C in biotin-BSA (Interchim, Montluçon, France) (0.5 mg/ml), rinsed again in PBS and then incubated in streptavidin (Interchim, Montluçon, France) (0.5 mg/ml) for 10 minutes. Finally, cantilevers were rinsed with PBS and set into a biotin-conA drop during 10 minutes then rinsed with PBS. This molecule allows binding of cancer cells to the cantilevers with a force larger than the cell-cell detachment force in our study: biotin-conA adheres to the cancer cell membrane with a detachment force of 2 nN [20], while the detachment force relevant in the interaction between cancer cell and EC is on the order of 1 nN.

Cancer cell capture

Cancer cells were grown in culture flasks, then were detached just before the AFM experiments, using a trypsin/EDTA solution (0.05% trypsin and 0.53 mM EDTA). RPMI medium with serum was added to the cells to block the effect of trypsin. Finally, cells were centrifuged and resuspended in medium without serum. Cancer cells were deposited in a Petri dish onto which an EC monolayer had been grown, and settled for a few seconds. Cell capture consisted in positioning the cantilever tip above a cancer cell (since cancer cells were fluorescent, they could be distinguished from ECs, see Figure 1), to come into contact with the cell during ten seconds with a force of 1 nN. Then the cantilever with the captured cell was retracted slowly at constant speed and the cell was kept in culture medium to rest for 15 minutes. Next, 1 ml of RPMI 1640 medium with serum was added. The cell was firmly bound to the cantilever and subsequently used to probe adhesion to ECs.

Force spectroscopy: analysis of cancer cell-EC interaction

First, the cancer cell was set above an EC. The cantilever was lowered at constant low speed (1 μm/s) to put the cancer cell in contact with the EC (above the nucleus). A compression force of 1 nN was applied to the EC during 10 seconds (Figure 1A) in order to create bonds and to reproduce firm adhesion. Finally, the cancer cell was retracted with a speed ranging between 0.5 μm/s to 20 μm/s. Measurement of the cantilever deflection during vertical motion was recorded during the different stages (Figure 1B). Typically, for one cancer cell-EC pair, a sequence of five force curves was obtained at five different retraction speeds (with a rest time of about 1 minute between each curve). Then the cancer cell was left at rest during ten minutes and moved above another EC to measure a sequence of five force curves again. Finally, each cancer cell was used three or four times, therefore fifteen or twenty such force curves (N = 15 or N = 20) were obtained. The measurements were then collected for various cancer cell lines, during similar experiments. A sketch of the typical retraction force in terms of the piezo displacement is presented in Figure 1C. The minimum point on the curve is the detachment force, i.e. the force necessary to separate the cancer cell from the EC. The detachment force is supported by the cell

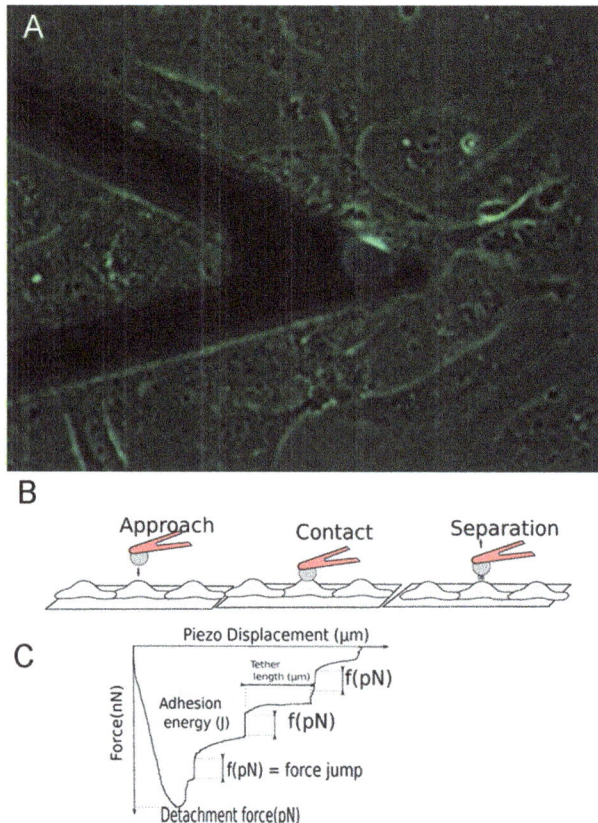

Figure 1. Interactions between cancer cells and ECs measured with AFM. A) Photograph of the cantilever with attached fluorescent cancer cell above the HUVEC monolayer. White scale bar corresponds to 20 µm. B) Sketch of the approach-retraction method and typical retraction force curve in terms of the piezo displacement. The cancer cell approaches the EC monolayer at constant speed. Then the cell comes into contact with the EC during 10 seconds (under 1 nN applied force) to create several bond complexes over the adhesion area. The cantilever is retracted at constant velocity in order to detach the adhesive bonds. The retraction curve shows force jumps corresponding to the rupture force (f) of bonds. The adhesive energy (shaded area) represents the detachment work done by the cantilever to completely detach the cell from the substrate. The detachment force is the force necessary to stretch the cancer cell and the EC until bonds start to detach. Note that some force jumps can follow a plateau corresponding to tether formation.

deformability, but also by the number and strength of adhesive bonds formed between cells. The different jumps in force correspond to the successive breakups of bonds involved during cell-cell interaction [24,25] and therefore represent rupture forces (i.e. receptor-ligand bonds). Note that a force jump can follow a plateau in force, corresponding to tether formation, whose extension is the plateau length. The retraction curve also provides information about the adhesion energy which is the work necessary to detach the cancer cell (shaded area in Figure 1C). This includes the work done to stretch the cells as well as the work done to break the molecular bonds [25]. All these parameters (detachment force, rupture force, adhesion energy) are obtained from the force curve using the Image Processing Software (JPK instrument, Berlin, Germany). For each set of conditions, AFM experiments were carried out about 9 times on 3 different days. Unless otherwise stated, data are reported as mean ± standard error of the mean. All statistical tests were performed using the R

software (2.14 release). Since the data are correlated, we used a Generalized Linear Mixed Model (GLMM). Differences between the parameters calculated on untreated and anti-ICAM-1-treated cells were tested by the mixed function of the afex package in R software.

Inhibition of ICAM-1 ligands on the ECs

Human monoclonal antibody to ICAM-1 [27] was used at a 30 µg/mL concentration. Before the AFM experiments, ECs were incubated for 15 minutes in the presence of the antibody at 37°C. Then cells were rinsed twice in PBS and incubated in 2 ml of culture medium.

Immobilization of ICAM-1 and BSA

A 20 µL aliquot of recombinant ICAM-1 (RD Systems, Lille, France) (25 µg/ml) in 0.1 M NaHCO$_3$ (pH 8.6) was adsorbed overnight at 4°C at the centre of the coverslip. Unbound proteins were removed by washing with PBS and 2 ml of complete RPMI 1640 medium were then added to the ICAM-1 coated dish before the AFM experiments.

For the BSA-coating protocol, a µL aliquot of BSA at 100 µg/ml in PBS was adsorbed 30 minutes at 37°C at the centre of the Petri dish. Unbound proteins were removed by washing with PBS and 2 ml of the complete RPMI medium were then added to the BSA coated dish before the AFM experiments.

Flow cytometry analysis of ICAM-1, MUC1 and CD43 expression and immunofluorescence staining

Expression levels of ICAM-1 (on the EC surface), MUC1 and CD43 (on the cancer cell surface) were analyzed by flow cytometry (Accuri C6 flow cytometer, BD Bio-sciences). Quantification was made by measuring the geometric mean fluorescence. For immunofluorescence staining, glass coverslips were coated with 25 µg/ml human fibronectin. Cells were fixed with 2% paraformaldehyde, and processed for indirect immunofluorescence microscopy.

For measuring expression levels of ICAM-1 and MUC1, ECs or cancer cells were incubated with the primary antibody and then with FITC-conjugated (goat anti-mouse IgG) secondary antibody (Jackson ImmunoResearch, USA). The primary antibodies are a Human monoclonal antibody to ICAM-1 [26] or an anti-MUC1 monoclonal antibody C595 (Santa Cruz Biotechnology, Santa Cruz, USA). The anti-MUC1 antibody recognizes a tetrapeptide motif within the protein core of the MUC1 molecule.

For CD43 expression level, cancer cells were incubated with a monoclonal antibody CD43-clone L10 labeled with FITC (Invitrogen, USA), which reacts with the extracellular domain.

Results

Adhesion of different cancer cell lines

To evaluate if cancer cell invasiveness is related to its adhesive properties, we carried out force spectroscopy measurements targeting the interaction between cancer cells (of different invasiveness) and ECs. The cancer cells arise from the following cell lines: RT112, T24 and J82. RT112 cells are the less invasive cells while T24 and J82 cells are the more invasive ones [21]. Force curves were performed between a cancer cell attached to the cantilever tip and a monolayer of ECs plated on a glass coverslip. Figure 2 shows typical force curves obtained during the interactions of the three cancer cell types (T24, J82 and RT112) with the ECs. Each retraction curve (retraction velocity V = 5 µm/s) shows several rupture events associated with the successive breaking of bonds involved during cell-cell interaction. Interestingly, the less invasive cells (RT112) present smaller rupture force steps as compared to most invasive cells (T24, J82). Moreover, the detachment force which is the minimum point (Figures 2A-B-C) of the curve is smaller for RT112 cells. Figures 2A-B-C also show the distribution of rupture forces detected for cancer cell interactions with ECs at V = 5 μm/s. These magnitudes [10–70 pN] are in the range of typical force values obtained for receptor-ligand bonds [23,27,28,29]. It is noteworthy that the three cell types exhibit different force values: measurements reveal an average rupture force of 29.6±0.8 pN for RT112, 34.0±0.9 pN for T24 and 44.2±1.1 pN for J82 (V = 5 μm/s). Note that the average rupture forces are smaller for RT112 cells which are the less invasive kind.

Adhesion energy and detachment force (cell level)

An important aspect to characterize the interaction of cancer cells to ECs is the adhesion energy which involves the whole cell contact area. The adhesion energy is derived through integration of the area below the curve F(z), where F is the force and z is the piezo displacement. The basis line is chosen as the final limiting value, after all bonds are detached. The JPK software allows to choose this value and then performs the integration. Therefore we investigated the adhesion energy as well as the detachment force (absolute value of the minimum force on retracting force curve, see Figure 1B) versus retraction speed (V). As shown in Figure 3, these two parameters increase with retraction speed. Regarding the adhesion energy, the most invasive J82 cells present larger values as compared to the T24 or RT112 cells. Moreover, this difference is confirmed by the detachment force values which are higher for J82 cells as compared to T24 and RT112 cells. In any case, detachment forces or adhesion energies are always smaller with the less invasive RT112 cell.

Effect of retraction speed on rupture force

The rupture force has been shown theoretically to depend on the logarithm of the loading rate of the cantilever [30]. To study the signature of each cancer cell line, one needs to analyze the force spectra of the three cancer cell types during their interaction with ECs (Figure 4). These spectra present force values depending

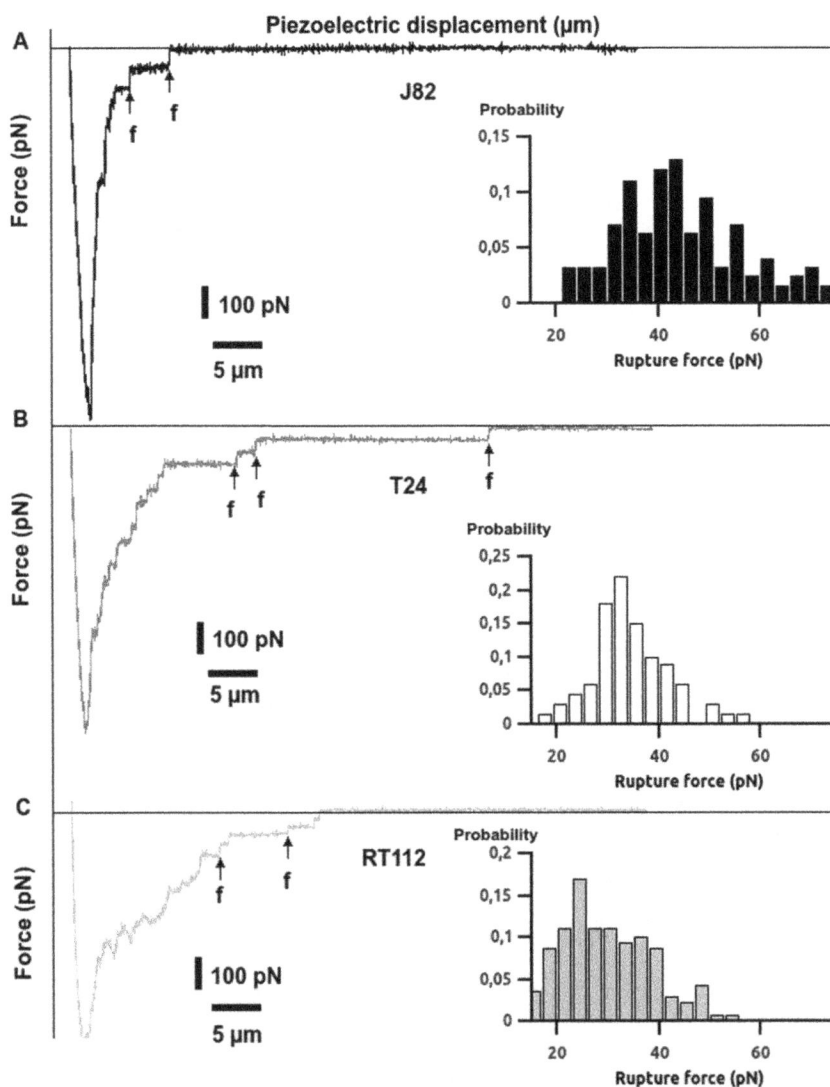

Figure 2. AFM force curves and rupture force histograms for different cancer cell lines. Typical force curves after 10s-contact between a TC and an EC on a HUVEC monolayer. Probability histograms with collected rupture forces f for J82 (A), T24 (B) and RT112 cells (C) at V = 5 μm/s. Vertical arrows denote examples of force jumps corresponding to breakup of receptor-ligand bonds.

A

B

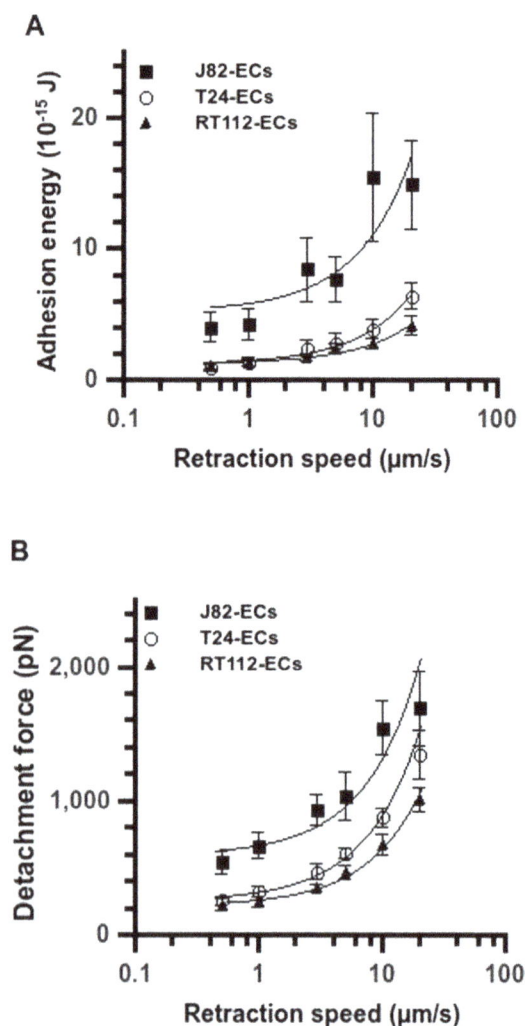

Figure 3. Adhesion energies and detachment forces for different cancer cell lines. Plot of the adhesion energy (A) and detachment force (B) vs. retraction speed after 10s-contact between a TC and an EC on a HUVEC monolayer. Three cancer cell lines: T24 (open circle), J82 (full square) and RT112 (full triangle). Data are plotted as mean ± standard error of the mean. The line is just a guide for the eye.

on the retraction speed or equivalently the loading rate r_f (N/s), equal to the product of the retraction speed V (m/s) times the spring constant k (N/m) of the cantilever, i.e. $r_f = kV$. Force values increase gradually with retraction speed and vary between 20.8±0.7 pN and 47.4±1.9 pN for RT112 cells, between 27.1±1.1 pN and 52.4±2.0 pN for T24 cells, and between 31.6±1.0 pN and 65.8±1.6 pN for J82 cells. For the three cancer cell lines, the average rupture force versus the logarithm of the retraction speed increases, but is not linear.

Measurement of specific and non specific adhesion forces for cancer cells

In a previous study, we showed that ICAM-1 was involved in TC extravasation [4]. To test the specific adhesion between cancer cells and ICAM-1 molecules, we carried out force spectroscopy experiments between a cancer cell attached to the tip of an AFM cantilever and immobilized ICAM-1 molecules on a glass dish. As shown in Figure 5, these measurements reveal that rupture forces are very close to the ones already obtained for cancer cell-EC

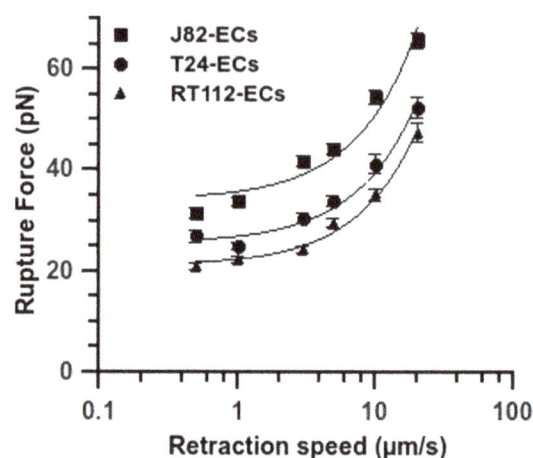

Figure 4. Rupture force vs. retraction velocity for different cancer cell lines. Relationship between rupture force and retraction speed after 10s-contact between a TC and an EC on a HUVEC monolayer. Three cancer cell lines: T24 (full circle), J82 (full square) and RT112 (full triangle) interacting with the endothelium. Data are plotted as mean ± standard error of the mean. The line is just a guide for the eye.

interaction [28]. The values are in the range of [20–70pN] for a retraction speed between 0.5 μm/s and 20 μm/s. To compare these values to the non specific adhesion forces, we also measured the rupture forces between TCs and a BSA-coated surface. The force level involved in the non specific adhesion is in the range of [10–45pN] which is much less important, around 40% to 70% of the specific binding force.

Role of the ICAM-1 receptor

As shown by confocal microscopy imaging (Figure 6A), the expression of ICAM-1 on unstimulated ECs is moderate. FACS analysis (Figure 6B) confirms the ICAM-1 expression level, when comparing the fluorescence levels of cells treated with an irrelevant antibody and with the anti-ICAM-1 antibody. To determine the relative contribution of the ICAM-1 receptor on cell-cell adhesion,

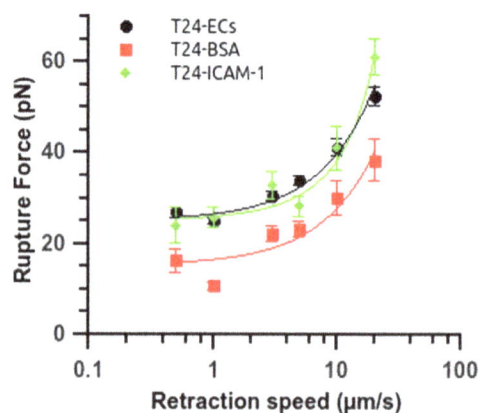

Figure 5. Control experiments for T24 cells interacting with recombinant ICAM-1 or BSA coated surfaces. Rupture force vs. retraction speed for T24 cells interacting either with a coated substrate or with ECs (circle). The substrate is coated with BSA 100 μg/ml (square) or recombinant ICAM-1 25 μg/ml (diamond). Data are plotted as mean ± standard error of the mean. The line is just a guide for the eye.

we examined the alteration of the adhesion forces when blocking this receptor with a specific monoclonal antibody. Figure 7 shows the effect of the antibody against ICAM-1 during the adhesion of the three cancer cell types with the ECs. Interestingly, inhibition of the EC ICAM-1 resulted in a significant decrease of the rupture forces for the more invasive cells only. For T24 cells, force averages varied between 27.1 pN and 52.4 pN (at different velocities) without blocking the ICAM-1 receptor, but between 14.4 pN and 35.7 pN, when blocking ICAM-1 (Figure 7A). This effect is also clearly visible on the box-whisker-plot obtained at a retraction speed of 5 μm/s (Figure 7 B). The anti-ICAM-1 antibody induces a significant decrease of the rupture force for T24 (from 34pN to 21.8 pN, see Figure 7B) and the value of 21.8 pN (+/−0.7) obtained after using of the antibody is comparable to the rupture force value of 23.3pN (+/−1.6) obtained for T24-BSA adhesion (see figure 7G). Therefore, after inhibition of ICAM-1, the rupture force level is typical of a non specific adhesion. This inhibition seems to be practically complete for T24 cells. For J82 cells, force averages vary between 31.6 pN and 65.8 pN without blocking ICAM-1 and between 17.7 pN and 58.1 pN when blocking ICAM-1. This effect of anti-ICAM-1 is clearly visible in the box-whisker plot of Figure 7D: the mean value decreases from 44.2 pN to 30.4 pN at a retraction speed of 5 μm/s. Finally, the adhesion of RT112 cells to ECs is not decreased in the presence of the anti-ICAM-1 antibody: the average values vary between 20.8 pN and 47.4 pN whereas they are between 21.1 pN and 58.6 pN when blocking ICAM-1. This non significant effect of the anti-ICAM-1 antibody is confirmed by the box-whisker plots (Figure 7F): the antibody does not induce any decrease in the rupture force. Therefore, an important reduction in binding forces for invasive cells (e.g. 35% for J82 and T24 cells) has been quantified here whatever the velocity, whereas there is no change in the case of the less invasive RT112 cell. This demonstrates clearly that ICAM-1 expressed by ECs plays a crucial role on the firm adhesion of the more invasive cells (J82 and T24).

Detailed analysis of rupture forces

Since we used average values of rupture forces which may hide the complexity of the adhesive bonds, a more detailed inspection of the force jumps (as shown using histograms) was carried out in order to gain more information. This analysis is given in Figure 8 where the TC-ECs or the TC-substrate (ICAM-1 or BSA) force jumps are recorded and presented using histograms, at a given velocity of 5 μm/s. Inspection of the histogram of T24-ECs rupture forces in Figure 8A (without the effect of anti-ICAM-1) reveals a Gaussian distribution centered at 32.9 pN (+/−5.8). Interestingly, this distribution of forces found for T24-EC interaction is quite similar to the one obtained during the interaction between T24 and the ICAM-1 coated-substrate (i.e. mean value = 28.8 pN +/− 5.1) (see histogram in Figure 8D). On the other hand, when the ECs have been treated with the anti-ICAM-1 antibody, the peak in Figure 8A almost disappears (the area under the curve is divided by a factor of ten). A new peak centered at 19 pN appears, similar to the value of 21.5 pN found for T24 interacting with the BSA-coated surface (Figure 8E) which can be attributed to non-specific interactions.

The histogram of J82-EC rupture forces reveals a distribution of a double Gaussian distribution: there are two peaks initially (42 pN and 70 pN) as can be seen by the large spectrum of force values. After incubation with the antibody, the last peak (70 pN) completely disappears whereas the first one (42 pN) is lowered by a factor of 3 (Figure 8B). We may conclude that ICAM-1 is expected to interact with two ligands on the J82 cell surface, and that the antibody inhibits both interactions, but preferentially one.

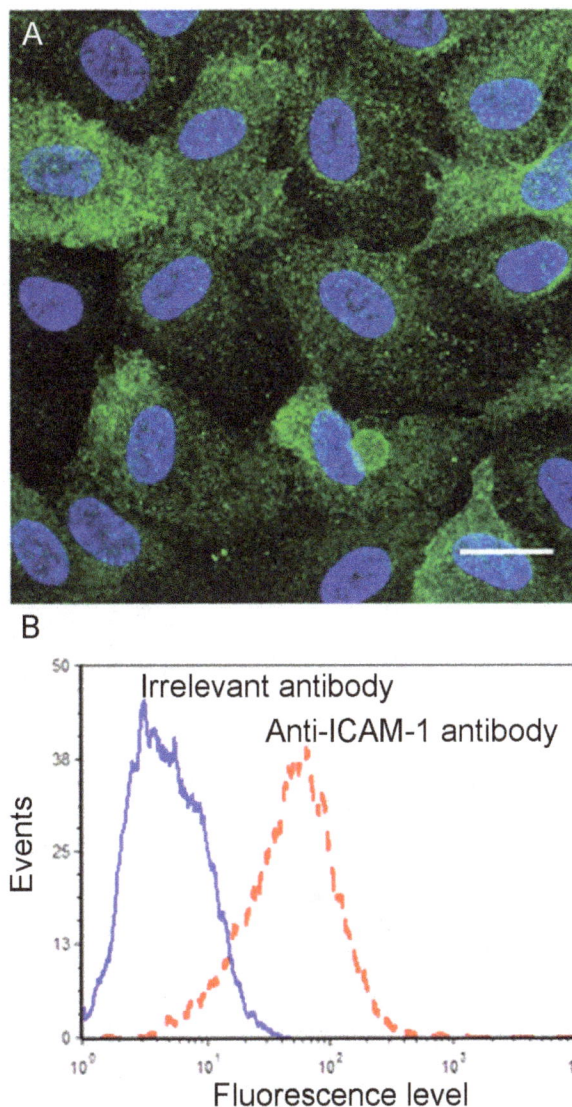

Figure 6. ICAM-1 expression on ECs. A) Confocal microscopy image of an EC monolayer stained for ICAM-1 (green). HUVECs were fixed with PFA. Nuclei are stained in blue using DAPI. **B)** Quantification of ICAM-1 levels by FACS analysis (dashed line) in comparison with an irrelevant antibody (solid line).

These bonds could be specific interactions with two different ligands for instance. In addition (Figure 8B), a new lower peak appears when using the antibody (≈28pN), whose value is very close to the one found for non-specific bonds.

The case of RT112 cell is different, as can be seen in Figure 8C. There is only one peak with and without the antibody located at similar levels (28 pN and 33 pN, no significant difference). The addition of anti-ICAM-1 antibody does not change the overall curve, therefore no clear effect is detected for RT112 cells, indicating that ICAM-1 is probably not involved in this adhesion process.

Analysis of ICAM-1 ligands (CD43 and MUC1) expression by invasive cells T24 and J82

Bladder cancer cells do not express the common ICAM-1 ligands, such as LFA-1 or Mac-1 [5]. On the other hand, the

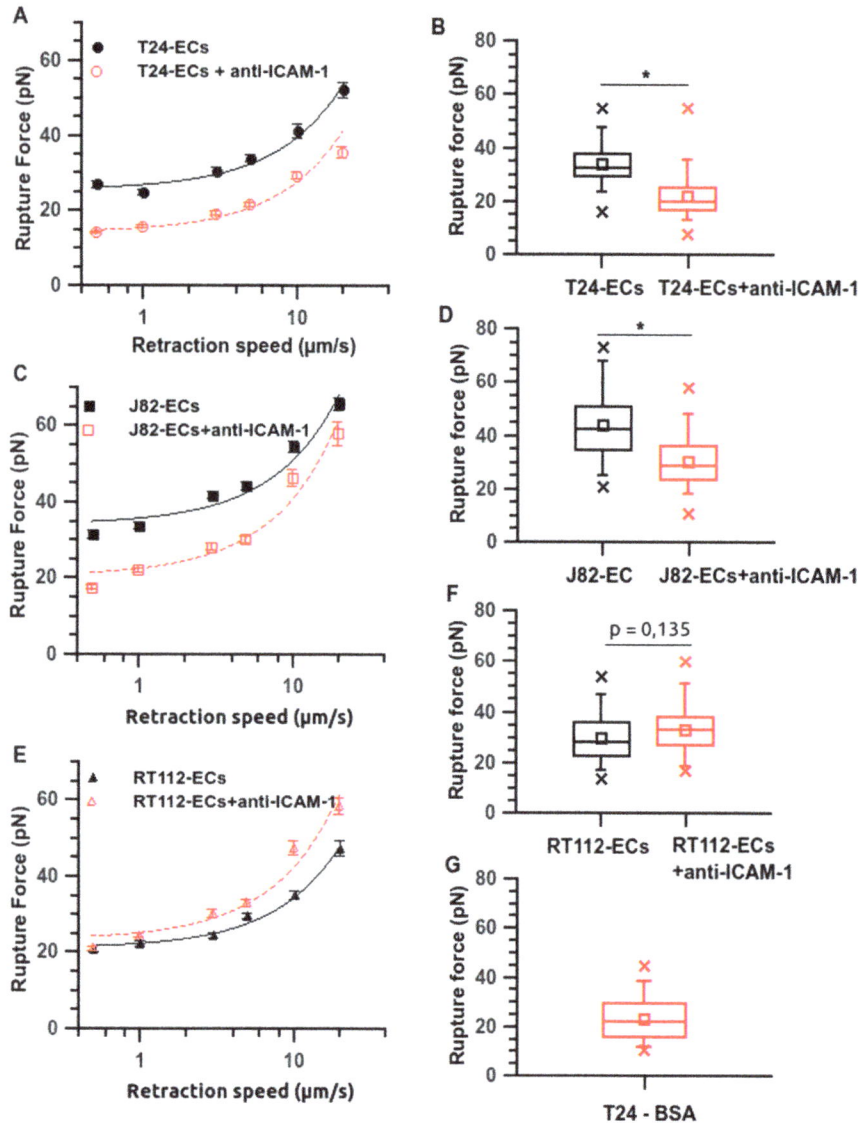

Figure 7. ICAM-1 is involved in the interaction between cancer cells and ECs. Rupture force vs. retraction speed after interaction between cancer cell and an EC, treated with an anti ICAM-1 antibody or not. Corresponding box-whisker plots show rupture forces at a retraction speed of 5 μm/s. (A, B) T24-EC, (C, D) J82-EC and (E, F) RT112-EC. As a comparison, the rupture force box plot is also shown for the T24-BSA interaction (panel G). For panels A, C and E, the line is just a guide for the eye. Data are plotted as mean ± standard error of the mean. Stars represent the p-value from GLMM statistical tests between parameters calculated on untreated and anti-ICAM-1-treated cells (*p≤0.05).

expression of MUC1 (Mucin 1) and CD43 (Leukosialin) were recently described as ICAM-1 ligands [31,10,9,32]. Therefore, we quantified their expression by flow cytometry. The results in Figure 9 show that T24 cells express only the CD43 ligand while J82 cells express both CD 43 and MUC1 ligands. Concerning RT112 cells, they express only the CD43 ligand. These results are discussed below.

Discussion

The mechanisms by which cells interact with the endothelium have been investigated in great details for leukocytes [20,33]. Experiments using AFM have proven to be very useful for studying these interactions allowing to quantify the adhesive forces between a single leukocyte and an endothelial monolayer. Moreover, this technique helps to identify the molecules involved

in the adhesion between cancer cells and the endothelium. Such experiments involving receptor-ligand bonds have been carried out by Zhang et al. [20,25] using leukocytes in contact with ECs to investigate the role of VCAM-1, ICAM-1, selectins, β_1 and β_3 integrins. A qualitative study on cancer cell-EC interactions using AFM was also made by Puech et al. [24] but they showed no detailed analysis about these kinds of interactions. Therefore, this work focuses on the possible adhesion molecules and forces involved during interactions between bladder cancer cells (T24, J82 and RT112) and an endothelial monolayer.

The method used here is similar to previous works [19,29,24], since we catch cancer cells with the cantilever and lower it to make contact with the ECs. Then we retract the cantilever, to capture the signature of receptor-ligand bonds from the force signals, as shown schematically in Figure 1 and in real experiments (Figure 2). One question here is to determine whether such receptor-ligand

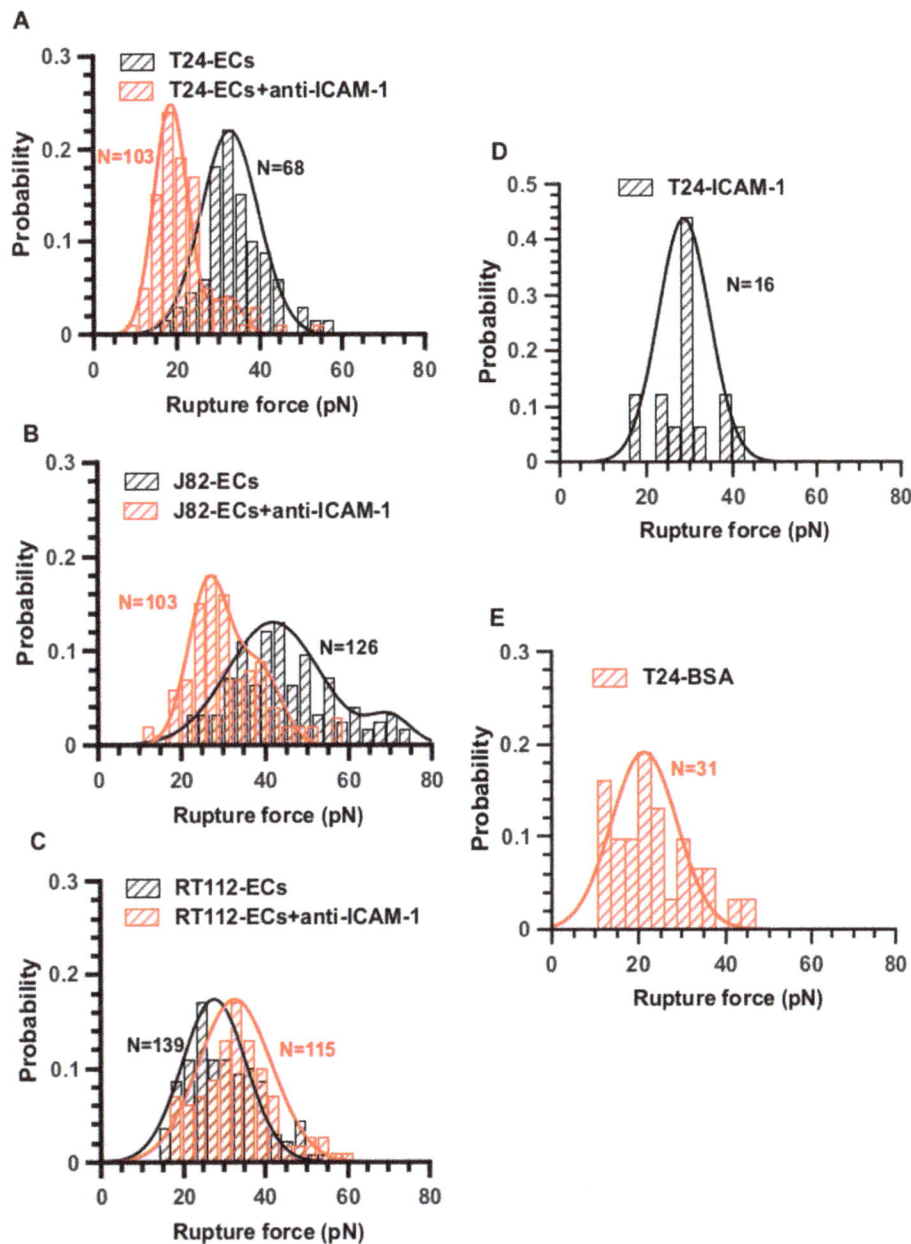

Figure 8. Distribution of rupture forces and effect of an anti-ICAM-1 antibody. Effect of an anti-ICAM-1 antibody on cancer-EC interactions. Rupture force distributions are Gaussian with one or two peaks revealing the presence of receptor/ligand bonds or non specific interactions. Probability histograms of rupture force (V = 5 μm/s) for (A) T24-HUVEC, (B) J82-HUVEC, (C) RT112-HUVEC. Black histograms represent interaction cancer-cell and EC without antibody whereas red ones show the force distribution after using the antibody. Panels D (T24-ICAM-1) and E (T24-BSA) show the rupture force probabilities for T24 cells in contact with coated substrates. The number N of events is indicated on the histograms.

bonds involve ICAM-1 when long tethers appear (Figure 1). Indeed Helenius et al. [28] showed that tethers usually correspond to the final part of the force curve, i.e. at long distances. Carpén et al. [34], on the other hand, showed possible connections of ICAM-1 to the cytoskeleton, suggesting the presence of bonds at shorter distances. In fact, this question still remains open as shown recently [35] since ICAM-1 can be found in filipodia, both on endothelial cells and on cells transfected with ICAM-1. This means that it is possible that tethers present ICAM-1 with or without any link with the cytoskeleton, and break far from the contact region, i.e. at large distances. Furthermore, it is possible that tethers may form on the cancer cell side. Finally, one may also consider the Jurkat

cell-endothelial cell case [20] where the formation of long tethers and high adhesion energies is attributed to the presence of adhesion molecules such as ICAM-1, which are inhibited by antibodies (around 40% inhibition for the anti-ICAM-1 antibody). Thus it will be considered here that most receptor-ligand bonds arise from the presence of ICAM-1.

In our experiments, values of the adhesion energies are exhibited (Figure 3) for the two cell lines RT112 and T24, very similar to other studies [20,25,36]. On the other hand, J82 cells show higher values ($\geq 4.0\ 10^{-15}$J) than the ones usually measured. This could be linked to the fact that they form two types of receptor-ligand bonds (Figures 8–9), as will be discussed below. In

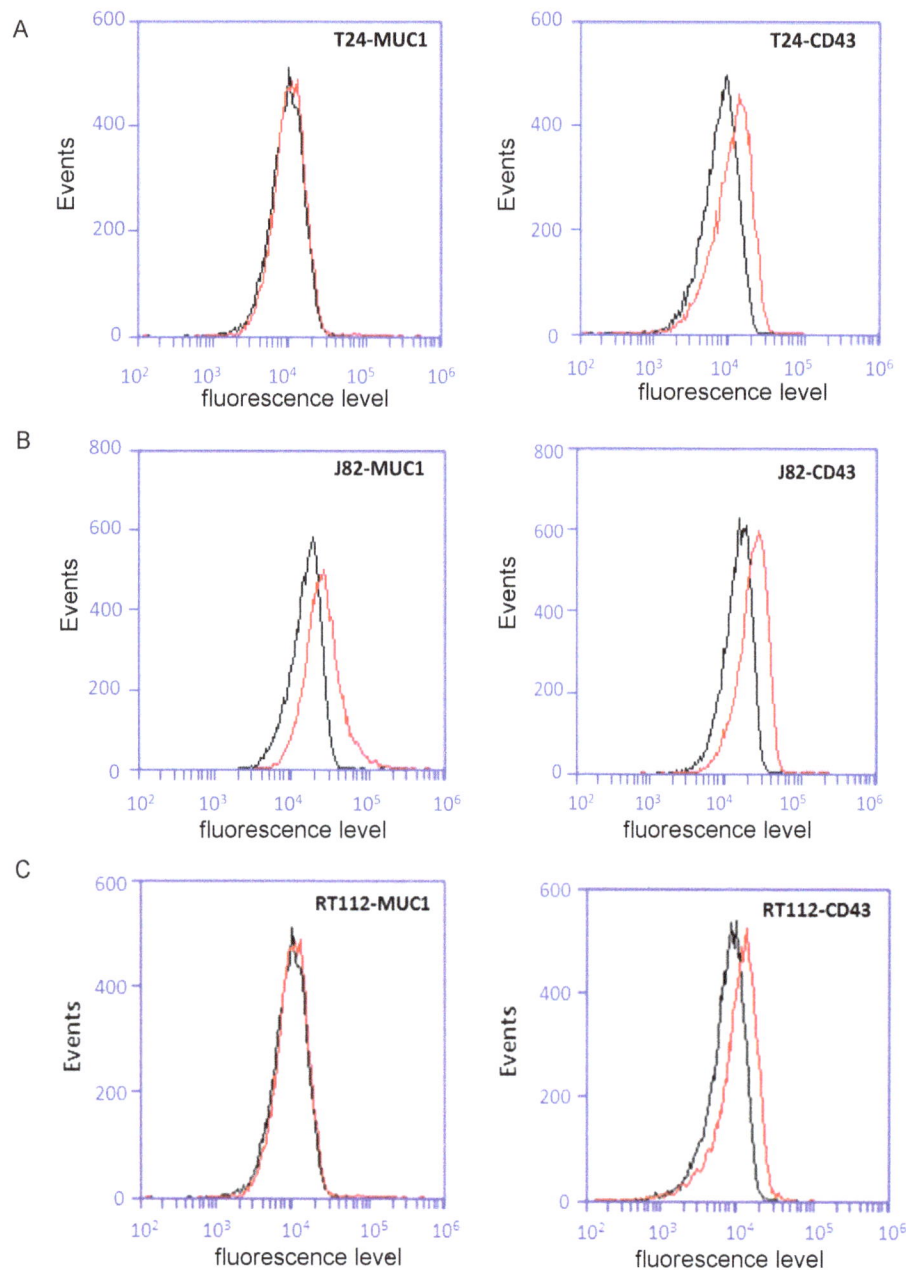

Figure 9. Expression of CD43 and MUC1 by the three bladder cell lines used in this study. Expression levels of CD43 and MUC1 (red line) by FACS analysis in comparison with an irrelevant antibody (black line): (A, D) T24 cells, (B, E) J82 cells and (C, F) RT112 cells.

addition, the detachment force increases with the retraction speed and is larger for the more invasive cells. This result shows that adhesion at the cell level is higher for the more invasive cells and does not depend on retraction speed. As mentioned in the literature, we may assume that these higher detachment forces obtained with the more invasive cells in AFM stretching experiments are associated with higher cell stiffness [37]. Indeed, complementary elasticity measurements (data not shown) on the cell body using a spherical AFM probe confirm that the more invasive cells are more rigid (elastic modulus $E = 493 \pm 138$ Pa for J82 cells, 351 ± 90 Pa for T24 cells and 246 ± 95 Pa for RT112 cells). But, as was discussed before, the contribution of adhesive events (breaking of receptor-ligand bonds) also plays a role in the global cell response.

Different levels of rupture forces are obtained (Figure 4), ranging between 20 and 70 pN. These values are similar to those previously obtained in other studies [28] for different types of receptor-ligand bonds like cadherin-cadherin [38,14], integrin-immunoglobulin [25,39] or selectin-mediated bonds [40]. It clearly appears that the cells with the higher metastatic capacity show higher rupture force levels. This difference in adhesion strength for the three cancer cell lines studied is valid whatever the retraction speed [0.5–20 μm/s]. These data suggest that for different types of cancer cells, either various receptor-ligand pairs are involved or these pairs are regulated differently with more or less affinity [41].

To shed light into these mechanisms, we investigated the distribution of rupture forces at different retraction speeds (i.e.

different loading rates), which exhibits multiple loading regimes, as seen by a continuous curve in the f-log(V) diagram (Figure 4). This behavior can be compared with the force-spectroscopy results obtained for leukocytes (expressing LFA-1) attached to substrates coated with ICAM-1 or ICAM-2 [42]. The meaning of the non-linear increase in rupture forces with retraction speed is related to the initial Bell's model [30] and its extensions by Evans and Richtie [43]. This theory predicts three different regimes of rupture force f vs. log(r_f). In the first regime, f increases slowly; then at intermediate velocities, the force increases linearly vs log(r_f) then we move into ultrafast regimes. Typically AFM data at classical velocities lie in the transition between the first two regimes where dependence is non-linear and increases monotonically. Only measurements on model systems (like streptavidin-biotin for example) exhibit a linear dependence. Usually with other receptor-ligand bonds, the response is always non-linear, and is more complex due to possible effects due to multiple types of bonds, leading to multiple barriers in the energy landscape [42]. Therefore the ICAM-1 receptor/ligand system presently characterized possibly involves multiple receptor-ligand types.

As shown by the values of the force jumps which are in the range [20pN–70pN], it appears that specific receptor-ligand bonds are present [28]. These interactions could involve endothelial adhesion molecules such as ICAM-1, VCAM-1 and E-selectin which have been shown to play an important role for the interactions between cancer cells and the endothelium monolayer [4,7]. Previously, we identified the role of ICAM-1 for cancer cell adhesion to the endothelium [4]; therefore, we investigated here the role of ICAM-1 expressed on ECs on these adhesion mechanisms by using a specific anti-ICAM-1 antibody (Figure 6). The use of anti-ICAM-1 led to a significant reduction of the rupture forces for the more invasive cells (reduction of 35% on average for T24 and J82 cells) but no significant inhibition was found for the less invasive RT112 cells (Figure 7A to 7E). This result confirms the implication of ICAM-1 in the adherence of T24 and J82 cancer cells to ECs. The rupture force levels obtained for T24 cells when the ICAM-1 antibody is used (Figure 7A and 7B) are mostly in the range [15–40pN] for increasing retraction speed, a low value probably corresponding to non-specific bonds. This is indeed confirmed by force spectroscopy experiments with BSA-coated substrates, giving similar numbers (Figure 5 and Figure 7G). On the other hand, the levels of forces obtained between T24 cells and an ICAM-1 coated surface are identical (within experimental error) to the rupture forces measured during T24-ECs interactions, confirming the presence of an interaction with ICAM-1.

Finally, to understand the details of these interactions, we analysed the rupture force distributions at a given retraction speed (5 μm/s) through histograms and box-whisker plots as presented in

Figure 8. First, this analysis is consistent with the previous results. The anti-ICAM-1 suppresses the specific interactions only for the more invasive cells: (i) the peak around 32.9 pN for T24 cells disappears when using the anti-ICAM-1 antibody (see Figure 8A) (ii) the high peak (70 pN) found for J82 cells completely disappears and the second one (42pN) is lowered by a factor 3 when using the antibody (see Figure 8B). Notably, the T24 cells and the J82 cells do not show the same number of peaks: this suggests that the ICAM-1 receptor on the EC interacts with one ligand on T24 cells and with 2 ligands on J82 cells.

Concerning the molecular structure linking cancer cells to the endothelium, since bladder cancer cells do not express common ICAM-1 ligands, such as LFA-1 or Mac-1, possible ligands on the cancer cell could very well be the MUC1 or CD43 ligands [31,32,44]. Geng *et al.* [44] demonstrated that efficient binding is possible between ICAM-1 and MUC1 whose expression increases with the invasivity of breast cancer cells [31]. Our measurements using flow cytometry demonstrated clearly that T24 cells express only MUC1 whereas J82 cells express MUC1 and CD43 (Figure 9). These results are in very close connection with the histogram analyses presented above, suggesting the presence of at least two ICAM-1 ligands on J82 cells and only one ligand on T24 cells. Note that for RT112 cells expressing only CD43, the endothelial ICAM-1 receptor does not seem to be involved, as shown by AFM spectroscopy.

To conclude, these experiments reveal the involvement of the endothelial ICAM-1 in the interactions between T24 and J82 TCs and ECs. The possible ICAM-1 ligands involved in this interaction are CD43 for T24 cells and both MUC1 and CD43 for J82 cells. Additional experiments are under way for studying the precise role of these two ICAM-1 ligands on these interactions. On the other hand, the less invasive RT112 cell does not adhere using this molecular scenario. This study provides a straightforward perspective for the understanding of the molecular mechanisms of the cancer cell-endothelium interactions. It leads to significant differences between cells of various metastatic potential and could provide interesting therapeutic means to block the extravasation process.

Acknowledgments

Special thanks goes to Aurélien Vesin for help for statistical analysis.

Author Contributions

Conceived and designed the experiments: VML AD CV. Performed the experiments: VML VSR. Analyzed the data: VML CV. Contributed reagents/materials/analysis tools: VML AD CV. Wrote the paper: VML AD CV.

References

1. Miles FL, Pruitt FL, van Golen KL, Cooper CR (2008) Stepping out of the flow: capillary extravasation in cancer metastasis. Clin Exp Metastasis 25: 305–324.
2. Steeg PS (2006) Tumor metastasis: mechanistic insights and clinical challenges. Nat Med. 12: 895–904.
3. Chotard-Ghodsnia R, Haddad O, Leyrat A, Drochon A, Verdier C, et al. (2007) Morphological analysis of tumor cell/endothelial cell interactions under shear flow. J Biomech 40: 335–344.
4. Haddad O, Chotard-Ghodsnia R, Verdier C, Duperray A (2010) Tumor cell/endothelial cell tight contact upregulates endothelial adhesion molecule expression mediated by NFkB: differential role of the shear stress. Exp. Cell Research 316: 615–626.
5. Strell C, Entschladen F (2008) Extravasation of leukocytes in comparison to tumor cells. Cell Commun Signal 6: 1–13.
6. Heyder C, Gloria-Maercker E, Hatzmann W, Niggemann B, Zänker K, et al. (2005) Role of the beta1-integrin subunit in the adhesion, extravasation and migration of T24 human bladder carcinoma cells. Clin Exp Metastasis 22: 99–106.
7. Yamada M, Yanaba K, Hasegawa M, Matsushita Y, Horikawa M, et al. (2006) Regulation of local and metastatic host-mediated anti-tumour mechanisms by L-selectin and intercellular adhesion molecule-1. Clin Exp Immunol 143: 216–227.
8. Roche Y, Pasquier D, Rambeaud J-J, Seigneurin D, Duperray A (2003) Fibrinogen mediates bladder cancer cell migration in an ICAM-1-dependent pathway. Thromb Haemost 89: 1089–1097.
9. Rosenstein Y, Park JK, Hahn WC, Rosen FS, Bierer BE, et al. (1991) CD43, a molecule defective in Wiskott-Aldrich syndrome, binds ICAM-1. Nature 354: 233–235.
10. Regimbald LH, Pilarski LM, Longenecker BM, Reddish MA, Zimmermann G, et al. (1996) The breast mucin MUCI as a novel adhesion ligand for endothelial intercellular adhesion molecule 1 in breast cancer. Cancer Res 56: 4244–4249.
11. Wheelock M, Shintani Y, Maeda M, Fukumoto Y, Johnson KR (2008) Cadherin switching. J Cell Sci 121: 727–735.

12. Lascombe I, Clairotte A, Fauconnet S, Bernardini S, Wallerand H, et al. (2006) N-cadherin as a novel prognostic marker of progression in superficial urothelial tumors. Clin Cancer Res 12: 2780–2787.

13. Laidler P, Gil D, Pituch-Noworolska A, Ciolczyk D, Ksiazek D, et al. (2000) Expression of beta1-integrins and N-cadherin in bladder cancer and melanoma cell lines. Acta Biochim Pol 47: 1159–1170.

14. Lekka M, Gil D, Dabroś W, Jaczewska J, Kulik A, et al. (2011) Characterization of N-cadherin unbinding properties in non-malignant (HCV29) and malignant (T24) bladder cells. J Mol Recognit 24: 833–842.

15. Schröder C, Witzel I, Müller V, Krenkel S, Wirtz R, et al. (2011) Prognostic value of intercellular adhesion molecule (ICAM-1) expression in breast cancer. J Cancer Res Clin Oncol 137: 1193–1201.

16. Buitrago D, Keutgen XM, Crowley M, Filicori F, Aldailami H (2012) Intercellular adhesion molecule-1 (ICAM-1) is upregulated in aggressive papillary thyroid carcinoma. Ann Surg Oncol 19: 973–980.

17. Pincet F, Husson J (2005) The solution to the streptavidin-biotin paradox: the influence of history on the strength of single molecular bonds. Biophys J 89: 4374–4381.

18. Litvinov R, Shuman H, Bennett J, Weisel J (2002) Binding strength and activation state of single fibrinogen-integrin pairs on living cells. Proc Natl Acad Sci USA 99: 7426–7431.

19. Benoit M, Gabriel D, Gerisch G, Gaub HE (2000) Discrete interactions in cell adhesion measured by single-molecule force spectroscopy. Nat Cell Biol 2: 313–317.

20. Zhang X, Wojcikiewicz E, Moy V (2006) Dynamic adhesion of T lymphocytes to endothelial cells revealed by atomic force microscopy. Exp Biol Med 231: 1306–1312.

21. Champelovier P, Simon A, Garrel C, Levacher G, Praloran V, et al. (2003) Is interferon gamma one key of metastatic potential increase in human bladder carcinoma? Clin Cancer Res 9: 4562–4569.

22. Hutter J, Bechhoefer J (1993) Calibration of atomic-force microscope tips. Rev Sci Instrum 64: 1868–1873.

23. Zhang X, Wojcikiewicz E, Moy V (2002) Force spectroscopy of the leukocyte function-associated antigen-1/intercellular adhesion molecule-1 interaction. Biophys J 83: 2270–2279.

24. Puech PH, Poole K, Knebel D, Muller D (2006) A new technical approach to quantify cell-cell adhesion forces by AFM. Ultramicroscopy 106: 637–644.

25. Zhang X, Chen A, Leon DD, Li H, Noiri E, et al. (2004) Atomic force microscopy measurement of leukocyte-endothelial interaction. Am J Physiol Heart Circ Physiol 286: H359–H367.

26. Sans E, Delachanal E, Duperray A (2001) Analysis of the roles of ICAM-1 in neutrophil transmigration using a reconstituted mammalian cell expression model: implication of ICAM-1 cytoplasmic domain and Rho-dependent signalling pathway. J Immunol 166: 544–551

27. Li F, Redick S, Erickson H, Moy V (2003) Force measurements of the alpha5beta1 integrin-fibronectin interaction. Biophys J 84: 1252–1262.

28. Helenius J, Heisenberg CP, Gaub H, Muller D (2008) Single-cell force spectroscopy. J Cell Sci 121: 1785–1791.

29. Pittet P, Lee K, Kulik AJ, Meister JJ, Hinz B (2008) Fibrogenic fibroblasts increase intercellular adhesion strength by reinforcing individual OB-cadherin bonds. J Cell Sci 121: 877–886.

30. Bell G (1978) Models for the specific adhesion of cells to cells. Science 200: 618–627.

31. Geng Y, Yeh K, Takatani T, King MR (2012) Three to tango: MUC1 as a ligand for both E-selectin and ICAM-1 in the breast cancer metastatic cascade. Front Oncol. 2: 1–8.

32. Santamaría M, López-Beltrán A, Toro M, Peña J, Molina IJ (1996) Specific monoclonal antibodies against leukocyte-restricted cell surface molecule CD43 react with nonhematopoietic tumor cells. Cancer Res 56: 3526–3529.

33. Barreiro O, Yanez-Mo M, Serrador JM, Montoya MC, Vicente-Manzanares M, et al. (2002) Dynamic interaction of VCAM-1 and ICAM-1 with moesin and ezrin in a novel endothelial docking structure for adherent leukocytes. J Cell Biol 157: 1233–1245.

34. Carpén O, Pallai P, Staunton DE, Springer TA (1992) Association of Intercellular Adhesion Molecule (ICAM-1) with Actin-containing Cytoskeleton and alpha-actinin. J Cell Biol 118: 1223–1234.

35. Van Buul JD, Van Rijssel J, Van Alphen FPJ, Hoogenboezem M, Tol S, et al. (2010) Inside-out regulation of ICAM-1 dynamics in TNF-alpha-activated endothelium. PLoS One 5: e11336.

36. Chu C, Celik E, Rico F, Moy VT (2013) Elongated membrane tethers, individually anchored by high affinity alpha4beta1/VCAM-1 complexes, are the quantal units of monocyte arrests. PLoS ONE 8: e64187.

37. Canetta E, Duperray A, Leyrat A, Verdier C (2005) Measuring cell viscoelastic properties using a force-spectrometer: influence of protein-cytoplasm interactions. Biorheology 42: 321–333.

38. Panorchan P, Thompson MS, Davis KJ, Tseng Y, Konstantopoulos K, et al. (2006) Single-molecule analysis of cadherin-mediated cell-cell adhesion. J Cell Sci 119: 66–74.

39. Wojcikiewicz E, Zhang X, Moy VT (2003) Force and Compliance Measurements on Living Cells Using Atomic Force Microscopy (AFM). Biol Proceed 6: 1–9.

40. Hanley WD, Wirtz D, Konstantopoulos K (2004) Distinct kinetic and mechanical properties govern selectin-leukocyte interactions. J Cell Sci 117: 2503–2511.

41. Klemke M, Weschenfelder T, Konstandin M, Samstag Y (2007) High affinity interaction of integrin alpha4-beta1 (VLA-4) and vascular cell adhesion molecule 1 (VCAM-1) enhances migration of human melanoma cells across activated endothelial cell layers. J Cell Physiol 212: 368–374.

42. Wojcikiewicz EP, Abdulreda MH, Zhang X, Moy VT (2006) Force spectroscopy of LFA-1 and its ligands, ICAM-1 and ICAM-2. Biomacromolecules 7: 3188–3195.

43. Evans E, Ritchie K (1997) Dynamic Strength of Molecular Adhesion Bonds. Biophys J 72: 1541–1555.

44. Geng Y, Marshall JR, King MR (2012) Glycomechanics of the metastatic cascade: tumor cell-endothelial cell interactions in the circulation. Ann Biomed Eng 40: 790–805.

12

Diabetes Mellitus and Risk of Bladder Cancer: A Meta-Analysis of Cohort Studies

Xin Xu, Jian Wu, Yeqing Mao, Yi Zhu, Zhenghui Hu, Xianglai Xu, Yiwei Lin, Hong Chen, Xiangyi Zheng, Jie Qin, Liping Xie*

Department of Urology, First Affiliated Hospital, Zhejiang University, Hangzhou, Zhejiang Province, China

Abstract

Objective: Diabetes is associated with increased risk of cancer at several sites, but its association with risk of bladder cancer is still controversial. We examined this association by conducting a systematic review and meta-analysis of cohort studies.

Methods: Studies were identified by searching PubMed, EMBASE, Scopus, Web of Science, Cochrane register, and Chinese National Knowledge Infrastructure (CNKI) databases through April 29, 2012. Summary relative risks (SRRs) with their corresponding 95% confidence intervals (CIs) were calculated using a random-effects model.

Results: A total of fifteen cohort studies were included in this meta-analysis. Analysis of all studies showed that diabetes was associated with a borderline statistically significant increased risk of bladder cancer (RR 1.11, 95% CI 1.00–1.23; p<0.001 for heterogeneity; $I^2 = 84\%$). When restricting the analysis to studies that had adjusted for cigarette smoking (n = 6) or more than three confounders (n = 7), the RRs were 1.32 (95% CI 1.18–1.49) and 1.20 (95% CI 1.02–1.42), respectively. There was no significant publication bias (p = 0.62 for Egger's regression asymmetry test).

Conclusions: Our findings support that diabetes was associated with an increased risk of bladder cancer. More future studies are warranted to get a better understanding of the association and to provide convincing evidence for clinical practice in bladder cancer prevention.

Editor: C. Mary Schooling, CUNY, United States of America

Funding: This study was supported by grants from National Key Clinical Specialty Construction Project of China, Key medical disciplines of Zhejiang province, Combination of traditional Chinese and Western medicine key disciplines of Zhejiang Province (2012-XK-A23), Health sector scientific research special project (201002010), National Natural Science Foundation of China (Grant No. 30900552) and Zhejiang Provincial Natural Science Foundation of China (Z2090356). The funders had no role in study design, data collection and analysis, decision to publish, or preparation of the manuscript.

Competing Interests: The authors have declared that no competing interests exist.

* E-mail: xielp@zjuem.zju.edu.cn

Introduction

Urinary bladder cancer ranks ninth in worldwide cancer incidence. It is the seventh most common malignancy in men and seventeenth in women [1]. An estimated 386,300 new cases and 150,200 deaths from bladder cancer occurred in 2008 worldwide. The highest incidence rates are found in the countries of Europe, North America, and Northern Africa [2]. Increasing evidence suggests a significant influence of genetic predisposition on bladder incidence [3]; the role of genetic factors in the etiology of bladder cancer is estimated to be about 31% [4]. Cigarette smoking, occupational exposure to arylamines, and schistosomal infection are the most established external risk factors for bladder cancer [5]. However, other independent risk factors are not clearly known and their roles in bladder cancer severity, progression and outcomes need further exploration.

Over the past few decades, the prevalence of diabetes mellitus has increased substantially and is highly suspected to be associated with an increased risk of some cancers. Considerable epidemiological studies and systematic reviews have shown positive associations between diabetes mellitus and the risk of biliary tract cancer [6], liver cancer [7], kidney cancer [8], pancreas cancer [9],

and colon and rectal cancer [10]. Likewise, relationships between diabetes and bladder cancer incidence have also been evaluated, yielding controversial results. Most studies have reported positive, but nonsignificant associations, which might be explained by the insufficient statistical power of individual studies.

A meta-analysis of the association between diabetes and bladder cancer risk published in 2006 concluded that diabetes was significantly associated with a higher risk (24%) of bladder cancer [11]. However, some limitations of this meta-analysis have to be mentioned, including a mixture of case–control and cohort studies, a mixture of bladder cancer incidence and mortality, lack of differentiation between type 1 and type 2 diabetes, and small numbers of bladder cancer case in most included studies. Since then, there are also many high-quality cohort studies on this association have been published [12–21], but controversy still reigns.

Given the inconsistency of the existing literature and the insufficient statistical power of primary studies, we performed a meta-analysis of all eligible cohort studies to derive a more precise estimation of the relationship between diabetes and risk of bladder cancer. Furthermore, we also examined whether the

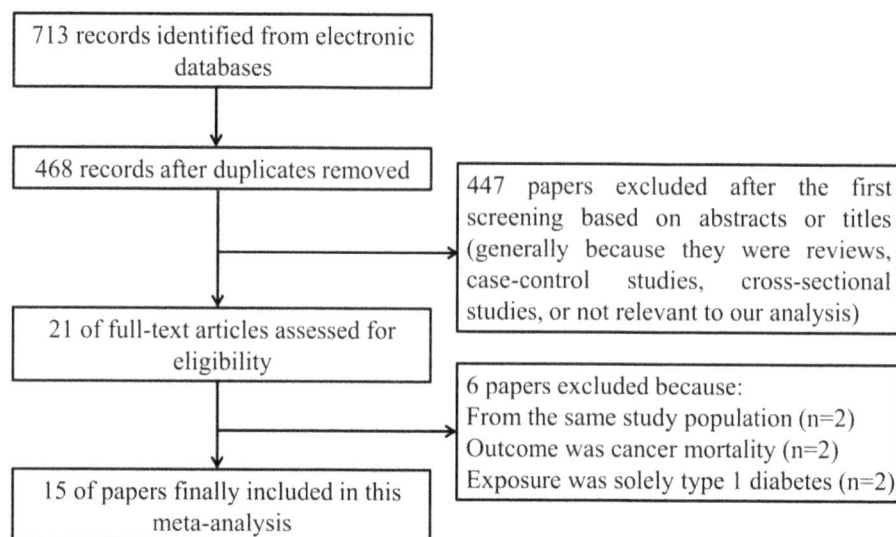

Figure 1. Flowchart of study assessment and selection.

association between them differs according to various study characteristics.

Materials and Methods

Publication Search

We carried out a search in PubMed, EMBASE, Scopus, Web of Science, Cochrane register, and Chinese National Knowledge Infrastructure (CNKI) databases, covering all the papers published from their inception to April 2012. The search strategy included terms for outcome (bladder neoplasm or bladder cancer or bladder tumor) and exposure (diabetes or diabetes mellitus). We evaluated potentially relevant publications by examining their titles and abstracts and all the studies matching the eligible criteria were retrieved. We also checked the references from retrieved articles and reviews to identify any additional relevant study.

Inclusion Criteria

Studies included in this meta-analysis had to meet all the following criteria: (a) they had a cohort design or nested case-control design; (b) one of the exposure of interest was diabetes mellitus; (c) one of the outcome of interest was incidence of bladder cancer; and (d) studies provided rate ratio, hazard ratio or standardized incidence ratio (SIR) with their 95% CIs, or data to calculate them. Studies on mortality rates from bladder cancer were not included, as it could be confounded by survival related factors. We also did not consider studies in which the exposure of interest was mainly or solely type 1 diabetes, which was defined as early-onset (age <30 years) of diabetes. If multiple publications from the same study population were available, the most recent and detailed study was eligible for inclusion in the meta-analysis.

Data Extraction

Data were extracted independently by two authors using a predefined data collection form, with disagreements being resolved by consensus. For each study, the following characteristics were collected: first author's name, year of publication, the country in which the study was carried out, participant characteristics (age and gender), year of study conducted, range for follow-up, sample size (cases and cohort size), methods of ascertainment

of diabetes and bladder cancer, estimate effects with their 95% CIs, and covariates adjusted for in the analysis. From each study, we extracted the RR estimate that was adjusted for the greatest number of potential confounders.

Statistical Methods

Studies that reported different measures of RR were included in this meta-analysis: rate ratio, hazard ratio and SIR. In practice, these three measures of effect yield similar estimates of RR because the absolute risk of bladder cancer is low.

Summary RR estimates with their corresponding 95% CIs were calculated with the DerSimonian and Laird [22] random effects models, which consider both within-study and between-study variation. Subgroup analyses were carried out by (a) geographic region, (b) smoking status, (c) the number of covariates adjusted for, (d) methods of ascertainment of diabetes. Only the studies based on rate ratio or hazard ratio were included for subgroup analysis.

Homogeneity of RRs across studies was tested by Q statistic (significance level at P<0.10) and the I^2 score. Publication bias was assessed using Begg's test (rank correlation method) [23] and Egger's test (linear regression method) [24]. P<0.05 was considered to be representative of a significant statistical publication bias. All of the statistical analyses were performed with STATA 11.0 (StataCorp, College Station, TX), using two-sided P-values.

Results

Literature Search

Figure 1 outlines our study selection process. Briefly, after removing duplications, the search strategy generated 468 articles. Of these, the majority were excluded after the first screening based on abstracts or titles, mainly because they were reviews, case-control studies, cross-sectional studies, or not relevant to our analysis.

After full-text review of 21 papers, 6 studies were excluded for the reasons as follows: overlapping publications from the same study population [25,26]; the outcome was cancer mortality [27,28]; the exposure was solely type 1 diabetes [29,30]. Thus,

Table 1. Characteristics of cohort studies of diabetes and bladder cancer based on rate ratio and hazard ratio.

Study	Year of study conducted	Follow up, years	Age/gender	Cases/Cohort	Diabetes assessment	Bladder cancer ascertainment	Adjustments
Lo et al./2012 (Taiwan)	1996–2009	3.5	All ages Male: 49.1%	4,311/1,790,868	Medical records (type 2)	Cancer registry	Sex, age, urbanization, hypertension and hyperlipidemia.
Attner et al./2012 (Sweden)	1998–2007	10	45–84 (86%) Male: 53%	19,756/167,080	Medical records (type 1 and 2)	Cancer registry	Age and gender
Atchison et al./2011 (USA)	1969–1996	10.5	18–100 Male: 100%	19,300/4,501,578	Medical records (type 2)	Medical records	Age, time, latency, race, number of hospital visits, alcohol-related conditions, obesity and chronic obstructive pulmonary disease
Woolcott et al./2011 (USA)	1993–2004	10.7	45–75 Male: 45%	818/185,816	Self-reported (type 1 and 2)	Cancer registry	Ethnicity, sex, smoking status, intensity and duration, and employment in a high risk Industry
Ogunleye et al./2009 (Scotland, UK)	1993–2004	3.9	All ages Male: 53%	68/9,577	Medical records (type 2)	Cancer registry	Age, sex and deprivation
Larsson et al./2008 (Sweden)	1997–2007	9.3	45–79 Male: 100%	414/45,906	Self-reported (type 1 and 2)	Cancer registry	Age, education, smoking status and pack-years of smoking
Inoue et al./2006 (Japan)	1988–1999	14	40–69 Male: 47.6%	135/97,771	Self-reported (type 1 and 2)	Cancer registry	Age, study area, history of cerebrovascular disease, history of ischemic heart disease, smoking, physical activity, BMI, alcohol intake, green vegetable intake, coffee
Khan et al./2006 (Japan)	1988–1997	18–20	40–79 Male: 41%	60/56,881	Self-reported (type 1 and 2)	Cancer registry	Age, smoking, BMI and alcohol
Jee et al./2005 (Korea)	1992–2002	10	30–95 Male: 64%	NA/829,770	Blood glucose level or medication use (type 2)	Cancer registry and medical records	Age, smoking and alcohol
Tripathi et al./2002 (USA)	1986–1998	13	55–69 Male: 0%	112/37,459	Self-reported (type 1 and 2)	Cancer registry	Age, smoking, regular physical activity, BMI, alcohol, married, occupation lifetime

NA, data not applicable; BMI, body mass index.

Table 2. Characteristics of cohort studies of diabetes and bladder cancer based on standardized incidence ratio.

Study	Year of study conducted	Follow up, years	Age/gender	Cases/Cohort	Diabetes assessment	Bladder cancer ascertainment	Adjustments
Wotton et al./2011 (UK)	1963-2008	NA	Male:54%	2,385/484,356	Medical records (estimated 90% type 2)	Medical records	Sex, age in 5-year bands, time period in single calendar years and district of residence
Hemminki et al./2010 (Sweden)	1964-2007	15	>39 Male: NA	483/125,126	Medical records (type 2)	Cancer registry	Age, sex, period, region and socioeconomic status
Swerdlow et al./2005 (UK)	1972-2003	18	30-49 Male:58.1%	20/5,066	Self-reported (estimated 36% type 1, 64% type 2)	Cancer registry	Age, sex, country of residence and calendar year
Wideroff et al./1997 (Denmark)	1977-1989	17	64(m); 69(f) Male: 49%	493/109,581	Medical records (type 1 and 2)	Cancer registry	Age, sex and calendar year
Ragozzino et al./1982 (USA)	1945-1969	8.6	61 Male: 53%	7/1,135	Blood glucose level (NA)	Histological verification	Age

NA, data not applicable; m, male; f, female.

a total of 15 cohort studies, which met the inclusion criteria, were included in this meta-analysis.

Study Characteristics

The characteristics of the 15 cohort studies are presented in Tables 1 and 2. Of these, 10 studies used rate ratio or hazard ratio as the measurement of RR [12–15,17,18,20,21,31,32] (Table 1), and 5 cohort studies used standardized incidence ratio as the measurement of RR [16,19,33–35] (Table 2). The studies were conducted in the following regions: Europe (n = 7) [14–16,19,21,33,35], Asia (n = 4) [12,13,20,31], and USA (n = 4) [17,18,32,34]. The study population in ten studies consisted of both sexes [12,15,16,18–21,33–35], four studies included men only [13,14,17,31] and one study included women only [32]. All included studies were published between 1982 and 2012, of which 66.7% (n = 10) [12–21] were published in 2006 or more recent years, and were not included in previous meta-analysis. The cohort ranged in size from 1,135 [34] to 4,501,578 [17]. Diabetes status was ascertained by self-reported history of diabetes mellitus, medical records or blood glucose level. Diagnosis of bladder cancer was based on medical record or cancer registry data, except one using histological verification [34]. Adjustments were made for potential confounders of one or more factors in all studies.

Diabetes Mellitus and Risk of Bladder Cancer

The overall RR with its 95% CI showed a borderline statistically significant association between diabetes mellitus and risk of bladder cancer (Fig. 2, RR 1.11, 95% CI 1.00–1.23). The summary RRs with 95% CIs were 1.01 (95% CI 0.82–1.24) for studies using standardized incidence ratio, and 1.19 (95% CI 1.04–1.36) for rate ratio or hazard ratio. There was statistically significant heterogeneity among studies (p<0.001 for heterogeneity; $I^2 = 84.0\%$).

Next, we conducted subgroup meta-analysis by various study characteristics (Table 3). In the subgroup analysis by geographical area, the association between diabetes and bladder cancer was more significant for studies conducted in Asia (RR 1.21, 95% CI 1.15–1.28; p = 0.658 for heterogeneity; $I^2 = 0\%$) than in Europe (RR 1.09, 95% CI 0.85–1.40; p = 0.189 for heterogeneity; $I^2 = 39.9\%$) or USA (RR 1.28, 95% CI 0.90–1.81; p<0.001 for heterogeneity; $I^2 = 88.6\%$). In further stratified analysis by the methods of ascertainment of diabetes, the summary RRs with 95% CIs were 1.34 (95% CI 1.11–1.62) for studies using self-report, and 1.11 (95% CI 0.95–1.31) for others methods.

We also investigated the impact of confounding factors on the estimates of relative risk (Table 3). Cigarette smoking is a risk factor for both diabetes and bladder cancer, and thus a potential confounder of the relationship between diabetes and risk of bladder cancer. Among the six studies that controlled for cigarette smoking, the pooled RR was 1.32 (95% CI 1.18–1.49; p = 0.467 for heterogeneity; $I^2 = 0\%$). Moreover, some studies in our analysis adjusted for more than three confounders. Therefore, we examined if more thoroughly adjusting for potential confounders affected the pooled RR and degree of heterogeneity (Table 3). The effect estimate for studies that adjusted for more than three confounders was RR, 1.20 (95% CI 1.02–1.42; p<0.001 for heterogeneity; $I^2 = 85.6\%$).

Publication Bias

There was no evidence of significant publication bias either with the Begg's test (P = 0.76) or with Egger's test (Fig. 3, P = 0.62).

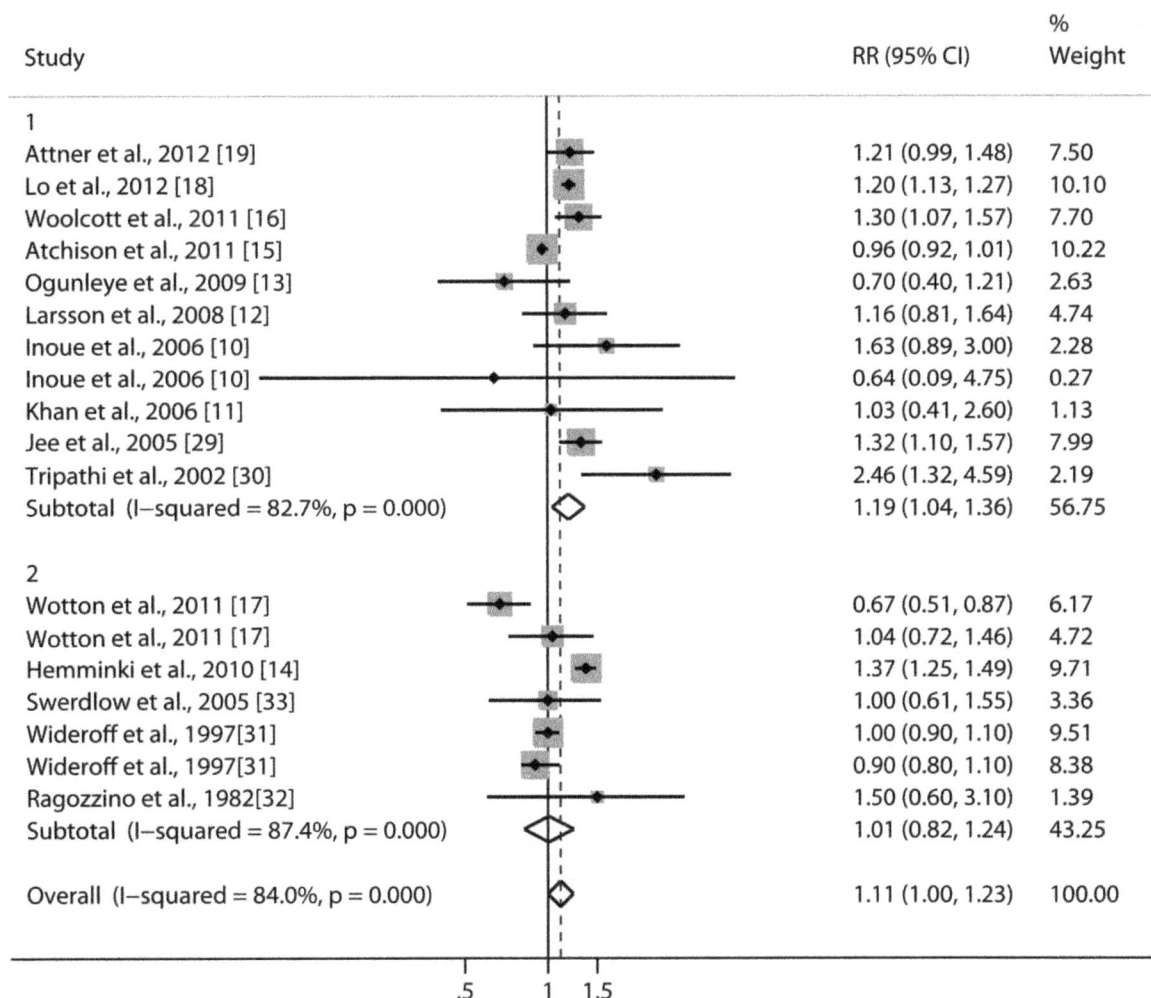

Figure 2. Relative risks for the association between diabetes and risk of bladder cancer in cohort studies. Studies are sub-grouped according to the measurements of relative risk. Diamonds represent study-specific relative risks or summary relative risks with 95% CIs; horizontal lines represent 95% confidence intervals (CIs). Test for heterogeneity among studies: p<0.001, I^2 =84.0%. 1, cohort studies (n = 10) use incidence rate as the measurement of relative risk. 2, cohort studies (n = 5) use standardized incidence rate as the measurement of relative risk.

Discussion

The findings of this meta-analysis of fifteen cohort studies indicate that diabetes is associated with an 11% increased risk of bladder cancer. It tended to be more remarkable for studies with a rate ratio or hazard ratio as the measure of relative risk than for studies with a standardized incidence ratio.

At present, whether diabetes is independently associated with incidence of bladder cancer remains controversial. Results from our subgroup analysis restricted to studies with control for smoking or adjusted for more than three confounders were more robust than that reported in the overall analysis, which indicated that the association may have been diluted by poor study methodologies and diabetes is probably an independent risk factor of bladder cancer.

Of note, the association between diabetes and bladder cancer was more pronounced in studies with a rate ratio or hazard ratio as the measure of relative risk than in studies with a standardized incidence ratio. Studies using standardized incidence ratio and standardized mortality ratio to estimate the relative risk may underestimate the true relative risk [36,37]. Because if the general population is taken to represent unexposed persons, it is almost inevitably biased in that it comprises all types of people including exposed ones [37]. Therefore, the summary RRs risk of this meta-analysis may have been attenuated by the results from studies using standardized incidence ratio as the measure of relative risk and the results of our meta-analysis were actually statistically robust.

The association between the duration of diabetes and risk of bladder cancer have been assessed in some studies, and inconsistent results were found [12,13,15–17,20,34]. In the study by Hemminki et al. [16], the standardized incidence ratio of bladder cancer declined from 1.37 with no latency period to 0.96 for a 5 year latency period, while Ogunleye et al. [15] reported that the RR between diabetes and bladder cancer was 0.70 (95% CI 0.40–1.21) when including all cases and 0.53 (95% CI 0.24–1.15) when excluding cases diagnosed within the first year of follow-up. The study conducted by Atchison et al. [17] also suggested the risk of bladder cancer declined over time. However, another three reports [12,13,20] found higher relative risks after excluding the first 2, 3.5 or 5 years of follow-up. Because of the inconsistent results, it remains unclear whether the duration of diabetes is directly associated with the risk of bladder cancer. Interestingly, we noticed that the studies reported risk reduction over time were

Table 3. Subgroup analysis of relative risks for the association between diabetes and bladder cancer.

Subgroup	References	RR (95% CI)	Heterogeneity test		
			Q	P	I^2 (%)
The measure of relative risk					
Standardized incidence ratio	16, 19, 33–35	1.01 (0.82, 1.24)	47.44	<0.001	87.4
Rate ratio or hazard ratio	12–15, 17, 18, 20, 21, 31, 32	1.19 (1.04, 1.36)	57.74	<0.001	82.7
Geographical region					
Europe	14, 15, 21	1.09 (0.85, 1.40)	3.33	0.189	39.9
USA	17, 18, 32	1.28 (0.90, 1.81)	17.47	<0.001	88.6
Asia	12, 13, 20, 31	1.21 (1.15, 1.28)	2.43	0.658	0.0
Adjustment for more than three confounders					
Yes	12–14, 17, 18, 20, 32	1.20 (1.02, 1.42)	48.45	<0.001	85.6
No	15, 21, 31	1.17 (0.94, 1.47)	4.62	0.099	56.7
Adjustment for smoking					
Yes	12–14, 18, 31, 32	1.32 (1.18, 1.49)	5.62	0.467	0.0
No	15, 17, 20, 21	1.07 (0.90, 1.27)	38.22	<0.001	92.2
Diabetes ascertainment					
Self-report	12–14, 18, 32	1.34 (1.11, 1.62)	5.62	0.345	11.0
Others methods	15, 17, 20, 21, 31	1.11 (0.95, 1.31)	44.32	<0.001	91.0

RR, relative risk; CI, confidence interval.

conducted in western countries, while higher relative risks for longer duration were suggested by studies from Asian countries. The mechanism behind this difference is not clear and should be further studied in the future.

A relationship between diabetes and risk of bladder cancer is biologically plausible. Type 2 diabetes is associated with insulin resistance, compensatory hyper-insulinemia, and up-regulated level of IGF-1. IGF-1 could stimulate cell proliferation and inhibit

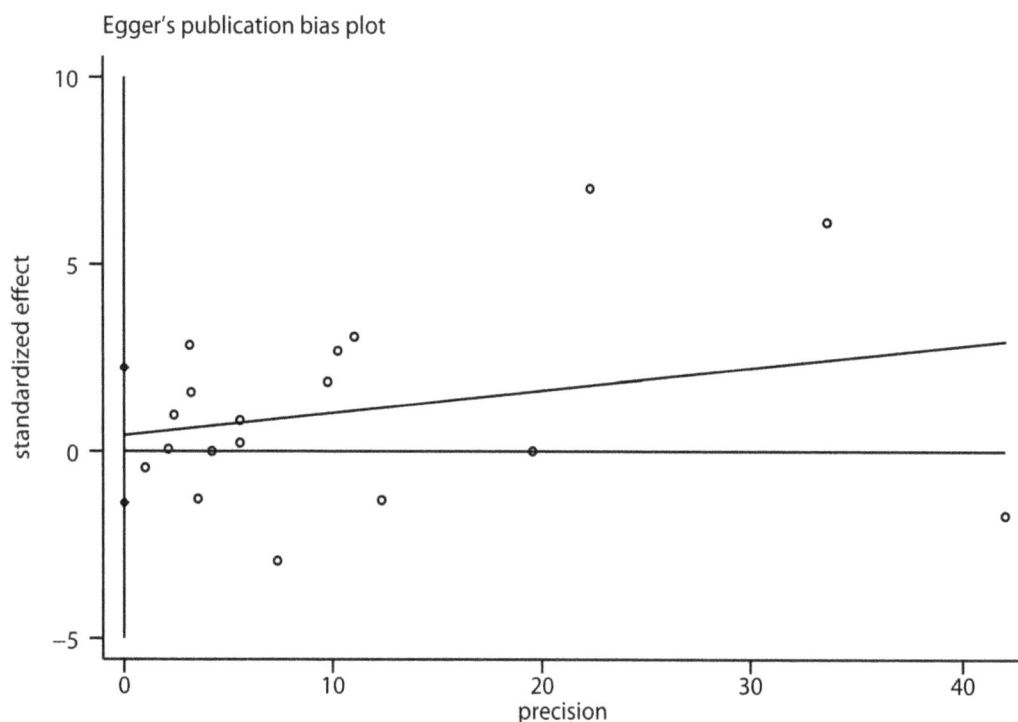

Figure 3. Funnel plot of cohort studies evaluating the association between diabetes and bladder cancer. Egger's regression asymmetry test (p = 0.62). Standardized effect was defined as the odds ratio divided by its standard error. Precision was defined as the inverse of the standard error.

apoptosis. Several epidemiological studies have implicated IGF-I in the development of breast and colorectal cancers [38,39]. A USA case-control study also has found statistically significantly higher circulating levels of IGF-I in bladder cancer cases than in controls [40]. An important role of IGF-I in the development of bladder cancer is also supported by studies in animals [41]. Additionally, diabetes is also associated with an increased risk of urinary tract infection [42] and urinary tract calculi [43], which have been related to various histologic types of bladder cancer, including transitional cell carcinoma, the predominant type [44,45].

Substantial heterogeneity was observed among studies of diabetes and bladder cancer risk, which may be due to different adjustment for confounding factors and different mixtures of type 1 and type 2 diabetic patients. Some studies included in this meta-analysis did not distinguish between type 1 and type 2 diabetes. As type-1 diabetes may not be related to bladder cancer risk [29,30], different proportions of type 1 and type 2 diabetic participants in the studies may in part account for the observed heterogeneity.

A major strength of our study is that with the accumulating evidence and enlarged sample size, we have enhanced statistical power to derive a more precise and reliable estimation of the relationship between diabetes and bladder cancer risk. Nonetheless, some limitations should be mentioned. One potential limitation of this meta-analysis was the various assessments of diabetes used between studies. Some studies used self-report as the method of diabetes ascertainment, which may lead to some misclassification of diabetic persons as non-diabetic persons. This underreporting may result in an underestimate of the magnitude of the association between diabetes and bladder cancer risk.

However, earlier studies have suggested that self-reported diabetes have good agreement with medical records [46,47]. A second limitation is the uncontrolled or unmeasured risk factors potentially produce biases. Although the magnitude of increased risk reported in studies adjusted for more than three confounders was more robust than that reported in the overall analysis, we still cannot rule out the possibility that residual confounding could affect the results. Recently, some studies reported that thiazolidinediones, particularly pioglitazone, were associated with an increased risk of bladder cancer [48,49]. However, most of the studies included in this meta-analysis did not provide the information of oral hypoglycemic use. Thus we failed to evaluate the therapeutic agents' influence on the association between the diabetes and bladder cancer risk. Finally, in any meta-analysis, the possibility of publication bias is of concern, because small studies with null results tend not to be published. However, we found no evidence of publication bias in this meta-analysis.

In summary, our findings support that diabetes was associated with the increased risk of bladder cancer. More future studies are warranted to get a better understanding of the association and to provide convincing evidence for clinical practice in bladder cancer prevention.

Author Contributions

Conceived and designed the experiments: LX XX JW. Performed the experiments: XX YL HC. Analyzed the data: JW YM YZ ZH. Contributed reagents/materials/analysis tools: XZ JQ LX. Wrote the paper: XX LX.

References

1. Ploeg M, Aben KK, Kiemeney LA (2009) The present and future burden of urinary bladder cancer in the world. World J Urol 27: 289–293.
2. Jemal A, Bray F, Center MM, Ferlay J, Ward E, et al. (2011) Global cancer statistics. CA Cancer J Clin 61: 69–90.
3. Burger M, Catto JW, Dalbagni G, Grossman HB, Herr H, et al. (2012) Epidemiology and Risk Factors of Urothelial Bladder Cancer. Eur Urol.
4. Lichtenstein P, Holm NV, Verkasalo PK, Iliadou A, Kaprio J, et al. (2000) Environmental and heritable factors in the causation of cancer–analyses of cohorts of twins from Sweden, Denmark, and Finland. N Engl J Med 343: 78–85.
5. Murta-Nascimento C, Schmitz-Drager BJ, Zeegers MP, Steineck G, Kogevinas M, et al. (2007) Epidemiology of urinary bladder cancer: from tumor development to patient's death. World J Urol 25: 285–295.
6. Ren HB, Yu T, Liu C, Li YQ (2011) Diabetes mellitus and increased risk of biliary tract cancer: systematic review and meta-analysis. Cancer Causes Control 22: 837–847.
7. Yang WS, Va P, Bray F, Gao S, Gao J, et al. (2011) The role of pre-existing diabetes mellitus on hepatocellular carcinoma occurrence and prognosis: a meta-analysis of prospective cohort studies. PLoS One 6: e27326.
8. Larsson SC, Wolk A (2011) Diabetes mellitus and incidence of kidney cancer: a meta-analysis of cohort studies. Diabetologia 54: 1013–1018.
9. Ben Q, Xu M, Ning X, Liu J, Hong S, et al. (2011) Diabetes mellitus and risk of pancreatic cancer: A meta-analysis of cohort studies. Eur J Cancer 47: 1928–1937.
10. Yuhara H, Steinmaus C, Cohen SE, Corley DA, Tei Y, et al. (2011) Is diabetes mellitus an independent risk factor for colon cancer and rectal cancer? Am J Gastroenterol 106: 1911–1921; quiz 1922.
11. Larsson SC, Orsini N, Brismar K, Wolk A (2006) Diabetes mellitus and risk of bladder cancer: a meta-analysis. Diabetologia 49: 2819–2823.
12. Inoue M, Iwasaki M, Otani T, Sasazuki S, Noda M, et al. (2006) Diabetes mellitus and the risk of cancer: results from a large-scale population-based cohort study in Japan. Arch Intern Med 166: 1871–1877.
13. Khan M, Mori M, Fujino Y, Shibata A, Sakauchi F, et al. (2006) Site-specific cancer risk due to diabetes mellitus history: evidence from the Japan Collaborative Cohort (JACC) Study. Asian Pac J Cancer Prev 7: 253–259.
14. Larsson SC, Andersson SO, Johansson JE, Wolk A (2008) Diabetes mellitus, body size and bladder cancer risk in a prospective study of Swedish men. Eur J Cancer 44: 2655–2660.
15. Ogunleye AA, Ogston SA, Morris AD, Evans JM (2009) A cohort study of the risk of cancer associated with type 2 diabetes. Br J Cancer 101: 1199–1201.

16. Hemminki K, Li X, Sundquist J, Sundquist K (2010) Risk of cancer following hospitalization for type 2 diabetes. Oncologist 15: 548–555.
17. Atchison EA, Gridley G, Carreon JD, Leitzmann MF, McGlynn KA (2011) Risk of cancer in a large cohort of U.S. veterans with diabetes. Int J Cancer 128: 635–643.
18. Woolcott CG, Maskarinec G, Haiman CA, Henderson BE, Kolonel LN (2011) Diabetes and urothelial cancer risk: the Multiethnic Cohort study. Cancer Epidemiol 35: 551–554.
19. Wotton CJ, Yeates DG, Goldacre MJ (2011) Cancer in patients admitted to hospital with diabetes mellitus aged 30 years and over: record linkage studies. Diabetologia 54: 527–534.
20. Lo SF, Chang SN, Muo CH, Chen SY, Liao FY, et al. (2012) Modest increase in risk of specific types of cancer types in type 2 diabetes mellitus patients. Int J Cancer.
21. Attner B, Landin-Olsson M, Lithman T, Noreen D, Olsson H (2012) Cancer among patients with diabetes, obesity and abnormal blood lipids: a population-based register study in Sweden. Cancer Causes Control 23: 769–777.
22. DerSimonian R, Laird N (1986) Meta-analysis in clinical trials. Control Clin Trials 7: 177–188.
23. Begg CB, Mazumdar M (1994) Operating characteristics of a rank correlation test for publication bias. Biometrics 50: 1088–1101.
24. Egger M, Davey Smith G, Schneider M, Minder C (1997) Bias in meta-analysis detected by a simple, graphical test. BMJ 315: 629–634.
25. Tseng CH (2011) Diabetes and risk of bladder cancer: a study using the National Health Insurance database in Taiwan. Diabetologia 54: 2009–2015.
26. Adami HO, McLaughlin J, Ekbom A, Berne C, Silverman D, et al. (1991) Cancer risk in patients with diabetes mellitus. Cancer Causes Control 2: 307–314.
27. Coughlin SS, Calle EE, Teras LR, Petrelli J, Thun MJ (2004) Diabetes mellitus as a predictor of cancer mortality in a large cohort of US adults. Am J Epidemiol 159: 1160–1167.
28. Tseng CH, Chong CK, Tseng CP, Chan TT (2009) Age-related risk of mortality from bladder cancer in diabetic patients: a 12-year follow-up of a national cohort in Taiwan. Ann Med 41: 371–379.
29. Zendehdel K, Nyren O, Ostenson CG, Adami HO, Ekbom A, et al. (2003) Cancer incidence in patients with type 1 diabetes mellitus: a population-based cohort study in Sweden. J Natl Cancer Inst 95: 1797–1800.
30. Shu X, Ji J, Li X, Sundquist J, Sundquist K, et al. (2010) Cancer risk among patients hospitalized for Type 1 diabetes mellitus: a population-based cohort study in Sweden. Diabet Med 27: 791–797.

31. Jee SH, Ohrr H, Sull JW, Yun JE, Ji M, et al. (2005) Fasting serum glucose level and cancer risk in Korean men and women. JAMA 293: 194–202.

32. Tripathi A, Folsom AR, Anderson KE (2002) Risk factors for urinary bladder carcinoma in postmenopausal women. The Iowa Women's Health Study. Cancer 95: 2316–2323.

33. Wideroff L, Gridley G, Mellemkjaer L, Chow WH, Linet M, et al. (1997) Cancer incidence in a population-based cohort of patients hospitalized with diabetes mellitus in Denmark. J Natl Cancer Inst 89: 1360–1365.

34. Ragozzino M, Melton LJ, 3rd, Chu CP, Palumbo PJ (1982) Subsequent cancer risk in the incidence cohort of Rochester, Minnesota, residents with diabetes mellitus. J Chronic Dis 35: 13–19.

35. Swerdlow AJ, Laing SP, Qiao Z, Slater SD, Burden AC, et al. (2005) Cancer incidence and mortality in patients with insulin-treated diabetes: a UK cohort study. Br J Cancer 92: 2070–2075.

36. Chaturvedi AK, Mbulaiteye SM, Engels EA (2008) Underestimation of relative risks by standardized incidence ratios for AIDS-related cancers. Ann Epidemiol 18: 230–234.

37. Jones ME, Swerdlow AJ (1998) Bias in the standardized mortality ratio when using general population rates to estimate expected number of deaths. Am J Epidemiol 148: 1012–1017.

38. Key TJ, Appleby PN, Reeves GK, Roddam AW (2010) Insulin-like growth factor 1 (IGF1), IGF binding protein 3 (IGFBP3), and breast cancer risk: pooled individual data analysis of 17 prospective studies. Lancet Oncol 11: 530–542.

39. Rinaldi S, Cleveland R, Norat T, Biessy C, Rohrmann S, et al. (2010) Serum levels of IGF-I, IGFBP-3 and colorectal cancer risk: results from the EPIC cohort, plus a meta-analysis of prospective studies. Int J Cancer 126: 1702–1715.

40. Zhao H, Grossman HB, Spitz MR, Lerner SP, Zhang K, et al. (2003) Plasma levels of insulin-like growth factor-1 and binding protein-3, and their association with bladder cancer risk. J Urol 169: 714–717.

41. Dunn SE, Kari FW, French J, Leininger JR, Travlos G, et al. (1997) Dietary restriction reduces insulin-like growth factor I levels, which modulates apoptosis, cell proliferation, and tumor progression in p53-deficient mice. Cancer Res 57: 4667–4672.

42. Funfstuck R, Nicolle LE, Hanefeld M, Naber KG (2012) Urinary tract infection in patients with diabetes mellitus. Clin Nephrol 77: 40–48.

43. Chen HS, Su LT, Lin SZ, Sung FC, Ko MC, et al. (2012) Increased risk of urinary tract calculi among patients with diabetes mellitus-a population-based cohort study. Urology 79: 86–92.

44. Jankovic S, Radosavljevic V (2007) Risk factors for bladder cancer. Tumori 93: 4–12.

45. Chow WH, Lindblad P, Gridley G, Nyren O, McLaughlin JK, et al. (1997) Risk of urinary tract cancers following kidney or ureter stones. J Natl Cancer Inst 89: 1453–1457.

46. Okura Y, Urban LH, Mahoney DW, Jacobsen SJ, Rodeheffer RJ (2004) Agreement between self-report questionnaires and medical record data was substantial for diabetes, hypertension, myocardial infarction and stroke but not for heart failure. J Clin Epidemiol 57: 1096–1103.

47. Margolis KL, Lihong Q, Brzyski R, Bonds DE, Howard BV, et al. (2008) Validity of diabetes self-reports in the Women's Health Initiative: comparison with medication inventories and fasting glucose measurements. Clin Trials 5: 240–247.

48. Neumann A, Weill A, Ricordeau P, Fagot JP, Alla F, et al. (2012) Pioglitazone and risk of bladder cancer among diabetic patients in France: a population-based cohort study. Diabetologia 55: 1953–1962.

49. Azoulay L, Yin H, Filion KB, Assayag J, Majdan A, et al. (2012) The use of pioglitazone and the risk of bladder cancer in people with type 2 diabetes: nested case-control study. BMJ 344: e3645.

13

Proline-Rich Tyrosine Kinase 2 (Pyk2) Regulates IGF-I-Induced Cell Motility and Invasion of Urothelial Carcinoma Cells

Marco Genua[1], Shi-Qiong Xu[1], Simone Buraschi[2], Stephen C. Peiper[2], Leonard G. Gomella[1], Antonino Belfiore[3], Renato V. Iozzo[2], Andrea Morrione[1]*

1 Endocrine Mechanisms and Hormone Action Program, Department of Urology, Kimmel Cancer Center, Thomas Jefferson University, Philadelphia, Pennsylvania, United States of America, 2 Cancer Cell Biology and Signaling Program, Department of Pathology, Anatomy and Cell Biology, Kimmel Cancer Center, Thomas Jefferson University, Philadelphia, Pennsylvania, United States of America, 3 Endocrinology, Department of Health, University of Catanzaro, Catanzaro, Italy

Abstract

The insulin-like growth factor receptor I (IGF-IR) plays an essential role in transformation by promoting cell growth and protecting cancer cells from apoptosis. We have recently demonstrated that the IGF-IR is overexpressed in invasive bladder cancer tissues and promotes motility and invasion of urothelial carcinoma cells. These effects require IGF-I-induced Akt- and MAPK-dependent activation of paxillin. The latter co-localizes with focal adhesion kinases (FAK) at dynamic focal adhesions and is critical for promoting motility of urothelial cancer cells. FAK and its homolog Proline-rich tyrosine kinase 2 (Pyk2) modulate paxillin activation; however, their role in regulating IGF-IR-dependent signaling and motility in bladder cancer has not been established. In this study we demonstrate that FAK was not required for IGF-IR-dependent signaling and motility of invasive urothelial carcinoma cells. On the contrary, Pyk2, which was strongly activated by IGF-I, was critical for IGF-IR-dependent motility and invasion and regulated IGF-I-dependent activation of the Akt and MAPK pathways. Using immunofluorescence and AQUA analysis we further discovered that Pyk2 was overexpressed in bladder cancer tissues as compared to normal tissue controls. Significantly, in urothelial carcinoma tissues there was increased Pyk2 localization in the nuclei as compared to normal tissue controls. These results provide the first evidence of a specific Pyk2 activity in regulating IGF-IR-dependent motility and invasion of bladder cancer cells suggesting that Pyk2 and the IGF-IR may play a critical role in the invasive phenotype in urothelial neoplasia. In addition, Pyk2 and the IGF-IR may serve as novel biomarkers with diagnostic and prognostic significance in bladder cancer.

Editor: Frederic Andre, Aix-Marseille University, France

Funding: This work has been supported by the Benjamin Perkins Bladder Cancer Fund, the Martin Greitzer Fund, AIRC grant IG-10625/2011, AIRC project Calabria 2011 and Fondazione Cassa di Risparmio di Calabria e Lucania (to A.B.) and National Institutes of Health Grants RO1 DK068419 (A.M.) and RO1 CA39481 and RO1 CA047282 (R.V.I.). The funders had no role in study design, data collection and analysis, decision to publish, or preparation of the manuscript.

Competing Interests: The authors have declared that no competing interests exist.

* E-mail: Andrea.Morrione@jefferson.edu

Introduction

Bladder cancer is a major epidemiological problem, whose incidence continues to rise. The most recent cancer statistic has estimated 73,510 new cases and 14,880 estimated deaths in the United States for 2012 [1]. The majority of bladder tumors (~70%) are low-grade noninvasive papillary tumors that do not penetrate the epithelial basement membrane (Ta stage). The remainder comprise tumors that have penetrated the basement membrane but not invaded the muscle layer of the bladder wall (T1 stage) and muscle-invasive tumors (T2, T3 and T4 stages) [2,3,4]. The prognosis for low-grade tumors is generally good, but about 10%–15% of these patients will later develop invasive disease. For invasive tumors the prognosis is much less favorable, with only 50% survival at 5 years. Invasive tumors frequently progress to life-threatening metastases, which is associated with a 5 year survival rate of 6% [3,4]. Thus, understanding the mechanisms that regulate bladder tumor invasion is critical to predict and treat this devastating condition in bladder cancer patients.

It is well established that the insulin-like growth factor receptor I (IGF-IR) plays a critical role in cell growth both *in vitro* [5] and *in vivo* [6]. Mice with targeted ablation of the *IGF-IR* gene have severe growth retardation, being only 45% the size of wild-type littermates [7,8]. Studies performed in mouse embryo fibroblasts derived from the *IGF-IR*-deficient mice (R-cells) have really underscored the essential role of the IGF-IR in transformation [9]. R-cells are indeed refractory to transformation induced by several tumorigenic agents (viral oncogenes such as Ras and SV40 large T Ag, as well as overexpressed PDGFR and EGFR, and various chemical agents) but are transformed upon IGF-IR re-expression [10,11]. Experiments on tumor cell lines and epidemiological studies have confirmed that activation of the IGF-IR is involved in the development of many common neoplastic diseases, including carcinomas of lung, prostate, pancreas, liver, colon and breast [10,12,13]. The transforming capability of the IGF-IR most likely depends on its ability to protect cancer cells from apoptosis [11,12,14,15,16].

We have recently demonstrated that the IGF-IR is upregulated in invasive and high-grade bladder cancer tumor tissues compared to low-grade and normal tissue controls and promotes motility and invasion of urothelial cancer cells [17,18]. Significantly, IGF-IR activation did not induce cell proliferation of bladder cancer cells, indicating that the IGF-IR acts as a "scatter factor" for urothelial carcinoma-derived cells and may regulate the transition to the invasive stage of bladder cancer [17]. We also showed that IGF-IR-dependent cell motility and invasion required the activation of the Akt and MAPK pathway [17,18] and Akt- and ERK-dependent activation of paxillin, which upon IGF-I-stimulation colocalized with focal adhesion kinase (FAK) in dynamic adhesions at the leading edge of migrating urothelial cancer cells and was critical for IGF-I-induced motility of these cells [17].

Here we show that while FAK was not required for IGF-IR-dependent signaling and motility of invasive urothelial carcinoma cells, the FAK-related Pyk2 [19,20] was strongly activated by IGF-I in urothelial carcinoma cells, was critical for IGF-IR-dependent motility and invasion and regulated IGF-I-dependent activation of the Akt and MAPK pathways. We also discovered that Pyk2 is overexpressed in bladder cancer tissues compared to normal tissue controls and that there is a striking increase in Pyk2 translocation to the nuclei of these malignant cells.

Collectively, these results provide novel information toward a better understanding of the mechanisms that regulate tumor progression in bladder cancer and suggest that Pyk2 and the IGF-IR may be critical for the transition to the invasive phenotype. In addition, these studies could potentially contribute to the identification of novel targets for therapeutic intervention in bladder tumors.

Results

FAK Activity in the Regulation of IGF-I-induced Migration, Invasion and Signaling

We recently discovered that paxillin plays an important role in regulating IGF-IR-dependent motility of urothelial carcinomas [17]. It is well established that FAK regulates paxillin activation [21] and the assembly/disassembly of focal adhesions (adhesion turnover) at the cell front of migrating cells [22]. However, it **is** not yet established whether FAK or its homolog Pyk2 [19,20], which is also expressed by urothelial cancer cells, may play a role in regulating IGF-I-induced motility of bladder cancer cells. Thus, we first employed small interfering RNA (siRNA) strategies to transiently deplete endogenous FAK in 5637 invasive urothelial carcinoma cells and then assessed FAK function in the regulation of IGF-I-induced motility and invasion. We reached a very significant depletion of endogenous FAK with the anti-FAK siRNA (Figure 1A). The oligos were specific for FAK insofar as there was no effect on Pyk2 expression levels (Figure 1A). Notably, FAK depletion did not induce a statistically-significant decrease in IGF-I-mediated migratory response in 5637 cells compared to either parental or scrambled oligos-transfected cells (Figure 1B). However, the invasive ability of 5637 cells was reduced, although at levels barely below statistical significance (P = 0.046) as compared to control oligos-transfected cells (Figure 1C). In addition, using immunoblot analysis with phospho-specific antibodies, we discovered that FAK depletion did not affect IGF-I-mediated activation of the MAPK or Akt pathways (Figure 1D), which are both necessary for IGF-IR-dependent motility and invasion of urothelial cancer cells [17,18].

Collectively, these results do not support a critical role for FAK in regulating IGF-IR-dependent motility and invasive capability of urothelial cancer cells.

Pyk2 is Critical for IGF-I-induced Motility, Invasion and Signaling

It is known that Pyk2 can promote both distinct and overlapping signaling events with FAK [23,24]. As we could not establish a major role for FAK in IGF-I-evoked motility of urothelial cancer cells, we considered the alternate hypothesis that Pyk2 is a predominant intracellular kinase that could mediate the downstream signaling pathway triggered by activation of the IGF-IR in urothelial cancer cells.

First, we discovered that IGF-I stimulation of 5637 cells induced a prolonged Pyk2 activation, which was sustained for up to 2 hours, as determined by immunoblot with anti-Phospho-Pyk2 antibody (Figure 2A). Second, we performed transient transfection assays in 5637 cells and determined that overexpression of wild type Pyk2 significantly increased IGF-I-induced migration, which was inhibited by the expression of a kinase-dead dominant negative Pyk2 (**P<0.01, compared to V-transfected cells) (Figure 2B). Proper expression of Flag-tagged wild-type or kinase-dead Pyk2 proteins was determined by immunoblot with anti-Flag antibodies (Figure 2C).

Next, to confirm Pyk2 function, we depleted endogenous Pyk2 in 5637 cells by siRNA approaches. Pyk2 depletion (Figure 3A) severely inhibited IGF-I-induced tumor cell migration (Figure 3B) and invasion through Matrigel™ (Figure 3C). Interestingly, Pyk2 depletion slightly upregulated FAK levels (Figure 3A), although FAK was unable to compensate for Pyk2 loss. In addition, Pyk2 knockdown in 5637 cells affected IGF-IR-downstream signaling and inhibited IGF-I-dependent activation of Akt and ERK1/2 and downstream effectors S6K and p90RSK (Figure 3D).

To corroborate our results on Pyk2 function, we transiently depleted by siRNA approaches endogenous Pyk2 in T24 cells, another IGF-I-responsive invasive urothelial cancer cell line [17,18]. We achieved a significant reduction in Pyk2 levels (Figure S1A) with a concurrent reduction in the ability of T24 cells to migrate (Figure S1B) and invade (Figure S1C) in response to IGF-I stimulation (*P<0.05, compared to either mock transfected or control oligo-transfected cells). In addition, Pyk2 ablation in T24 cells was associated with reduced IGF-I-dependent activation of ERK1/2 and S6K, while Akt and p90RSK activation was not affected (Figure S1D).

Collectively, our findings reveal an essential role for Pyk2 in the IGF-IR functional regulation of tumor cell motility and invasion, key properties of the aggressive cancer phenotype.

Pyk2 colocalizes with the IGF-IR and Complexes with IRS-1/2 and Grb2 in Urothelial Cancer Cells

To determine whether Pyk2 may interact with the IGF-IR in 5637 cells, we initially performed co-immunoprecipitation assays but we were unable to detect an interaction between endogenous IGF-IR and Pyk2 proteins. Thus, we used confocal microscopy analysis to determine whether Pyk2 may colocalize with the IGF-IR in 5637 urothelial cancer cells. While in serum-starved 5637 cells Pyk2 did not colocalize with the IGF-IR (Figure 4A), 30 minutes of IGF-I stimulation induced significant colocalization of endogenous Pyk2 and IGF-IR proteins (Figure 4A) suggesting that Pyk2 may be recruited to the IGF-IR upon ligand stimulation.

Next, to investigate the mechanisms by which Pyk2 regulates IGF-IR downstream signaling, we performed co-immunoprecipitation assays in both 5637 and T24 cells. The main goal of these studies was to determine whether Pyk2 would complex with the docking proteins IRS-1 and/or IRS-2 or Grb2 adaptors, known to regulate IGF-IR-dependent activation of the Akt and MAPK pathways, respectively [25,26,27]. In 5637 cells, IRS-1 was

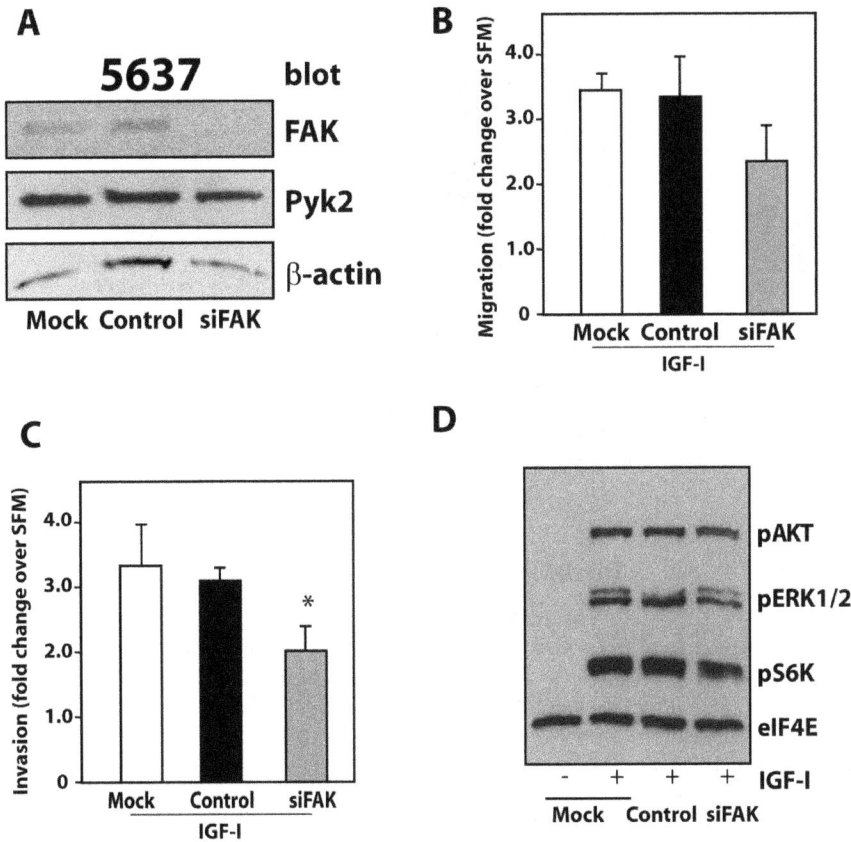

Figure 1. FAK is not important for IGF-I-mediated motility and signaling of invasive urothelial cancer cells. (A) 5637 cells were transfected with the FAK siGenome pool or control oligos. After 72 hours FAK and Pyk2 expression was detected by immunoblot with specific antibodies. Blot is representative of three independent experiments with an average FAK depletion level of 93.3±3.5 (arbitrary units) as assessed by densitometric analysis (B and C) Migration and invasion assays of 5637 cells were performed as described in Materials and Methods and assessed after 16 hours of IGF-I stimulation. Values are expressed as fold change over SFM and represent mean ± SD. *$P = 0.046$. (D) FAK-depleted 5637 cells were tested for Akt and MAPK activation after 10 minutes of IGF-I stimulation using a mix of phospho-specific antibodies (PathScan Cocktail I). eIF4E monitors protein loads. Blot is representative of three independent experiments.

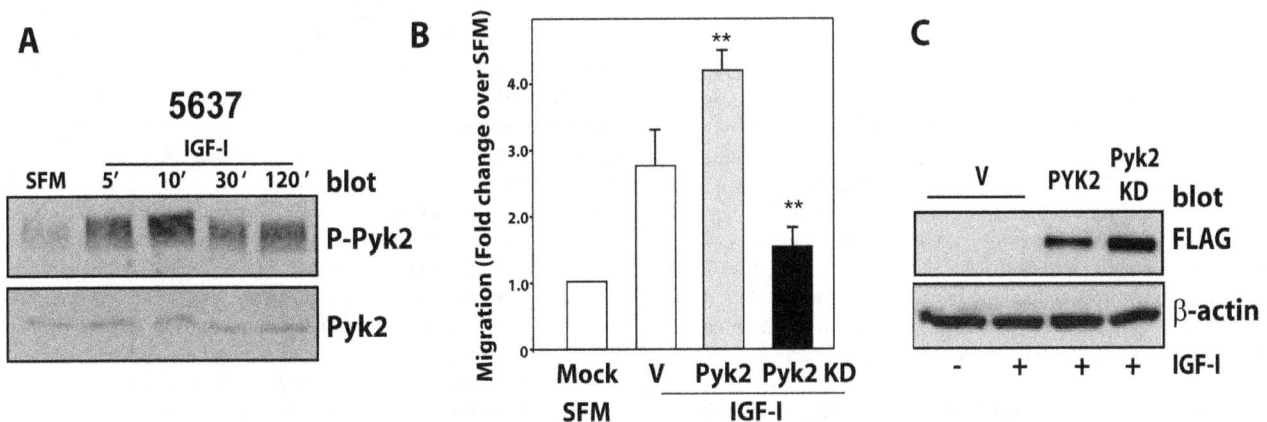

Figure 2. IGF-I-activated Pyk2 is critical for IGF-IR-dependent motility of invasive urothelial cancer cells. (A) Serum-starved 5637 cells were stimulated with 50 ng/ml of IGF-I for the indicated time points. Pyk2 phosphorylation was detected by immunoblot using anti-phospho-Pyk2 (Tyr402) antibodies, while total Pyk2 protein level was assessed using anti-Pyk2 polyclonal antibodies. Blot is representative of two independent experiments. (B) Migration of 5637 cells transiently transfected with either Flag-tagged wild type (PYK2 WT) or a dominant negative (KD PYK2) Pyk2 proteins was assessed after 16 hours of IGF-I stimulation. Values are expressed as fold change over SFM and represent mean ± SD. ** $P<0.01$. (C) Expression levels of transiently transfected Pyk2 proteins were assessed by immunoblot with anti-flag M2 antibodies. Blot is representative of two independent experiments.

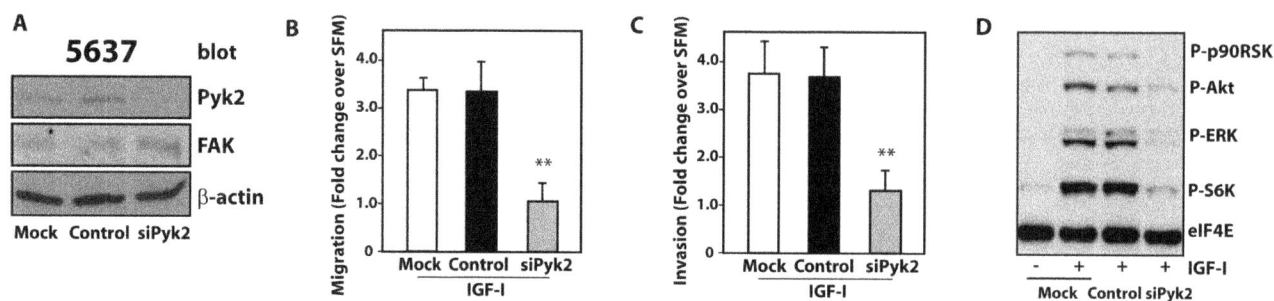

Figure 3. Pyk2 is critical for IGF-IR-induced motility, invasion and signaling of invasive urothelial cancer cells. (A) 5637 cells were transfected with the Pyk2 siGenome pool or control. After 72 hours Pyk2 and FAK expression was detected by immunoblot with specific antibodies. Blot is representative of three independent experiments with an average Pyk2 depletion level of 92.6±3 (arbitrary units) as assessed by densitometric analysis (B and C) Migration and invasion of 5637 cells were assessed as described in Materials and Methods after 16 hours of IGF-I stimulation. Values are expressed as fold change over SFM and represent mean ± SD. *$P<0.05$; **$P<0.01$. (D) Pyk2-depleted 5637 cells were tested for the activation of the Akt and MAPK pathways after 10 min of IGF-I stimulation using a mix of phospho-specific antibodies (PathScan Cocktail I). eIF4E monitors protein loads. Blot is representative of three independent experiments.

detectable in complex with Pyk2 in unstimulated cells but uncoupled from Pyk2 after 30 minutes of IGF-I stimulation (Figure 4B). In contrast, IRS-2 binding to Pyk2 was barely detectable in serum-starved 5637 cells but strongly increased after IGF-I stimulation (Figure 4B). Grb2 recruitment to Pyk2 was detectable in unstimulated 5637 cells but it was strongly enhanced after ligand stimulation (Figure 4B). The same results were recapitulated in T24 cells with only some differences in the levels of IRS-1, IRS-2 and Grb2 detectable in Pyk2 co-immunoprecipitates (Figure 4C). These qualitative differences may be likely due to differences in the relative abundance of these proteins in 5637 and T24 cells as in fact 5637 cells express higher level of Pyk2 proteins compared to T4 (data not shown). In addition, the interaction between Pyk2, IRS-1 and IRS-2 could be indirect and mediated by additional associated proteins, which may differ between 5637 and T24 cells.

These results indicate that Pyk2, by recruiting IRS-2 and Grb2, could play a critical role in regulating IGF-IR-dependent activation of downstream signaling pathways required for motility and invasion of urothelial cancer cells.

Pyk2 is Overexpressed in Bladder Cancer Tissues

We have recently shown that the IGF-IR is overexpressed in invasive bladder cancer tissues compared to normal tissue controls [17] and IGF-IR levels increase with bladder cancer progression [18]. Thus, we determined the expression of Pyk2 in a well annotated bladder cancer tissue microarray using immunofluorescence and AQUA analysis (Automated Quantitative Analysis) [28]. Pyk2 expression significantly increased in various bladder cancer tissues types (Figure 5A and B) as compared to normal tissue controls. In addition, the AQUA analysis for Pyk2 expression in various cellular compartments revealed that there was a significantly higher level of Pyk2 expression in the nuclei of urothelial cancer tissue cells when compared to cells in normal tissues (*$P=0.012$, Figure 5C).

Nuclear Pyk2 staining is better visualized at higher magnification of selected field of normal and urothelial carcinoma tissues (Figure S2).

Collectively, our results have identified a novel protein in the IGF-IR pathway that may be critical for bladder cancer. They also provide the first evidence that Pyk2 may translocate into the nuclei of bladder cancer cells. In addition, Pyk2 may serve in conjunction with the IGF-IR as a novel diagnostic and possibly prognostic biomarker for bladder cancer.

Discussion

The molecular mechanisms that determine malignant transformation of urothelial cells in the bladder are still very poorly characterized. In addition, there is an urgent need to identify proteins that may play a key role in driving the progression to the invasive and possibly metastatic phenotype in bladder neoplasia [2,3,4].

We have recently established that activation of the IGF-IR does not evoke *in vitro* cell proliferation but promotes motility and invasion of urothelial cancer cells [17,18]. These results support the hypothesis that the IGF-IR may not be so critical for bladder cancer initiation, but may play a prominent role during progression to the invasive and possibly metastatic stage of bladder cancer.

Based on our previous observation that upon IGF-I-stimulation FAK localizes with paxillin at dynamic adhesion sites of migrating cells [17], we investigated whether FAK, or its homolog Pyk2, would modulate IGF-IR action in urothelial cancer cells. We demonstrate that: (i) Depletion of endogenous FAK protein by siRNA strategies does not affect IGF-I-dependent motility and signaling of 5637 urothelial cancer cells. (ii) The FAK homolog Pyk2 is activated upon IGF-I stimulation of 5637 cells. (iii) Transient expression of wild type Pyk2 enhances IGF-I-induced migration, which is severely inhibited instead by the expression of a dominant-negative kinase-dead Pyk2 mutant. (iv) Pyk2 depletion by siRNA approaches inhibits IGF-I-dependent migration and invasive ability of 5637 and T24 cells and affects IGF-IR downstream signaling. (v) Upon IGF-I stimulation Pyk2 complex with IRS-2 and Grb2 in 5637 and T24 urothelial cancer cells. (vi) Pyk2 is overexpressed in various bladder cancer tissue types compared to normal tissue controls. (vii) Pyk2 expression increases in the nuclei of urothelial cancer tissue cells compared to normal tissue cells.

FAK and Pyk2 are related tyrosine-kinases involved in the dynamic regulation of the actin cytoskeleton, a process critical for cell motility, mitosis and tumor progression [24,29]. FAK and Pyk2 share a conserved molecular architecture and exhibit an overall 45% sequence identity with the greatest sequence identity (60%) in the kinase domain [24,29]. FAK is ubiquitously expressed while Pyk2 expression has a more limited tissue distribution with the highest Pyk2 expression levels detected in cells of the central nervous system and in hematopoietic lineage [29]. In addition, FAK and Pyk2 differs for their intracellular distribution, with FAK

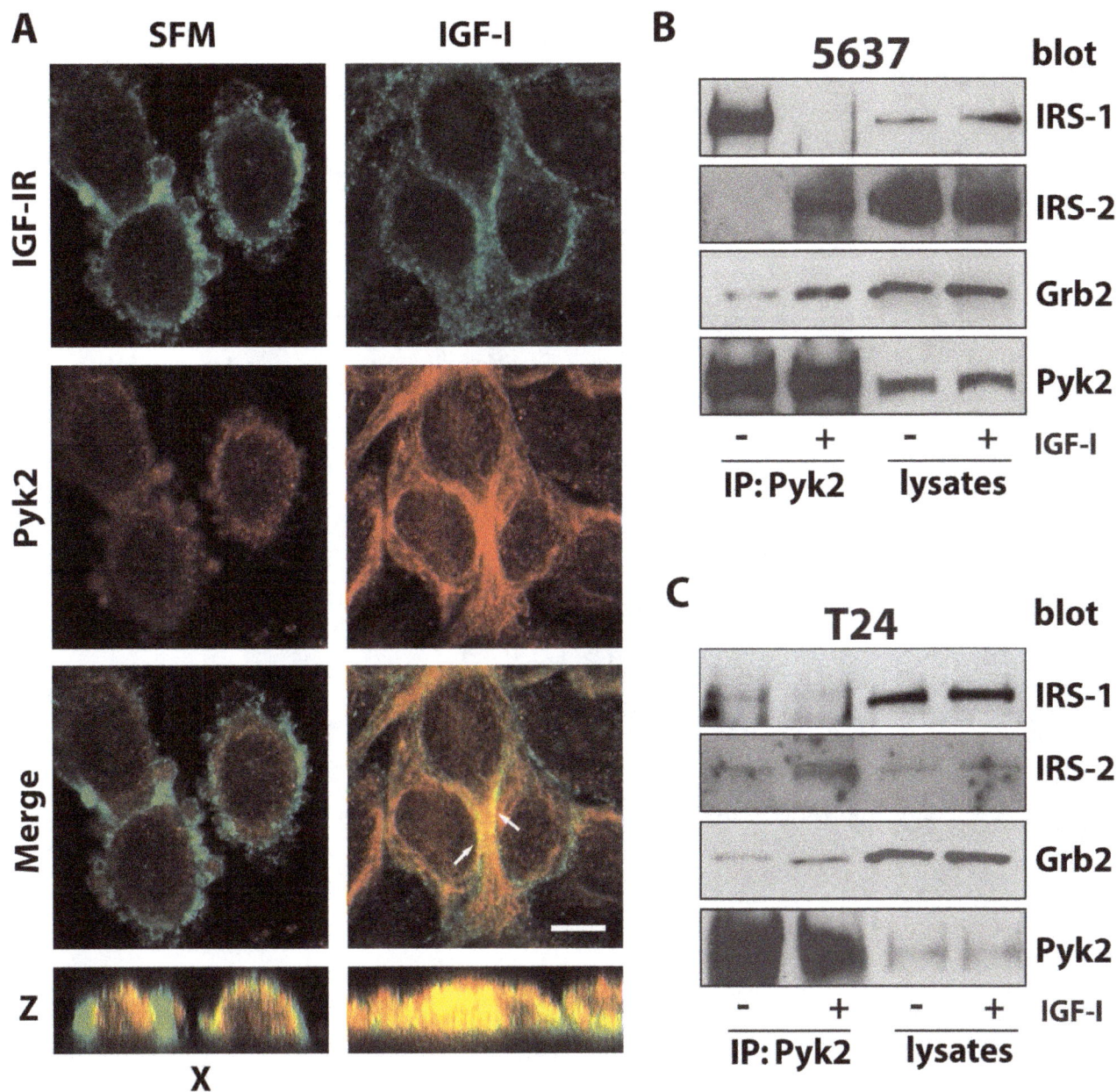

Figure 4. Pyk2 colocalizes with the IGF-IR and complexes with IRS-2 and Grb2 after IGF-I stimulation of urothelial cancer cells. (A) 5637 cells were serum-starved over night and then treated with 50 ng/ml of IGF-I for 30 minutes. After fixation, cells were labeled with a monoclonal anti-IGF-IR (green) and a polyclonal anti-Pyk2 (red) and imaged by confocal microscopy. The pictures of merged fields show colocalization (yellow) of IGF-IR and Pyk2 in the IGF-I treated cells (arrows) but not in unstimulated control cells. The distinct co-localization of Pyk2 and IGF-IR is detectable in the Z stacks (yellow staining, bottom panel). Pictures are representative of at least 10 independent fields from two independent experiments. An average of 300 cells was examined for each condition. Bar: 10 μm. (B) 5637 and(C) T24 bladder cancer cells were serum-starved for 24 hours and then stimulated with 50 ng/ml of IGF-I for 30 minutes. Two mg of cell lysates were immunoprecipitated with anti-Pyk2 polyclonal antibodies. IRS-1, IRS-2, Grb2 and Pyk2 levels were assessed by immunoblot with specific polyclonal antibodies. Blots are representatives of three independent experiments.

prevalently expressed at focal adhesions while Pyk2 expression is more distributed throughout the cell and sometimes enriched in perinuclear regions [29].

We have recently shown that IGF-I stimulation of invasive urothelial cells induces paxillin phosphorylation at Tyrosine 31 [17], a process mediated by FAK in other cellular models [21]. We further showed that paxillin localizes with FAK at the leading edge of migrating cells [17]. Because in other tumor models FAK is required for PI3K- and Ras-dependent tumorigenesis [30] and the

integrins/FAK complex activates Ras signaling to MAPK [31,32] a plausible mechanism by which IGF-I promotes migration and invasion of bladder cancer cells would be by activating FAK and the signaling cascade leading to Akt, MAPK and paxillin activation. Surprisingly, FAK depletion in 5637 cells had no effect in modulating both IGF-I-induced migration and IGF-IR-dependent activation of the Akt and MAPK pathways. The modest inhibitory effect on invasion detected in FAK-depleted 5637 cells in the absence of MAPK and Akt inhibition suggest that additional

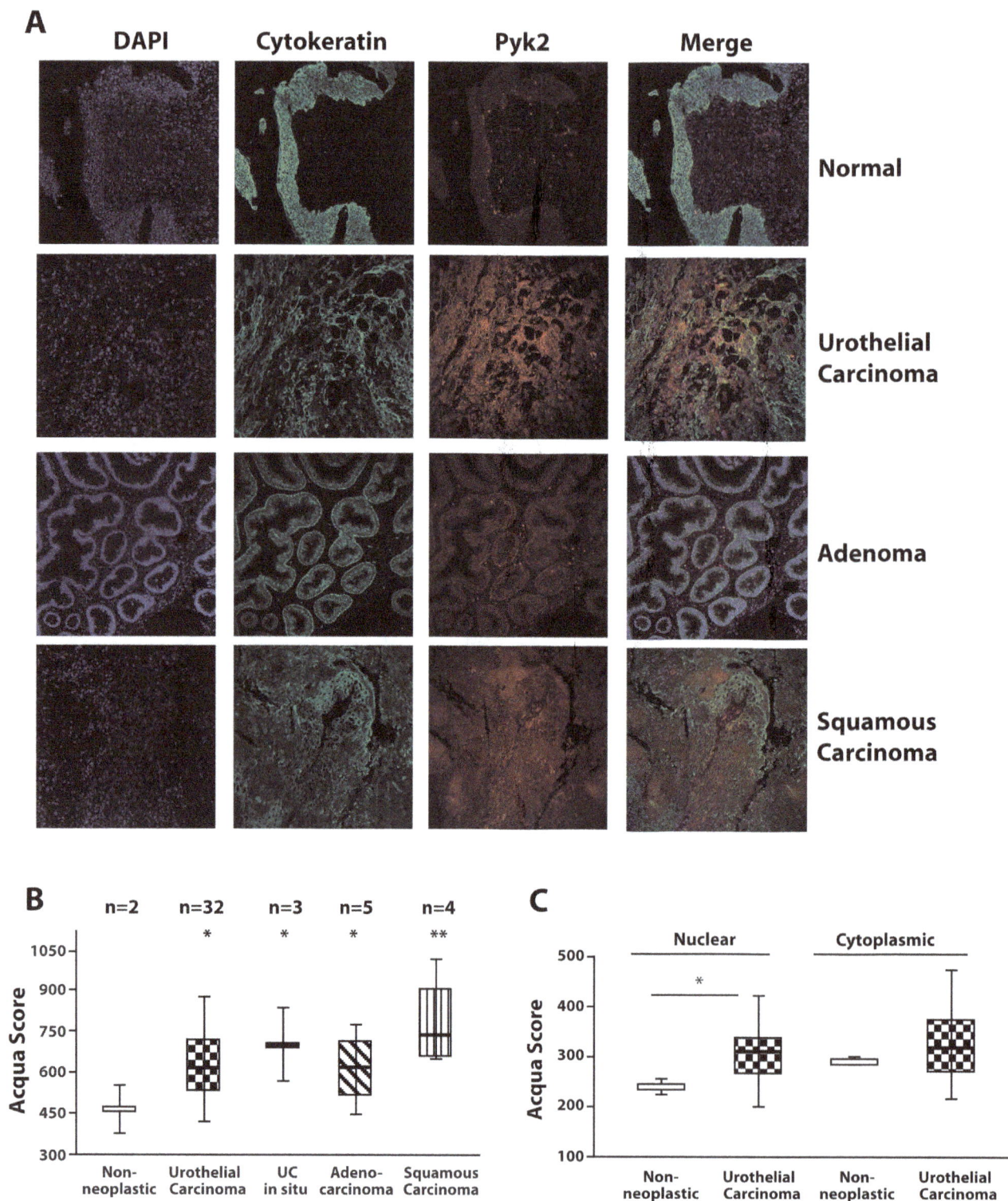

Figure 5. Pyk2 is up-regulated in bladder cancer tissues. (A) Pyk2 expression on a bladder cancer tissue microarray was determined by immunofluorescence and AQUA analysis using the AQUA PM-2000 system (HistoRx, Inc). Automated quantification and statistics on the different types of bladder cancer tumor tissues (B) and in the cytoplasmic and nuclear fractions of urothelial carcinoma cells (C) was calculated by AQUA Software. (B) *$P<0.05$. **$P<0.01$ compared to normal tissue controls. (C) *$P = 0.012$ compared to non-neoplastic nuclear fraction.

MAPK- and Akt-independent pathways may partially contribute to FAK-dependent invasive signaling in these cells.

However, we discovered that altering Pyk2 expression by transient overexpression of either wild type or dominant-negative Pyk2 proteins, or by siRNA-mediated Pyk2 depletion, had a major effect on IGF-I-induced motility and invasive ability of 5637 and T24 urothelial cancer cells. These functional assays were further corroborated by biochemical assays showing a significant inhibition of IGF-IR-activation of downstream signaling when intracellular Pyk2 levels were reduced. Thus, these results suggest that Pyk2 may have a more prevalent role than FAK in regulating IGF-IR-dependent biological responses in invasive urothelial cancer cells.

As Pyk2 depletion severely inhibits IGF-I-induced signaling, it could be argued that the effects of Pyk suppression on migration are a consequence of reduced proliferation/survival. However, we have previously shown that in both 5637 and T24 urothelial cancer cells the ability of IGF-I to induce motility (migration and invasion) is totally independent from the IGF-IR ability to sustain proliferation/survival, as in fact IGF-I does not enhance cell growth in these cells, which proliferate in the absence of serum [17].

To investigate the mechanisms by which Pyk2 may regulate IGF-I-dependent biological responses in urothelial cells, we initially assessed by confocal microscopy whether upon IGF-I-stimulation Pyk2 colocalized with paxillin in focal adhesions. However, in both serum-starved and IGF-I-stimulated 5637 and T24 cells we could not detect any colocalization of Pyk2 and paxillin, and Pyk2 staining was more diffuse throughout the cytoplasm and not enriched in focal adhesions (not shown). In addition, we performed co-immunoprepitation experiments in which we failed to detect a Pyk2/paxillin complex (not shown). These results strongly indicate that Pyk2 action in regulating IGF-I-dependent motility of urothelial cancer cells can be separated from paxillin function at focal adhesions.

Ligand-dependent recruitment of IRS-1/2 and Grb2 proteins to the IGF-IR is a critical step in the activation of the Akt and MAPK pathways in various IGF-IR-dependent biological responses [25,33,34,35,36]. Interestingly, IGF-I stimulation of 5637 and T24 urothelial cancer cells evoked the formation of a complex containing Pyk2, IRS-2 and Grb2 suggesting that in urothelial cancer cells Pyk2 may work as a critical signaling hub downstream of the IGF-IR. Whether Pyk2 binds directly to the IGF-IR and mediates the recruitment of IRS-2 and Grb2 to the receptor has not been demonstrated. So far we have not being able to detect an interaction between the IGF-IR and Pyk2 by co-immunoprecipitation experiments in 5637 cells but this negative result could be likely attributed to the relative low level of endogenous proteins. On the other hand, this result could also indicate that the IGF-IR and Pyk2 may interact indirectly in a complex with other signaling molecules of the IGF-IR system, such as IRS-1 and IRS-2. However, we have demonstrated by confocal microscopy that the IGF-IR and Pyk2 colocalize in ligand-dependent fashion suggesting that Pyk2 upon IGF-I stimulation may complex with the IGF-IR and facilitate the recruitment of signaling molecules to the receptor.

Recent experiments in vascular smooth muscle cells have demonstrated that upon IGF-I stimulation Pyk2 mediates the recruitment of Grb2 to the signaling SHP-1/SHP2/Src complex thus promoting MAPK activation and cell proliferation [37]. However, whether a similar mechanism may be conserved in urothelial cancer cells remains to be elucidated.

Our recent data have demonstrated that the IGF-IR is overexpressed in invasive bladder cancer tissues compared to normal tissue controls [17] and IGF-IR levels increase with bladder cancer progression [18]. The AQUA analysis we performed shows that Pyk2 expression is significantly upregulated in various bladder cancer tissue subtypes compared to normal controls but we could not detect a statistically significant difference in Pyk2 expression levels associated with different stages of urothelial carcinoma. A study with a larger sampling representing different stages of urothelial carcinoma is required to clearly establish whether Pyk2 may work as a prognostic marker for bladder cancer progression. Interestingly, in urothelial carcinoma cells the AQUA analysis revealed a statistically significant increase in the fraction of Pyk2 detected in the nucleus compared to cells in normal controls. Pyk2 localization in the nucleus has been previously demonstrated [38,39] but the function of Pyk2 in the nucleus has not been characterized. Our results provide the first evidence of increased levels of nuclear Pyk2 in bladder cancer cells thereby suggesting the novel hypothesis that in bladder cancer cells IGF-I-activated Pyk2 may act not only in the cytoplasm but also translocate into the nucleus, where it might work as a transcription factor. Significantly, IRS-1 and IRS-2 proteins have been shown to translocate to the nucleus in several cancer cell models [40,41,42,43], where they regulate gene expression [43,44]. In addition IRS-1 level in the nucleus predicts tamoxifen response in patients with early breast cancer [45], Thus, our results suggest the attractive hypothesis that IRS-1 or IRS-2 proteins may play a role in regulating Pyk2 translocation and/or interact with Pyk2 in the nucleus.

Experiments are currently under way to determine whether Pyk2 nuclear translocation is detectable in various urothelial cancer cell lines and is mediated by IGF-I. Future experiments will also determine IRS-1 or IRS-2 action in regulating Pyk2 nuclear translocation and function.

In conclusion, we have identified Pyk2 as a novel critical regulator of IGF-IR-dependent motility and invasion of urothelial cancer cells. These studies will greatly contribute to the identification of novel targets for therapeutic intervention in bladder tumors. In addition IGF-IR and Pyk2 may work as novel biological markers for bladder cancer progression.

Materials and Methods

Cells and Materials

Urothelial carcinoma-derived human 5637 and T24 cells were obtained from ATCC (Manassas, VA, USA. 5637 and T24 cells were maintained in RPMI medium supplemented with 10% fetal bovine serum (FBS). Serum-free medium (SFM) is DMEM supplemented with 0.1% bovine serum albumin and 50 μg/mL of transferrin (Sigma-Aldrich, St Louis, MO, USA). Recombinant IGF-I was purchased from Calbiochem (San Diego, CA, USA).

siRNA-mediated Gene Silencing

To silence FAK or Pyk2 we used RNA interference by using small-interfering RNA (siRNA). 5637 and T24 cells were transfected with vehicle (DEPC-treated water), control siRNA (scrambled), or siRNA specific oligos (200–400 pmol/L) using the TransIT-siTKO reagent (Mirus Bio LLC, Madison, WI, USA). Both scrambled and anti-FAK or anti-PYK2 siRNA oligos were from Thermo Scientific Dharmacon (siGenome Smartpool siRNA) (Lafayette, CO, USA). Cells were analyzed for motility and signaling 72 hours post-transfection. siRNA efficiency was detected by immunobloting using anti-FAK (#3285) and anti-Pyk2 (#3090) polyclonal antibodies (both from Cell Signaling Technology, Beverly, MA, USA). ß-actin was detected using anti-ß-actin polyclonal antibody (Sigma-Aldrich). Densitometric analysis was performed using the ImageJ program (rsbweb.nih.gov/ij/).

Transient Transfection Assays

5637 cells were transiently transfected using the TransIT®-Prostate Transfection Kit (Mirus BIO LLC) with the expression plasmid pShCMV.3X FLAG expressing either wild type or kinase-dead (K457A) Pyk2 mutant protein. Forty-eight hours post transfection, cells were serum-starved for additional 24 hours and then stimulated or not with 50 ng/mL of IGF-I. Migration was determined after 18 hours of incubation with the ligand, as stated below. In parallel, cells were lysed with cold RIPA buffer and the expression of the transfected plasmids was detected by western blot analyses using an anti-FLAG antibody (Santa Cruz Biotechnologies, Inc.).

Migration and Invasion Assays

5637 or T24 cells were plated in duplicate at a density of 3×10^4 cells/35-mm^2 plates in serum-supplemented medium. After 24 hours, cells were transferred to SFM or SFM supplemented with 50 ng/mL of IGF-I. Migration or invasion experiments were carried on for 4 hours or 16 hours, depending on the cell line used (T24 or 5637, respectively). Migration experiments were performed using HTS FluoroBloks^{TM} inserts (BD, San Jose, CA, USA) as previously described [17,18,46,47]. Membranes were mounted on a slide and migrated cells were counted and photographed with a Zeiss Axiovert 200 M cell live microscope at the Kimmel Cancer Center Bioimaging Facility. Cell invasion through a 3D-extracellular matrix was assessed using BD Matrigel^{TM}-coated Invasion Chambers (BD Biocoat) [17,18,47]. After 24 hours filters were washed, fixed, and stained with Coomassie Brilliant Blue. Cells that had invaded to the lower surface of the filter were counted under the microscope.

Analyses of Protein/Protein Interactions

5637 or T24 cells were serum-starved for 24 hours and then stimulated with IGF-I (50 ng/mL) for 30 minutes. Cells were lysed in cold RIPA buffer without sodium deoxycholate. The insoluble material was separated by centrifugation and the supernatants were incubated at 4°C under rotation for 18 hours with anti-Pyk2 polyclonal antibody (Sigma-Aldrich). At the end of the incubation, immunocomplexes were separated by adding 30 μL of mix protein A/G-Sepharose for additional 30 minutes. The resolved proteins were reduced in 40 μL of Laemmli buffer and subjected to SDS-PAGE. IRS-1 and IRS-2 interactions were determined by immunoblot using Anti-IRS-1 and Anti-IRS-2 polyclonal antibodies from Millipore (Burlington, MA, USA). The anti-Grb2 monoclonal antibody is from BD Biosciences. Blots are representative of three independent experiments.

Detection of Activated Signaling Pathways

5637 or T24 cells were serum-starved for 24 hours and then stimulated with IGF-I (50 ng/mL) for 5, 10, 30 and 120 minutes. Pyk2 phosphorylation was detected by immunoblot using anti-phospho-Pyk2 (Tyr-402) antibodies (Cell Signaling Technology). The activation of p90RSK, Akt, ERK1/2 and S6 Ribosomal Protein was analyzed by western immunoblot using the PathScan Multiplex Western Cocktail I (Cell Signaling Technology). EIF4E protein is used as control to monitor the loading of the samples.

Confocal Microscopy

5637 cells were plated onto 4-well chamber slides (BD Biosciences) and serum-starved over night prior to treatment with 50 ng/ml of IGF-I for 10, 30 and 60 minutes. Cells were then washed with 1X PBS and fixed with 4% PFA for 30 minutes at room temperature. Subsequently, slides were subjected to immunofluorescence and confocal analysis as previously described [18,46,48,49,50]. Primary antibodies were anti-IGF-IR monoclonal (Calbiochem) and anti-Pyk2 polyclonal antibodies (Santa Cruz Biotechnologies). Secondary antibodies were goat anti-mouse IgG Alexa Fluor$^®$ 488 and goat anti-rabbit IgG Alexa

Fluor$^®$ 594 antibodies (Invitrogen). Confocal analysis was performed on a Zeiss LSM810 microscope. The filters were set to 488 and 594 nm for dual channel imaging. All the images were then analyzed using Image J and Adobe Photoshop CS3 (Adobe Systems, San Jose, CA) software.

Pyk2 Expression in Bladder Cancer Tissues

Pyk2 expression levels in bladder cancer tissue were determined by AQUA analysis (Automated Quantitative Analysis) [28] on an Accumax bladder cancer tissue microarray (TMA #A215), composed by 4 non neoplastic spots and 45 different bladder cancer tissues (n = 33 urothelial carcinoma, n = 5 adenocarcinoma, n = 4 squamous carcinoma and n = 3 urothelial carcinoma in situ, two spots for each case). Detailed information regarding the TMA used is available on Accumax website. The antibodies used for immunofluorescence were rabbit pan-cytokeratin antibody (Cy2 conjugated, DAKO), Pyk2 antibody (Rabbit monoclonal YE353, Abcam) and DAPI. Pyk2 antibody was conjugated with Cy5 since it is outside the auto-fluorescence spectrum of tissue. Nuclear and cytoplasmic mask were automatically defined by AQUA Software, and applied to quantify Pyk2 expression on TMA. The analysis was performed at the Kimmel Cancer Center Translational Core Facility using an AQUA PM-2000 system (HistoRx, Inc). Automated quantification and statistics was calculated by AQUA Software. *$P<0.05$. **$P<0.01$ compared to normal.

Statistical Analysis

Experiments were carried out in triplicate and repeated at least three times. Results are expressed as mean ± SD. All statistical analyses were carried out with PRISM GraphPad Software, v.5. Results were compared using the two-sided Student's t test. Differences were considered statistically significant at $P<0.05$.

Supporting Information

Figure S1 Pyk2 is critical for IGF-IR-induced motility, invasion and signaling of invasive urothelial cancer cells. (A) T24 cells were transfected with the Pyk2 siGenome pool or control. After 72 hours Pyk2 and FAK expression was detected by immunoblot with specific antibodies. Blot is representative of three independent experiments with an average Pyk2 depletion level of 93.4±3.5 (arbitrary units) as assessed by densitometric analysis (B and C) Migration and invasion of T24 cells were assessed as described in Materials and Methods after 4 hours of IGF-I stimulation. Values are expressed as fold change over SFM and represent mean ± SD. *$P<0.05$. (D) Pyk2-depleted T24 cells were tested for the activation of the Akt and MAPK pathways after 10 min of IGF-I stimulation using a mix of phosphor-specific antibodies (Pathscan cocktail I). eIF4E monitors protein loads. Blot is representative of three independent experiments.

Figure S2 Pyk2 is up-regulated in urothelial carcinoma. Pyk2 expression on a bladder cancer tissue microarray was determined by immunofluorescence and AQUA analysis using the AQUA PM-2000 system (HistoRx, Inc). Higher magnification images from the same normal and urothelial carcinoma tissue samples shown in Figure 5 were acquired using a LEICA DM5500B microscope equipped with Leica Application Suite, Advanced Fluorescence 1.8 software (Leica Mycrosystem, Inc.) using a 63X Objective. Pictures are representative of at least 10 independent fields. Bar ~10 μm.

Acknowledgments

We thank Dr. Joseph C. Loftus, Mayo Clinic Arizona, for generously providing wild-type and Pyk2 mutated constructs.

Author Contributions

Conceived and designed the experiments: MG RVI AB AM. Performed the experiments: MG SQX SB. Analyzed the data: MG AB RVI AM. Contributed reagents/materials/analysis tools: SCP LGG AB RVI AM. Wrote the paper: RVI AM.

References

1. Siegel R, Naishadham D, Jemal A (2012) Cancer statistics, 2012. CA: A Cancer Journal for Clinicians 62: 10–29.
2. Mitra AP, Cote RJ (2009) Molecular Pathogenesis and Diagnostics of Bladder Cancer. Annu Rev Pathol 4: 251–285.
3. Knowles MA (2008) Molecular pathogenesis of bladder cancer. Int J Clin Oncol 13: 287–297.
4. Goebell PJ, Knowles MA (2010) Bladder cancer or bladder cancers? Genetically distinct malignant conditions of the urothelium. Urol Oncol 28: 409–428.
5. Scher CD, Stone ME, Stiles CD (1979) Platelet-derived growth factor prevents G0 growth arrest. Nature 281: 390–392.
6. Baserga R (1995) The insulin-like growth factor I receptor: a key to tumor growth? Cancer Res 55: 249–252.
7. Baker J, Liu JP, Robertson EJ, Efstratiadis A (1993) Role of insulin-like growth factors in embryonic and postnatal growth. Cell 75: 73–82.
8. Eggenschwiler J, Ludwig T, Fisher P, Leighton PA, Tilghman SM, et al. (1997) Mouse mutant embryos overexpressing IGF-II exhibit phenotypic features of the Beckwith-Wiedemann and Simpson-Golabi-Behmel syndromes. Genes Dev 11: 3128–3142.
9. Sell C, Dumenil G, Deveaud C, Miura M, Coppola D, et al. (1994) Effect of a null mutation of the insulin-like growth factor I receptor gene on growth and transformation of mouse embryo fibroblasts. Mol Cell Biol 14: 3604–3612.
10. Surmacz E (2003) Growth factor receptors as therapeutic targets: strategies to inhibit the insulin-like growth factor I receptor. Oncogene 22: 6589–6597.
11. Baserga R, Morrione A (1999) Differentiation and malignant transformation: two roads diverged in a wood. J Cell Biochem 75: 68–75.
12. Pollak MN, Schernhammer ES, Hankinson SE (2004) Insulin-like growth factors and neoplasia. Nat Rev Cancer 4: 505–518.
13. Le Roith D, Karas M, Yakar S, Qu BH, Wu Y, et al. (1999) The role of the insulin-like growth factors in cancer. Isr Med Assoc J 1: 25–30.
14. Baserga R (2000) The contradictions of the insulin-like growth factor 1 receptor. Oncogene 19: 5574–5581.
15. Baserga R, Hongo A, Rubini M, Prisco M, Valentinis B (1997) The IGF-I receptor in cell growth, transformation and apoptosis. Biochim Biophys Acta 1332: F105–126.
16. Le Roith D (2000) Regulation of proliferation and apoptosis by the insulin-like growth factor I receptor. Growth Horm IGF Res 10 Suppl A: S12–13.
17. Metalli D, Lovat F, Tripodi F, Genua M, Xu SQ, et al. (2010) The insulin-like growth factor receptor I promotes motility and invasion of bladder cancer cells through Akt- and mitogen-activated protein kinase-dependent activation of paxillin. Am J Pathol 176: 2997–3006.
18. Iozzo RV, Buraschi S, Genua M, Xu SQ, Solomides CC, et al. (2011) Decorin antagonizes IGF-IR function by interfering with IGF-IR activity and attenuating downstream signaling. J Biol Chem 286: 34712–34721.
19. Lev S, Moreno H, Martinez R, Canoll P, Peles E, et al. (1995) Protein tyrosine kinase PYK2 involved in Ca(2+)-induced regulation of ion channel and MAP kinase functions. Nature 376: 737–745.
20. Yu H, Li X, Marchetto GS, Dy R, Hunter D, et al. (1996) Activation of a novel calcium-dependent protein-tyrosine kinase. Correlation with c-Jun N-terminal kinase but not mitogen-activated protein kinase activation. J Biol Chem 271: 29993–29998.
21. Zhao J, Guan JL (2009) Signal transduction by focal adhesion kinase in cancer. Cancer Metastasis Rev 28: 35–49.
22. Webb DJ, Donais K, Whitmore LA, Thomas SM, Turner CE, et al. (2004) FAK-Src signalling through paxillin, ERK and MLCK regulates adhesion disassembly. Nat Cell Biol 6: 154–161.
23. Weis SM, Lim ST, Lutu-Fuga KM, Barnes LA, Chen XL, et al. (2008) Compensatory role for Pyk2 during angiogenesis in adult mice lacking endothelial cell FAK. J Cell Biol 181: 43–50.
24. Lipinsky CA, FLoftus JC (2010) The Pyk2 FERM domain: a Novel Therapeutic Target. Expert Opin Ther Targets 14: 95–108.
25. Morrione A, Romano G, Navarro M, Reiss K, Valentinis B, et al. (2000) Insulin-like growth factor I receptor signaling in differentiation of neuronal H19–7 cells. Cancer Res 60: 2263–2272.
26. Peruzzi F, Prisco M, Dews M, Salomoni P, Grassilli E, et al. (1999) Multiple signaling pathways of the insulin-like growth factor 1 receptor in protection from apoptosis. Mol Cell Biol 19: 7203–7215.
27. Peruzzi F, Prisco M, Morrione A, Valentinis B, Baserga R (2001) Anti-apoptotic signaling of the insulin-like growth factor-I receptor through mitochondrial translocation of c-Raf and Nedd4. J Biol Chem 276: 25990–25996.
28. Rubin MA, Zerkowski MP, Camp RL, Kuefer R, Hofer MD, et al. (2004) Quantitative determination of expression of the prostate cancer protein alpha-methylacyl-CoA racemase using automated quantitative analysis (AQUA): a novel paradigm for automated and continuous biomarker measurements. Am J Pathol 164: 831–840.
29. Schaller MD (2010) Cellular functions of FAK kinases: insight into molecular mechanisms and novel functions. J Cell Sci 123: 1007–1013.
30. Pylayeva Y, Gillen KM, Gerald W, Beggs HE, Reichardt LF, et al. (2009) Ras- and PI3K-dependent breast tumorigenesis in mice and humans requires focal adhesion kinase signaling. J Clin Invest 119: 252–266.
31. Guo W, Giancotti FG (2004) Integrin signalling during tumour progression. Nat Rev Mol Cell Biol 5: 816–826.
32. Bao W, Stromblad S (2004) Integrin alphav-mediated inactivation of p53 controls a MEK1-dependent melanoma cell survival pathway in three-dimensional collagen. J Cell Biol 167: 745–756.
33. Valentinis B, Romano G, Peruzzi F, Morrione A, Prisco M, et al. (1999) Growth and differentiation signals by the insulin-like growth factor 1 receptor in hemopoietic cells are mediated through different pathways. J Biol Chem 274: 12423–12430.
34. Valentinis B, Navarro M, Zanocco-Marani T, Edmonds P, McCormick J, et al. (2000) Insulin receptor substrate-1, p70S6K, and cell size in transformation and differentiation of hemopoietic cells. J Biol Chem 275: 25451–25459.
35. Morrione A, Navarro M, Romano G, Dews M, Reiss K, et al. (2001) The role of the insulin receptor substrate-1 in the differentiation of rat hippocampal neuronal cells. Oncogene 20: 4842–4852.
36. Dews M, Prisco M, Peruzzi F, Romano G, Morrione A, et al. (2000) Domains of the insulin-like growth factor I receptor required for the activation of extracellular signal-regulated kinases. Endocrinology 141: 1289–1300.
37. Shen X, Xi G, Radhakrishnan Y, Clemmons DR (2010) Recruitment of Pyk2 to SHPS-1 signaling complex is required for IGF-I-dependent mitogenic signaling in vascular smooth muscle cells. Cell Mol Life Sci 67: 3893–3903.
38. Farshori PQ, Shah BH, Arora KK, Martinez-Fuentes A, Catt KJ (2003) Activation and nuclear translocation of PKCdelta, Pyk2 and ERK1/2 by gonadotropin releasing hormone in HEK293 cells. J Steroid Biochem 85: 337–347.
39. Aoto H, Sasaki H, Ishino M, Sasaki T (2002) Nuclear translocation of cell adhesion kinase beta/proline-rich tyrosine kinase 2. Cell Struct Funct 27: 47–61.
40. Lassak A, Del Valle L, Peruzzi F, Wang JY, Enam S, et al. (2002) Insulin receptor substrate 1 translocation to the nucleus by the human JC virus T-antigen, J Biol Chem 277: 17231–17238.
41. Wu A, Sciacca L, Baserga R (2003) Nuclear translocation of insulin receptor substrate-1 by the insulin receptor in mouse embryo fibroblasts. Journal of Cellular Physiology 195: 453–460.
42. Sun H, Tu X, Prisco M, Wu A, Casiburi I, et al. (2003) Insulin-like growth factor I receptor signaling and nuclear translocation of insulin receptor substrates 1 and 2. Molecular Endocrinology 17: 472–486.
43. Reiss K, Del Valle L, Lassak A, Trojanek J (2011) Nuclear IRS-1 and cancer. J Cell Physiol 227: 2992–3000.
44. Wu A, Chen J, Baserga R (2008) Nuclear insulin receptor substrate-1 activates promoters of cell cycle progression genes. Oncogene 27: 397–403.
45. Migliaccio I, Wu MF, Gutierrez C, Malorni L, Mohsin SK, et al. (2010) Nuclear IRS-1 predicts tamoxifen response in patients with early breast cancer. Breast Cancer Res Treat 123: 651–660.
46. Monami G, Emiliozzi V, Bitto A, Lovat F, Xu SQ, et al. (2009) Proepithelin regulates prostate cancer cell biology by promoting cell growth, migration, and anchorage-independent growth. Am J Pathol 174: 1037–1047.
47. Lovat F, Bitto A, Xu SQ, Fassan M, Goldoni S, et al. (2009) Proepithelin is an autocrine growth factor for bladder cancer. Carcinogenesis 30: 861–868.
48. Monami G, Emiliozzi V, Morrione A (2008) Grb10/Nedd4-mediated multi-ubiquitination of the insulin-like growth factor receptor regulates receptor internalization. J Cell Physiol 216: 426–437.
49. Monami G, Gonzalez EM, Hellman M, Gomella LG, Baffa R, et al. (2006) Proepithelin promotes migration and invasion of 5637 bladder cancer cells through the activation of ERK1/2 and the formation of a paxillin/FAK/ERK complex. Cancer Res 66: 7103–7110.
50. Buraschi S, Pal N, Tyler-Rubinstein N, Owens RT, Neill T, et al. (2010) Decorin antagonizes Met receptor activity and down-regulates {beta}-catenin and Myc levels. J Biol Chem 285: 42075–42085.

14

Proteomic Analysis of Bladder Cancer Indicates Prx-I as a Key Molecule in BI-TK/GCV Treatment System

Li Jiang[1], Xiao Xiao[1], Jin Ren[1], YongYong Tang[1], HongQing Weng[1], Qi Yang[1], MingJun Wu[2], Wei Tang[1]*

1 Department of Urology, The First Affiliated Hospital of Chongqing Medical University, Chongqing, China, **2** Institute of Life Science, Chongqing Medical University, Chongqing, China

Abstract

In order to understand the molecular mechanisms of Bifidobacterium infantis thymidine kinase/nucleoside analogue ganciclovir (BI-TK/GCV) treatment system which was proven to exhibit sustainable anti-tumor growth activity and induce apoptosis in bladder cancer, a proteomic approach of isobaric tags for relative and absolute quantification (iTRAQ), followed by liquid chromatography-tandem mass spectrometry (LC-MS/MS) was used. 192 down-regulated and 210 up-regulated proteins were identified after treatment with BI-TK/GCV system in Sprague-Dawley (SD) rats. Western blot analysis and immunohistochemistry analysis confirmed that Peroxiredoxin-I (Prx-I) was significantly down-regulated in bladder cancer after treatment. Prx-I silencing by transfection of Prx-I shRNA significantly suppressed growth, promoted apoptosis and regulated the cell cycle in T24 cells and reduced the phospho-NF-κB p50 and p65 protein expression which revealed the links between Prx-I and NF-κB pathway implied by Ingenuity pathway analysis (IPA). These findings yield new insights into the therapy of bladder cancer, revealing Prx-I as a new therapeutic target and indicating BI-TK/GCV system as a prospective therapy by down-regulation of Prx-I through NF-κB signaling pathway.

Editor: Hari K Koul, Louisiana State University Health Sciences center, United States of America

Funding: This work was supported in part by the research grant from the Natural Scientific Foundation of China (No. 81072087/H1619). The URL for National Natural Science Foundation of China: http://www.nsfc.gov.cn/publish/portal0/default.htm. The funders had no role in study design, data collection and analysis, decision to publish, or preparation of the manuscript. No additional external funding received for this study.

Competing Interests: The authors have declared that no competing interests exist.

* E-mail: tangwei2060@163.com

Introduction

Bladder cancer is the most common urological cancer in Asia and its clinical management is extremely expensive [1]. In 2014, about 74,690 new cases of bladder cancer are expected to be diagnosed, and about 15,580 of them will die [2]. Bladder cancer can be divided into two major clinical and pathological subtypes: superficial non-muscle-invasive type and advanced muscle-invasive type [3]. In general, superficial bladder cancer is treated with endoscopic resection with favorable prognosis, but it sometimes reoccurs with grade progression [4]. The management of advanced bladder cancer is a major challenge, and these patients have a less favorable prognosis with a very low 5-year survival rate; therefore, more aggressive therapeutic options are necessary such as radical cystectomy and urinary diversion [5]. Further, bladder cancer especially the advanced type reoccurs in a substantial number of patients, and even results in death, and therefore, preferably less aggressive approaches should be developed to combat the disease.

Herpes simplex virus thymidine kinase (HSV-TK)–mediated suicide gene therapy as a widely accepted strategy for bladder cancer can convert the nontoxic nucleoside analog ganciclovir (GCV) into a toxic triphosphorylated form, which subsequently causes the death of rapidly dividing cells [6]. We previously resorted to *Bifidobacterium infantis* (BI) which is a tumor-targeting bacterium, because it selectively localizes and proliferates within the hypoxic regions of tumors as a non-pathogenic and anaerobic bacterium [7,8]. We found that the BI and TK/GCV (BI-TK/ GCV) system exhibited a sustainable anti-tumor growth activity in the rodent bladder cancer model in vivo, which involved both extrinsic and intrinsic apoptosis pathways [9].

In an effort to understand the underlying molecular mechanisms and identify the potential target protein molecule of this safe and effective treatment system, we resorted to mass spectrometry (MS)-based isobaric tags for relative and absolute quantification (iTRAQ) to obtain comprehensive differential protein profiles. Furthermore, we investigated the molecular pathway of Peroxiredoxin-I (Prx-I), one of the identified down-regulated proteins in bladder cancer identified by iTRAQ after treatment with BI-TK/ GCV.

Materials and Methods

Materials

The BI-TK/GCV treatment system was constructed successfully by our research group (Chongqing, China) [9].

Experimental animals

Seventy female Sprague–Dawley rats (6–8 weeks old, weighing 180–200 g) were purchased from Chongqing National Biological Industry Base of Experimental Animal Center (China) and housed under specific pathogen-free condition at 23–27°C and humidity 55–65% with 12-h light–dark cycles. All animal procedures were approved by the Animal Use and Care Committee of Chongqing Medical University. A rat bladder tumor model was built by perfusion of N-methyl-nitrosourea (MNU)(Sigma, USA). MNU was diluted into 20 g/l by a citric acid buffer solution. Each bladder was perfused with 0.1 ml once every 2 weeks, for a total of four perfusions.

Studies in vivo

Sixty tumor-bearing Sprague-Dawley rats were randomly divided into four groups (each $n = 15$): a normal saline group, a BI group, a BI/PGEX-1 group, and a BI-TK group. After the bifidobacterium was concentrated, about 0.5 ml of the corresponding interventions was injected via the tail vein (bacterium count, 4.4×10^9) once a week for 4 weeks. All groups received daily intraperitoneal injection of GCV (50 mg/kg) for 28 days. All the rats were sacrificed under anesthesia with sodium pentobarbital. Part of the bladder cancer tissues from the four groups were preserved in paraffin for immunohistochemical (IHC) analysis, and the rest of the tissues were kept at $-80°C$ for further analysis.

Protein sample preparation and iTRAQ labeling

The tissues were lysed in a lysis buffer (7 m urea, 1 mg/ml DNaseI, 1 mmNa$_3$VO$_4$, and 1 mm phenylmethane sulfonylfluoride, PMSF) and centrifugated at 6000 g and 4°C for 30 min. The supernatant was collected and the total protein content was measured using 2D Quantification Kit (Amersham Biosciences, Uppsala, Sweden). Each sample was digested with 20 µl of 0.1 µg/µl trypsin solution (Promega, Madison, USA) at 37°C overnight and then labeled with the iTRAQ tags as follows: (i) normal saline group, 114 tags; (ii) BI-TK group, 115 tags; (iii) BI/PGEX-1 group, 116 tags; (iv) BI group, 117 tags. The labeled samples were pooled prior to further analysis.

Strong cation exchange (SCX) chromatography

To reduce the sample complexity for liquid chromatography (LC)-MS/MS analysis, the pooled samples were diluted 10-fold with an SCX buffer A (10 mm KH$_2$PO$_4$ in 25% acetonitrile at pH 3.0) and utilized to a 2.1×200 mm polysulfoethyl A SCX column (PolyLC; Columbia, USA). The column was eluted with a gradient of 0–25% SCX buffer B (10 mM KH$_2$PO$_4$ at pH 3.0 in 25% acetonitrile containing 350 mM KCl) over 30 min, followed by a gradient of 25–100% SCX buffer B over 40 min. These SCX fractions were lyophilized in a vacuum concentrator and subjected to C-18 clean-up using extraction column (100 mg capacity, Supelco; Sigma-Aldrich, St. Louis, USA).

Electrospray ion-quadrupole time-of-flight MS (ESI-Q-TOF-MS) Analysis

MS was performed using a nano-LC coupled online to a QStar Elite mass spectrometer (Applied Biosystems). The LC eluent was directed to an ESI source for Q-TOF-MS analysis. The mass spectrometer was set to perform information dependent acquisition (IDA) in the positive ion mode, with a selected mass range of 300–2,000 m/z. Peptides with +2 to +4 charge states were selected for tandem mass spectrometry, and the time of summation of MS/MS events was set to 3 s. Relative quantification of proteins, in case of iTRAQ, was performed on the MS/MS scans and was the ratio of the areas under the peaks at 113, 114, 115, and 116 Da, which were the masses of the tags that correspond to the iTRAQ reagents.

Proteomic analysis

The bioinformatic processes and molecular function of the identified proteins in the BI-TK group after treatment were classified by the PANTHER classification system (www.pantherdb.org). The pathways of differentially expressed proteins identified by iTRAQ were analyzed by the Ingenuity pathway analysis (IPA) program (http://www.ingenuity.com). On the software Ingenuity, the data were used to extract interactive networks among the proteins in the International Protein Index (IPI) database. A network with a score higher than 2 is usually considered valid.

Validation by Western blot and IHC

Western blotting and IHC were used to confirm the expression of Prx-I. T The protein samples (about 20 mg) were separated using SDS–PAGE. After SDS–PAGE electrophoresis, proteins were transferred to PVDF membranes. Subsequently, the lysates were incubated with a primary anti-Prx-I rabbit monoclonal antibody (1:1500) (Abcam, USA). The immunoreactive signals were detected by enhanced chemiluminescence kit (Amersham Biosciences, Sweden). The procedures were conducted according to the manufacturer's instructions. Bladder cancer tissues from four groups were incubated overnight with primary antibodies. The tissues were incubated with secondary antibodies for 2 h. The cell nuclei were counterstained with hematoxylin. The proportion of positively stained tumor cells was determined by Image-Pro Plus (IPP) 6.0 and was graded as follows: 0, negative; 1, <10%; 2, 10–50%; 3, >50%. The immunostaining intensity was scored as follows: 0, absent; 1, light yellow; 2, yellowish brown; 3, brown. The protein in bladder cancer tissues was evaluated using the staining index (SI): SI = proportion × intensity of positive tumor cells.

Prx-1 Knockdown by shRNA

T24 cells were subjected to Prx1 knockdown. Short hairpin RNA (shRNA) was exprssed with GV102 system (GeneChem, China). The three pairs of sense and antisense sequences of oligonucleotides targeting human Prx1(GeneBank_ID: NM_002574) were as follows: PRDX1-RNAi (sh-1) sense strand 5'-GATCCCGCTTTCAGTGA-TAGGGCAGAACTCGAGTTCTGCCCTATCACTGAAAGC-TTTTTGGAT-3', PRDX1-RNAi (sh-1) antisense strand 5'-AG-CTATCCAAAAAGCTTTCAGTGATAGGGCAGAACTCGAG-TTCTGCCCTATCACTGAAAGCGG-3'; PRDX1-RNAi (sh-2) sense strand 5'-GATCCCGATGAGACTTTGAGACTAGTTCT-CGAGAACTAGTCTCAAAGTCTCATCTTTTTGGAT-3', PRDX1-RNAi (sh-2) antisense strand 5'-AGCTATCCAAAAA-GATGAGACTTTGAGACTAGTTCTCGAGAACTAGTCTCA-AAGTCTCATCGG-3'; PRDX1-RNAi(sh-3) sense strand 5'-GATCCCCCATGAACATTCCTTTGGTATCTCGAGATAC-CAAAGGAATGTTCATGGTTTTTGGAT-3', PRDX1-RNA-i(sh-3) antisense strand 5'-AGCTATCCAAAAACCATGAA-CATTCCTTTGGTATCTCGAGATACCAAAGGAATGTTCA-TGGGG-3'.A scrambled sequence of the Prx-I target was used as a negative control (con sh). T24 cells were transiently transfected with the Prx1-shRNA expression vectors by using Lipofectamine 2000 (Invitrogen, USA). Non-infected T24 cells (parental) and Prx-I control shRNA infected T24 cells (con sh) were also used. The highest efficiency of knockdown by shRNA vectors in T24 cells was determined by quantitative real-time polymerase chain reaction (qRT-PCR). The primer sequences for Prx-I were 5'-AGCCT-GTCTGACTACAAAG-3' (forward) and 5'-TCTGCCCTAT-CACTGAAAG-3' (reverse), which yielded a 104 bp product. The primer sequences for the internal control GAPDH were 5'-CACCCACTCCTCCACCTTTG-3' (forward) and 5'-CCAC-CACCCTGTTGCTGTAG-3' (reverse), which yielded a 110 bp product. The expression value of Prx-I compared with that of GAPDH was calculated as 2-ΔΔCt. All reactions were conducted in triplicate. Then the expressions of Prx-I in T24 cells knocked down by shRNAs were measured by Western blotting.

Cell proliferation assay

After transfection with Prx-I shRNA for 24 h, the T24 cells were seeded into 96-well culture plates at a density of 4×10^3 cells in a final volume of 100 μl/well, and the untransfected cells were used as a control. The cell proliferation rate was calculated at different time points (24, 48 and 72 h) using Cell Counting Kit-8 (CCK-8) (Sigma, USA). Experiments were performed according the manufacturer's protocol. The absorbance at 450/630 nm was measured with a Thermo spectrophotometer (Waltham, USA). The average absorbance from six wells per group was calculated.

Flow cytometric analysis

After transfection for 48 h, the cells were trypsinized and centrifuged at 1500 rpm for 5 min. The cells were harvested and washed with PBS twice. After stained with 50 μg/ml Annexin V-fluorescein isothiocyanate (FITC) (BD Biosciences, USA) and 20 μl of 500 μg/ml propidium iodide (PI) (Sigma, USA) for apoptosis detection, the cells were incubated in dark at room temperature for 15 min and subjected to flow cytometry analysis (FACS). Then the cells were collected, washed with PBS, fixed with 75% ethanol at $-20°C$ overnight. The fixed cells were washed with cold PBS twice, added 500 μL DNA staining solution (including 200 μg/mL RNase A and 20 μg/mL propidium iodide staining solution) and incubated for 30 minutes. Finally, the cells were subjected to cell cycle analysis by FACS. The data were analyzed and evaluated on the program ModFit (Topsham, USA).

Effect of Prx-I on phospho-NF-κB p50 and p65

The link between Prx-I and the NF-kappa-B (NF-κB) complex signaling had been implied in the protein pathway of IPA. Therefore, in order to explore whether the effect of Prx-I on apoptotic signaling proteins was attributable to NF-κB inhibition, we evaluated nuclear levels of phospho-NF-κB p50 and p65 (Abcam, USA) by Western blot.

Statistical analysis

The data were expressed as mean ± standard deviation (SD) and compared using analysis of variance. The level of significant difference was defined as $p < 0.05$. All analyses were performed on SPSS 18.0 (SPSS, Chicago, USA) for Windows.

Results

Quantification and identification of differentially expressed proteins by iTRAQ

A total of 2343 unique proteins were identified with 95% confidence by the ProteinPilot search algorithm against the IPI rat protein database v3.49. A strict cutoff value of a 1.3-fold change resulted in a final set of 402 differentially expressed proteins, including 192 down-regulated proteins and 210 up-regulated proteins in the BI-TK group after treatment. Strikingly, a novel molecule Prx- I drew our particular attention, with a 0.52-fold decrease in the BI-TK group versus the normal saline group. A schematic diagram of iTRAQ is shown in Figure 1A, and the MS/MS spectrum of Prx- I (peptide sequence: VVGDHVEVHAR) is shown in Figure 1B. The iTRAQ tags are as follows: (i) the normal saline group, 114 tags; (ii) the BI-TK group, 115 tags; (iii) the BI/PGEX-1 group, 116 tags; (iv) the BI group, 117 tags. The protein ID in IPI, name and main functions with abundance changes are epitomized in Table S1.

Bioinformatic functional analysis of differentially expressed proteins after treatment with BI-TK/GCV

To probe into their biological roles in the curative effect of BI-TK/GCV on bladder cancer, the differentially expressed proteins were categorized into various processes and function classes based on PANTHER classification system. In biological process analysis, the largest proportion of differentially expressed proteins was in metabolic process, followed by cellular process and cell communication process (Figure 2A). Notably, the proteins involved in catalytic activity, binding, structural molecule activity, enzyme regulator activity, and receptor activity were the top five molecular function categories (Figure 2B). Moreover, proteins involved in antioxidant activity accounted for 1.3%, respectively. Figure 2C depicts the primary pathways generated by IPA of the differentially expressed proteins. This network scored 36 and consisted of 37 proteins involved in apoptosis, oxidative stress, and metabolism. In particular, Prx-I, the markedly down-expressed protein after treatment, is directly linked to transcription factor NF-kappa-B (NF-κB) complex pathway in this network, indicating that Prx-I may play an important role in the apoptosis of bladder cancer by BI-TK/GCV system partly through the NF-κB signaling pathway.

Validation of Prx-I by Western blot and IHC

The differential expression levels of Prx- I identified by iTRAQ approach were validated by Western blot (Figure 3A). Compared with the normal saline group, expression of Prx-I is down-regulated in the other three groups (especially in the BI-TK group), which is similar to the results obtained by iTRAQ. Moreover, the Prx-I expression in the tumor tissues was verified by IHC analysis (Figure 3B). The Prx-I content in bladder cancer cells of BI-TK group was significantly lower than that in the other groups ($p < 0.05$, Figure 3B), which is consistent with the results obtained by iTRAQ and Western blot.

qPCR and Western blot for the interfering efficiency in T24 cells

First, the Prx-I mRNA levels from four shRNA vectors transfected for 48 h in the T24 cell lines were measured by qPCR using Lipofectamine 2000. The Prx-I expression decreased by ~40%, 26%, 18% and 1% in the sh-1, sh-2, sh-3 and con sh groups, respectively compared to the parental group (Figure 4A). To confirm this interfering efficiency, the protein expression levels of Prx-I in T24 cells after transfection were examined by Western blot. Results showed that Prx-I levels decreased significantly by ~48%, 30%, 18% and 3% from baseline in the sh-1, sh-2, sh-3 and con sh groups respectively (Figure 4B), indicating that the highest interfering efficiency in T24 cells was in the sh-1 group.

Prx-I knockdown inhibited T-24 cell growth

The effects of Prx-I shRNA transfection on T24 cell growth were investigated through CCK8 assays. A slight inhibition in growth was observed at 24 h after transfection. Furthermore, obvious inhibitory effects on cell proliferation were observed in Prx-I knockdown-cells at 48 and 72 h, compared with the parental and con sh groups (Figure 5, $p < 0.05$), suggesting that the inhibition of Prx-I could suppress T24 cell growth in vitro.

Effect of Prx-I shRNA transfection on the apoptosis and cell cycle of T-24 cell

The effects of Prx-I knockdown on apoptosis and cell cycle of T24 cell were investigated. After 48 h of transfection, the apoptosis rate in the sh-1 group ($21.99 \pm 1.10\%$) was significantly higher compared with the con shRNA group ($4.51 \pm 0.73\%$) and parental

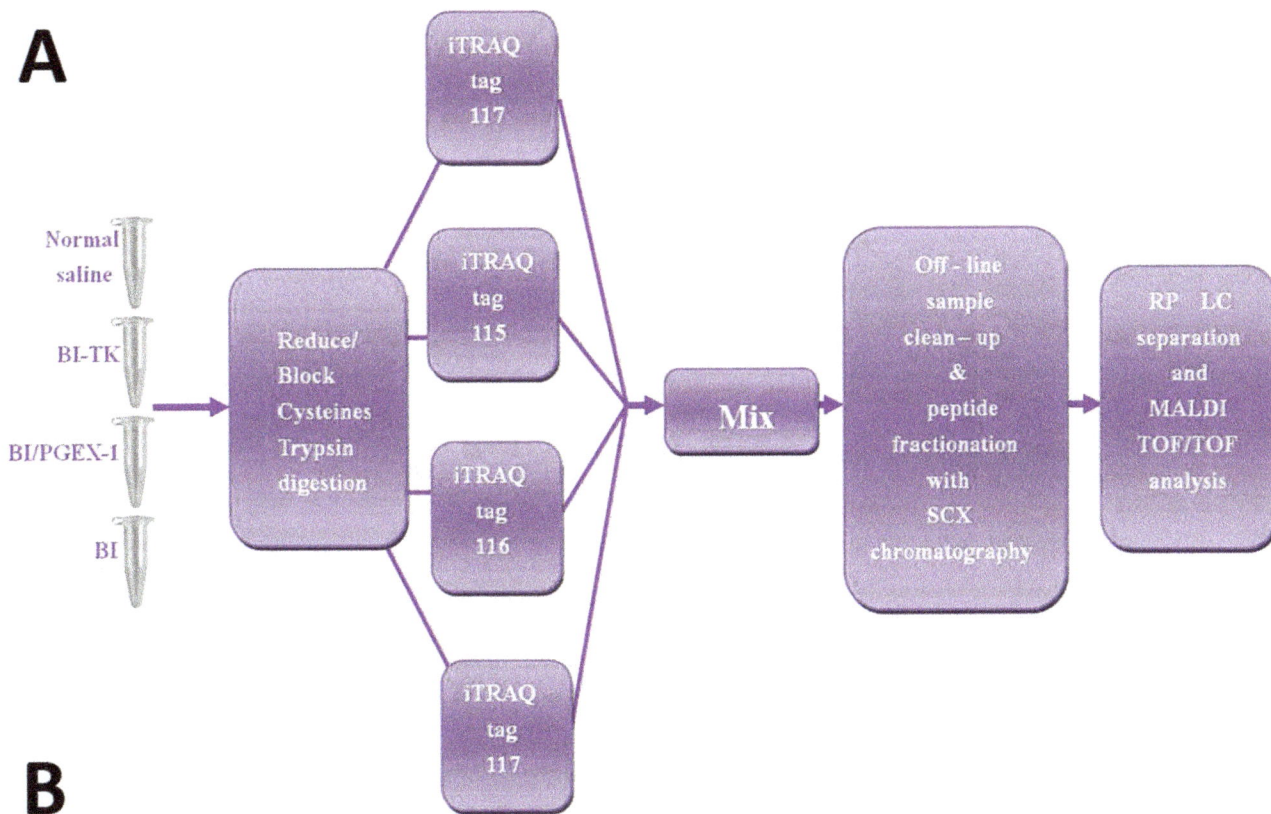

Figure 1. Experimental design of proteome analysis after treatment using iTRAQ labeling. A: Schematic diagram showing the workflow of iTRAQ. B: MS/MS spectrum showing the peptides of Prx-I (peptide sequence: VVGGDHVEVHAR). The 4 peak contours describe that the sample volumes are the same which guarantees the results are authentic and reliable.

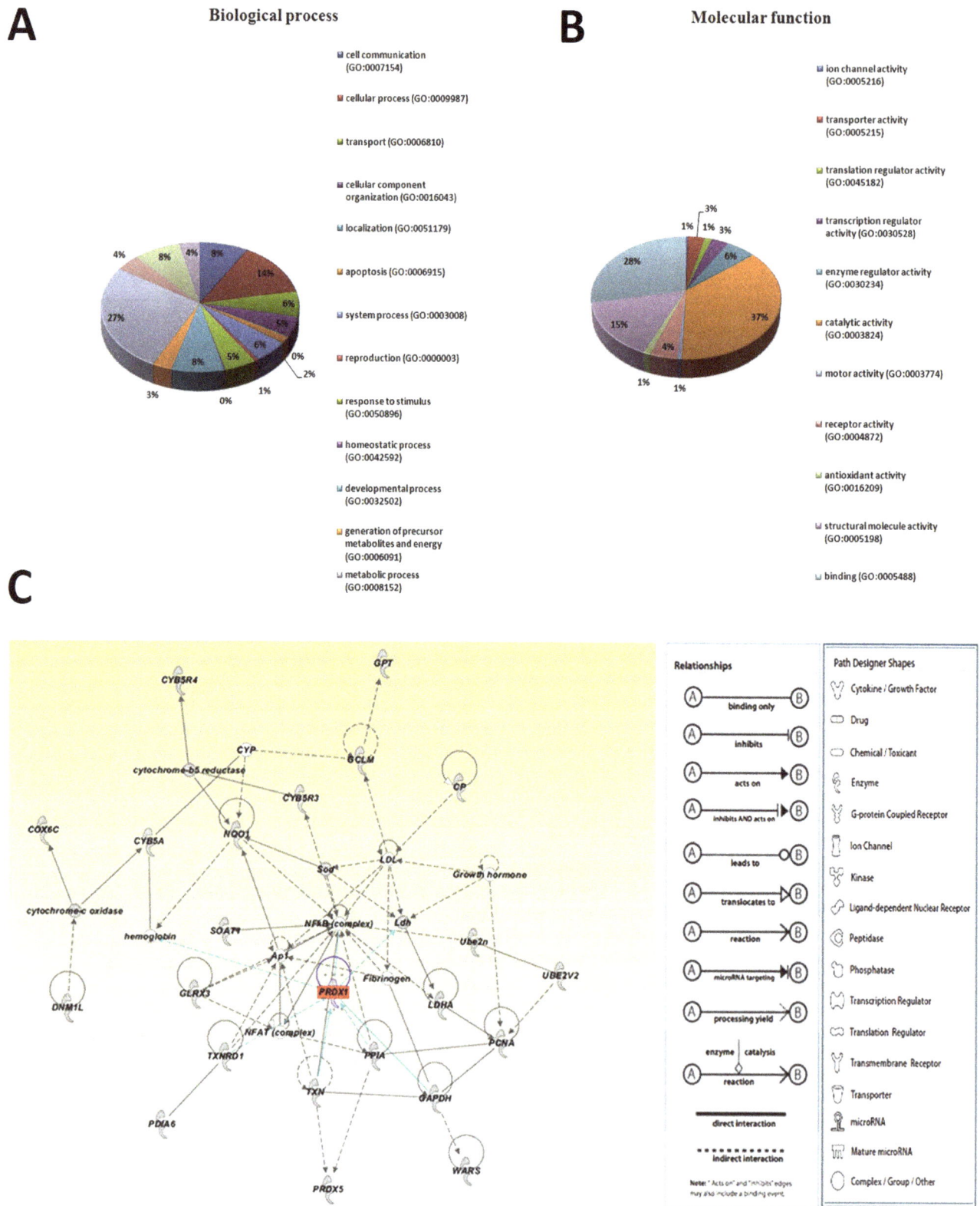

Figure 2. Bioinformatic analysis of differentially expressed proteins after treatment with BI-TK/GCV. PANTHER classification of proteins based on (A) Biological process and (B) molecular function. (C) Interplaying network of proteins with abundance change generated by Ingenuity pathway analysis (IPA). The network implied the connection of Prx-I and NF-κB complex.

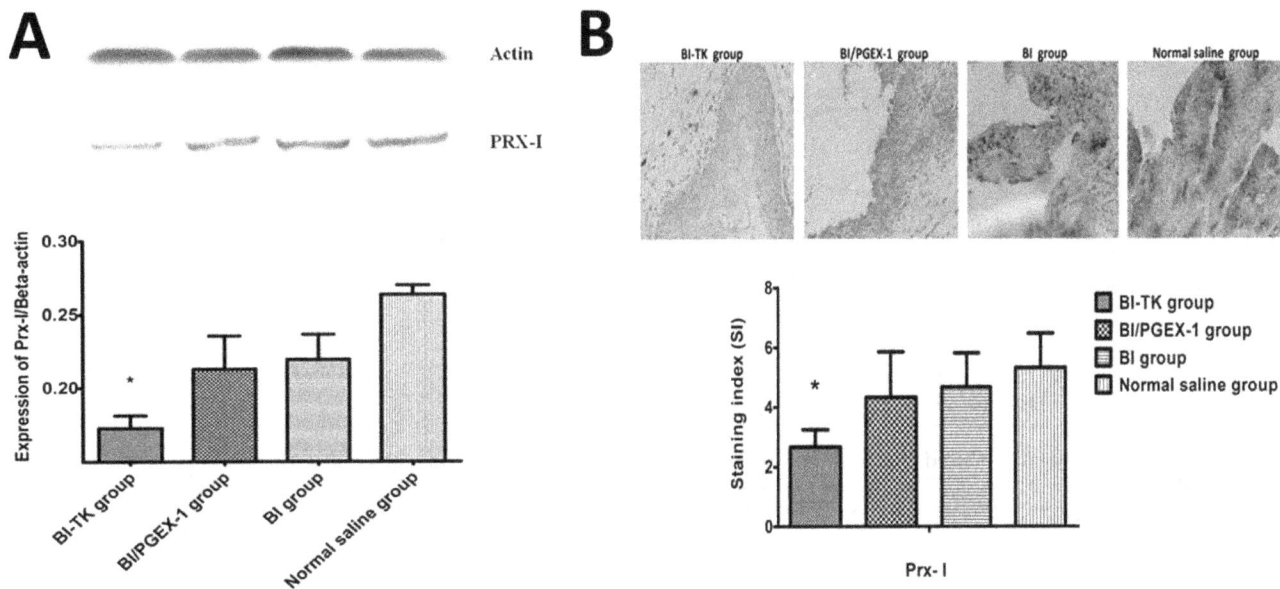

Figure 3. Validation of Prx-I by Western blot and immunohistochemical (IHC) analysis. A: Expressions of Prx-I in four groups by Western blot analysis. Beta-actin was used as a loading control. B: Representative images showing the immunoexpression of Prx-I in tumor tissues of four groups. Compared with the normal saline group, expression of Prx-I is down-regulated in the other three groups (especially in the BI-TK group), which is similar to the results obtained by iTRAQ. (Asterisk (*) indicates P<0.05 in BI-TK group versus normal saline group)

group (4.96±0.46%) (P<0.05) (Figure 6A). Cell cycle analysis showed that G0/G1 phase ratio in the sh-1 group (61.13±.50%) was significantly higher compared with the con sh group (49.62±0.84%) and parental group (48.03±1.17%) (P<0.05) (Figure 6B).

Effect of Prx-I on NF-κB pathway

As described above, Prx-I is directly linked to NF-κB complex, which has been implied in the protein pathway (Figure 2C). To

explore whether the effects of Prx-I on apoptotic signaling proteins were attributable to NF-kB inhibition, the activated forms of phospho-NF-κB p50 and p65 were examined by Western blot after transfection with Prx-I shRNA in T24 cells. A significant decrease (P<0·05) in the protein expression of both phospho-NF-κB p50 and p65 was observed in sh-1 group (Figure 7), compared with the con sh and parental groups, indicating that Prx-I knockdown inhibited activation of NF-κB P50 and P65 in T24 cells.

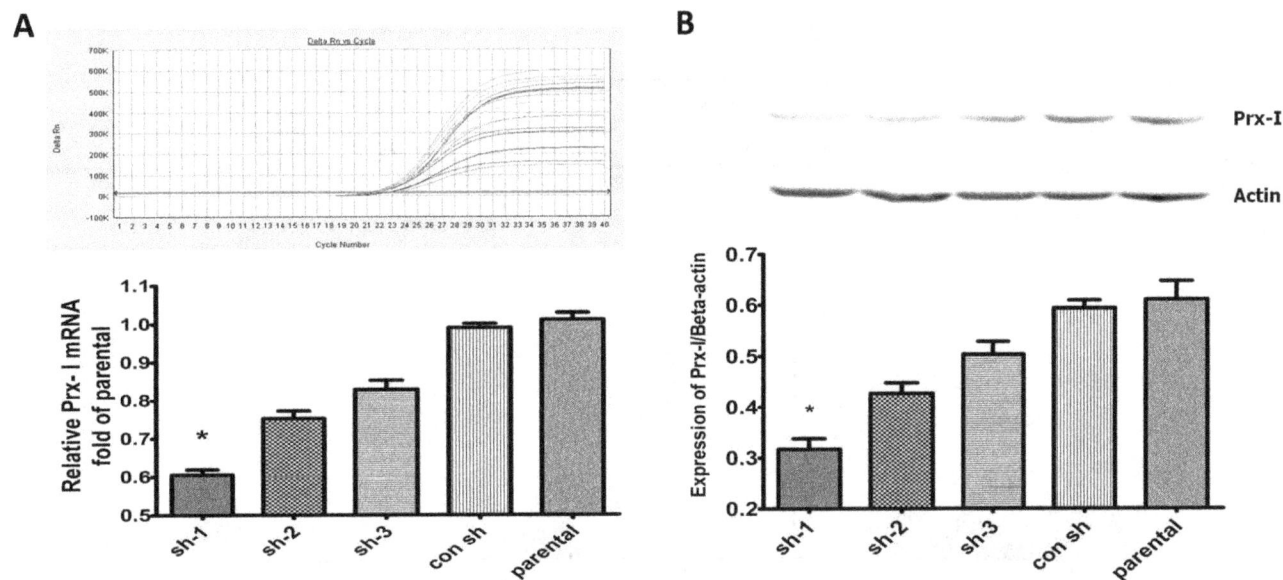

Figure 4. Suppression of Prx-I expression with the shRNA vectors in T24 cells. A: The expression of Prx-I mRNA was examined by qPCR. GAPDH served as an internal control. B: The Prx-I protein levels were analyzed by Western blot after transfection. Sh-1 treatment led to a significant reduction in Prx-I protein expression in T-24 cells. (Asterisk (*) indicates P<0.05 in sh-1 group versus parental group)

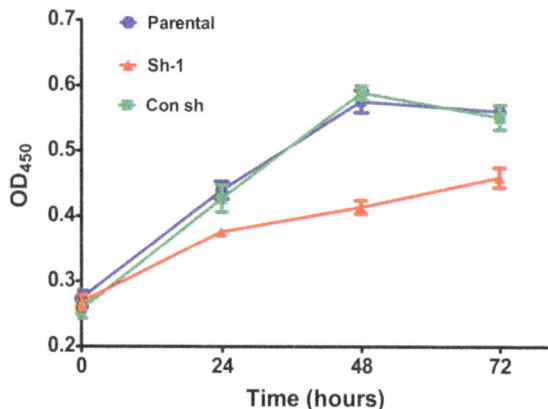

Figure 5. Prx-I knockdown inhibited the proliferation of T24 cells in vitro. The growth rates in Prx-I knockdown group was significantly reduced, compared with the parental and con sh groups, measured by CCK8 assay.

Discussion

In our previous study, BI-TK/GCV was constructed and proved effective in inhibiting the progressive growth of bladder tumor which was related to apoptosis in vivo [9,10], indicating that BI-TK/GCV was a successful treatment system and might provide a novel strategy for treatment of advanced or metastatic bladder cancer in future.

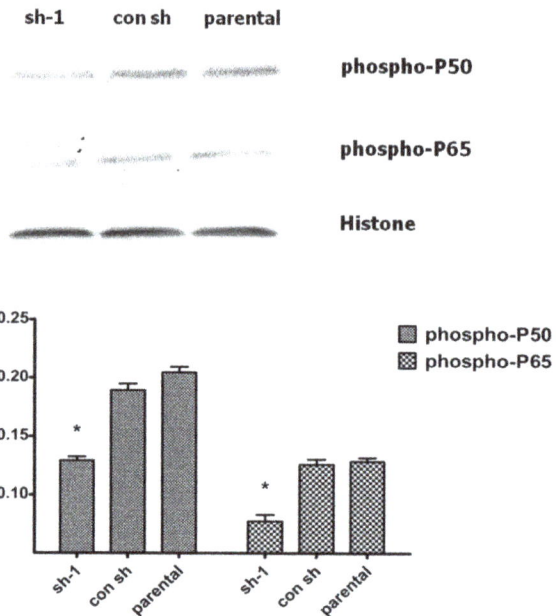

Figure 7. Effect of Prx-I-shRNA transfection on protein expression of phospho-NF-κB p50 and p65 in T24 cells by Western blots. A significant decrease in the protein expression of both phospho-NF-κB p50 and p65 in sh-1 group. (Asterisk (*)indicates $P<0.05$ in sh-1 group versus parental group)

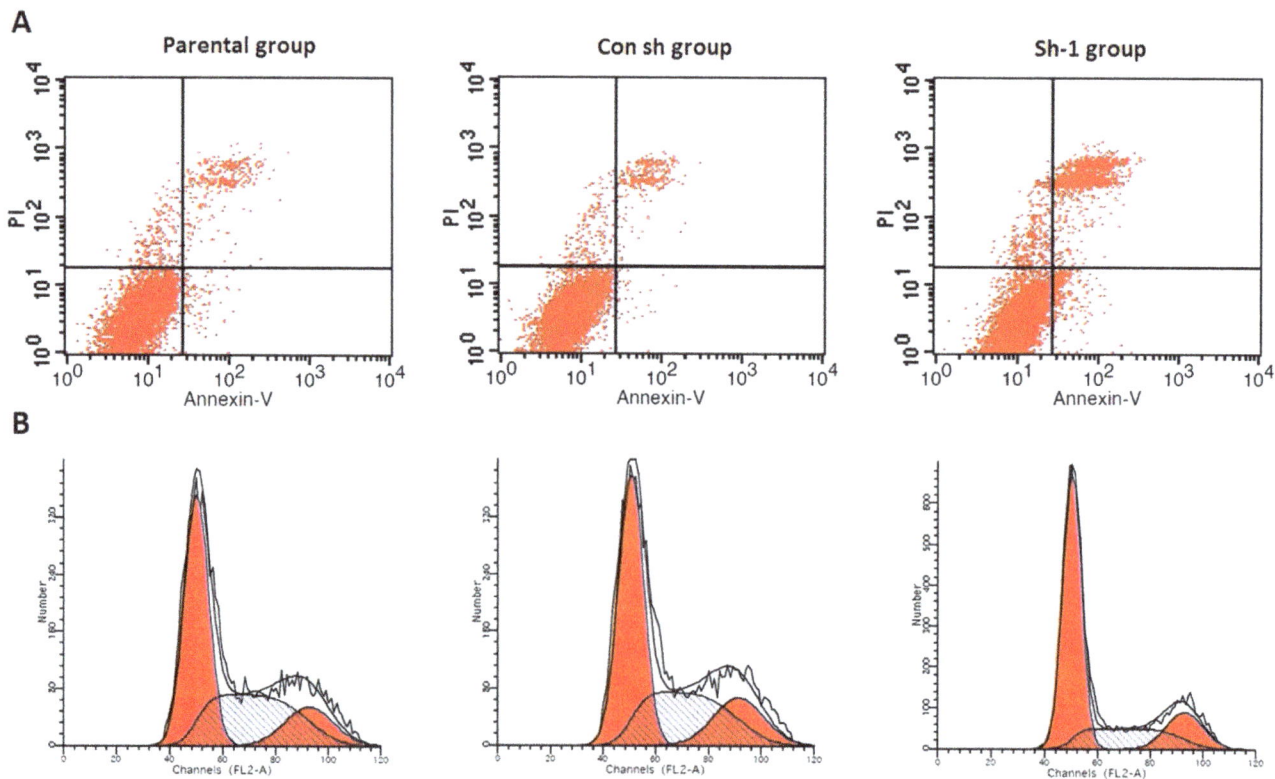

Figure 6. Effect of Prx-I-shRNA transfection on the apoptosis and cell cycle of T24 cells. A: Prx-I knockdown induced apoptosis in T24 cells. B: Representative pictures of FACS analysis showing Prx-I knockdown induced G0/G1 cell cycle arrest in T24 cells with a corresponding decrease in S-phase cells ($P<0.05$).

In this study, a proteomic approach iTRAQ was used to identify differentially expressed proteins, aiming to reveal the molecular mechanisms and provide theoretical support for the effectiveness of BI-TK/GCV system. iTRAQ identified 402 differentially expressed proteins in bladder cancer tissues after treatment, including 192 downregulated proteins and 210 upregulated proteins. The targeting proteins with differential abundance (Table S1) played pivotal roles in a number of cellular pathways, including metabolism, apoptosis, antioxidant activity, cell cycle, proliferation, signal transduction and cell adhesion. Although the exact mechanism by which BI-TK/GCV reaches its intracellular targets is unclear, the targeting proteins of BI-TK/GCV are supposed to participate in the proliferation and apoptosis of bladder cancer cells, and provide novel targets for future therapy.

Prx-I stood out in our proteomic analysis because it had rarely been linked directly with bladder cancer although it has been shown to down-express in bladder cancer tissues after treatment with BI-TK/GCV. The mammalian peroxiredoxin (Prx) family which consists of six proteins is H_2O_2-scavenging enzymes present in procaryotic and eucaryotic cells [11–13]. Prx-I belongs to typical-2-Cys and is the most abundant and ubiquitously distributed isoform of PRDX [14,15], which has been closely interrelated with cell proliferation and differentiation, intracellular redox signaling, and apoptosis [16–19]. Prx-I is highly expressed in solid organs and in tissues of some cancers [20–23], and is also positively associated with the recurrence and progression rates of bladder cancer [24,25]. Similarly, Prx-I over-expression is associated with diminished overall survival, poor clinical outcome, and resistance of cancer cells to radiotherapy and chemotherapy [26–28], while the down-expression of Prx-I by RNAi is associated with therapeutic challenges for liver cancer, esophageal cancer, and thyroid cancer [29–31]. Actually, based on the iTRAQ analysis (Table S1), Western blot (Fig. 3A) and IHC analysis (Fig. 3B) in the present study, Prx-I expression significantly decreased in bladder cancer tissues after treatment with BI-TK/GCV, indicating that Prx-I may contribute to the effect of BI-TK/GCV treatment on anti-growth and pro-apoptosis of bladder cancer. Knockdown of Prx-I gene by shRNA significantly suppressed growth, promoted apoptosis and regulated the cell cycle in bladder cancer cells (Figure 6, 7). These results demonstrate the positive role of Prx-I in the development of bladder cancer. We presume that BI-TK/GCV treatment system is able to prevent tumor growth and induce apoptosis in the rodent bladder cancer model by down-regulating Prx-I expression. But what signaling pathway it is through?

Fortunately, the links between Prk-I and the NF-κB complex signaling have been implied in the protein pathway of IPA (Figure 2C), which lead us to find the clue. Prxs have been implicated as key regulatory factors in redox signaling [32–34]. Prxs can quench the second messenger H_2O_2 and inhibit signal transduction by activating the metabolism of H_2O_2. Overoxidation of Prx from a cysteine-sulfenic acid (Cys-SOH) to a cysteinesulfinic acid (Cys-SO_2H) can stop the metabolism of H_2O_2, allowing the accumulation of H_2O_2 concentration and the propagation of signal transduction. Reduction of Cys-SO2H to Cys-SOH is achieved through the actions of sulfiredoxin, which restores Prx-mediated H_2O_2 metabolism [35–37]. Cytoplasmic Prx1 regulates H_2O_2-dependent NF-κB activation and nuclear translocation, and nuclear Prx1 regulates NF-κB/DNA binding through elimination of H_2O_2 as a p50 subunit oxidant [38]. Prx1 enhances p65-mediated cyclooxygenase (COX)-2 gene expression in estrogen receptor (ER) deficient human breast cancer cells (MDA-MB-231), and knockdown of Prx-I can attenuate COX-2 expression by reducing the occupancy of NF-κB at its upstream promoter element, indicating that Prx-I acts as a chaperone to enhance the transactivation potential of NF-kappaB in ER-deficient-breast cancer cells [39]. Actually, in the present study, knockdown of Prx-I reduced protein expressions of phospho-NF-κB p50 and p65, and thus it suppressed growth, promoted apoptosis and regulated the cell cycle of bladder cancer cells by inhibiting the NF-κB pathway, which conformed to the IPA network (Figure 2C).

Conclusions

Taken together, we identified that Prx-I along with the NF-κB pathway contributed to bladder cancer for the first time. The BI-TK/GCV treatment system exhibited a sustainable anti-tumor growth activity and induced apoptosis in bladder cancer tissues by inhibition of Prx-I through the NF-κB pathway. Our research provides a new insight into bladder cancer treatment and indicates that BI-TK/GCV treatment system by targeting at Prx-I can be a novel therapeutic strategy in the future.

Author Contributions

Conceived and designed the experiments: LJ. Performed the experiments: XX JR YYT. Analyzed the data: LJ. Contributed reagents/materials/analysis tools: HQW QY MJW. Wrote the paper: WT.

References

1. Siegel R, Naishadham D, Jemal A (2012) Cancer statistics. CA Cancer J Clin 62: 10–29.
2. American Cancer Society (ACS) (2014) Cancer Facts & Figures 2014. American Cancer Society, Atlanta, GA.
3. Goebell PJ, Knowles MA (2010) Bladder cancer or bladder cancers? Genetically distinct malignant conditions of the urothelium. Urol Oncol 28: 409–428.
4. Pasin E, Josephson DY, Mitra AP, Cote RJ, Stein JP (2008) Superficial bladder cancer: an update on etiology, molecular development, classification, and natural history. Rev Urol 10: 31–43.
5. Jemal A, Siegel R, Xu J, Ward E (2010) Cancer statistics, 2010. CA Cancer J Clin 60: 277–300.
6. Sharma A, Tandon M, Bangari DS, Mittal SK (2009) denoviral vector-based strategies for cancer therapy. Curr Drug ther 4: 117–138.
7. Kimura NT, Taniguchi S, Aoki K, Baba T (1980) Selective localization and growth of Bifidobacterium bifidum in mouse tumors following intravenous administration. Cancer Res 40: 2061–2068.
8. Yazawa K, Fujimori M, Amano J, Kano Y, Taniguchi S (2000) Bifidobacterium longum as a delivery system for cancer gene therapy: selective localization and growth in hypoxic tumors. Cancer Gene Ther 7: 269–274.
9. Yin X, Yu B, Tang Z, He B, Ren J, et al. (2013) Bifidobacterium infantis-mediated HSV-TK/GCV suicide gene therapy induces both extrinsic and intrinsic apoptosis in a rat model of bladder cancer. Cancer Gene Ther 20: 77–81.
10. Tang W, He Y, Zhou S, Ma Y, Liu G (2009) A novel Bifidobacterium infantis-mediated TK/GCV suicide gene therapy system exhibits antitumor activity in a rat model of bladder cancer. J Exp Clin Cancer Res 28: 155.
11. Zhang B, Wang Y, Su Y (2009) Peroxiredoxins a novel target in cancer radiotherapy. Cancer Lett 286: 154–160.
12. Knoops B, Loumaye E, Van Der Eecken V (2007) Evolution of the peroxiredoxins. Subcell Biochem 44: 27–40.
13. Edgar RS, Green EW, Zhao Y, van Ooijen G, Olmedo M, et al. (2012) Peroxiredoxins are conserved markers of circadian rhythms. Nature 486: 459–464.

14. Chae HZ, Oubrahim H, Park JW, Rhee SG, Chock PB (2012) Protein glutathionylation in the regulation of peroxiredoxins: a family of thiol-specific peroxidases that function as antioxidants, molecular chaperones, and signal modulators. Antioxid Redox Signal 16: 506–523.

15. Lowther WT, Haynes AC (2011) Reduction of cysteine sulfinic acid in eukaryotic, typical 2-Cys peroxiredoxins by sulfiredoxin. Antioxid Redox Signal 15: 99–109.

16. Immenschuh S, Baumgart Vogt E (2005) Peroxiredoxins, oxidative stress, and cell proliferation. Antioxid Redox Signal 7: 768–777.

17. Neumann CA, Cao J, Manevich Y (2009) Peroxiredoxin 1 and its role in cell signaling. Cell Cycle 15: 4072–4078.

18. Du ZX, Yan Y, Zhang HY, Liu BQ, Gao YY, et al. (2010) Suppression of MG132-mediated cell death by peroxiredoxin 1 through influence on ASK1 activation in human thyroid cancer cells. Endocr Relat Cancer 17: 553–560.

19. Kim H, Lee TH, Park ES, Suh JM, Park SJ, et al. (2000) Role of peroxiredoxins in regulating intracellular hydrogen peroxide and hydrogen peroxide-induced apoptosis in thyroid cells. J Biol Chem 275: 18266–18270.

20. Fujii J, Ikeda Y (2002) Advances in our understanding of peroxiredoxin, a multifunctional, mammalian redox protein. Redox Rep 7: 123–130.

21. Kinnula VL, Lehtonen S, Sormunen R, Kaarteenaho Wiik R, Kang SW, et al. (2002) Overexpression of peroxiredoxins I, II, III, V, and VI in malignant mesothelioma. J Pathol 196: 316–323.

22. Lehtonen ST, Svensk AM, Soini Y, Pääkkö P, Hirvikoski P, et al. (2004) Peroxiredoxins, a novel protein family in lung cancer. Int J Cancer 111: 514–521.

23. Noh DY, Ahn SJ, Lee RA, Kim SW, Park IA, et al. (2001) Overexpression of peroxiredoxin in human breast cancer. Anticancer Res 21: 2085–2090.

24. Quan C, Cha EJ, Lee HL, Han KH, Lee KM, et al. (2006) Enhanced expression of peroxiredoxin I and VI correlates with development, recurrence and progression of human bladder cancer. J Urol 174: 1512–1516.

25. Soini Y, Haapasaari KM, Vaarala MH (2011) 8-hydroxydeguanosine and nitrotyrosine are prognostic factors in urinary bladder carcinoma. Int J Clin Exp Pathol 4: 267–275.

26. Yanagawa T, Ishikawa T, Ishii T, Tabuchi K, Iwasa S, et al. (1999) Peroxiredoxin I expression in human thyroid tumors. Cancer Lett 145: 127–132.

27. Yanagawa T, Omura K, Harada H (2005) Peroxiredoxin I expression in tongue squamous cell carcinomas as involved in tumor recurrence. Int J Oral Maxillofac Surg 34: 915–920.

28. Kim HJ, Chae HZ, Kim YJ, Kim YH, Hwangs TS, et al. (2003) Preferential elevation of Prx I and Trx expression in lung cancer cells following hypoxia and in human lung cancer tissues. Cell Biol Toxicol 19: 285–298.

29. Aguilar-Melero P, Prieto-Álamo MJ, Jurado J, Holmgren A, Pueyo C, et al. (2013) Proteomics in HepG2 hepatocarcinoma cells with stably silenced expression of PRDX1. J Proteomics 79: 161–171.

30. Gao MC, Jia XD, Wu QF, Cheng Y, Chen FR, et al. (2011) Silencing Prx1 and/or Prx5 sensitizes human esophageal cancer cells to ionizing radiation and increases apoptosis via intracellular ROS accumulation. Acta Pharmacol Sin 32: 528–536.

31. Riddell JR, Bshara W, Moser MT, Spernyak JA, Foster BA, et al. (2011) Peroxiredoxin 1 controls prostate cancer growth through Toll-like receptor 4-dependent regulation of tumor vasculature. Cancer Res 71: 1637–1646.

32. Woo HA, Chae HZ, Hwang SC, Yang KS, Kang SW, et al. (2003) Reversing the inactivation of peroxiredoxins caused by cysteine sulfinic acid formation. Science 300: 653–656.

33. Hanschmann EM, Godoy JR, Berndt C (2013) Thioredoxins, glutaredoxins, and peroxiredoxins-molecular mechanisms and health significance: from cofactors to antioxidants to redox signaling. Antioxid Redox Signal 19: 1539–1605.

34. Chang TS, Jeong W, Woo HA, Lee SM, Park S, et al. (2004) Characterization of mammalian sulfiredoxin and its reactivation of hyperoxidized peroxiredoxin through reduction of cysteine sulfinic acid in the active site to cysteine. J Biol Chem 279: 50994–51001.

35. Poole LB, Hall A, Nelson KJ (2011) Overview of peroxiredoxins in oxidant defense and redox regulation. Curr Protoc Toxicol Chapter 7:Unit7.9.

36. Rhee SG, Kang SW, Jeong W (2005) Intracellular messenger function of hydrogen peroxide and its regulation by peroxiredoxins. Curr Opin Cell Biol 17: 183–189.

37. Haynes AC, Qian J, Reisz JA, Furdui CM, Lowther WT, et al. (2013) Molecular basis for the resistance of human mitochondrial 2-cys peroxiredoxin 3 to hyperoxidation. J Biol Chem 288: 29714–29723.

38. Hansen JM, Moriarty Craige S, Jones DP (2007) Nuclear and cytoplasmic peroxiredoxin-1 differentially regulate NF-kappaB activities. Free Radic Biol Med 43: 282–288.

39. Wang X, He S, Sun JM (2010) Selective association of peroxiredoxin 1 with genomic DNA and COX-2 upstream promoter elements in estrogen receptor negative breast cancer cells. Mol Biol Cell 21: 2987–2995.

15

A Quantitative Proteomic Analysis Uncovers the Relevance of CUL3 in Bladder Cancer Aggressiveness

Laura Grau[1][9], Jose L. Luque-Garcia[2][9], Pilar González-Peramato[3], Dan Theodorescu[4], Joan Palou[5], Jesus M. Fernandez-Gomez[6], Marta Sánchez-Carbayo[1]*

1 Tumor Markers Group, Spanish National Cancer Research Center, Madrid, Spain, 2 Department of Analytical Chemistry, Complutense University of Madrid, Madrid, Spain, 3 Pathology Department, Hospital Universitario La Paz, Madrid, Spain, 4 Mellon Urologic Cancer Institute, University of Virginia, Charlottesville, Virginia, United States of America, 5 Urology Department, Fundacio Puigvert, Barcelona, Spain, 6 Urology Department, Hospital Central de Asturias, Oviedo, Spain

Abstract

To identify aggressiveness-associated molecular mechanisms and biomarker candidates in bladder cancer, we performed a SILAC (Stable Isotope Labelling by Amino acids in Cell culture) proteomic analysis comparing an invasive T24 and an aggressive metastatic derived T24T bladder cancer cell line. A total of 289 proteins were identified differentially expressed between these cells with high confidence. Complementary and validation analyses included comparison of protein SILAC data with mRNA expression ratios obtained from oligonucleotide microarrays, and immunoblotting. Cul3, an overexpressed protein in T24T, involved in the ubiquitination and subsequent proteasomal degradation of target proteins, was selected for further investigation. Functional analyses revealed that Cul3 silencing diminished proliferative, migration and invasive rates of T24T cells, and restored the expression of cytoskeleton proteins identified to be underexpressed in T24T cells by SILAC, such as ezrin, moesin, filamin or caveolin. Cul3 immunohistochemical protein patterns performed on bladder tumours spotted onto tissue microarrays (n = 284), were associated with tumor staging, lymph node metastasis and disease-specific survival. Thus, the SILAC approach identified that Cul3 modulated the aggressive phenotype of T24T cells by modifying the expression of cytoskeleton proteins involved in bladder cancer aggressiveness; and played a biomarker role for bladder cancer progression, nodal metastasis and clinical outcome assessment.

Editor: John Matthew Koomen, Moffitt Cancer Center, United States of America

Funding: This work was supported by a grant (SAF2009-13035) from the Spanish Ministry of Education and Culture (to M.S.-C.). J.L.L.-G. was supported by the "Ramón y Cajal" program, and the CTQ2010-18644 grant from the Spanish Ministry of Economy and Competitiveness. The funders had no role in study design, data collection and analysis, decision to publish, or preparation of the manuscript.

Competing Interests: The authors have declared that no competing interests exist.

* E-mail: mscarbayo@cnio.es

[9] These authors contributed equally to this work.

Introduction

Bladder cancer represents the 4th most common malignancy among men and the 8th most frequent cause of male cancer deaths [1]. Clinically, approximately 75% of transitional cell carcinomas (TCC) are non-muscle invasive (TIS, Ta, and T1), 20% muscle infiltrating (T2–T4), and 5% metastatic at the time of diagnosis [1]. Low-grade tumors are papillary and usually non-invasive, while high-grade tumors can be either papillary or non-papillary, and often invasive. Patients diagnosed with localized TCC have a 5-year survival rate above 90%. However, patients with regional and distant metastatic disease have a 5-year survival rate below 50% and 10%, respectively [1]. Bladder cancer progression follows complex sequential steps, not completely understood [2–4]. Differences in aggressiveness behaviour have been described between the invasive T24 bladder cancer cell line and the more aggressive T24T variant that develops metastases after tail vein injection [5–9]. Identification of differentially expressed proteins between these cells might uncover molecular mechanisms associated with tumor aggressiveness in vitro potentially leading to metastasis. Proteins participating in such pathways could serve as biomarkers for either early identification of aggressive outcome and/or potentially be therapeutically targetable.

Quantitative proteomics contributes to the discovery of candidate disease-specific target and biomarkers. While protein and antibody arrays permit differential quantification of known proteins [10,11], mass spectrometry techniques lead for protein identification [12]. Stable isotope labelling by amino acids in cell culture (SILAC) involves the addition of (12)C- and (13)C-labeled amino acids to growth media of separately cultured cells, giving rise to cells containing "light" or "heavy" proteins, respectively [12–31]. To our knowledge, SILAC has not been reported in bladder cancer. Here, a quantitative proteomic analysis was applied to T24 and T24T cells to identify proteins and pathways related to their differential aggressiveness following our experimental design (Figure 1).

Materials and Methods

1. Functional analysis of T24 and T24T bladder cancer cells

Cell culture. T24 was obtained from the American Type Culture Collection and cultured as previously described [32,33].

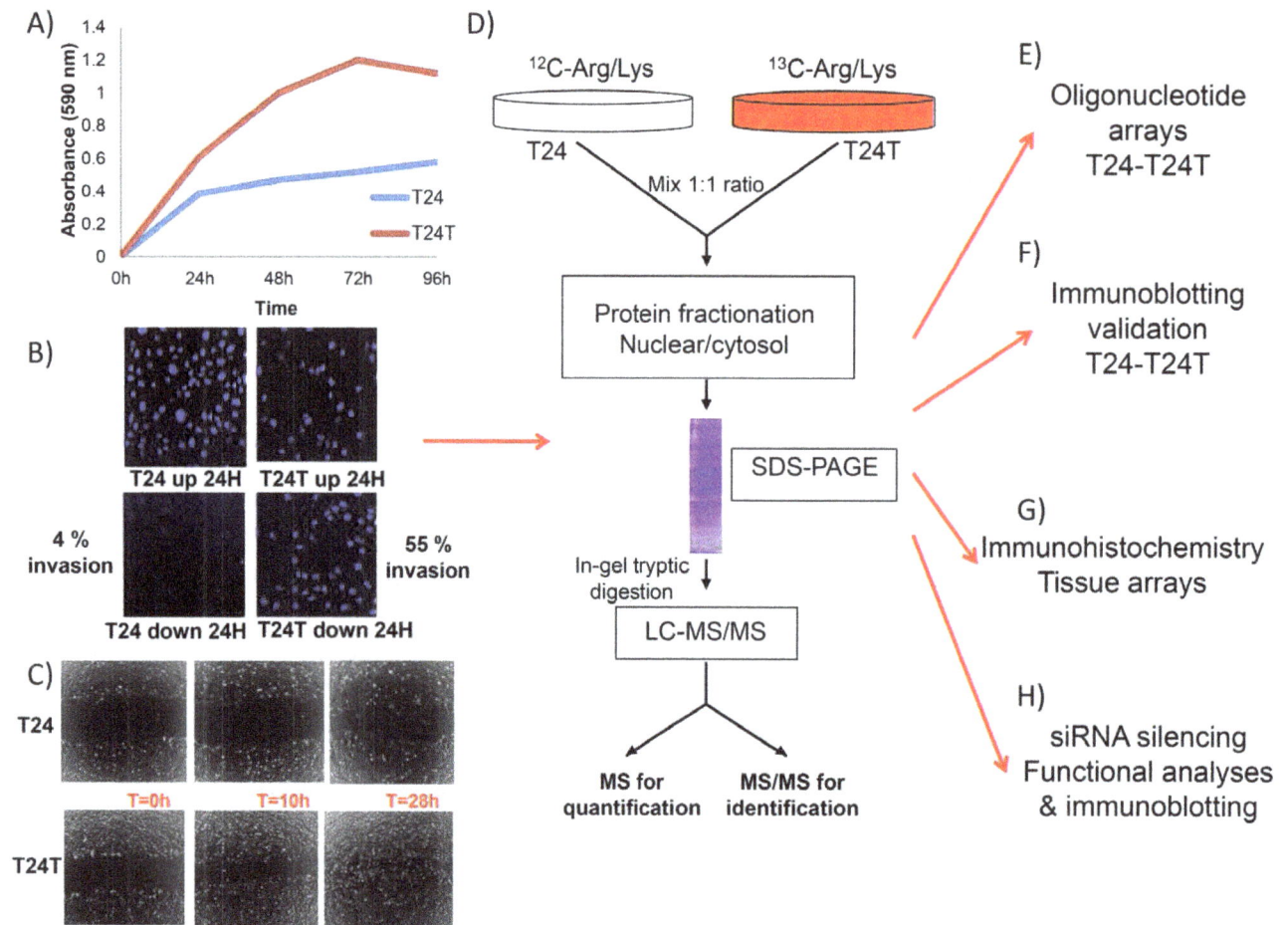

Figure 1. Cell line phenotypes and experimental design. Functional analyses were performed to assess the differential aggressive phenotype of T24 and T24T bladder cancer cells on: **A**) proliferation, **B**) invasion, and **C**) migration. The average of duplicate experiments for each functional assay of these cells at several timepoints is represented in each panel. **D**) Schematic diagram showing the workflow used for the multiplexed SILAC-based experiments. Internal labelling was performed *in vitro*, the protein extracts were fractionated via SDS-PAGE, digested with trypsin in gel, and tryptic digests were analyzed by LC-MS/MS to both identify and quantify the proteins present. **E**) Comparison of the protein changes identified by SILAC was performed with those observed by oligonucleotide arrays. **F**) Validation of the protein changes identified by SILAC in Western blots of protein extracts obtained from T24-T24T cells. **G**) Immunohistochemistry on tissue arrays containing bladder tumors served to validate associations of identified proteins with clinicopathological variables in bladder cancer. **H**) siRNA silencing of identified proteins and subsequent functional analyses and immunoblotting validation served to evaluate the impact of identified candidates on the aggressive phenotype of T24T and the regulation of other differentially expressed proteins identified by SILAC.

T24T was derived from T24 at Dr Theodorescu's laboratory [5–9]. Cells were grown for 4–6 passages and harvested at 75%-90% confluency. Cell pellets were washed three times in cold PBS, and frozen at -20°C before RNA and protein extraction.

Proliferation assay

1.2×10^4 cells per well were seeded in 96-well plates in triplicate in DMEM containing 10% FBS. After culturing for 24, 48, 72 and 96 hours, proliferation was measured with the MTT assay (Roche, Mannheim, Germany).

Wound healing assay. 3.5×10^5 cells were seeded in 6-well plates, and a wound was made in the monolayer using a sterile pipette tip once the cells reached confluency. Photographs of cells invading the wound were taken at the indicated times.

Invasion assay. Cell culture 24-well plates inserts (pore size 8 μm, BD Biosciences, San José, CA) were seeded with 2.5×10^4 T24 and T24T cells, and also with T24T cells after 24 and 48 hours post-transfection with Cul3 siRNA (50 nM) in 500 μL of DMEM medium with 0.1% FBS in the upper chamber. Medium

with 10% FBS (500 μL) was added to the lower chamber as a chemotactic agent. Matrigel invasion chambers (BD) were maintained for 24 hours in a humidified incubator at 37°C, 5% CO_2 atmosphere. Cells on both sides of the matrigel chamber were fixed with 4% paraformaldehyde for 10 minutes, washed with PBS, stained with 1μg/mL 4'-6-Diamidino-2-phenylindole (DAPI: Sigma, St Louis, MO) for 10 minutes, and analysed by confocal microscopy (Leica TCS-SP5, Wetzlar, Germany). The number of invading cells was assessed with the Imaris software (Bit Plane, Zurich, Switzerland), estimating the percentage of invasion as: number of invading cells/number of total cells×100.

Cul3 silencing. Cul3 knocked-down was performed in T24T by transient transfection with Lipofectamine (Invitrogen, Carlsbad, CA) using control (not-targeting) small interfering double-stranded RNA (siRNA) and the smart pool siRNA targeted against Cul3 (both from Dharmacon, Waltham, MA). Cul3 silencing transfectants exposed to 50nM and 100Nm of targeted siRNA were collected at 24h and 48h for proliferation, migration or invasion assays, as described above. Cul3 silencing was confirmed by immunoblotting.

2. SILAC protein profiling

Cell Culture and Metabolic Labeling.   T24 and T24T cells were maintained in lysine and arginine-depleted DMEM (Millipore, Billerica, MA) supplemented with 10% dialyzed FBS (Invitrogen, Carlsbad, CA), 100 units/mL of penicillin/streptomycin (Invitrogen) and either naturally-occurring isotope abundances ("light") (T24) or stable isotope-labelled ("heavy") $^{13}C_6$ lysine and $^{13}C_6$ arginine amino acids (Cambridge Isotope Labs, Andover, MA) (T24T). Culture media were refreshed every 2 days by removing half of the volume present on each plate and replacing it with fresh medium. Cells were grown for at least 6 doublings to allow full incorporation of labelled amino acids. Two large-scale SILAC replicates (2×10^7 cells per condition) were performed. Complete incorporation of ^{13}C-Arg and ^{13}C-Lys into T24 and T24T cells after six cell divisions in isotopically heavy medium (direct and reverse labeling) was verified by MS of a protein digest.

Protein Fractionation.   To reduce the complexity of the sample, a nuclear/cytosol fractionation was performed. Cells were lysed in a lysis buffer (20 mM HEPES, pH 7.0, 10 mM KCl, 2 mM MgCl, 0.5% Nonidet P40, 1 mM Na_3VO_4, 1 mM PMSF, 0.15 U mL^{-1} aprotinin) and homogenized by 30 strokes in a Dounce homogenizer. The homogenate was centrifuged at 1,500 g for 5 min to sediment the nuclei. The supernatant was then resedimented at 15,000 g for 5 min, and the resulting supernatant formed the non-nuclear or cytosol fraction. The nuclear pellet was washed three times and resuspended in the same buffer containing 0.5 M NaCl. The extracted material was sedimented at 15,000 g for 10 min and the resulting supernatant was termed the nuclear fraction.

SDS-PAGE and in-gel digestion.   Proteins in cytosolic and nuclear fractions were separated by SDS-PAGE on 10% SDS-polyacrylamide gels. A total of 80 µg of protein was loaded per lane. After electrophoresis, proteins were visualized by Coomassie blue staining and the gel lane was cut horizontally into 20 sections. Excised gel bands were cut into small pieces and destained in 50:50 25 mM ammonium bicarbonate/acetonitrile, dehydrated with acetonitrile and dried. Gel pieces were rehydrated with 30 µL of 12.5 ng/mL trypsin solution in 25 mM ammonium bicarbonate and incubated overnight at 37°C. Peptides were extracted using acetonitrile and 5% formic acid, dried by vacuum centrifugation and resuspended in 15 µL of 2% acetonitrile in 0.1% formic acid. All samples were sonicated for 10 min before MS analysis.

Nanoflow LC-MS/MS.   The peptide mixture from in-gel tryptic digestions (using 30 µL of trypsin at 12.5 ng/mL) was analyzed using nanoflow LC-MS/MS. Peptides were loaded onto a trap column (Reprosil C_{18}, 3 µm particle size, 0,3×10 mm, 120 Å pore size, SGE) and then eluted to the analytical column (Acclaim PepMap 100, C_{18}, 3 µm particle size, 75 µm×15 cm, 100 Å pore size, Dionex, LC Packings) with a linear gradient of 5–80% acetonitrile in 0.1% formic acid. Sample was delivered over 120 min by a nano-LC ultra 1D plus system (Eksigent) at a 200 nL/min flow-rate to a stainless steel nano-bore emitter (OD 150 µm, ID 30 µm, Proxeon, Odense, Denmark). Peptides were scanned and fragmented with an LTQ XL linear ion trap mass spectrometer (Thermo, San Jose, CA) operated in data-dependent ZoomScan and MS/MS switching mode using the three most intense precursors detected in a survey scan from 400 to 1600 u (three µscans). ZoomScan mass window was set to 12 Da enabling monitoring of the entire ^{12}C/^{13}C isotopic envelope of most doubly and triply charged peptides. Singly charged ions were excluded for

MS/MS analysis. Normalized collision energy was set to 35% and dynamic exclusion was applied during 3 min periods to avoid repetitive fragmentation ions.

Protein identification and quantitation.   Generated .raw files were converted to .mgf files for MASCOT database search. A database containing the NCBInr Homo Sapiens sequences containing 34180 protein entries (as of 04-03-2008) was searched using MASCOT Software (version 2.3 Matrix Science) for protein identification. Search criteria included trypsin specificity with one missed cleavage allowed, and methionine oxidation, ^{13}C-Arg and ^{13}C-Lys as variable modifications. A minimum precursor fragment-ion mass accuracy of 1.2 and 0.3 Da, respectively, and a requirement of at least two bold red (unique peptides) per protein were required for protein quantitation. Cut-off values for MASCOT scores of peptides and proteins were set to 39 ($p<0.05$) and 46 ($p<0.01$), respectively, to consider them as accurate identifications. The false positive rate was calculated searching the same spectra against the NCBInr Homo Sapiens decoy randomized database. Relative quantification ratios of identified proteins were calculated using QuiXoT (version 1.3.26). SILAC T24T/T24 ratios were defined by the intensities of the heavy peptides (C^{13}) divided by the intensities of the light peptides (C^{12}). Protein ratios obtained by QuiXoT were manually verified for all peptides. A proportion of $^{13}C_6$-Arg was converted to $^{13}C_5$-Pro leading to a reduction in the intensity of the isotope-labeled peptide peak; this was corrected for all peptides containing one or more proline residues by adding the intensity found for the peptide containing $^{13}C_6$-Arg $^{13}C_5$-Pro or $^{13}C_6$-Lys $^{13}C_5$-Pro to the intensity of the peak containing only $^{13}C_6$-Arg or $^{13}C_6$-Lys. A combined list of proteins identified in all experiments was condensed at 80% homology using the ProteinCenter software package (Proxeon Bioinformatics AS, Odense, Denmark) to remove redundant IDs such as human orthologous sequences, redundant database entries, and indistinguishable isoforms based on observed peptide coverage. Subcellular localization and functional processes of the proteins identified by SILAC were assigned based on the biological knowledge available in Gene Ontology (GO) annotations. The Ingenuity Pathway (IPA) software was also used to provide insight into biological networks [33,34].

3. Gene Expression Profiling with Oligonucleotide Arrays

RNA extraction.   Total RNA was isolated using TRIzol (Life Technologies, Carlsbad, CA) followed by RNeasy purification. RNA quality was evaluated based on 260:280 ratios of absorbance, and integrity was checked by gel electrophoresis using the 2100 Bioanalyzer (Agilent, Palo Alto, CA) [32,34].

Gene arrays.   Complementary DNA was synthesized by *in vitro* transcription from 1.5 µg of the total RNA purified using a T7-oligo(dT) Promoter Primer Assay (Affymetrix, Santa Clara, CA), labeled with biotinylated nucleotides (Enzo Biochem, Farmingdale, NY), and hybridized to test GeneChips (Affymetrix), to assess sample quality before hybridizing onto the U133A human GeneChips containing 22,283 probes representing known genes and expression sequence tags (Affymetrix) [34].

Data analysis.   Scanned image files were visually inspected for artifacts and analyzed using the Affymetrix Microarray Suite 5.0 (MAS 5.0). Differential expression was evaluated using signal as the main response measure extracted for each gene in every sample, as determined by the default settings of the MAS 5.0. Correlations between gene and protein ratios were analyzed using Kendall's tau test. To compare SILAC and oligonucleotide arrays results, the cumulative probability of expected and observed results were represented over the range of differential expression ratios.

4. Validation by immunoblotting

Total protein was extracted from bladder cancer cells using RIPA lysis buffer and quantified with the Bradford assay using BSA as standard (Protein Assay, Bio-Rad, Hercules, CA). Total protein extracts (50 μg) were mixed with 5x SDS sample buffer (62.5 mM TrisHCl [pH 6.8], 2% SDS, 10% glycerol, 5% β-mercaptoethanol, 0.005% bromophenol blue) and resolved by SDS-PAGE on 10% acrylamide gels. Proteins were electrotransferred onto PVDF membranes (Millipore, Bedford, MC) and activation with methanol. Membranes were blocked with 5% non-fat dry milk in PBS and 0.1% Tween-20 for 1 hour at room temperature and incubated overnight at 4 °C with primary antibodies against: Annexin2 (39 kDa, mouse, 1:2000, #610068, BD Transduction Laboratories, San José, CA US), Bcas2 (26 kDa, mouse, 1:6000, #H00010286-M01, Abnova, Heidelberg, Germany), L-Caldesmon (80kDa, mouse, 1:100, #C56520, BD Transduction Laboratories), calreticulin (48 kDa, rabbit, 1:5000, #C4606, Sigma, St. Louis, MO, US), Caveolin1 (20–22 kDa, mouse, 1:100, #C37120, BD Transduction Laboratories), cdc2 (34 kDa, rabbit, 1:1000, #sc-954, Santa Cruz, Santa Cruz, CA, US), CD44 (80 kDa, mouse, 1:50, #NCL-CD44v3, Novocastra, Wetzlar, Germany), Copine3 (38 kDa, rabbit,1:100, kindly supplied by Dr. Piris, located at CNIO, Madrid, Spain), Cul3 (89 kDa, rabbit, 1:100, #RB1575PCS, NeoMarkers, Fremont, CA, US), Cytokeratin18 (48 kDa, mouse, 1:100, #IF14, Oncogene-MERCK, Darmstad, Germany), DDX21 (87 kDa, rabbit,1:3500, #10528-1-AP, Proteintech, US), DNMT1 (183 kDa, mouse, 1:100, #IMG-261, IMGENEX, San Diego, CA, US), Dynactin p50 (44 kDa, mouse,1:100, #D74620, BD Transduction Laboratories), Dynamin (mouse, 97 kDa, 1:5000, #D25520, BD Transduction Laboratories,), EGFR (175 kDa, mouse, 1:100, #GRO1, Oncogene-MERCK), Ezrin (80 kDa, mouse, 1:7000, #E8897, Sigma), Filamin A (250 kDa, mouse, 1:50, #NCL-FIL, Novocastra, UK), gelsolin (47 kDa, mouse,1:100, #G4896, Sigma), HSP70 (70 kDa, mouse, 1:200, #SC-66048, Santa Cruz), importin 9 (116 kDa, goat, 1:100, sc-103567, Santa Cruz), MCM6 (92 kDa, rabbit, 1:200, kindly supplied by Dr. Mendez, located at CNIO, Madrid, Spain), MAPK-4 (65 kDa, rabbit,1:1000, sc-68169, Santa Cruz), Moesin (68–77 kDa, mouse,1:50, #MS-727-P0, NeoMarkers), MSH6 (152 kDa, mouse,1:200, #610918, BD transduction Laboratories), Nucleophosmin/B23 (32kDa, mouse, 1:5000, #18-7288, Zymed, SF, CA, US), NUP133 (133 kDa, mouse,1:500, #SC-101290, Santa Cruz), Rab14 (23 kDa, rabbit, 1:100, #PRO-873, Avivasybio, San Diego, CA), RCC1 (44 kDa, goat, 1:300, #SC-1161, Santa Cruz), VDAC (30 kDa, rabbit, 1:100, #4866, Cell Signaling, Beverly, MA). Blots were washed in PBS and 0.1% Tween-20, and incubated with horseradish peroxidase-conjugated secondary antibodies for 1 h at room temperature: anti-mouse (1:1000), anti-rabbit (1:2000) and anti-goat (1:2000, all Dako, Glostrup, Denmark). Antibody binding was visualised using an enhanced chemiluminescent immunoblotting detection system (ECL, GE Healthcare). α-tubulin (50kDa, mouse, 1:4000, #T5168, Sigma) was used as loading and normalizing control. Immunoblots were scanned and analyzed using the ImageJ1.43u software (Wayne Rasband, National Institute of Health).

5. Clinical evaluation of the expression of metastases related biomarkers

Tissue samples and microarrays. Seven custom-made bladder cancer tissue microarrays were constructed at the Tumor Markers Group including triplicate or quadriplicate cores (1.0 mm) of primary bladder tumors (n = 284) following randomized designs. Paraffin-embedded tumors for tissue array construction were collected and handled anonymously following ethical and legal protection guidelines of human subjects after written consent approval and Institutional Review Board (IRB) approved protocols corresponding to the research project SAF2009-13035 at collaborating institutions: Fundacio Puigvert and Hospital Central de Asturias. Demographic information indicated the presence of 251 males and 33 females, with a median age of 66.0 years (range:25–81). Tumor stage distribution was: pT1 (n = 87), pT2 (n = 121), pT3 (n = 48) and pT4 (n = 28), and tumor grade distribution was: low-grade (n = 58) and high-grade (n = 226), defined according to consensus criteria [35]. Two of these tissue microarrays including a set of 71 muscle-invasive (pT2+) high grade TCC bladder tumors with known lymph node metastatic status (N0 = 37, N+ = 34). Clinicopathologic and annotated follow-up information allowed associations of Cul3 with histopathology and outcome.

Immunohistochemistry. Protein expression of Cul3 was assessed by immunohistochemistry on tissue microarrays using avidin-biotin immunoperoxidase procedures. Antigen retrieval (0.01% citric acid for 15 minutes under microwave) was employed prior to incubation overnight at 4 °C with the Cul3 rabbit antibody used in immunoblotting (1:300 dilution). Antibody binding was detected with a biotinylated goat anti-rabbit secondary antibody (1:1000, Vector Laboratories). Absence of primary antibody was used as negative control. Testis was utilized as positive control. Diaminobenzidine was utilized as the final chromogen and hematoxylin as the nuclear counterstain [32–34].

Statistical Analysis. Means of findings from two independent observers of all cores from each tumor sample arrayed were used for statistical analyses. Associations of Cul3 expression by immunohistochemistry with histopathologic stage and tumor grade were evaluated using the non-parametric Wilcoxon-Mann-Whitney and Kruskall-Wallis tests [36]. Cul3 expression was evaluated as a continuous variable based on the number of cells expressing the protein in the nucleus. The intensity of the staining was categorized as negative (−) to low (+), intermediate (++) and high (+++). In addition to the intracellular localization, it was also evaluated whether the protein was present or not in the extracellular matrix surrounding neoplastic cells. Cul3 cutoff level for prognostic evaluation was selected on the basis of median expression values among groups under analyses. Association of Cul3 with disease-specific survival was evaluated using the log-rank test in cases with available follow-up. Disease-specific survival time was defined as the months elapsed between transurethral resection or cystectomy and death as a result of disease (or the last follow-up date). Patients alive at the last follow-up or lost to follow-up were censored. Survival curves were plotted using Kaplan-Meier methodology [36]. Statistical analyses were performed using SPSS statistical package (version 17.0).

Results

Functional analyses *in vitro*

Several aggressiveness aspects of T24-T24T cells were initially analysed. T24T had significant higher proliferation rates than T24 at the four time points studied (p<0.05, Figure 1A). Invasion assays indicated that T24 were on average 50% less invasive than T24T cells at 48h (Figure 1B). Wound healing assays revealed significantly faster migration rate for T24T (Figure 1C). *In vitro* assays suggested that T24T cells had more aggressive phenotypes.

Changes in protein abundance between T24 and T24T cells using SILAC

A total of 1830 proteins were identified in the two SILAC experiments, from which 831 were simultaneously identified in both replicates and passed the criteria established for protein quantitation. The overall false discovery rate was 2.1% being estimated by the number of hits against the reverse sequence/total hits (p<0.01). The mean relative standard deviation (SD) of the ratios obtained from replicates was 0.24, indicating good agreement between experiments.

Regarding SILAC ratios distribution, most of the proteins identified were within the SILAC ratio range between 1.5 and 0.67, as expected when analysing closely related cell lines in a 1:1 protein mixture (Figure 2A). Using 1.5 as the threshold ratio, 289 proteins were differentially expressed between the two cell lines, 88 of which were more abundant in T24T. Among the 289 differentially expressed proteins (Table S1), Table 1 includes those proteins previously related to bladder cancer metastases, and those validated by immunoblotting. The full list of proteins identified in both replicates (n = 831) using SILAC is in Table S2.

Functional classification of the proteins identified

The functional annotation of the 289 differentially expressed proteins in T24 and T24T cells was initially assigned using the Protein Center software. Three main types of annotations were obtained from GO consortium website: cellular components, molecular functions, and biological processes (Figure 2B, C, D). A GOslim approach defined specifically for ProteinCenter reduced the multiple GO annotations to a manageable set of approximately 20 high-level terms that were used to filter the information into percentage estimations. Major molecular functions included protein binding (78%) or catalytic activity (67%). Metabolic processes (84%) and cellular organization and biogenesis (54%) were frequent biological processes. Protein annotation distribution supported the *in vitro* functional assays described above linking cellular reorganization with migration and invasion phenotypes (Figure 1). A high number of proteins localized to the cytoplasm (87%) was found as compared to the nucleus (48%). This observation led us to focus on proteins that could play a relevant role in cytoskeletal reorganization and the aggressive phenotype of T24T.

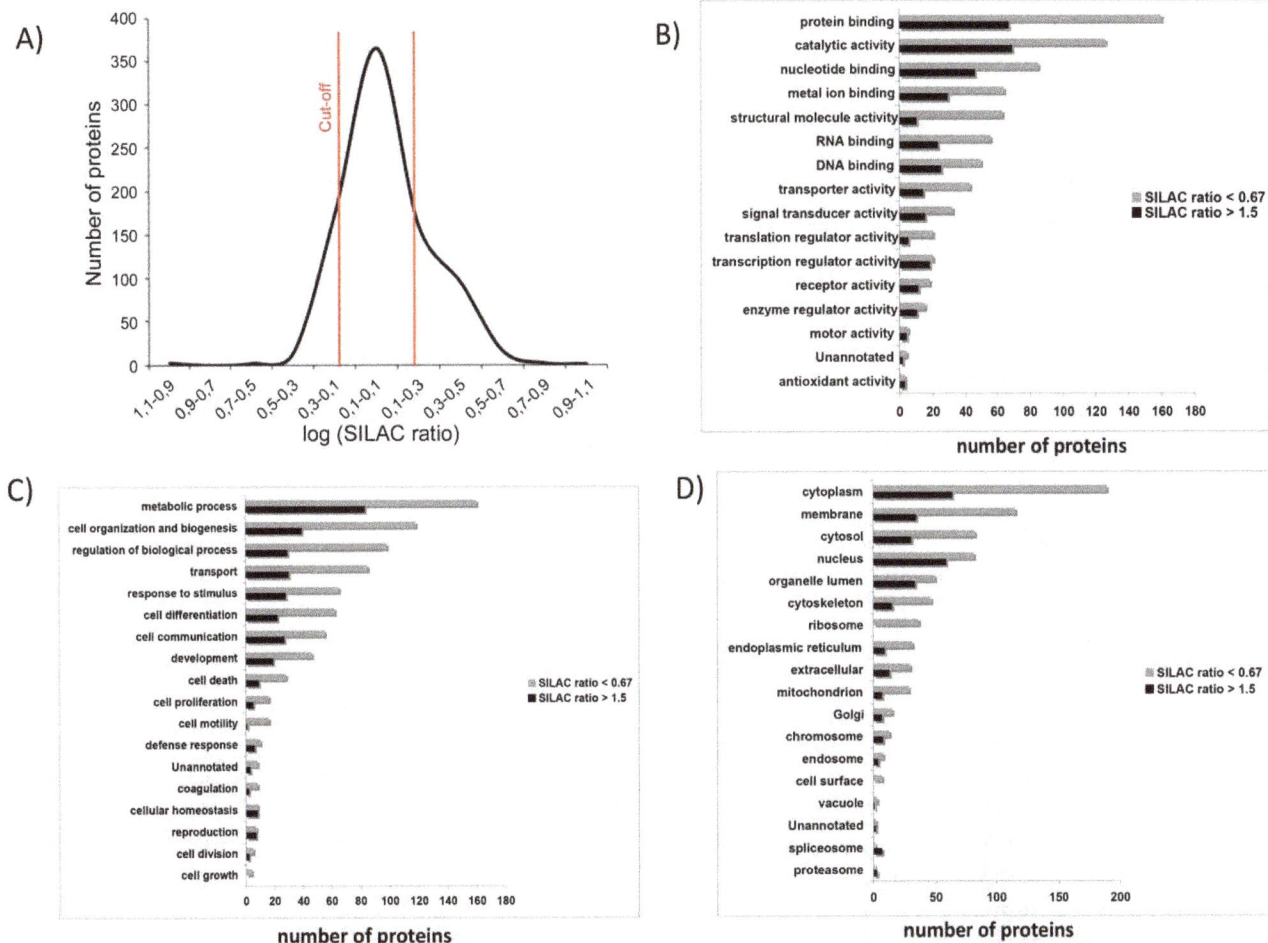

Figure 2. A) Distribution of SILAC T24T/T24 ratios: The log of the SILAC ratio for each protein (*n* = 2) represents the difference in relative expression between highly metastatic (T24T) and invasive (T24) bladder cancer cells. Proteins were sorted and plotted by SILAC ratio. As expected for a 1:1 mixture, most proteins showed a SILAC ratio within the 1.5 and 0.67 cutoffs. Classification of the proteins identified based on their functional annotations using the Gene Ontology: **B**) Molecular function, **C**) Biological processes and **D**) Cellular components. These analyses were performed with the 289 proteins found to be differentially expressed. When more than one assignment was available for a given protein, all the functional annotations were considered in the analyses. These classifications were redundant (over 100%) as proteins could be annotated in more than one assignment.

Table 1. Selected proteins with altered abundance in bladder cancer metastatic T24T versus T24 cells.

Accession number (gi)	Protein Name	Common name/ Abbreviation	Molecular weight (Kda)	Gene Array T24T/T24 Ratio	SILAC T24T/T24 Ratio	SD[1]
4507951	tyrosine 3-monooxygenase/tryptophan 5-monooxygenase activation protein, eta polypeptide	YWHAH	30	0.92	9.44	0.09
122939159	peptidyl arginine deiminase, type II	PADI2	75	–	8.35	0.69
41872631	fatty acid synthase	FASN	273	–	3.85	0.14
4504165	gelsolin isoform a precursor	GSN*	90	10.20	3.61	0.73
32171238	BAI1-associated protein 2-like 1	BAIAP2L1	56	–	3.03	0.05
4505591	peroxiredoxin 1	PRDX1	22	–	2.88	0.13
148298764	hydroxymethylglutaryl-CoA synthase 1	HMGCS1	57	1.17	2.83	0.25
38569421	ATP citrate lyase isoform 1	ACLY	120	10.74	2.54	0.17
10864011	sulfide dehydrogenase like	SQRDL	50	–	2.50	0.13
4507835	uridine monophosphate synthase	UMPS	52	1.18	2.34	0.20
4503165	cullin 3	Cul3*	89	1.00	2.26	0.18
4504169	glutathione synthetase	GSS	52	1.12	2.24	0.20
4503377	dihydropyrimidinase-like 2	DPYSL2	67	1.15	2.19	0.18
29789090	regulator of chromosome condensation 2	RCC2	56	–	2.19	0.28
20127454	5-aminoimidazole-4-carboxamide ribonucleotide formyltransferase/IMP cyclohydrolase	ATIC	64	–	2.15	0.20
21361709	regulation of nuclear pre-mRNA domain containing 1A	RPRD1A	35	–	2.09	0.25
47933397	lanosterol synthase	LSS	83	–	2.06	0.18
39777597	transglutaminase 2 isoform a	TGM2	77	1.04	2.01	0.04
116734860	amylo-1, 6-glucosidase, 4-alpha-glucanotransferase isoform 1	AGL	174	11.93	1.95	0.17
14150139	within bgcn homolog isoform 1	WIBG	22	–	1.94	0.06
20070384	phosphoglycerate mutase family member 5	PGAM5	32	–	1.92	0.18
4506903	splicing factor, arginine/serine-rich 9	SFRS9	25	1.04	1.9	0.05
gi|48255933	high-mobility group nucleosome binding domain 1	HMGN1	10	–	1.87	0.13
24308013	peptidase (mitochondrial processing) alpha	PMPCA	16	–	1.84	0.10
21361659	importin 9	IPO9*	116	1.09	1.83	0.17
29725609	**epidermal growth factor receptor isoform a precursor**	**EGFR***	175	9.96	1.82	0.12
26051235	nucleoporin 133kDa	NUP133*	133	1.06	1.78	0.21
4507877	**vinculin isoform VCL**	**VCL**	123	0.09	0.67	0.03
48255935	**CD44 antigen isoform 1 precursor**	**CD44***	80	0.83	0.66	0.06
4504047	**GNAS complex locus GNASL**	**GNAS**	45	1.03	0.61	0.08
161702986	Ezrin	EZR*	80	0.72	0.58	0.04
4504183	**glutathione transferase**	**GSTP1**	23	0.94	0.58	0.05
103472005	**antigen identified by monoclonal antibody Ki-67**	**MKI67**	358	–	0.56	0.05
4505257	Moesin	MSN*	68–77	0.89	0.54	0.04
55770844	**catenin, alpha 1**	**CTNNA1**	100	1.01	0.47	0.01
50845388	annexin A2 isoform 1	ANXA2*	39	0.97	0.42	0.04
4503015	copine III	CPNE3*	38	0.96	0.40	0.05
116063573	filamin A, alpha isoform 1	FLNA*	250	0.92	0.38	0.04
5031815	lysyl-tRNA synthetase isoform 2	KARS	68	1.04	0.31	0.03
156071459	solute carrier family 25, member 5	SLC25A5	35	0.98	0.30	0.06
19920317	cytoskeleton-associated protein 4	CKAP4	66	–	0.28	0.04
33620775	kinectin 1 isoform a	KTN1	14	1.03	0.26	0.04
209862851	plastin 3	PLS3	16	0.01	0.26	0.02
71773415	annexin VI isoform 2	ANXA6	75	0.90	0.24	0.01
105990514	filamin B, beta (actin binding protein 278)	FLNB	278	–	0.23	0.03
116805322	gamma filamin isoform a	FLNC	291	0.75	0.23	0.04

Table 1. Cont.

Accession number (gi)	Protein Name	Common name/ Abbreviation	Molecular weight (Kda)	Gene Array T24T/T24 Ratio	SILAC T24T/T24 Ratio	SD[1]
4507813	*UDP-glucose dehydrogenase*	*UGDH*	55	9.11	0.23	0.03
16753203	ubiquilin 1 isoform 1	UBQLN1	62	–	0.22	0.01
15451856	*caveolin 1*	*CAV1**	20–22	0.96	0.21	0.04
7305053	myoferlin isoform a	MYOF	234	–	0.21	0.05
156104878	*Glutaminase*	*GLS*	73	1.05	0.20	0.03
42734430	polymerase I and transcript release factor	PTRF	43	–	0.20	0.03
157694492	MYB binding protein 1a isoform 2	MYBBP1A	133	1.12	0.20	0.14
63252913	*gelsolin-like capping protein*	CAPG	38	0.83	0.16	0.04
21071056	*SWI/SNF-related matrix-associated actin-dependent regulator of chromatin a4 isoform B*	SMARCA4	184	0.74	0.16	0.08
5453555	ras-related nuclear protein	RAN	24	–	0.07	0.11

All proteins were identified at >99% confidence (corresponding to a Mascot score >46). The table includes the accession number (gi), protein name, molecular weight (in kD), gene array ratio, SILAC ratios (T24T/T24), and the standard deviation (SD, n = 2). All proteins were identified in the two SILAC replicates with at least two unique peptides. Proteins previously described to be involved in cancer metastases are highlighted in italics, while those reported to be related to bladder cancer metastases are highlighted in bold. Proteins validated in immunoblots are highlighted with an asterisk. The absence of values in the "Gene Array Ratio" column, highlighted as "-", indicates absence of the specific probe on the array. The complete set of differentially expressed proteins identified is provided in Table S1.

Comparison of gene and protein expression ratios

SILAC protein expression ratios were compared with mRNA expression provided by oligonucleotide microarrays for the candidates identified by both methods (n = 438) (Table 1, Table S3). A positive correlation coefficient (Kendalls tau) of 0.206 (p<0.0005) was obtained (Figure S1A). Importantly, the median SILAC protein expression ratio was 0.98 for these candidates (range: 0.16–9.44), which was similar to the median of 1.02 observed for oligonucleotide arrays (range: 0.01–100.80). Excluding two outliers detected by both techniques increased the correlation coefficient to 0.210 (p<0.0005, N = 438: Figure S1B). To interpret the differences between the expected and the observed correlations between RNA and protein expression, the cumulative probability of the observed ratio for differential expression was represented against the expected ratio for both techniques (Figure S1C, D). The figures highlighted the wider ranges of differential expression observed in oligonucleotide arrays when compared to the same candidates in SILAC analyses.

Validation of SILAC identified candidates using immunoblotting

To validate SILAC expression ratios of proteins identified in both replicates, immunoblotting was performed (Figure 3). Increased expression in T24T was observed for gelsolin, Cul3, importins, nucleoporins and EGFR, and decreased expression was found for ezrin, moesin, filamin, caveolin or CD44, among others. Immunoblots were quantified to correlate with expression ratios obtained by SILAC and in gene arrays. Based on the good agreement of these observations for Cul3, a protein known to be involved in the ubiquitination and subsequent degradation of target proteins, it was selected for further analyses to: a) evaluate its clinical relevance as a biomarker candidate to assess aggressive clinical behaviour, and b) to evaluate Cul3 impact on the aggressive phenotype of T24T and on modulating expression of other differentially expressed proteins identified by SILAC. Figure S2 showed the additional validation by immunoblots of candidates differentially expressed in T24T cells in oligonucleotide arrays that were not quantified by SILAC, and *vice versa*, for which antibodies

were available. We did not observe major differences in experimental molecular weights as compared to predicted sizes.

Molecular pathways associated with aggressiveness

To understand the mechanisms by which differentially expressed proteins contribute to bladder cancer aggressiveness, the dataset containing the differentially expressed proteins (N = 289) was uploaded into the IPA software. An interaction map grouped 31 of the differentially expressed proteins to which Cul3 was added (Figure S3). An independent analysis was performed importing the top ten selected differentially expressed proteins in both SILAC and gene arrays, and validated in immunoblots (Figure S4). This analysis highlighted that validated proteins contributing to this network participated in the following critical neoplastic-related annotated biological functions: cellular assembly and organization, cancer, cell movement, cell morphology, and cell function and maintenance.

Cul3 is differentially expressed in bladder tumors and associated with bladder cancer aggressiveness

Protein expression patterns of Cul3 by immunohistochemistry were optimized and assessed on tissue arrays. Differential expression was observed for Cul3 among the bladder tumors tested. Significant statistical associations were found between Cul3 nuclear over-expression and increasing tumor stage when comparing non-invasive (Figure 4A) versus muscle-invasive (Figure 4B) bladder tumors (p = 0.001, n = 284). Moreover, Cul3 over-expression was associated with poor disease-specific survival (log-rank, p = 0.002), (Figure 4C). Primary invasive bladder tumors that developed lymph node metastases showed higher expression levels of Cul3 as compared to those with negative lymph nodes (p = 0.025). A high intensity and the presence of Cul3 in the extracellular matrix were also associated with increasing stage (p = 0.004, and p = 0.005, respectively), and with the presence of lymph node metastasis (p = 0.002, and p = 0.001). These observations indicated that Cul3 over-expression could be associated with tumor staging and the metastatic phenotype. Overall, expression patterns of Cul3 in bladder

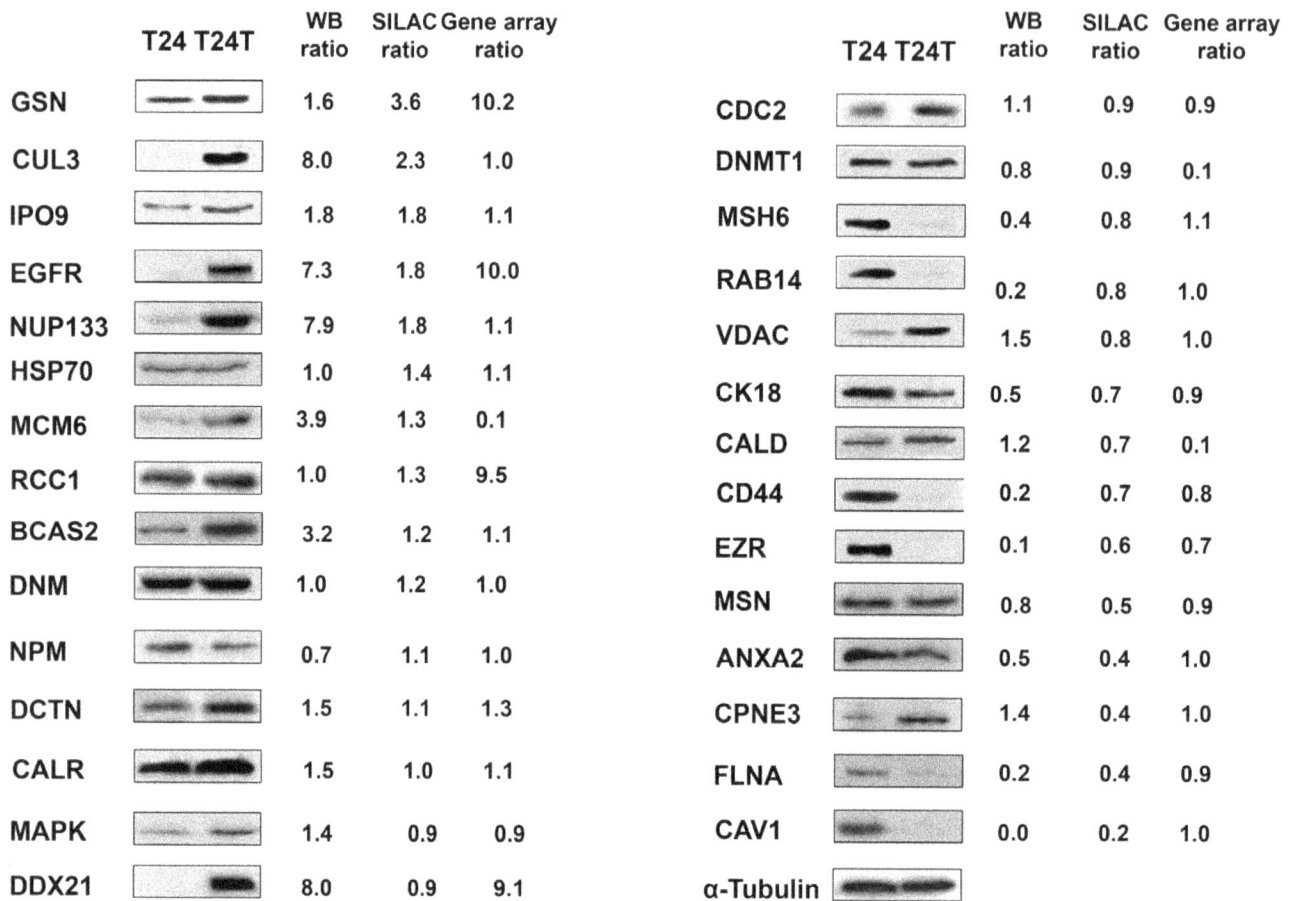

	T24 T24T	WB ratio	SILAC ratio	Gene array ratio		T24 T24T	WB ratio	SILAC ratio	Gene array ratio
GSN		1.6	3.6	10.2	CDC2		1.1	0.9	0.9
CUL3		8.0	2.3	1.0	DNMT1		0.8	0.9	0.1
IPO9		1.8	1.8	1.1	MSH6		0.4	0.8	1.1
EGFR		7.3	1.8	10.0	RAB14		0.2	0.8	1.0
NUP133		7.9	1.8	1.1	VDAC		1.5	0.8	1.0
HSP70		1.0	1.4	1.1	CK18		0.5	0.7	0.9
MCM6		3.9	1.3	0.1	CALD		1.2	0.7	0.1
RCC1		1.0	1.3	9.5	CD44		0.2	0.7	0.8
BCAS2		3.2	1.2	1.1	EZR		0.1	0.6	0.7
DNM		1.0	1.2	1.0	MSN		0.8	0.5	0.9
NPM		0.7	1.1	1.0	ANXA2		0.5	0.4	1.0
DCTN		1.5	1.1	1.3	CPNE3		1.4	0.4	1.0
CALR		1.5	1.0	1.1	FLNA		0.2	0.4	0.9
MAPK		1.4	0.9	0.9	CAV1		0.0	0.2	1.0
DDX21		8.0	0.9	9.1	α-Tubulin				

Figure 3. Verification of the expression of the proteins identified. (A) Validation of the SILAC results of selected proteins in immunoblots of protein extracts from the bladder cancer cells analyzed. The results validated the expression levels of proteins identified by the proteomic approach, including differentially and non-differentially expressed candidates. Antibodies displaying a single predominant band at the expected molecular weights were accepted: and α-tubulin, was used as the loading control. GSN, Gelsolin; Cul3, Cullin 3; IPO9. Importin 9; EGFR, Epidermal Growth Factor Receptor; NUP133, Nucleoporin 133; HSP70, Heat Shock Protein 70kDa; MCM6, Minichromosome Maintenance Complex Component 6; RCC1, Regulator of Chromosome Condensation 1; BCAS2, Breast Carcinoma Amplified Sequence 2; DNM, Dynamin; NPM, Nucleophosmin; DCTN, Dynactin; CALR, Calreticulin; MAPK, Mitogen-Activated Protein Kinase; DDX21, DEAD (Asp-Glu-Ala-Asp) box polypeptide 21; CDC2: Cell Division Cycle 2; DNMT1, DNA (cytosine-5)-Methyltransferase 1; MSH6, MutS Homolog 6; RAB14, GTPase Rab14; VDAC, Voltage-Dependent Anion Channel; CK18, Cytokeratin 18; CALD, Caldesmon; CD44, CD44 antigen isoform 1 precursor 2; EZR, Ezrin; MSN, Moesin; ANXA2, Annexin A2; CPNE3, Copine 3; FLNA, Filamin A; CAV1, Caveolin 1. Western Blots were scanned and analyzed using α-tubulin as normalizing control.

tumors suggested its role as a biomarker for tumor stratification, metastasis and clinical outcome prognosis.

Functional and immunoblotting analyses upon Cul3 silencing

The impact of knocking down Cul3 expression using siRNA at 50nM and 100nM in the aggressive phenotype of T24T cells was assessed *in vitro*. Proliferation diminished at 24 and 48 hours after Cul3 silencing (p<0.05) (Figure 5A). Wound healing assays revealed the slower migration rate of T24T cells lacking Cul3 expression (Figure 5B). Invasion assays indicated that T24T cells silenced for Cul3 were on average 50% less invasive at both time points than the control siRNA (Figure 5C). Using Cul3 siRNAs at 100nM showed similar invasion rates as 50 nM (data not shown). The impact of Cul3 silencing on the expression of other proteins found differentially expressed by SILAC was tested by immunoblots (Figure 5D). Cul3 silencing restored the expression of cytoskeleton adhesion proteins such as filamin A, ezrin, caveolin1 or moesin. Overall, functional analyses and immunoblotting validation upon Cul3 silencing revealed that Cul3 modulated the

aggressive phenotype of T24T, and modified the expression of cytoskeleton proteins also identified differentially expressed by SILAC.

Discussion

A SILAC approach was designed to identify pathways associated with bladder cancer aggressiveness. Cul3 was revealed as a candidate contributing to the aggressive phenotype of T24T modifying cytoskeleton remodelling and as a bladder cancer biomarker correlating with poor outcome. Our comparative functional analyses of T24-T24T were complementary and agreed with previous *in vitro* results describing a more aggressive phenotype of T24T cells. By contrast to earlier analyses [5], we performed proliferation by seeding cells at a three-fold higher density, plus wound healing and invasion assays. These data highlighted the ability of T24T cells to grow on top of each other, in contrast to the contact inhibition previously described for T24 cells. These results further suggested that T24T cells have a greater potential for proliferation, motility and potentially to metastasize,

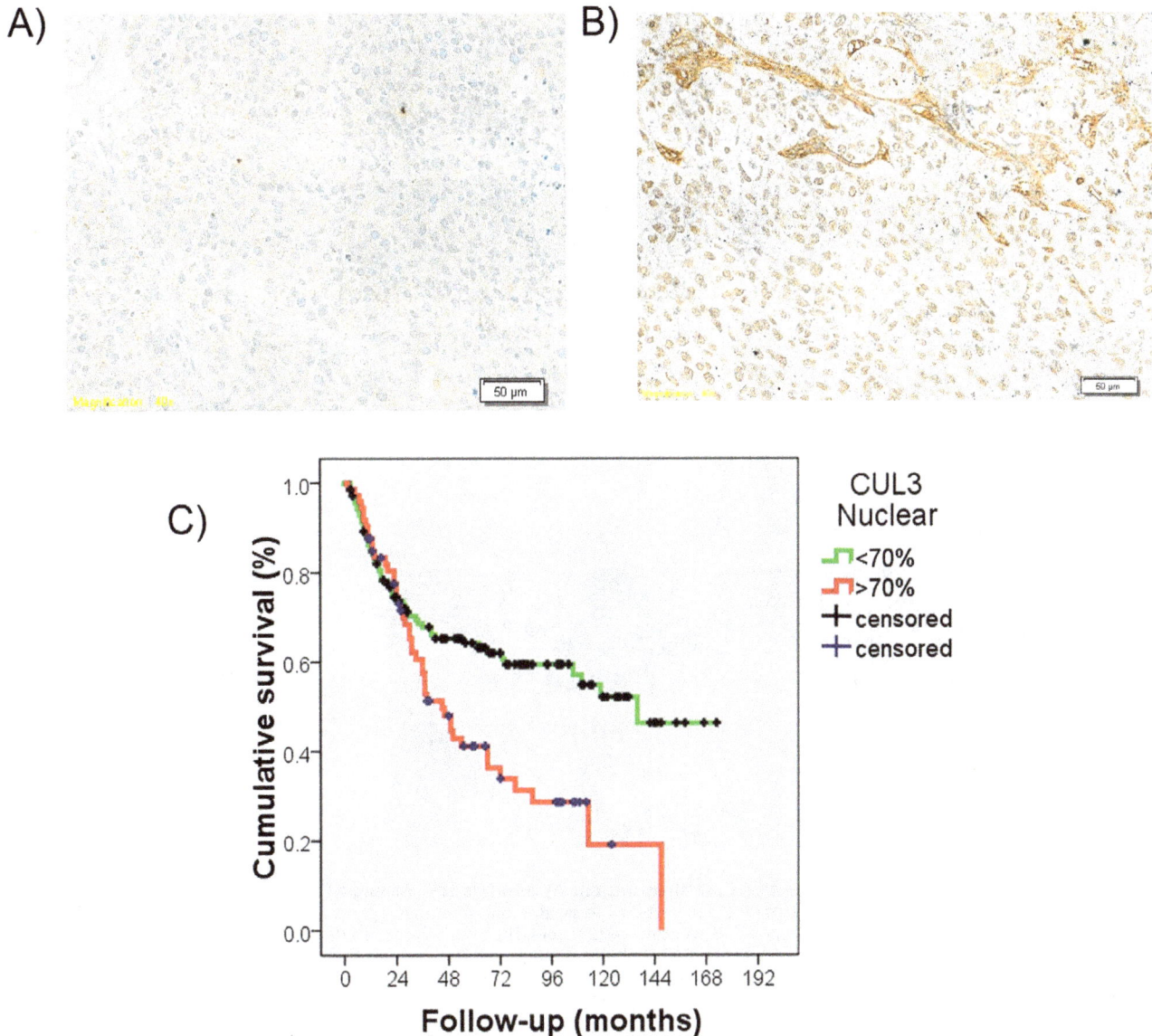

Figure 4. Clinical validation analyses of the differential expression of Cul3 in bladder cancer progression. (A, B) Representative immunohistochemistry expression patterns of Cul3 in non-invasive (A) and invasive (B) bladder tumors contained in tissue arrays. Strong expression of Cul3 was observed in invasive bladder tumors when compared to non-invasive lesions. Cul3 can also be observed in the extracellular matrix in B. There was a significant difference regarding the expression of Cul3 regarding tumor stage (p = 0.001: Original magnifications: x200). **(C)** Kaplan-Meier curve survival analysis indicating that increased nuclear Cul3 protein expression assessed by immunohistochemistry in tissue arrays was significantly associated with poor disease-specific survival (p = 0.002).

as demonstrated *in vivo* [6–9]. A high number of proteins were found differentially expressed between T24-T24T, with biological network annotations supporting the functional differences observed *in vitro*. Furthermore, proteins were shown differentially expressed using oligonucleotide arrays and by selected immunoblotting. Immunostaining of tissue arrays containing independent series of bladder cancer patients served to assess the associations of a selected protein, Cul3, with clinicopathological variables. Functional analyses and immunoblotting validation upon Cul3 silencing highlighted its impact in the aggressive phenotype of T24T cells and at modulating other cytoskeleton proteins identified by SILAC. Thus, combination of -omic approaches, functional and clinical analyses identified Cul3 as a novel candidate related to bladder cancer aggressiveness.

The extent of the proteomic profile defined in this study was comparable to other SILAC studies [13–29]. On the basis of the identity and biological abundance of the proteins identified, SILAC exhibited a satisfactory dynamic range in profiling both high- and low-abundance proteins. The broad spectrum of proteins observed reflects SILAC suitability for proteomic studies of cancer cells. Subcellular fractionation reduced sample complexity and increased the probability of detecting less abundant proteins. The level of ambiguity for a protein ratio was estimated taking into account the SDs within each protein because every SILAC ratio was calculated as a mean of at least 2 peptide values with their associated SDs. We selected 1.5 and 0.67 as cutoffs, also frequently used in SILAC-related studies [13,16,23,30]. When comparing two closely-related cell lines, it is expected that most of

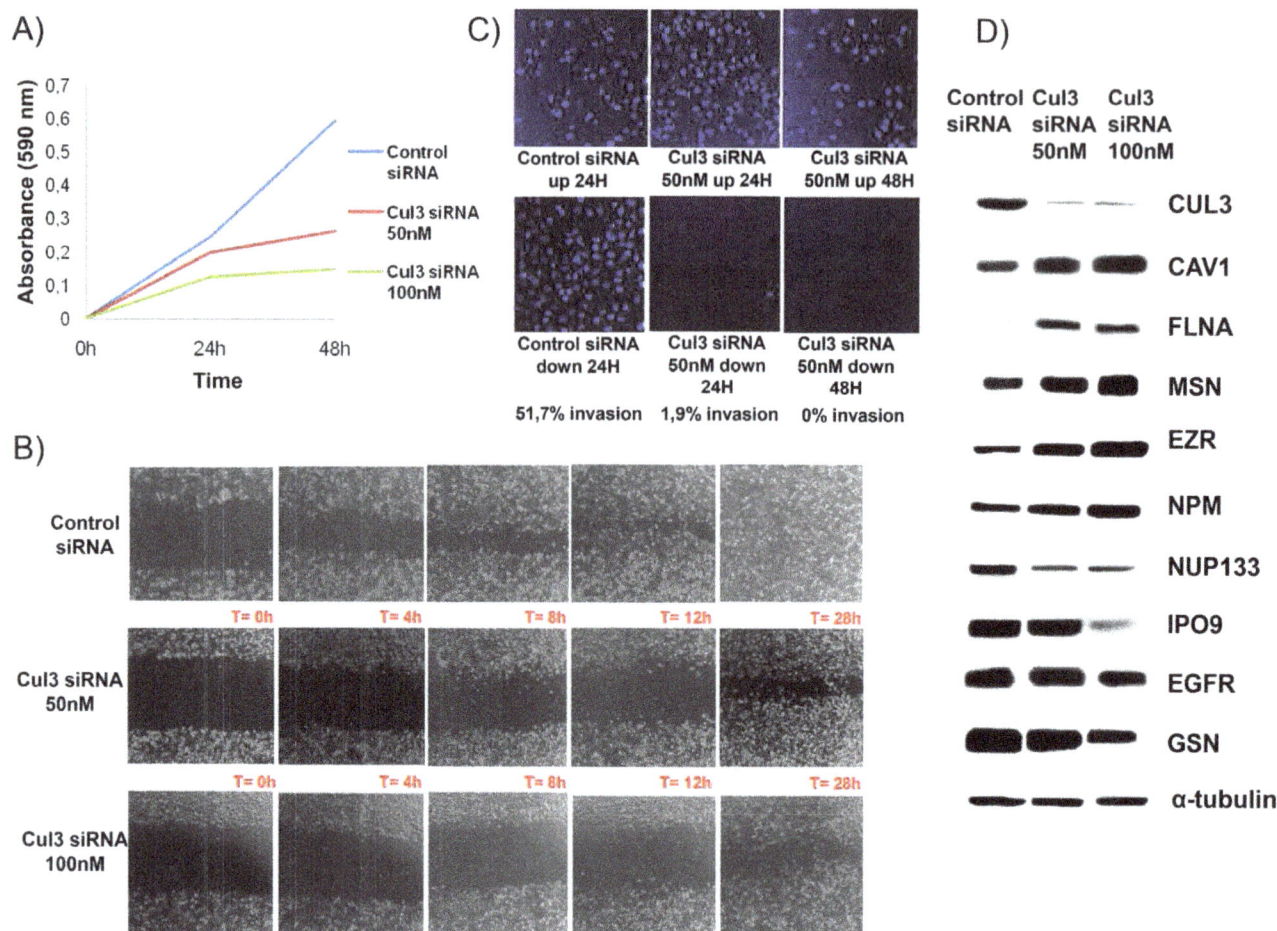

Figure 5. Functional analyses of the impact of Cul3 silencing on: A) proliferation, B) migration, and C) invasion. The average of duplicate experiments of each functional assay with siRNAs against Cul3 versus the control siRNA is represented in each panel. **D)** Immunoblotting of proteins found differentially expressed by SILAC upon Cul3 silencing on T24T cells. The results suggested that the differential expression of several of these proteins would be likely regulated by Cul3. Antibodies displaying a single predominant band at the expected molecular weights were accepted: Cul3, Cullin 3; CAV1, Caveolin 1; FLNA, Filamin A; MSN, Moesin; EZR, Ezrin; NPM, Nucleophosmin; NUP133, Nucleoporin 133; IPO9. Importin 9; EGFR, Epidermal Growth Factor Receptor; GSN, Gelsolin; and α-tubulin, was used as the loading control.

the proteins are expressed at similar levels. Indeed, most of the SILAC ratios were within the 0.67–1.5 range, apart from those related with the difference between these cells at their steady states (that could be attributed to their different phenotype). In SILAC, normalization was performed using the original mixture of the cells at a 1:1 ratio and reaching 100% labeling efficiency for both cell populations.

The limitation of selecting a threshold of expression to consider proteins to be differentially expressed requires a follow-up validation analysis for key data. Verification of changes by two independent analytical methods, and using independent *in vitro* strategies and clinical material provided confidence that the experimental design permitted significant changes in abundance to be validated. The limited correlation between transcript and protein expression at their steady state was similar to the 0.28 previously reported in pancreatic cells [14]. This could be attributed to the wider range of ratios of expression measured by gene arrays while the majority of the SILAC ratios were in the low range. SILAC ratios were more limited due to the internal labelling and the characteristic 1:1 mixture of the protein extracts analyzed. The weak correlation between the gene array and SILAC ratios highlighted the

relevance of quantitative proteomic approaches to estimate the expression of proteins of interest (not always predictable based on transcript levels), in concordance with previous reports [14]. There were missing data between both techniques because not all the coding products of the genes measured by the early version of the Affymetrix oligonucleotide array (U133A) were detected by SILAC. Similarly, genes coding for the 831 proteins identified by SILAC duplicates were not included among the probes contained in the commercial U133 oligonucleotide array. Availability of both transcript and protein expression levels could also be utilized to uncover potential regulatory mechanisms modifying translation or protein degradation. Immunoblotting validation was closely correlated to the SILAC results, and also served to validate candidates identified in oligonucleotide arrays (Figure S2).

Cul3 was selected from the top over-expressed candidates in T24T not previously characterized in bladder cancer for which we had available reagents for further studies. Cul3 was differentially expressed in T24T using three different methodologies: SILAC, gene arrays and immunoblotting. Cul3 is one of the four members of the cullin protein family [37,38]. It belongs to the core component of multiple ubiquitin-protein ligase complexes that mediate the ubiquitination and subsequent proteasomal degradation of their target proteins [39,40]. Cul3 acts as a scaffolding protein in a heterodimeric complex playing a central role in the specificity of polyubiquitinization of these proteins, positioning the substrate and the ubiquitin-conjugating enzyme [38,41]. Although the full list of targets whose ubiquitination and degradation is mediated by Cul3 remains unknown, cancer-related proteins reported include cyclin E [42], or Rho [43], among others [42–45]. In concordance with the interaction network shown in Figure S3, it could be proposed that Cul3 would be involved in the proteasomal degradation of adhesion associated cytoskeletal proteins such as filamin A, ezrin, caveolin1 or moesin. Indeed, the expression of these proteins increased upon Cul3 silencing, observations highlighting the impact of Cul3 expression not only on the aggressive phenotype of T24T shown by functional assays, but also modifying the expression of other proteins identified by SILAC. It remains to be characterized whether Cul3 might be directly involved in the proteasomal degradation of cytoskeleton proteins, potentially regulating the migration and invasive aggressiveness properties of T24T cells. Regarding therapeutic implications, members of the cullin family are covalently modified by NEDD8, where Cul3 ubiquitating ligase functioned as a NEDD8-bound heterodimer [46]. Neddylation and deneddylation may regulate Cul3 protein accumulation [47], suggesting new approaches to treat cancer by inhibiting the NEDD8-activated-cullin ligases [48]. To our knowledge, this is the first study evaluating Cul3 by immunohistochemistry, not only in bladder cancer but also in human tumors. Our findings were innovative and clinically relevant since Cul3 expression was linked to the invasive/metastatic phenotype in human bladder tumors, and also revealed that this protein can be secreted to the extracellular matrix. Our results highlighted the impact of the ubiquitin-proteasome pathway in bladder cancer aggressiveness, uncovering a novel biomarker and pathway potentially exploited therapeutically. Further focused designed studies are warranted to dissect the clinical relevance of Cul3 expression patterns in specific bladder cancer subgroups and address their specific clinical outcome endpoints.

The proteomic approach identified differential expression of proteins previously linked with aggressive clinical outcome in bladder tumors: gelsolin [49], moesin [32], Ezrin [50], caveolin [32], Filamin A [33]. The large number of differentially expressed proteins localized to the cytoplasm highlighted the relevance of adhesion molecules and cytoskeletal reorganization in bladder cancer aggressiveness (suported also by the IPA analysis), which could justify the higher proliferative, migration and invasive rate of T24T. Cul3 was uncovered as a clinically and biologically relevant candidate, which could promote cancer aggressiveness by regulating the expression of other critical cancer-related proteins [48–50]. Further research is warranted to define how cytoskeleton remodelling of these proteins specifically contribute to bladder cancer aggressiveness.

Concluding Remarks

The SILAC approach served to identify potential candidates involved in bladder cancer aggressiveness in vitro. Functional and clinical validation analyses served to uncover the roles of Cul3 at regulating cytoskeleton remodelling, and as a progression and clinical outcome stratification biomarker.

Supporting Information

Figure S1 Comparison of the metastatic profile using gene profiling of a oligonucleotide array and SILAC. (A)

Dispersion plot of the ratios of expression (represented as circles) observed between the oligonucleotide arrays and SILAC considering the 438 candidates defined by both techniques. The outliers represent candidates with very high differential ratios by oligonucleotide arrays (around 100) and SILAC (around 10). **(B)** Dispersion plot of the ratios of expression (represented as circles) observed between the oligonucleotide arrays and SILAC, excluding the outliers with high expression in the oligonucleotide arrays (>100) and in the SILAC (>9). Even after excluding the outliers, while the range of expression of the ratios for oligonucleotide microarrays was extensive, in SILAC analyses the majority of the differential expression was mild in the low range of ratios. **(C)** Cumulative probabilities (represented as circles) of the observed differential expression ratio against the expected ratio for oligonucleotide arrays. **(A)** Cumulative probabilities (represented as circles) of the observed differential expression ratio against the expected ratio for SILAC approach.

Figure S2 Western blotting validation of differentially expressed proteins in T24T when compared to T24 on the basis of the oligonucleotide arrays and that were not quantified using SILAC. MMP2, Matrix Metalloproteinase 2; EphA1, Ephrin type-A receptor 1; MAGE 1, Melanoma associated antigen 1; IGFBP2, Insulin-like growth factor-binding protein 2; SOX9, Transcription factor SOX-9; PMF-1, Poly-amine-modulated factor 1; SIVA, Apoptosis regulatory protein Siva; XRCC1, X-ray repair cross-complementing protein 1; ZYX, Zyxin; RAB6, Ras-related protein 6; MMP1, Matrix Metalloproteinase 1; CK2, Cytokeratin 2; FGFR1, Fibroblast growth factor receptor 1; CDK4, Cyclin-Dependent Kinase 4; REG1, Lithostathine 1; CLDN3, Claudin 3; SDC, Syndecan; KISS1, Metastasis-suppressor KiSS-1; SYP, Synaptophysin; SOX4, Transcription factor SOX-4; ANXA1, Annexin A1; GGT-1, Gamma-glutamyltranspeptidase 1; BDNF-1, Brain-derived neurotrophic factor; NUP62, Nucleoporin 62; GAL3, Galectin 3; GRB2, Growth factor receptor-bound protein 2; COX2, Cyclooxigenase2. The antibodies were raised against the following protein (and the dilutions used in immunoblots are shown): Annexin1 (38 kDa, mouse, 1:2000, #610066, BD Transduction Laboratories), BDNF (14–27 kDa, mouse, 1:50, #MAB248, R&D Systems, Minneapolis, MN, US), CDK4 (30 kDa, rabbit, 1:500, #SC-260, Santa Cruz), Claudin-3 (22kDa, rabbit, 1:1000, #18-7340, Zymed, Paisley, UK), Cox2 (70 kDa, mouse, 1:500, #35-8200, Zymed), Cytokeratin 2 (66 kDa, mouse, 1:100, #65177, Progen Biotechnik GmbH, Heidelberg), EphA1 (24 kDa, rabbit,1:50, #34-3300, Zymed), FGF Receptor (110 kDa, mouse,1:100, #13-3100, Zymed), Galectin-3 (18 kDa, rabbit, 1:40, #18-0393, Zymed), GGT-1 (30–35 kDa, mouse, 1:200, #H00002678-M01, clone 1F9, Abnova), GRB2 (25kDa, mouse, #610112, BD Transduction Laboratories) IGFBP-2 (35 kDa, mouse, 1:200, #MAB674, R&D Systems), KISS1 (16 kDa, rabbit, 1:50, #3590, Biovision, CA, USA), MAGE1 (46 kDa, mouse, 1:100, #MA454, Abcam, Cambridge, UK), MMP1 (54 kDa, mouse, 1:2000, #IM35, MERCK), MMP2 (64–72 kDa, mouse, 1:100, #MAB9021, clone 101721, R&D Systems), NUP62 (62 kDa, mouse, 1:100, #N43620, BD Transduction Laboratories), PMF-1 (23 kDa, mouse, 1:100, #P24620, BD Transduction Laboratories,), RAB6 (25 kDa, rabbit, 1:100, #SC-310, Santa Cruz), Reg1 (rabbit, 20 kDa, 1:1000 dilution, kindly supplied by Dr. Iovanna, located at Inserm, Marseille, France), SOX9 (65 KDa, goat, 1:250, #AF3075, R&D Systems,), SOX4 (40–46 kDa, mouse, 1:500, #H00006659-A01, Abnova), Synaptophysin (38 kDa, rabbit, 1:100, #18-0130, Zymed), Syndecan (90 kDa, rabbit, 1:100, #36-2900, Zymed), SIVA (37,5 kDa, goat, 1:1000, #HM1334,

Hypromatrix, Worcester, MA), XRCC1 (70 kDa, mouse, 1:50, #SC-56254, Santa Cruz), Zyxin (83 kDa, mouse, 1:100, #Z45420, BD). Western Blots were scanned and analyzed using α-tubulin as normalizing loading control.

Figure S3 Functional networks of the proteins identified: in silico protein interaction analysis. Molecular network obtained using the IPA software selected from the networks of differentially expressed proteins identified as it contained the highest number of the proteins identified by SILAC (n = 31). Addition of Cul3, the validated candidate, to this molecular network served to generate an interaction map connecting the novel candidate with other proteins identified through their previously described biological interactions. In this network, genes or gene products are represented as nodes, and the biological relationship between two nodes is represented as an edge. All edges are supported by at least one publication from the information stored in the Ingenuity knowledge database.

Figure S4 Functional networks of the proteins identified: in silico protein interaction analysis. Biological interaction networking highlighted on the map of the top ten differentially expressed proteins in SILAC and oligonucleotide arrays, and validated in Western blots, including Cul3. Accession number and T24T/T24 ratio values for the proteins identified in Table 1 were imported into IPA software to generate different molecular networks. In this network, genes or gene products are represented as nodes, and the biological relationship between two nodes is represented as an edge. All edges are supported by at least one publication from the information stored in the Ingenuity knowledge database. The intensity of the node colour indicates the degree of over- (red) or under- (green) expression in T24T when compared to T24. The legend of the interaction network and the relationships between molecules is also provided.

Table S1 Proteins with altered abundance in bladder cancer metastatic cells. All proteins were identified at >99% confidence (corresponding to a Mascot score >46). The table includes accession number (gi), protein name, molecular weight (in kD), gene array ratio, SILAC ratios and the standard deviation (SD, n = 2). All proteins were identified in the two SILAC

replicates with at least two unique peptides. Proteins previously described to be involved in cancer metastases are highlighted in italics, while those reported to be related to bladder cancer metastases are highlighted in bold.

Table S2 Protein ID and quantification. Proteins are listed alphabetically according to Protein Name. Proteins were identified according to the NCBI human databases (NCBI GI #s given for each ID). The table includes the corresponding UniProt and IPI accession numbers where available, Mascot scores corresponding to the highest scoring occurrence of a given protein or peptide, and GO annotations. T24T/T24 SILAC ratio = Intensity of the heavy peptide (C^{13})/Intensity of the light peptide (C^{12}).

Table S3 Detailed information of ratios obtained from the proteins identified by SILAC (831 proteins, first sheet) and those measured simultaneously by oligonucleotide arrays (438 proteins, second sheet), including probe identification and gene description of the oligonucleotide arrays.

Acknowledgments

The authors would like to thank all members of the Tumor Markers Group, especially Marta Herreros and Esteban Orenes and the Proteomics Unit for their technical support and constructive suggestions in the preparation of this manuscript. We would also like to acknowledge the members of our clinical collaborators at the different institutions contributing to this study (Fundacio Puigvert, Hospital del Mar, Instituto Catala de Oncologia, and Hospital Central de Asturias), as well as the members of the Spanish Oncology Group of Genitourinary Cancer (SOGUG), for their support in facilitating the tumor specimens and the information regarding the clinical follow-up of the bladder cancer cases analyzed in this study.

Author Contributions

Conceived and designed the experiments: MS-C. Performed the experiments: LG JLL-G PGP DT JP JMFG MSC. Analyzed the data: LG JLL-G PGP DT JP JMFG MSC. Contributed reagents/materials/analysis tools: PGP DT JP JMFG. Wrote the paper: LG JLL-G MSC.

References

1. Jemal A, Siegel R, Ward E, Hao Y, Xu J, et al. (2009) Cancer statistics 2009. CA Cancer J Clin 59: 225–49.
2. Sánchez-Carbayo M, Cordon-Cardó C (2007) Molecular alterations associated with bladder cancer progression. Semin Oncol. 34, 75–84.
3. Smith SC, Theodorescu D (2009) The Ral GTPase pathway in metastatic bladder cancer: key mediator and therapeutic target. Urol Oncol 27: 42–7.
4. Apolo AB, Milowsky M, Bajorin DF (2009) Clinical states model for biomarkers in bladder cancer. Future Oncol 5: 977–92.
5. Gildea JJ, Golden WL., Harding MA, Theodorescu D (2000) Genetic and phenotypic changes associated with the acquisition of tumorigenicity in human bladder cancer. Genes Chromosomes Cancer 27: 252–263.
6. Seraj MJ, Harding MA, Gildea JJ, Welch DR, Theodorescu D (2001) The relationship of BRMS1 and RhoGDI2 gene expression to metastatic potential in lineage related human bladder cancer cell lines. Clin. Experim. Metastasis 18: 519–525.
7. Harding MA, Arden KC, Gildea JW, Gildea JJ, Perlman EJ, et al. (2002) Functional genomic comparison of lineage-related human bladder cancer cell lines with differing tumorigenic and metastatic potentials by spectral karyotyping, comparative genomic hybridization, and a novel method of positional expression profiling. Cancer Res 62: 6981–6989.
8. Gildea JJ, Herlevsen M, Harding MA, Gulding KM, Moskaluk CA, et al. (2004) PTEN can inhibit in vitro organotypic and in vivo orthotopic invasion of human bladder cancer cells even in the absence of its lipid phosphatase activity. Oncogene 23: 6788–6797.

9. Wu Y, McRoberts K, Berr SS, Frierson Jr HF, Conaway M, et al. (2007) Neuromedin U is regulated by the metastasis suppressor RhoGDI2 and is a novel promoter of tumor formation, lung metastasis and cancer cachexia. Oncogene 6: 765–773.
10. Sanchez-Carbayo M, Socci ND, Lozano JJ, Haab BB, Cordon-Cardo C (2006) Profiling bladder cancer using targeted antibody arrays. Am J Pathol 168: 93–103.
11. Orenes-Piñero E, Barderas R, Rico D, Casal JI, Gonzalez-Pisano D, et al. (2010) Serum and tissue profiling in bladder cancer combining protein and tissue arrays. J Proteome Res. 9:164–73.
12. Ong SE, Blagoev B, Kratchmarova I, Kristensen DB, Steen H, et al. (2002) Stable isotope labelling by amino acids in cell culture SILAC as a simple and accurate approach to expression proteomics. Mol Cell Proteomics 1: 376–386.
13. Luque-García JL, Martinez-Torrecuadrada JL, Epifano C, Cañamero M, Babel I, et al. (2010) Differential protein expression on the cell surface of colorectal cancer cells associated to tumor metastasis. Proteomics 10:940–52.
14. Gronborg M, Kristiansen TZ, Iwahori A, Chang R, Reddy R, et al. (2006) Biomarker discovery from pancreatic cancer secretome using a differential proteomic approach. Mol. Cell. Proteomics 5: 157–171.
15. Everyley PA, Krijgsveld J, Zetter BR, Gygi SP (2004) Quantitative cancer prpteomics: stable isotope labelling with amino acids in cell culture (SILAC) as a tool for prostate cancer research. Mol. Cell. Proteomics 3: 729–735.
16. Zhang G, Fenyo D, Neubert TA (2008) Screening for EphB signalling effectors using SILAC with a linear ion trap-orbitrap mass spectrometer. J. Proteome Res 7: 4725–4726.

17. Dobreva I, Fielding A, Foster LJ, Dedhar S (2008) Mapping the integrin-linked kinase interactome using SILAC. J. Proteome Res 7: 1740–1749.
18. Qiu H, Wang Y (2008) Quantitative analysis of surface plasma membrane proteins of prmary and metastatic melanoma cells. J Proteome Res 7:1904–1915.
19. Chen N, Sun W, Deng X, Hao Y, Chen X, et al. (2006) Quantitative proteome analysis of HCC cell lines with different metastatic potentials by SILAC. Proteomics 8: 5108–5118.
20. Pijnappel WP, Kolkman A, Baltissen MP, Heck AJ, Timmers HM (2009) Quantitative mass spectrometry of TATA binding protein-containing complexes and subunit phosphorylations during the cell cycle. Proteome Sci. 7: 46.
21. Lam YW, Evans VC, Heesom KJ, Lamond AI, Matthews DA (2010) Proteomics analysis of the nucleolus in adenovirus-infected cells Mol Cell Proteomics 9: 117–130.
22. Rangiah K, Tippornwong M, Sangar V, Austin D, Tetreault MP, et al. (2009) Differential secreted proteome approach in murine model for candidate biomarker discovery in colon cancer. J Proteome Res 8: 5153–5164.
23. Zhang G, Spellman DS, Skolnik EY, Neubert TA (2006) Quantitative phosphotyrosine proteomics of EphB2 signaling by stable isotope labelling by amino acids in cell culture (SILAC) J. Proteome Res 5: 581–588.
24. Lund R, Leth-Larsen R, Jensen ON, Ditzel HJ (2009) Efficient isolation and quantitative proteomic analysis of cancer cell plasma membrane proteins for identification of metastasis-associated cell surface markers. J Proteome Res 8: 3078–3090.
25. Ong SE, Mann M (2006) A practical recipe for stable isotope labelling by amino acids in cell culture (SILAC) Nat Protoc 1: 2650–2660.
26. Mann M (2006) Functional and quantitative proteomics using SILAC. Nat. Rev. Mol Cell Biol 7: 952–958.
27. Guha U, Chaerkady R, Marimuthi A, Patterson AS, Kashyap MK, et al. (2008) Comparisons of tyrosine phosphorylated proteins in cells expressing lung cancer-specific alleles of EGFR and KRAS. Proc Natl Acad Sci USA 105: 14112–14117.
28. Sun Y, Mi W, Cai J, Ying W, Liu F, et al. (2008) Quantitative proteomic signature of liver cancer cells: tissue transglutaminase 2 could be a novel protein candidate of human hepatocellular carcinoma. J. Proteome Res 7: 3847–3859.
29. Pan C, Olsen JV, Daub H, Mann M (2009) Global effects of kinase inhibitors on signalling networks revealed by quantitative phosphoproteomics. Mol Cell Proteomics 8: 2796–2808.
30. Spellman DS, Deinhardt K, Darie CC, Chao MV, Neubert TA (2008) Stable isotopic labelling by amino acids in cultured primary neurons: application to brain-derived neurotrophic factor-dependent phosphotyrosine-associated signalling. Mol. Cell. Proteomics 7: 1067–1076.
31. Selbach M, Schwanhäusser B, Thierfelder N, Fang Z, Khanin R, et al. (2008) Widespread changes in protein synthesis induced by microRNAs. Nature 455:58–63.
32. Sánchez-Carbayo M, Socci ND, Charytonowicz E, Lu M, Prystowsky M, et al. (2002) Molecular profiling of bladder cancer using cDNA microarrays: defining histogenesis and biological phenotypes. Cancer Res 62: 6973–6980.
33. Ruppen I, Grau L, Orenes-Piñero E, Ashman K, et al. Differential protein expression profiling by iTRAQ-two-dimensional LC-MS/MS of human bladder cancer EJ138 cells transfected with the metastasis suppressor KiSS-1 gene. Mol Cell Proteomics. 2010, 9: 2276–91.
34. Sanchez-Carbayo M, Socci ND, Lozano J, Saint F, Cordon-Cardo C (2006) Defining molecular profiles of poor outcome in patients with invasive bladder cancer using oligonucleotide microarrays. J Clin Oncol 24:778–89.
35. American Joint Committee on Cancer: Staging of cancer at genitourinary sites (1988) In:American Joint Committee on Cancer: Manual for Staging of Cancer, 3rd Edition. Philadelphia: J. B., Lippincott, Co. 194–195.
36. Dawson-Saunders B, Trapp RG (1994) Basic & Clinical Biostatistics. 2nd edition, Norwalk, Connecticut, Appleton & Lange.
37. Du M, Sansores-Garcia L, Zu Z, Wu KK (1998) Cloning and expression analysis of a novel salicylate suppressible gene, Hs-CUL-3, a member of cullin/Cdc53 family. J Biol Chem 273:24289–24292.
38. Furukawa M, He YJ, Borchers C, Xiong Y (2003) Targeting of protein ubiquitination by BTB–Cullin 3–Roc1 ubiquitin ligases. Nature Cell Biol 5: 1001–1007.
39. Petroski MD, Deshaies RJ. (2005) Function and regulation of cullin–RING ubiquitin ligases. Nature Rev. Mol. Cell Biol 6: 9–20.
40. Van den Heuvel S (2004) Protein degradation: CUL-3 and BTB – partners in proteolysis. Curr Biol 14: R59–R61.
41. Singer JD, Gurian-West M, Clurman B, Roberts JM (1999) Cullin-3 targets cyclin E for ubiquitination and controls S phase in mammalian cells. Genes Dev 13:2375–2387.
42. Wilkins A, Ping Q, Carpenter CL (2004) RhoBTB2 is a substrate of the mammalian CUL-3 ubiquitin ligase complex. Genes Dev 18:856–61.
43. Lee DF, Kuo HP, Liu M, Chou CK, Xia W, et al. (2009) KEAP1 E3 ligase-mediated downregulation of NF-kappaB signaling by targeting IKKbeta. Mol Cell 36: 131–40.
44. Pintard L, Willis JH, Willems A, Johnson JL, Srayko M, et al. (2003) The BTB protein MEL-26 is a substrate-specific adaptor of the CUL-3 ubiquitin-ligase. Nature 425: 311–316.
45. Hori T, Osaka F, Chiba T, Miyamoto C, Okabayashi K, et al. (1999) Covalent modification of all members of human cullin family proteins by NEDD8. Oncogene 18:6829–6834.
46. Wu JT, Lin HC, Hu YC, Chien CT (2005) Neddylation and deneddylation regulate CUL1 and cul-3 protein accumulation. Nat Cell Biol 7:1014–1020.
47. Soucy TA, Smith PG, Milhollen MA, Berger AJ, Gavin JM, et al. (2009) An inhibitor of NEDD8-activating enzyme as a new approach to treat cancer. Nature 458:732–736.
48. Mani A, Gelmann, E. P. (2005) The ubiquitin-proteasome pathway and its role in cancer. J. Clin Oncol. 23: 4776–4789.
49. Sanchez-Carbayo M, Socci ND, Richstone L, Corton M, Behrendt N, et al. (2007) Genomic and proteomic profiles reveal the association of gelsolin to TP53 status and bladder cancer progression. Am J Pathol 171:1650–8.
50. Palou J, Algaba F, Vera I, Rodriguez O, Villavicencio H, et al. (2009) Protein Expression Patterns of Ezrin Are Predictors of Progression in T1G3 Bladder Tumours Treated with Nonmaintenance Bacillus Calmette-Guérin. Eur Urol. 56: 829–836.

16

Long Interspersed Nuclear Element-1 Hypomethylation and Oxidative Stress: Correlation and Bladder Cancer Diagnostic Potential

Maturada Patchsung[1,9]**, Chanchai Boonla**[1,9]**, Passakorn Amnattrakul**[2]**, Thasinas Dissayabutra**[1]**, Apiwat Mutirangura**[3]**, Piyaratana Tosukhowong**[1]*

1 Department of Biochemistry, Faculty of Medicine, Chulalongkorn University, Bangkok, Thailand, 2 Department of Surgery, Faculty of Medicine, Chulalongkorn University, Bangkok, Thailand, 3 Department of Anatomy, Faculty of Medicine, Chulalongkorn University, Bangkok, Thailand

Abstract

Although, increased oxidative stress and hypomethylation of long interspersed nuclear element-1 (LINE-1) associate with bladder cancer (BCa) development, the relationship between these alterations is unknown. We evaluated the oxidative stress and hypomethylation of the LINE-1 in 61 BCa patients and 45 normal individuals. To measure the methylation levels and to differentiate the LINE-1 loci into hypermethylated, partially methylated and hypomethylated, peripheral blood cells, urinary exfoliated cells and cancerous tissues were evaluated by combined bisulfite restriction analysis PCR. The urinary total antioxidant status (TAS) and plasma protein carbonyl content were determined. The LINE-1 methylation levels and patterns, especially hypomethylated loci, in the blood and urine cells of the BCa patients were different from the levels and patterns in the healthy controls. The urinary TAS was decreased, whereas the plasma protein carbonyl content was increased in the BCa patients relative to the controls. A positive correlation between the methylation of LINE-1 in the blood-derived DNA and urinary TAS was found in both the BCa and control groups. The urinary hypomethylated LINE-1 loci and the plasma protein carbonyl content provided the best diagnostic potential for BCa prediction. Based on post-diagnostic samples, the combination test improved the diagnostic power to a sensitivity of 96% and a specificity of 96%. In conclusion, decreased LINE-1 methylation is associated with increased oxidative stress both in healthy and BCa subjects across the various tissue types, implying a dose-response association. Increases in the LINE-1 hypomethylation levels and the number of hypomethylated loci in both the blood- and urine-derived cells and increase in the oxidative stress were found in the BCa patients. The combination test of the urinary hypomethylated LINE-1 loci and the plasma protein carbonyl content may be useful for BCa screening and monitoring of treatment.

Editor: Kin Mang Lau, The Chinese University of Hong Kong, Hong Kong

Funding: This work was supported by Ratchadapisake Sompote Fund, Chulalongkorn University (to PT), by the Biochemistry and Molecular Biology of Metabolic Diseases Research Unit and by the Higher Education Research Promotion and National Research University Project of Thailand, Office of the Higher Education Commission and the Ratchadaphiseksomphot Endowment Fund (HR 1162A). AM is supported by Research Chair Grant 2011, National Science and Technology Development Agency (NSTDA), Thailand, and the Four Seasons Hotel Bangkok's 4th Cancer Care charity fun run in coordination with the Thai Red Cross Society and Center of Excellence in Molecular Genetics of Cancer and Human Diseases, Chulalongkorn University. The funders had no role in study design, data collection and analysis, decision to publish, or preparation of the manuscript.

Competing Interests: The authors have declared that no competing interests exist.

* E-mail: piyaratana_t@yahoo.com

9 These authors contributed equally to this work.

Introduction

Carcinogenesis of the urinary bladder is complex because both genetic mutations and epigenetic alterations play important roles. Furthermore, inflammation and oxidative stress critically contribute to development of bladder cancer (BCa) [1–3]. Various lines of evidence report an increased oxidative stress in patients with BCa [3–6]. Oxidative stress is a condition of the excessive production of reactive oxygen species (ROS) and/or a reduction of antioxidants. ROS directly damages the cellular DNA and promotes tumor development not only through genetic mutations but also through epigenetic alterations [7]. Common epigenetic alterations in human cancers include global hypomethylation and regional (site-specific CpG island promoter) hypermethylation of the tumor suppressor genes [8,9]. Hypomethylation of the cancer genome

occurs on the repetitive sequences and retrotransposable elements [10], which accelerates the genomic instability [10–13] and alters gene expression [14]. The best characterized and most abundant retrotransposon in the mammalian genome is the long interspersed nuclear element-1 (LINE-1 or L1), and it is known that LINE-1 hypomethylation is associated with many malignancies [15,16].

In urothelial cancer, the hypomethylation of LINE-1 was first demonstrated in urothelial cell lines and tumor tissues by Schulz and colleagues based on experiments using methylation-sensitive restriction enzymes (*Hpa*II/*Msp*I) and Southern blotting [17,18]. The LINE-1 hypomethylation corresponded well with an increase in the LINE-1 transcripts and a decrease in gene containing LINE-1 mRNA [14]. Later, our group employed a combined bisulfite restriction analysis (COBRA) PCR to demonstrate LINE-1 hypomethylation in various carcinomas tissues including bladder cancer [15]. Choi et al. used bisulfite-PCR pyrosequencing and showed an obvious hypomethylation of LINE-1 in bladder tumor tissues relative to the adjacent normal tissues [19]. The reduction of 5-methylcytosine levels in leukocyte DNA was shown in Spanish patients with bladder cancer relative to the matched controls [20]. Recently, the hypomethylation of LINE-1 in peripheral blood cells was associated with an increased risk for bladder cancer, especially in women [21]. Among nonsmoking Chinese, similar result that LINE-1 hypomethylation in lymphocytes was associated with increased risk for bladder cancer was demonstrated [22]. Previously, the methylation of LINE-1 in urinary exfoliated cells and its implication in bladder cancer has not been investigated. Even though LINE-1 hypomethylation and increased oxidative stress are well recognized in BCa patients, the association between these two phenomena has not been explored.

To date, the most commonly used techniques for measuring LINE-1 methylation level are pyrosequencing and COBRA PCR. These two methods had have similar efficacy in the detection of methylation levels and have limited margins of error [23]. The pyrosequencing of LINE-1 detects a few more CpG dinucleotides, usually three CpGs, [24] than the COBRA PCR detects (usually two CpGs). However, the LINE-1 methylation of each locus is not homogenous [23,25], which can influence expression and stability of the genome in cis [16]. Consequently, the LINE-1 methylation levels do not precisely represent the biological roles of the epigenomic modification [16]. To improve LINE-1 methylation evaluation, in addition to overall methylation level, we used COBRA PCR of LINE-1 to classify the genome-wide LINE-1 loci into four groups, $^{m}C^{m}C$ (hypermethylated), $^{u}C^{u}C$ (hypomethylated), $^{m}C^{u}C$ and $^{u}C^{m}C$ (partial methylated), and calculate the percentages of each group (Fig. 1) [26]. Of note, certain LINE-1 methylation assays have a positive methylation control base which can be use to determine the efficacy of the bisulfite treatment.

To evaluate the association between oxidative stress and LINE-1 hypomethylation, we determined the methylation levels of LINE-1 in the blood and urine cells obtained from the BCa patients and from the healthy individuals. Oxidative stress, indicated by the urinary total antioxidant status (TAS) and plasma protein carbonyl content, was compared between the two groups. The association of the LINE-1 methylation levels with the oxidative stress status was evaluated, and the usefulness of LINE-1 hypomethylation detection in the urinary exfoliated cells and the overall oxidative stress as markers for BCa diagnosis was assessed.

Materials and Methods

Participants

Sixty-one patients with BCa that were admitted to the King Chulalongkorn Memorial Hospital, Bangkok, Thailand between 2009 and 2010 were recruited for the study. All of the patients had histological proof of a superficial transitional cell carcinoma. Any BCa patients that presented with a muscle invasive phenotype were excluded from this study. Age- and gender-matched healthy individuals (n = 45) were used as controls. The controls were selected from members of the healthy elderly community at Lumpini Park, Bangkok, where they came everyday to do exercise. The healthy condition was confirmed by direct interview and their annual medical check-up to ensure that there was no history of urinary disorders and any malignancies. All subjects voluntarily participated in the study. The study protocol was reviewed and approved by the Ethics Committee of the Faculty of Medicine, Chulalongkorn University, Bangkok, Thailand. Written informed consents were obtained from all participants.

Specimen collection and DNA extraction

Heparinized blood and midstream spot morning urine (between 8:00 am and 12:00 pm) were collected from all participants. The blood samples were centrifuged to collect the plasma and buffy coat. The plasma samples were kept at $-80°C$ until testing. The buffy coat samples were immediately subjected to DNA extraction. To isolate the urinary exfoliated cells, 50 ml of the urine samples was centrifuged at 4,000 rpm for 20 min at 4°C. The cell pellet was collected and stored in RNA stabilizer (QIAGEN, Germany) at $-80°C$ until analysis. Of the 61 BCa patients, 14 had available cancerous tissues, which were obtained during the operation of transurethral resection, immediately stored in RNA stabilizer and kept at $-80°C$ for the LINE-1 measurement. Due to low amount of nucleated cells in urines, especially in healthy urines, DNAs from urinary exfoliated cells were successfully extracted from 30 BCa patients and 14 healthy controls. The DNA was extracted from peripheral blood buffy coats, urinary exfoliated cells and cancerous tissues using the High Pure PCR Template Preparation Kit (Roche Diagnostics, Indianapolis, USA). The incomplete specimen collection was considered as a weakness of the study. In BCA group, the blood, urinary exfoliated cells and cancerous tissues were accounted for 61 (100%), 30 (49.18%) and 14 (22.95%), respectively. Fourteen BCa patients (22.95%) had all types of specimens for analysis. In healthy control group, 45 (100%) blood and 14 (31.11%) urinary exfoliated cells samples were analyzed. Fourteen control subjects (31.11%) had both specimens for analysis. The power to detect the correlation observed for an n = 14 was calculated using the G*Power 3.1.3 software [27], and the output displayed the power of 0.66 (inputs: two-tails, effect size = 0.56, α = 0.05, total sample size = 14).

LINE-1 methylation by COBRA PCR

In brief, genomic DNAs (250 ng) derived from blood, urine and cancerous tissue samples were treated with sodium bisulfite as previously described [15]. The bisulfite-treated DNA was subjected to 35 cycles of PCR with LINE-1-F (5′-CCGT AAG GGGTTAGGGAGTTTTT-3′) and LINE-1-R (5′-RTAAAACCCTCCRAACCAAAT ATAAA-3′) primers with an annealing temperature of 50°C to generate 160 bp PCR amplicons. The amplicons were further digested with TaqI (2 U) (sticky end) and TasI (2 U) (sticky end) in NEB3 buffer (MBI Fermentas, Glen Burnie, MD) at 65°C overnight. The digested products were then electrophoresed in an 8% nondenaturing polyacrylamide gel and subsequently stained with SYBR green. The experiment was performed in duplicate.

The intensities of the COBRA LINE-1 fragments in the polyacrylamide gel were quantified using a phosphoimager and ImageQuant Software (Molecular Dynamics, GE Healthcare, Slough, UK). As detected by COBRA, methylation status of the 2 CpG dinucleotides of LINE-1 loci was classified into four groups as follows: (1) LINE-1 loci containing 2 unmethylated CpGs ($^{u}C^{u}C$); (2) LINE-1 loci containing 2 methylated CpGs ($^{m}C^{m}C$); (3) LINE-1 loci containing 5′-methylated and 3′-unmethylated CpGs ($^{m}C^{u}C$); and (4) LINE-1 loci containing 5′-unmethylated and 3′-methylated CpGs ($^{u}C^{m}C$). The details for band intensity quantitation was fully described elsewhere [28]. In brief, four bands that differed in their states of methylation, including 98 bp ($^{u}C^{u}C$), 160 ($^{m}C^{u}C$), 80 (^{m}C) and 62 (^{u}C) bp, were quantified (Fig. 1). The intensity of each band was divided by its paired length as followed: 160 bp/160 (A), 98 bp/94 (B), 80 bp/79 (C) and 62 bp/62 (D). The LINE-1 methylation level (overall or total) was calculated as the percent of the methylated bands (^{m}C) intensity divided by the sum of the ^{m}C and unmethylated bands (^{u}C) intensities, (C+A)/(C+A+A+B+D)×100. The percent of $^{u}C^{u}C$

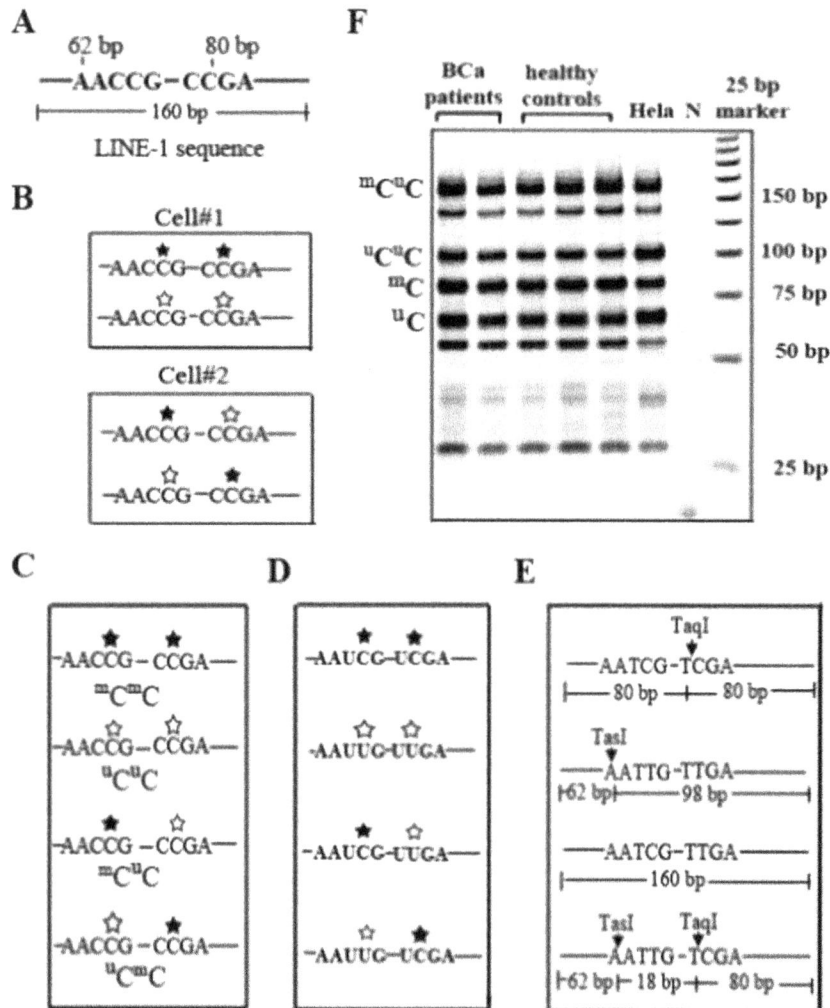

Figure 1. The methylation patterns of LINE-1 detected by COBRA PCR. A: The detecting 5′ UTR of the LINE-1 sequence contains two CpG dinucleotide loci, and the PCR amplicon size of LINE-1 is 160 bp. B: There are 4 possible methylation patterns of the LINE-1 sequence (one cell contains two alleles). The solid stars represent methylated cytosines and the hollow stars represent unmethylated cytosines. C: COBRA LINE-1 separated the detecting region into four products: $^{m}C^{m}C$, $^{u}C^{u}C$, $^{m}C^{u}C$ and $^{u}C^{m}C$. D: After the bisulfite treatment, the unmethylatated cytosine residues are converted to uracil, but the methylated cytosine residues are unaltered. This leads to retention or loss of CpG containing restriction enzyme sites, respectively. E: The PCR products are digested with TaqI (recognition sequence: TCGA) and TasI (recognition sequence: AATT) restriction enzymes. A TaqI positive digest yields two 80-bp DNA fragments, while a TasI positive digest yields a 62- and a 98-bp fragment. F: Representative gel image for COBRA LINE-1 assay. Lanes 1–2: DNAs from BCa patients, Lanes 3–5: DNAs from healthy controls, Lane 6: DNA from HeLa cells as positive control and normalizing sample, Lane 7: negative (N) control, Lane 8: 25 bp markers.

(hypomethylated loci) was calculated from the followed equation: $B/(((C-D+B)/2)+A+D)\times100$. The $^{m}C^{u}C$ (partial methylated loci) was computed from the equation: $A/(((C-D+B)/2)+A+D)\times100$. The $^{m}C^{m}C$ (hypermethylated loci) was computed from the equation: $((C-D+B)/2)/(((C-D+B)/2)+D+A)\times100$. The CV of the LINE-1 methylation levels in blood, urinary exfoliated cells and cancerous tissues DNAs were 7.31% (range: 2.33–12.91%), 7.64% (range: 2.50–13.17%) and 8.00% (range: 3.56–10.54%), respectively. DNA from HeLa cells was used as a control to normalize the inter-assay methylation variation for all of the experiments (Fig. 1F). The percent of LINE-1 methylation detected in HeLa DNAs was 28.59%, and this value was used for normalization between the runs. The mean of LINE-1 methylation in HeLa DNAs was 27.74±2.33%, and the between-run CV was 8.41%.

Total antioxidant status (TAS)

The 2, 2-diphenyl-1-picryl-hydrazyl (DPPH) reduction assay was performed to determine the TAS in urine samples. Briefly, a urine sample (20 µL) was added to of 400 µL of 10 mM phosphate buffered saline (PBS, pH 7.4) and 400 µL of freshly prepared 0.1 mM DPPH in methanol. The reaction tubes were incubated at room temperature for 20 min in the dark. The optical density (OD) at 520 nm was measured. The antioxidant capacity of the sample was calculated based on the % inhibition of DPPH radicals using the following equation: % inhibition $=(OD_{blank}-OD_{sample}/OD_{blank})\times100$. L-ascorbic acid (vitamin C) was used at concentrations of 0.25, 0.5 and 1 mM to generate a standard curve (% inhibition vs. concentration). The TAS value of the urine sample was expressed as the vitamin C equivalent antioxidant capacity (VCEAC mM). All experiments were done in duplicate. The CV for urinary TAS determination was 7.81% (range: 1.02–14.59%).

Protein carbonyl determination

The protein carbonyl content was used as an indicator of protein oxidation by ROS in plasma. A plasma sample was diluted (1:20) with PBS (10 mM, pH 7.4) and then centrifuged at 10,000 rpm for 10 min. The plasma supernatant (250 μL) was added to 1 mL of 10 mM 2,4-dinitrophenylhydrazine (DNPH) in 2N HCl. For a reagent blank control, 1 mL of 2N HCl was added to 250 μL of the plasma supernatant. The mixtures were incubated at room temperature in the dark for 45 min and were vortexed at 10-min intervals. Then, 1.2 mL of 20% cold trichloroacetic acid was added and incubated for 10 min on ice; this was followed by centrifugation at 3,000 rpm for 15 min to collect the protein pellets. The pellets were washed three times with 2.5 mL of ethanol/ethyl acetate (1:1, v/v) each to remove non-reacted DNPH. The washed pellets containing 2,4-dinitrophenylhydrazone were resuspended in 6 M guanidine hydrochloride/0.5 M potassium phosphate monobasic, pH 2.5, at 37°C for 15 min with vortexing. The absorbance at 375 nm was measured using the corresponding reagent blank for a zero setting. The extinction coefficient for the 2,4-dinitrophenylhydrazone at 375 nm is 22,000 M^{-1} cm^{-1} and the protein carbonyl concentration (nMol/mL) was calculated as the absorbance x 45.45 [29]. The content of protein carbonyl in the plasma was expressed per mg of total proteins (measured by the dye-binding method). The CV for determination of plasma protein carbonyl content was 8.43% (range: 2.72–13.80%).

Statistical analysis

The data with normal distribution were presented as the mean ± standard deviation, and the data with skewed distribution were presented as median (interquartile range, IQR). For comparisons between two independent groups, the independent sample t-test was used for normally distributed data, and the Mann-Whitney test was used for skewed data. Pearson's correlation test was used to assess the correlation between continuous variables. A receiver operating characteristic (ROC) analysis was performed to test the ability of the COBRA LINE-1 methylation test to differentiate BCa subjects from healthy subjects. An area under the ROC curve (AUC) of 1.0 indicates perfect accuracy, whereas an AUC of 0.5 indicates that the test lacks discriminatory power. A cutoff value was selected for computing the diagnostic values. SPSS version 17.0 (SPSS Inc., Chicago, IL) and STATA version 8.0 (StataCorp, College Station, Texas) were used for all calculations. A P value<0.05 was considered statistically significant.

Results

The BCa patients (n = 61) were between 42 and 89 years of age (65.11±12.16 years) and consisted of 52 (85.25%) males and 9 (14.75%) females. In the control group, there were 45 healthy subjects between 46 and 81 years of age (61.00±13.25 years); this group had 37 (82.22%) males and 8 (17.78%) females. Mean body mass index (BMI) of the patient and control groups were 22.24±3.71 and 23.15±2.45 (kg/m²), respectively. The sex distribution, age and BMI between the two groups were not significantly different.

The methylation level of LINE-1 was measured in DNA derived from peripheral blood, urinary exfoliated cells and cancerous tissues. The percentage of LINE-1 methylation in the peripheral blood cells from the BCa patients was significantly lower than that of the healthy controls (P = 0.001) (Fig. 2A). Likewise, the LINE-1

methylation levels in the urinary exfoliated cells from the BCa patients were significantly lower than those of the healthy controls (P = 0.044) (Fig. 2B). The LINE-1 methylation levels in the BCa cancerous tissues were significantly lower than those in the urinary exfoliated cells of the BCa (P = 0.038) and healthy (P = 0.001) subjects (Fig. 2B). The percentage of $^{u}C^{u}C$ loci in the peripheral blood cells and urinary exfoliated cells of the BCa patients was significantly greater than the controls (P = 0.013 and <0.001, respectively) (Fig. 2C and 2D). The number of $^{m}C^{u}C$ loci from the urinary exfoliated cells of the BCa patients was significantly lower than that of the controls (P = 0.006), but the levels of $^{m}C^{u}C$ loci in the peripheral blood cells from the BCa and healthy groups were not different (P = 0.133) (Figure S1). These data confirmed the presence of LINE-1 hypomethylation in bladder cancer and showed similar results to those previously reported for oral cancer [26] that demonstrated the specificity of $^{u}C^{u}C$ loci to cancer DNA.

The determinations of the urinary TAS and plasma protein carbonyl content were performed in both healthy and BCa groups. A significant reduction in the urinary TAS level in the BCA patients relative to the healthy controls was observed (P<0.001) (Fig. 3A). The plasma protein carbonyl content in the BCa patients was significantly higher than that in healthy controls (P<0.001) (Fig. 3B). Our findings indicated an increase in the oxidative stress in the BCa patients.

In the BCa patients, we found a strong, positive and linear correlation between the urinary TAS and LINE-1 methylation in circulating blood cells (regression coefficient = 8.017) (r = 0.618, P<0.001) (Fig. 4A). Moreover, a significant positive correlation between the urinary TAS and cancerous tissue LINE-1 methylation levels was observed (regression coefficient = 5.519) (r = 0.567, P = 0.034) (Fig. 4B). Interestingly, we also found a positive correlation between the urinary TAS and the level of LINE-1 methylation in the peripheral blood cells of the healthy individuals (regression coefficient = 8.937) (r = 0.469, P = 0.001) (Fig. 4C). The correlations between urinary TAS and the other patterns of LINE-1 methylation ($^{m}C^{m}C$, $^{u}C^{u}C$, $^{u}C^{m}C$ and $^{m}C^{u}C$) were evaluated (Figure S2). The significant inverse correlations between urinary TAS and the $^{u}C^{u}C$ levels in BCa peripheral blood cells (r = −0.440, P = 0.001), BCa cancerous tissues (r = −0.440, P = 0.001) and peripheral blood cells of healthy controls (r = −0.315, P = 0.035) were observed.

Using one-way ANOVA test, significant differences of LINE-1 methylation levels in blood, urine and cancerous tissue DNAs were not observed among BCa patients with different smoking status (non-smokers, current smokers and quitted smokers) (P = 0.477, 0.711 and 0.964, respectively). Likewise, levels of urinary TAS and plasma protein carbonyl content among the different smoking status were not significantly different (P = 0.053 and 0.093, respectively). Urinary TAS (P = 0.055 for healthy, P = 0.879 for BCa) and plasma protein carbonyl content (P = 0.634 for healthy, P = 0.072 for BCa) were not significantly different between males and females both in healthy and BCa groups. However, positive correlation between urinary TAS and age in healthy group (r = 0.374, P = 0.011) and negative correlation between plasma protein carbonyl content and BMI in BCa group (r = −0.261, P = 0.044) were revealed.

A ROC analysis was performed to evaluate how well the determination of the LINE-1 methylation can discriminate between the BCa patients and healthy individuals. Among the various patterns of LINE-1 methylation, the $^{u}C^{u}C$ level in the urinary exfoliated cells had the greatest diagnostic value with the highest AUC at 0.848 (95% CI: 0.719–0.977) (Table 1 and Fig. 5A). At a 38.43% cutoff, sensitivity, specificity and accuracy of the urinary $^{u}C^{u}C$ determination were 80.00%, 85.00% and

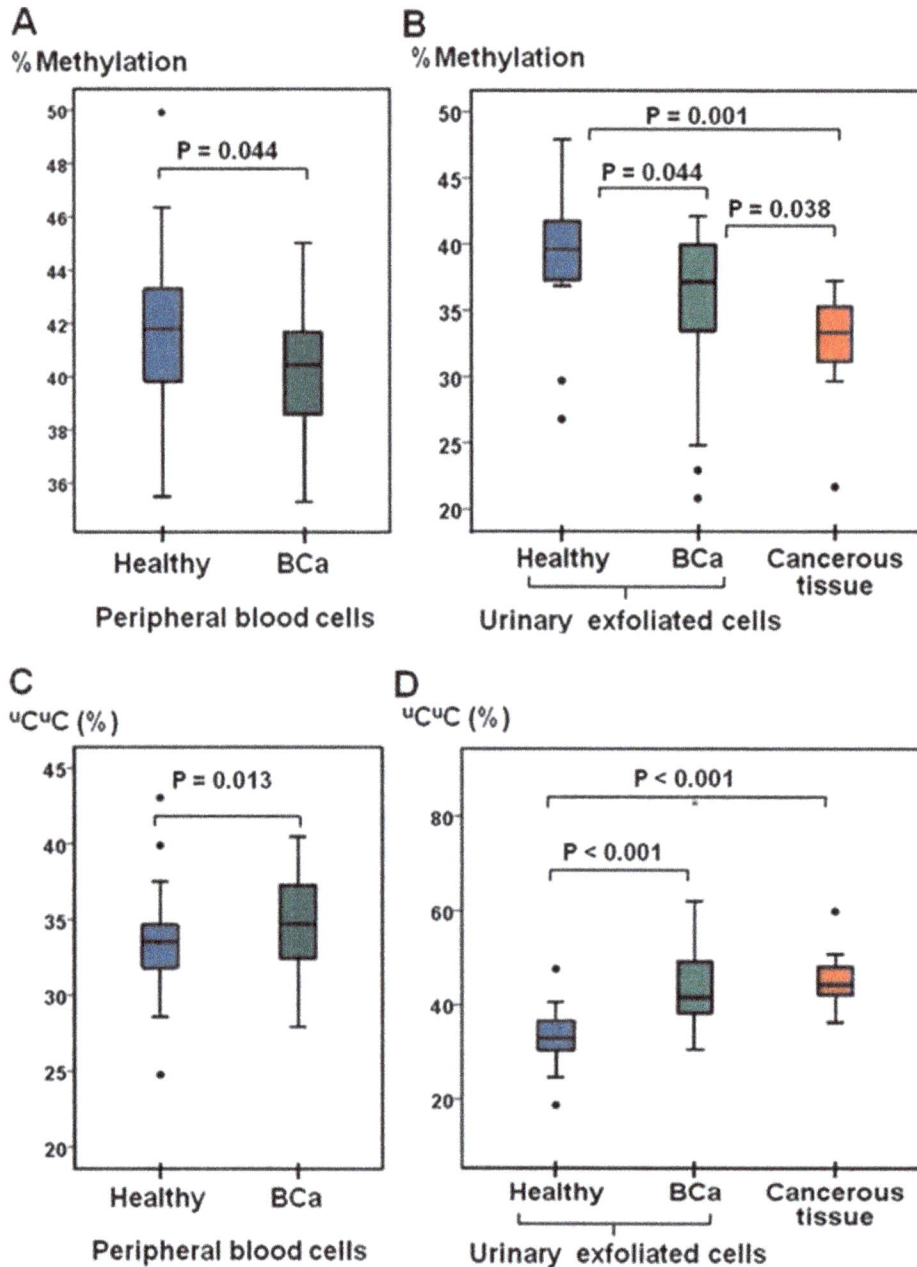

Figure 2. The LINE-1 methylation and $^{u}C^{u}C$ levels compared between the BCa and healthy groups. A: The percentage of LINE-1 methylation levels in the peripheral blood DNA from BCa patients (n = 61) was significantly lower than that from the healthy controls (n = 45). B: The LINE-1 methylation levels in the DNA derived from the urinary exfoliated cells from BCa patients (n = 30) were significantly decreased relative to those from the healthy controls (n = 14). The LINE-1 methylation levels in the cancerous tissues (n = 14) were significantly lower than the LINE-1 methylation levels in the urinary exfoliated cells from both BCa and healthy subjects. C: The $^{u}C^{u}C$ levels in the peripheral blood DNA from BCa patients were significantly higher than those from the healthy controls. D: The $^{u}C^{u}C$ levels in the urinary exfoliated cells of BCa patients were significantly increased compared to those from the healthy controls. The cancerous tissue $^{u}C^{u}C$ levels were not significantly different from the $^{u}C^{u}C$ levels from the BCa urinary exfoliated cells (P = 0.721), but they were significantly higher than those from the urinary exfoliated cells of healthy controls.

81.82%, respectively. The AUC values of the % methylation in both the blood (0.684) and the urine (0.691) cells were lower than that of urinary $^{u}C^{u}C$ (Figure S3). Thus, the determination of $^{u}C^{u}C$ in the urinary exfoliated cells provided the highest diagnostic potential relative to the other forms of methylation.

The ROC curves of the urinary TAS and plasma protein carbonyl content were also generated. The urinary TAS had an AUC of 0.800 (95% CI: 0.711–0.888) and had sensitivity,

specificity and accuracy of 88.52%, 60.00%, and 76.42%, respectively, at a cutoff of 1.32 VCEAC mM (Table 1 and Fig. 5B). An AUC value for the plasma protein carbonyl content was 0.819 (95% CI: 0.733–0.905), and its sensitivity, specificity and accuracy, at a cutoff of 0.44 nMol/mg of protein, were 81.97%, 73.33% and 78.30%, respectively (Table 1 and Fig. 5C).

We further evaluated whether the combination of $^{u}C^{u}C$ in the urinary exfoliated cells and the plasma protein carbonyl content

A Urinary TAS (VCEAC mM)

B Plasma protein carbonyl (mg/mg protein)

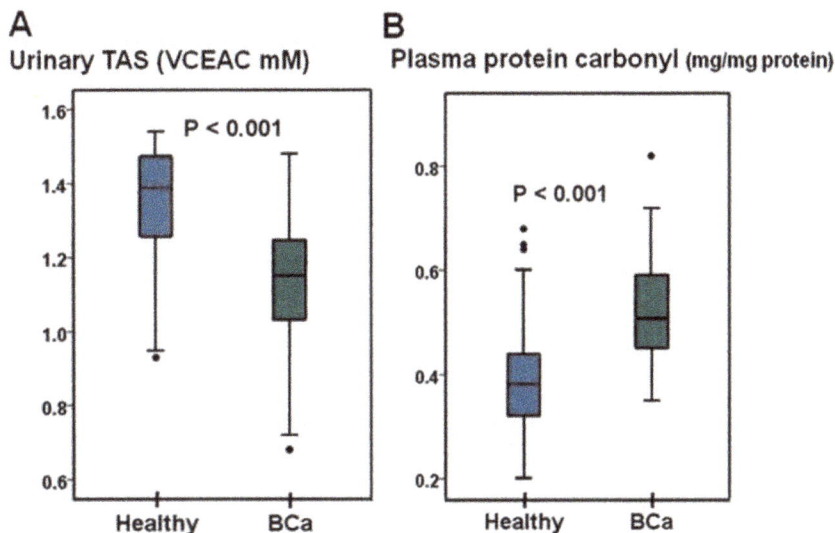

Figure 3. The oxidative stress biomarkers in patients with BCa. A: The level of urinary TAS in the BCa patients was significantly lower than that in the healthy controls. B: The level of the plasma protein carbonyl content in the BCa patients was significantly greater than that from the healthy controls.

would improve the diagnostic potential for BCa. The test criteria revealed that two positive results showed a higher specificity (96.00% with sensitivity of 65.58%) and a higher sensitivity (96.39% with specificity of 62.33%) when at least one marker was positive (Fig. 6).

Discussion

The loss of DNA methylation in the LINE-1 elements is suggested to be a cardinal event in cancer development because it promotes genomic instability and alters gene expression [12–16]. The mechanism that causes this loss of DNA methylation is unknown. The evaluation of the correlation of LINE-1 methylation levels between several loci suggested that the LINE-1

hypomethylation mechanism is generalized [23]. The timing of DNA methylation and bladder cancer is not yet clear. Rather, it has been shown to be a biomarker in post-diagnostic sample analyses, however, this relationship has not been shown in using pre-diagnostic samples, and it is not yet clear whether the lower methylation observed was caused by the carcinogenic process itself [30]. In the present study, we demonstrated here for the first time a significant positive correlation between LINE-1 hypomethylation and oxidative stress not only in cancer patients but also in healthy individuals. Therefore, oxidative stress may be one of the causes or consequences of LINE-1 hypomethylation.

Currently, to our knowledge, there is no biochemical mechanism that implies how LINE-1 hypomethylation can produce ROS. However, the mechanism of how oxidative stress reduces

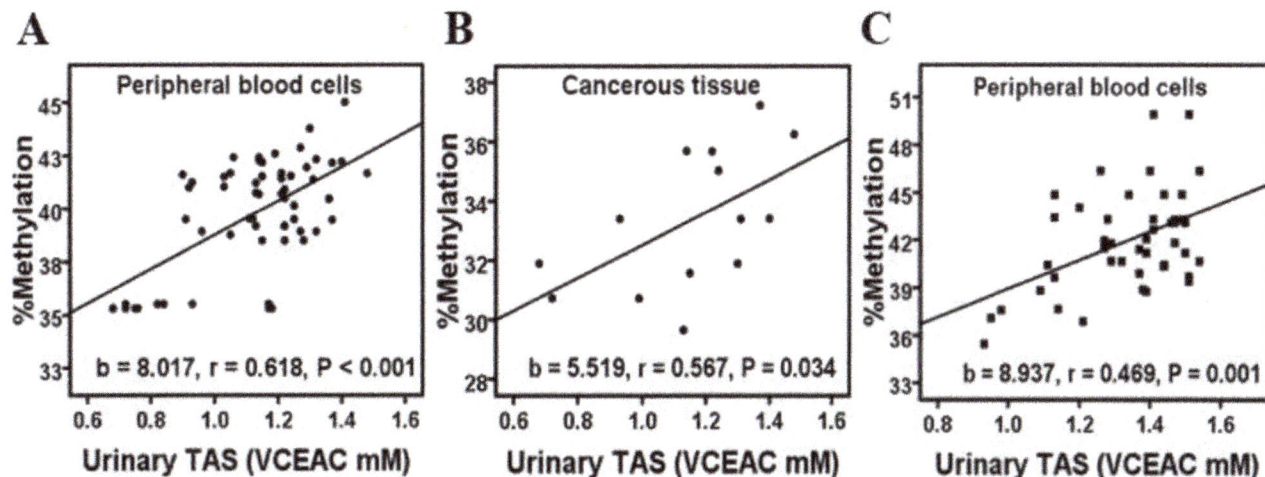

Figure 4. A univariate correlation analysis between the levels of urinary TAS and LINE-1 methylation. A: The urinary TAS was linearly correlated with the LINE-1 methylation levels in the peripheral blood cells of the BCa patients. B: The urinary TAS was linearly correlated with the LINE-1 methylation levels in the cancerous tissue obtained from the BCa patients. C: In the healthy group, the urinary TAS was also linearly correlated with the LINE-1 methylation levels in the peripheral blood cells. b: regression coefficient, r: Pearson's correlation coefficient. The displayed P values are from the Pearson's correlation test.

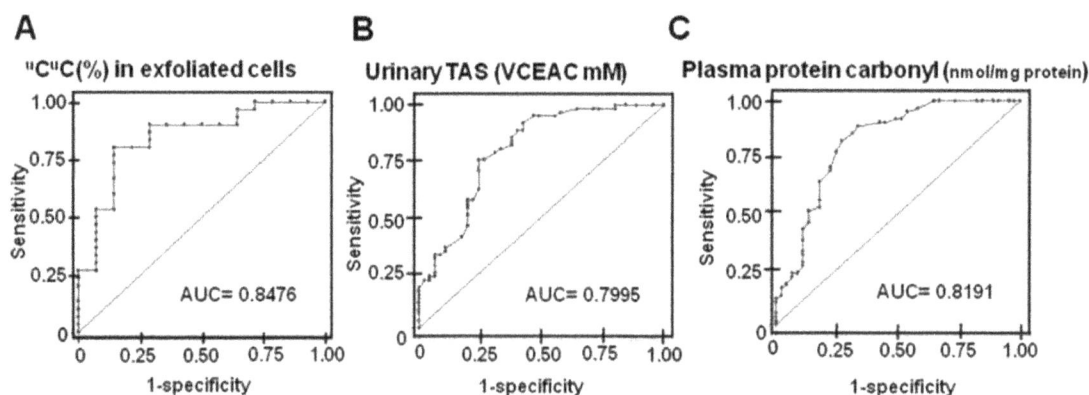

Figure 5. The ROC curves of $^uC^uC$ determination, the urinary TAS and the plasma protein carbonyl content. A: The % $^uC^uC$ in the urinary exfoliated cells. B: The urinary TAS. C: The plasma protein carbonyl content. The determination of $^uC^uC$ in the urinary exfoliated cells had the highest AUC, which suggests the highest diagnostic potential.

DNA methylation has been proposed [31], and the oxidative stress-induced DNA methylation change appears to be temporal [32,33]. Oxidized DNA lesions that are induced by ROS, such as 8-OHdG (in CpG dinucleotides), can strongly inhibit the methylation by a DNA methyltransferase at the adjacent C residues [34]. Additionally, an unfixed 8-OHdG may introduce a G-T transversion resulting in the loss of CpG dinucleotides [35]. Additionally, in an oxidative stress condition, the resynthesis of glutathione (GSH) in response to GSH depletion through the methionine cycle in one-carbon metabolism pathway is increased. This pathway requires S-adenosylmethionine (SAM) for synthesizing the homocysteine to be used for the GSH synthesis, leading to a decreased availability of SAM for DNA methylation [36]. The agents and conditions that induce GSH depletion have been demonstrated to impair DNA methylation [37,38]. Therefore, oxidative stress is thought to alter the methylation of DNA, which leads to changes in the gene expression that could contribute to tumor development [7]. In addition to decreased availability of SAM, depletion of methyl pool in folate-deficient models has been shown to cause DNA hypomethylation [39,40].

The LINE-1 methylation levels have been studied in several sources of DNA to improve cancer diagnosis. Unfortunately, there are tissue specific methylation levels and that these differ depending upon the methylation biomarker used to measure methylation [15]. In clinical specimens both cancerous and normal cells are usually coexisted, which means that based only on the LINE-1 methylation levels cancer DNA cannot be

effectively detected when the DNA sources are contaminated with DNA from various types of normal cells. For detection of noninvasive BCa by DNA examination, blood and urine are the common sources of DNA. Although cancer cells are present in both sources, the contamination with various types of normal cells is usually inevitable. Previously, we tested the DNA from both an oral rinse and from the white blood cells of patients with oral cancer and found that the percentage of hypomethylated loci or $^uC^uC$ was more specific to the cancer DNA than the overall LINE-1 methylation levels [26,41]. Moreover, the LINE-1 methylation levels between the cell types (oral epithelial and blood cells) were different because of the number of partial LINE-1 methylation loci. Here, we showed similar data in BCa; the number of LINE-1 hypomethylated loci in urinary exfoliated cells is a better tumor marker than the overall LINE-1 methylation level.

The increase in oxidative stress in BCa is well recognized and is believed to be critically involved in urothelial carcinogenesis [3–6]. The study results support this association; there still need to be experiments or analyses conducted using pre-diagnostic samples to confirm the temporality of the association observed here. The plasma protein carbonyl content was increased in the patients with BCa relative to the levels in the healthy controls [42]. The total antioxidant activity measured in the plasma of urothelial bladder carcinoma patients was lower than that in healthy controls [43]. In this study, we used the urinary TAS to reflect the overall antioxidant capacity in the body because the urinary TAS is a well-accepted marker for estimating the total antioxidants in biological

Table 1. The ROC analysis and diagnostic values of the measurements of the LINE-1 methylation and $^uC^uC$ levels as well as oxidative stress biomarkers.

Samples	Measurements	AUC	Cutoff	Sensitivity (%)	Specificity (%)	Accuracy (%)
Peripheral blood cells	Methylation (%)	0.684	42.87	96.67	40.00	72.38
	$^uC^uC$ (%)	0.641	34.64	50.00	77.78	61.90
Urinary exfoliated cells	Methylation (%)	0.691	42.15	100.00	21.43	75.00
	$^uC^uC$ (%)	0.848	38.43	80.00	85.00	81.82
Urine	TAS (VCEAC mM)	0.800	1.32	88.52	60.00	76.42
Plasma	Protein carbonyl (nMol/mg proteins)	0.820	0.44	81.97	73.33	78.30

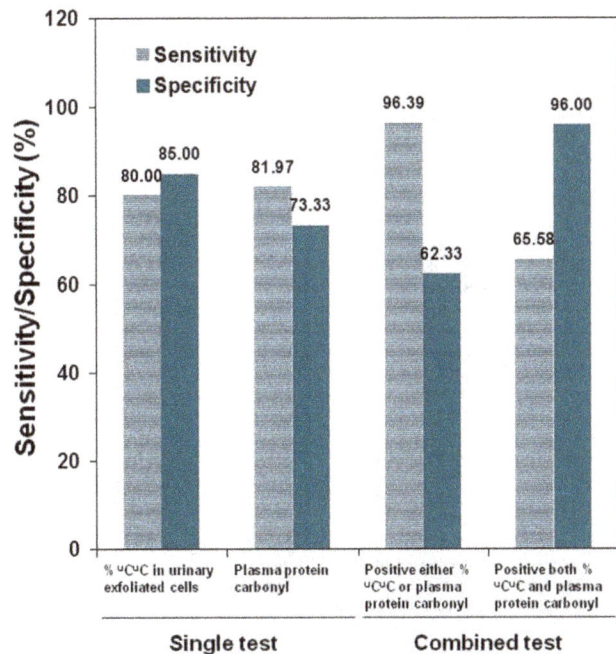

Figure 6. The sensitivity and specificity of the combined test of % $^{u}C^{u}C$ in the urinary exfoliated cells and the plasma protein carbonyl content. An increased sensitivity (96.39%) was achieved when either the % $^{u}C^{u}C$ in urinary exfoliated cells or the plasma protein carbonyl content was positive. Additionally, an increased specificity (96.00%) of the test was achieved when at least one of both markers was positive.

fluids [44]. Based on our findings, we conclude that the patients with BCa had an increase in oxidative stress. When combined with the LINE-1 hypomethylation levels, we hypothesize that the deprivation of antioxidants or an increase in oxidative stress may influence the global hypomethylation that promotes carcinogenesis.

The ROC analysis revealed the promising diagnostic potential of the measurements for the plasma protein carbonyl content and the LINE-1 hypomethylated loci in urinary exfoliated cells. The combination of these two tests increased the sensitivity and specificity of the diagnostic values to 96%. This association needs to be evaluated in pre-diagnostic samples. To date, there is no biomarker that can replace the need for cystoscopy, and the discovery of a new BCa biomarker is still a challenge for the field [45]. Although many urinary biomarkers have been reported to detect BCa with high sensitivity, their specificity is much lower than the urine cytology (95–100%) [45,46]. A meta-analysis reported that the sensitivity of urine cytology is only 34% [47]. Thus, a novel, noninvasive test with a high sensitivity and specificity that is comparable to that of urine cytology is required. Relative to the previously reported biomarkers for detecting BCa [45–48], the current combination tests have shown to have a diagnostic potential in the pre-diagnostic samples.

In conclusion, we found a positive correlation between the LINE-1 hypomethylation of urine exfoliative cells and the oxidative stress in both normal individuals and BCa patients.

ROS is hypothesized to be one of the candidate mechanisms that can reduce LINE-1 methylation. Moreover, the ROS generation and LINE-1 methylation levels and patterns in the blood, urinary exfoliated cells and cancer cells from patients were significantly changed relative to healthy controls. The combined information from these two tests demonstrated a very high sensitivity and specificity for BCa diagnosis, however, it needs to be confirmed using pre-diagnostic samples, prior to implementation in cancer diagnosis. Further studies of global hypomethylation and ROS will not only improve our knowledge of carcinogenic mechanisms but will also improve our management of the disease.

Statement of translational relevance

Patients with bladder cancer have increased oxidative stress and LINE-1 hypomethylation relative to healthy controls. LINE-1 hypomethylation is correlated with an increased ROS generation in both normal and cancer subjects, indicating a reverse association between LINE1 methylation and oxidative stress. LINE-1 hypomethylation is known to promote genome instability, alter gene expression and contribute to tumor progression. Thus, the treatment that effectively reduces the oxidative stress in the patients may attenuate the LINE-1 hypomethylation and decelerate the progression of the tumor. Until now, there has been no noninvasive biomarker for detecting a bladder tumor that can replace the need for cystoscopy. Based on pre-diagnostic samples, the determination of the hypomethylated loci of LINE-1 in urinary exfoliated cells combined with the plasma protein carbonyl content show high sensitivity and specificity for bladder cancer prediction. This combination test may be clinically useful for bladder cancer diagnosis and monitoring of treatment thus reducing the frequency of invasive cystoscopic procedures. However, the test should be performed in pre-diagnostic samples before the actual diagnostic power of the test can be evaluated.

Supporting Information

Figure S1 Comparison of partial methylation loci of LINE-1 in blood and urinary exfoliated cells as well as cancerous tissues of bladder cancer patients and healthy controls.

Figure S2 Correlations between urinary TAS and LINE-1 methylation patterns ($^{m}C^{m}C$, $^{u}C^{u}C$, $^{u}C^{m}C$ and $^{m}C^{u}C$) in peripheral blood cells (A–D and I–L) and cancerous tissues (E–H) of the patients with BCa (A–H) and healthy controls (I–L).

Figure S3 ROC curves of various forms of LINE-1 methylation in blood and urine cells.

Author Contributions

Conceived and designed the experiments: PT CB AM. Performed the experiments: MP CB TD. Analyzed the data: CB MP. Contributed reagents/materials/analysis tools: PT AM CB. Wrote the paper: CB MP AM. Patient recruitment and specimen collection: PA PT MP. Read revised manuscript for typing errors: TD PT AM CB. Read revised manuscript and comments: AM CB PT TD.

References

1. Kawai K, Yamamoto M, Kameyama S, Kawamata H, Rademaker A, et al. (1993) Enhancement of rat urinary bladder tumorigenesis by lipopolysaccharide-induced inflammation. Cancer Res 53: 5172–5175.

2. Michaud DS (2007) Chronic inflammation and bladder cancer. Urol Oncol 25: 260–268.

3. Opanuraks J, Boonla C, Saelim C, Kittikowit W, Sumpatanukul P, et al. (2010) Elevated urinary total sialic acid and increased oxidative stress in patients with bladder cancer. Asian Biomedicine 4: 703–710.

4. Akcay T, Saygili I, Andican G, Yalcin V (2003) Increased formation of 8-hydroxy-2′-deoxyguanosine in peripheral blood leukocytes in bladder cancer. Urol Int 71: 271–274.

5. Salim EI, Morimura K, Menesi A, El-Lity M, Fukushima S, et al. (2008) Elevated oxidative stress and DNA damage and repair levels in urinary bladder carcinomas associated with schistosomiasis. Int J Cancer 123: 601–608.

6. Soini Y, Haapasaari KM, Vaarala MH, Turpeenniemi-Hujanen T, Karja V, et al. (2011) 8-hydroxydeguanosine and nitrotyrosine are prognostic factors in urinary bladder carcinoma. Int J Clin Exp Pathol 4: 267–275.

7. Wachsman JT (1997) DNA methylation and the association between genetic and epigenetic changes: relation to carcinogenesis. Mutat Res 375: 1–8.

8. Esteller M (2008) Epigenetics in cancer. N Engl J Med 358: 1148–1159.

9. Rodriguez-Paredes M, Esteller M (2011) Cancer epigenetics reaches mainstream oncology. Nat Med 17: 330–339.

10. Wilson AS, Power BE, Molloy PL (2007) DNA hypomethylation and human diseases. Biochim Biophys Acta 1775: 138–162.

11. Hatziapostolou M, Iliopoulos D (2011) Epigenetic aberrations during oncogenesis. Cell Mol Life Sci 68: 1681–1702.

12. Pornthanakasem W, Kongruttanachok N, Phuangphairoj C, Suyarnsestakorn C, Sanghangthum T, et al. (2008) LINE-1 methylation status of endogenous DNA double-strand breaks. Nucleic acids research 36: 3667–3675.

13. Kongruttanachok N, Phuangphairoj C, Thongnak A, Ponyeam W, Rattanatanyong P, et al. (2010) Replication independent DNA double-strand break retention may prevent genomic instability. Molecular cancer 9: 70.

14. Aporntewan C, Phokaew C, Piriyapongsa J, Ngamphiw C, Ittiwut C, et al. (2011) Hypomethylation of intragenic LINE-1 represses transcription in cancer cells through AGO2. PloS one 6: e17934.

15. Chalitchagorn K, Shuangshoti S, Hourpai N, Kongruttanachok N, Tangkijvanich P, et al. (2004) Distinctive pattern of LINE-1 methylation level in normal tissues and the association with carcinogenesis. Oncogene 23: 8841–8846.

16. Kitkumthorn N, Mutirangura A (2011) Long interspersed nuclear element-1 hypomethylation in cancer: biology and clinical applications. Clin Epigenet doi:10.1007/s13148-13011-10032-13148.

17. Florl AR, Lower R, Schmitz-Drager BJ, Schulz WA (1999) DNA methylation and expression of LINE-1 and HERV-K provirus sequences in urothelial and renal cell carcinomas. Br J Cancer 80: 1312–1321.

18. Jurgens B, Schmitz-Drager BJ, Schulz WA (1996) Hypomethylation of L1 LINE sequences prevailing in human urothelial carcinoma. Cancer Res 56: 5698–5703.

19. Choi SH, Worswick S, Byun HM, Shear T, Soussa JC, et al. (2009) Changes in DNA methylation of tandem DNA repeats are different from interspersed repeats in cancer. Int J Cancer 125: 723–729.

20. Moore LE, Pfeiffer RM, Poscablo C, Real FX, Kogevinas M, et al. (2008) Genomic DNA hypomethylation as a biomarker for bladder cancer susceptibility in the Spanish Bladder Cancer Study: a case-control study. Lancet Oncol 9: 359–366.

21. Wilhelm CS, Kelsey KT, Butler R, Plaza S, Gagne L, et al. (2010) Implications of LINE1 methylation for bladder cancer risk in women. Clin Cancer Res 16: 1682–1689.

22. Cash HL, Tao L, Yuan JM, Marsit CJ, Houseman EA, et al. (2012) LINE-1 hypomethylation is associated with bladder cancer risk among nonsmoking Chinese. Int J Cancer 130: 1151–1159.

23. Phokaew C, Kowudtitham S, Subbalekha K, Shuangshoti S, Mutirangura A (2008) LINE-1 methylation patterns of different loci in normal and cancerous cells. Nucleic acids research 36: 5704–5712.

24. Baba Y, Huttenhower C, Nosho K, Tanaka N, Shima K, et al. (2010) Epigenomic diversity of colorectal cancer indicated by LINE-1 methylation in a database of 869 tumors. Molecular cancer 9: 125.

25. Singer H, Walier M, Nusgen N, Meesters C, Schreiner F, et al. (2012) Methylation of L1Hs promoters is lower on the inactive X, has a tendency of being higher on autosomes in smaller genomes and shows inter-individual variability at some loci. Human molecular genetics 21: 219–235.

26. Pobsook T, Subbalekha K, Sannikorn P, Mutirangura A (2011) Improved measurement of LINE-1 sequence methylation for cancer detection. Clin Chim Acta 412: 314–321.

27. Faul F, Erdfelder E, Buchner A, Lang AG (2009) Statistical power analyses using G*Power 3.1: tests for correlation and regression analyses. Behavior research methods 41: 1149–1160.

28. Kitkumthorn N, Tuangsintanakul T, Rattanatanyong P, Tiwawech D, Mutirangura A LINE-1 methylation in the peripheral blood mononuclear cells of cancer patients. Clin Chim Acta. 2012 Feb 1. http://dx.doi.org/10.1016/j.cca.2012.01.024.

29. Castegna A, Drake J, Pocernich C, Butterfield DA (2003) Protein Carbonyl Levels—An Assessment of Protein Oxidation. Methods in Biological Oxidative Stress. In: Hensley K, Floyd RA, editors: Humana Press. pp 161–168.

30. Nelson HH, Marsit CJ, Kelsey KT (2011) Global methylation in exposure biology and translational medical science. Environmental health perspectives 119: 1528–1533.

31. Franco R, Schoneveld O, Georgakilas AG, Panayiotidis MI (2008) Oxidative stress, DNA methylation and carcinogenesis. Cancer Lett 266: 6–11.

32. Campos AC, Molognoni F, Melo FH, Galdieri LC, Carneiro CR, et al. (2007) Oxidative stress modulates DNA methylation during melanocyte anchorage blockade associated with malignant transformation. Neoplasia 9: 1111–1121.

33. Hartnett L, Egan LJ (2012) Inflammation, DNA methylation and colitis-associated cancer. Carcinogenesis.

34. Weitzman SA, Turk PW, Milkowski DH, Kozlowski K (1994) Free radical adducts induce alterations in DNA cytosine methylation. Proceedings of the National Academy of Sciences of the United States of America 91: 1261–1264.

35. Kuchino Y, Mori F, Kasai H, Inoue H, Iwai S, et al. (1987) Misreading of DNA templates containing 8-hydroxydeoxyguanosine at the modified base and at adjacent residues. Nature 327: 77–79.

36. Hitchler MJ, Domann FE (2007) An epigenetic perspective on the free radical theory of development. Free radical biology & medicine 43: 1023–1036.

37. Lertratanangkoon K, Orkiszewski RS, Scimeca JM (1996) Methyl-donor deficiency due to chemically induced glutathione depletion. Cancer research 56: 995–1005.

38. Lertratanangkoon K, Wu CJ, Savaraj N, Thomas ML (1997) Alterations of DNA methylation by glutathione depletion. Cancer letters 120: 149–156.

39. Miller JW, Borowsky AD, Marple TC, McGoldrick ET, Dillard-Telm L, et al. (2008) Folate, DNA methylation, and mouse models of breast tumorigenesis. Nutrition reviews 66 Suppl 1: S59–64.

40. Miller JW, Nadeau MR, Smith J, Smith D, Selhub J (1994) Folate-deficiency-induced homocysteinaemia in rats: disruption of S-adenosylmethionine's co-ordinate regulation of homocysteine metabolism. The Biochemical journal 298 (Pt 2): 415–419.

41. Subbalekha K, Pimkhaokham A, Pavasant P, Chindavijak S, Phokaew C, et al. (2009) Detection of LINE-1s hypomethylation in oral rinses of oral squamous cell carcinoma patients. Oral oncology 45: 184–191.

42. Yilmaz IA, Akcay T, Cakatay U, Telci A, Ataus S, et al. (2003) Relation between bladder cancer and protein oxidation. Int Urol Nephrol 35: 345–350.

43. Badjatia N, Satyam A, Singh P, Seth A, Sharma A (2010) Altered antioxidant status and lipid peroxidation in Indian patients with urothelial bladder carcinoma. Urol Oncol 28: 360–367.

44. Bartosz G (2003) Total antioxidant capacity. Advances in clinical chemistry 37: 219–292.

45. Dey P (2004) Urinary markers of bladder carcinoma. Clinica chimica acta; international journal of clinical chemistry 340: 57–65.

46. Vrooman OP, Witjes JA (2008) Urinary markers in bladder cancer. European urology 53: 909–916.

47. Mitra AP, Cote RJ (2010) Molecular screening for bladder cancer: progress and potential. Nat Rev Urol 7: 11–20.

48. Van Tilborg AA, Bangma CH, Zwarthoff EC (2009) Bladder cancer biomarkers and their role in surveillance and screening. International journal of urology: official journal of the Japanese Urological Association 16: 23–30.

17

High Expression of HuR in Cytoplasm, but not Nuclei, is Associated with Malignant Aggressiveness and Prognosis in Bladder Cancer

Yasuyoshi Miyata*, Shin-ichi Watanabe, Yuji Sagara, Kensuke Mitsunari, Tomohiro Matsuo, Kojiro Ohba, Hideki Sakai

Department of Nephro-Urology, Nagasaki University Graduate School of Biomedical Sciences, Nagasaki, Japan

Abstract

Introduction: Human antigen R (HuR) regulates the stability of mRNA and is associated with cell proliferation, angiogenesis, and lymphangiogenesis. However, the clinical significance and pathological role of HuR in bladder cancer remains unclear. The main objective of this investigation was to clarify the relationships between HuR expression and clinical significance and cancer cell proliferation, angiogenesis, lymphangiogenesis, and expressions of cyclooxygenase (COX)-2 and vascular endothelial growth factor (VEGF)-A, -C, and -D.

Methods: All expressions were examined by immunohistochemical techniques in 122 formalin-fixed specimens of bladder cancer patients. HuR expression was evaluated separately with cytoplasmic and nuclear staining. Cell proliferation, angiogenesis and lymphangiogenesis were measured as the percentage of Ki-67-positive cell (proliferation index, PI), CD34-stained vessels (microvessel density, MVD), and D2-40-stained vessels (lymph vessel density, LVD). Relationships between each HuR expression and clinicopathological features, prognosis, and expressions of COX-2 and VEGFs were analyzed by multi-variate analyses. HuR expression was also investigated in 10 mice of N-Butyl-N-[4-hydroxybutil] nitrosamine (BBN) induced bladder cancer model.

Results: In human tissues, high cytoplasmic expression was seen in 5% and 25.4% of normal and cancer cells, respectively. Nuclear HuR expression bore no significant relationship to any pathological features. However, cytoplasmic HuR expression appeared positively associated with pT stage and grade ($P<0.001$). In mouse tissues, similar trends were confirmed. Cytoplasmic expression correlated with PI, MVD, and LVD, as well as expression of VEGF-A and -C, but not VEGF-D. High cytoplasmic expression of HuR was a significant predictor of metastasis and cause-specific survival, and was identified as a prognostic correlative factor for metastasis (hazard ratio, 4.75; $P = 0.028$) in a multivariate analysis model that included pathological features.

Conclusions: Cytoplasmic HuR appears to play important roles in cell proliferation, progression, and survival of bladder cancer patients. Its expression was associated with angiogenesis, lymphangiogenesis, and expressions of VEGF-A and –C.

Editor: Kaustubh Datta, University of Nebraska Medical Center, United States of America

Funding: This research was supported in part by a Grant-in-Aid from the Japan Society for the Promotion of Science (No. 22591771). However, the funders had no role in study design, data collection and analysis, decision to publish, or preparation of the manuscript. No additional external funding was received for this study.

Competing Interests: The authors have declared that no competing interests exist.

* E-mail: int.doc.miya@m3.dion.ne.jp

Introduction

Regulation of mRNA decay is an essential mechanism for controlling gene expression. The control of mRNA stability depends on sequences in the transcript itself and on RNA-binding proteins that dynamically bind to these sequences. Human antigen R (HuR) is a member of the embryonic-lethal, abnormal vision (ELAV)-like protein family of RNA-binding proteins, and is reported to be a multifunctional protein that has been implicated in the regulation of various aspects of RNA metabolism. That is, HuR is involved in post-transcriptional regulation of the turnover and stability of RNA [1].

HuR is also reported to regulate cell proliferation and tumor-associated inflammation [2,3]. In addition, HuR has been found to be involved in the regulation of angiogenesis by interacting with the transcripts of numerous angiogenesis-promoting factors, and is also known to correlate with lymphangiogenesis in a variety of pathological conditions, including cancer [3,4]. Based on these facts, it has been suggested that HuR plays important roles in carcinogenesis, tumor growth, metastasis, and prognosis in malignancies. Actually, several reports have described HuR expression showing positive associations with malignant aggressiveness and serving as a prognostic factor for poor clinical outcome in various cancers [5–7]. On the other hand, markedly different findings have been reported in patients with breast cancer

[8]. The pathological roles and prognostic value of HuR expression in cancer patients thus remain contentious, and the clinical significance and predictive value for prognosis in patients with bladder cancer has yet to be clarified.

As mechanisms for these pathological activities, vascular endothelial growth factors (VEGFs) and cyclooxygenase (COX)-2 are the most well-known HuR-associated factors [5,7,9–11]. These proteins have also been reported to be associated with malignant aggressiveness and prognosis in patients with bladder cancer [12,13]. However, little information has been accumulated regarding the relationship between HuR expression, VEGF-A, -C, and -D, and COX-2 in human bladder cancer tissues.

The intracellular location of HuR has been reported to be predominantly nuclear in many types of cancer cells [14,15]. However, HuR shuttles from the nucleus to cytoplasm in response to various stimuli, prolonging mRNA half-life and facilitating the efficient translation of proteins [15]. Given these facts, investigation as to the clinical, pathological, and prognostic roles of nuclear and cytoplasmic expression of HuR is warranted.

The main purpose of this study was to clarify the pathological significance and prognostic value of nuclear and cytoplasmic HuR expression in patients with bladder cancer. To confirm the pathological significance of HuR under a given tissue microenvironment, chemically induced bladder cancer mouse model was used for additional experiments. In addition, relationships between these HuR expressions, angiogenesis and lymphangiogenesis, and VEGF-A, -C, -D, and COX-2 expressions were also examined in patients with bladder cancer.

Materials and Methods

Ethics Approval

The study was conducted according to the Helsinki II declaration and it was approved by the Ethics Review Committee of the Nagasaki University Hospital, Nagasaki, Japan.

Written informed consent was obtained from the patients involved in our study before their enrollment. Animals in this study were handled according to the Guidelines for Animal Experiments of Nagasaki University, and the Regulations of Animal Care and Use Committee approved the study protocol.

Patients

All slides of 122 bladder cancer specimens obtained from transurethral resection (TUR) at our hospital between 1993 and 2004 were reviewed. All patients had been clinically diagnosed with non-muscle invasive bladder cancer (NMIBC) without metastasis. We excluded patients who had received neoadjuvant therapy. In addition, specimens that cancer cell number was under 500 were also excluded from this study. On the other hand, among the 122 patients, adjuvant therapy including systematic chemotherapy, intravesical chemotherapy, and intravesical bacillus-Calmette-Guérin were performed in 14 (11.5%), 67 (54.9%), and 19 patients (15.6%), respectively. All patients were evaluated by chest radiography, ultrasonography, and computed tomography (CT) of the urinary bladder and abdomen, and cystoscopy. In addition, CT of the lung or brain, magnetic resonance imaging (MRI), drip-infusion pyelography, and bone scans were performed as deemed necessary. Tumors were staged according to the American Joint Committee on Cancer and graded according to the World Health Organization and International Society for Urological Pathology classification system. In the present study, tumors were grouped for statistical analysis into the following groups: low- (pTa+1) and high-stage (≥T2); or low- (grades 1 and 2) and high-grade (grade 3). We also examined 20 tissue samples of

normal urinary bladder obtained from apparently normal areas of the bladder of patients with transitional cell carcinoma of the upper urinary tract. All of control patients showed G1 and non-muscle invasive disease, and they showed recurrence within a follow-up period of 10–17 years. The median duration of follow-up was 51 months (range, 2–182 months).

Animal

HuR expression was examined in 10 samples of normal urothelial cells (without BBN), 5 of NMIBC (BBN solution for 14 weeks), and 5 of muscle invasive bladder cancer (MIBC) (for 24 weeks) of chemical induced bladder cancer mouse model. This model was used in a previous report [16].

Immunohistochemistry

Immunohistochemical examinations were performed using formalin-fixed, paraffin-embedded sections. We used anti-HuR antibody (Santa Cruz Biotechnology, Santa Cruz, CA) as the primary antibody (rabbit polyclonal, reactive for both of human and mouse HuR). Five-micrometer-thick sections were deparaffinized in xylene and rehydrated in graded solutions of ethanol. Antigen retrieval was performed at 100°C for 15 min. in 0.01 M sodium citrate buffer (pH 6.0). All sections were then immersed in 3% hydrogen peroxide for 30 min to block endogenous peroxidase activity. Sections were incubated overnight with the primary antibody at 4°C, then washed in 0.05% Tween 20 in phosphate-buffered saline (PBS). Next, sections were incubated with peroxidase using the labeled polymer method with Dako EnVision+^{TM} Peroxidase, (Dako, Carpinteria, CA) for 60 min. The peroxidase reaction was visualized with the liquid 3,3'-diaminobenzidine tetrahydrochloride (DAB) substrate kit (Invitrogen Corporation, Carlsbad, CA). Sections were counterstained using hematoxylin. Other methods were performed as described previously [13,17,18]. Briefly, we also evaluated VEGF-A, -C, and -D and COX-2 expressions in similar specimens using immunohistochemical techniques. In addition, microvessel density (MVD) and lymph vessel density (LVD) were estimated using CD34-positive lumina and D2-40-positive lumina, respectively. Details of the methods for determining MVD and LVD were as described previously [13]. We performed all evaluation anew for this study. A variety of cancer specimens that had been confirmed in preliminary studies as immunoreactive for the studied antigens were used as positive controls for HuR (liver), VEGFs (renal cell carcinoma), COX-2 (colon), D2-40 (tonsil), and CD34 (kidney). The specificities of these specimens as positive controls were confirmed in our previous reports [13,17,18]. A consecutive section from each sample processed without the primary antibody was used as a negative control. Positive and negative controls were set up for each batch of experiments. In addition, to confirm the specificity of HuR immunoreactivity, we performed similar investigation by using goat polyclonal antibody (Santa Cruz Biotechnology, Santa Cruz, CA) in samples of human (n = 40) and mouse tissues (n = 20), and they were also incubated with blocking peptide for this anti-HuR antibody (Santa Cruz Biotechnology, Santa Cruz, CA).

Evaluation

HuR expression was evaluated by immunoreactive score as reported previously [19]. Briefly, cytoplasmic and nuclear staining patterns were scored using the following scales: 0, no staining; 1, weak and/or focal staining (<10% of cells); 2, moderate or strong staining (10–50% of cells); and 3, moderate or strong staining (>50% of cells). Scores 0 and 1 were judged as low expression, and scores 2 and 3 were judged as high expression. This evaluation method was used for mouse tissues. With regard to other expressions, results were considered positive if staining intensity was strong, and the percentage of positively stained cancer cells was determined using a continuous scale according to previous reports [13,17]. Briefly, expression levels were assessed semi-quantitatively from the percentage of expressing carcinoma cells (from ≥500 carcinoma cells). These cells were examined using an E-400 microscope (Nikon, Tokyo, Japan) and digital images were captured (DU100; Nikon). In addition, we used a computer-aided image analysis system (Win ROOF version 5.0; Mitani, Fukui, Japan) to calculate statistical variables. Two investigators (S.W. and Y.M.), blinded to clinical features and survival data, independently performed semi-quantitative analyses and immunostaining interpretations. The rate of disagreement in analysis between these two investigators was <10% and the mean density was used for statistical analyses.

Statistical Analysis

Data are expressed as means (standard deviation [SD]). Student's t-test was used for analysis of continuous variables. The chi-square test and Fisher's exact test were used for comparisons of categorical data. Spearman's correlation coefficient was used to determine associations between two continuous variables. Crude and adjusted effects were estimated by logistic regression analysis and described as odds ratios (OR) with 95% confidence intervals (95%CIs), together with P-values. Survival analysis was evaluated using Kaplan-Meier analysis and the log-rank test, and variables that achieved statistical significance ($P<0.050$) in univariate analyses were subsequently entered into a multivariate analysis using Cox proportional hazards analysis (described as hazard ratio [HR] with 95%CI, together with the P-values) (Model A). In addition, to examine the predictive value of HuR expression in greater detail, the analysis included a multivariate model including all risk factors (Model B). All statistical tests were two-sided and significance was defined as $P<0.050$. All statistical analyses were performed on a personal computer with StatView for Windows version 5.0 software (Abacus Concepts, Berkeley, CA).

Results

Localization and Expression of HuR

In normal urothelial cells, weak to moderate nuclear HuR expression was detected, along with absent to weak cytoplasmic expression (Fig. 1A). Finally, 90% (18/20) was judged as showing high nuclear expression in normal urothelial cells. In contrast, high cytoplasmic expression was seen in only 5% (1/20) of normal tissues. With regard to nuclear HuR expression in cancer cells, expression was high in 88 specimens (72.1%; score 2, n = 64; score 3, n = 24) and low in 34 (27.9%; score 0, n = 1; score 1, n = 33). On the other hand, with regard to cytoplasmic expression in cancer cells, expression was high in 31 specimens (25.4%; score 2, n = 24; score 3, n = 7) and low in 91 (74.6%; score 0, n = 37; score 1, n = 54). Representative examples of low and high HuR expression in cancer tissue are shown in Figure 1B and C, respectively.

In animal experiments, high nuclear expression was found in 80% (8/10) and 70% (7/10) of normal urothelial and cancer cells, respectively. On the other hand, high cytoplasmic expression in normal cells was detected in 10% (1/10). In cancer cells, high expression in NMIBC and MIBC was detected in 40% (2/5) and 80% (4/5), respectively. Representative examples of HuR expression in mice tissues were showed in Figure 2A and B. Importantly, similar results were obtained using another anti-HuR antibody and its staining was reduced by competition with blocking peptide.

Clinical and Pathological Significance of HuR Expression

Relationships between pathological features and HuR expression in the nucleus and cytoplasm are shown in Table 1. Nuclear HuR expression showed no significant relationship to pT stage or grade ($P=0.471$ and $P=0.773$, respectively). Conversely, cytoplasmic HuR expression was positively associated with pT stage ($P<0.001$) and grade ($P<0.001$).

As shown in Table 2, cytoplasmic HuR expression was positively associated with expressions of COX-2 ($P=0.011$), VEGF-A ($P=0.021$) and VEGF-C ($P=0.004$), but not with VEGF-D expression ($P=0.134$). In addition, cytoplasmic HuR expression also displayed positive correlations with MVD ($P=0.010$) and LVD ($P=0.023$). On the other hand, nuclear expression of HuR showed no significant correlation with any of these expressions or variables (Table 2). Thus, representative examples for these significant molecules are shown in the high HuR expression sample (Figure 1D–F).

Relationships between HuR-related Molecules and Angiogenesis or Lymphangiogenesis

In our study population, MVD was closely associated with VEGF-A (r = 0.40, $P<0.001$), VEGF-C (r = 0.41, $P<0.001$), and COX-2 expression (r = 0.31, $P<0.001$), but not with VEGF-D (r = 0.17, P = 0.652). Similarly, LVD was also associated with VEGF-A (r = 0.39, $P<0.001$), VEGF-C (r = 0.58, $P<0.001$), and VEGF-D (r = 0.53, $P<0.001$), but not with COX-2 expression (r = 0.15, P = 0.103). The schema of such correlations was shown in Figure 3.

To clarify the significance of expressions of VEGF-A, VEGF-C, and COX-2 for MVD and LVD in greater detail, multivariate analysis was performed with models including these factors, pT stage, and grade. With regard to MVD, although VEGF-C and COX-2 were associated with MVD (OR = 1.05, 95%CI = 1.02–1.08, P = 0.002 and OR = 1.05, 95%CI = 1.00–1.11, P = 0.043, respectively), VEGF-A expression showed the strongest association (OR = 1.05, 95%CI = 1.03–1.11, $P<0.001$). Similar analysis showed that VEGF-C was most closely associated with LVD (OR = 1.05, 95%CI = 1.01–1.08, P = 0.001), while VEGF-A expression was also associated (OR = 1.05, 95%CI = 1.01–1.08, P = 0.011).

Survival Analyses

Nuclear HuR expression was not identified as a significant predictor of recurrence in the urinary tract, metastasis, or cause-specific survival (log-rank P = 0.156, P = 0.058, and P = 0.940, respectively). Conversely, high cytoplasmic HuR expression was a significant predictor for each of these parameters (Fig. 4 A–C). To show more detailed values of predictive factors, similar analyses were also performed for pathological features and adjuvant therapy. In addition, we showed multivariate analysis models including all these factors (Model A) and cytoplasmic HuR expression and pathological features (Model B) are showed in Table 3. In both models, HuR expression was identified as a prognostic factor for metastasis, but not for recurrence into the urinary tract (HR = 2.00, 95%CI = 0.98–4.11, P = 0.057 in Model A and HR = 1.82, 95%CI = 0.90–3.72, P = 0.094 in Model B) and cause-specific survival (HR = 5.42, 95%CI = 0.29–6.71, P = 0.688 in Model A and HR = 1.26, 95%CI = 0.42–3.75, P = 0.683 in Model B).

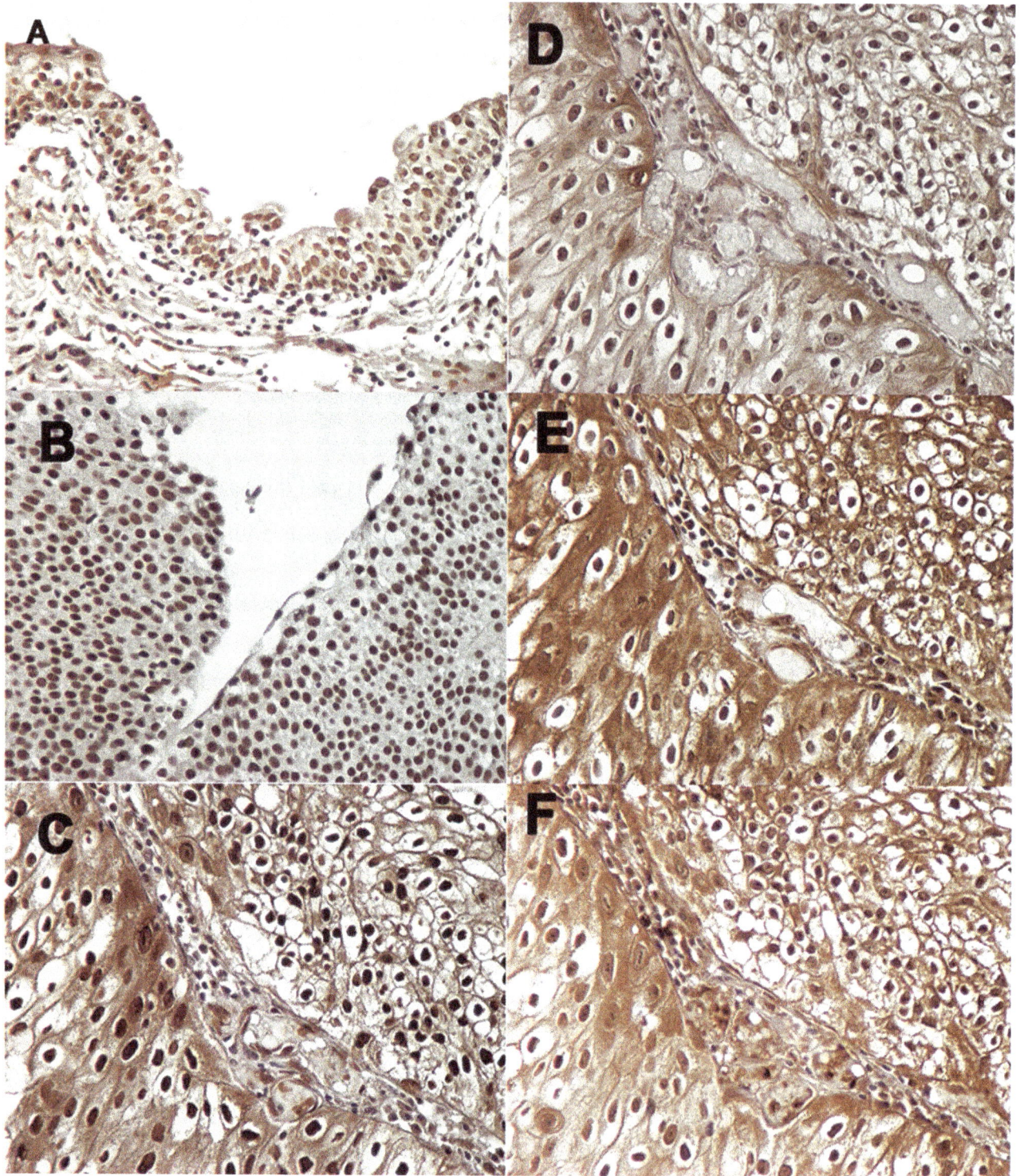

Figure 1. Representative examples of HuR immunoreactivity in normal urothelial cells (A; magnification, ×200.) and cancer cells (B and C; magnification, ×400.). HuR was mainly detected in nuclei of both normal and cancer cells in bladder tissues. Moderate or strong cytoplasmic expression was evident in cancer cells (C), but was rare in normal urothelial cells (A). Some cancer cells are also showed weak cytoplasmic expression although nuclear expression was detected (B). In addition, we showed representative figures of HuR expression (C) and factors related thereto; (D) cyclooxygenase-2, (E) vascular endothelial growth factor-A, (F) vascular endothelial growth factor-C in same area. (all magnification, x400).

Discussion

The present study demonstrated that cytoplasmic HuR expression was closely associated with malignant potential, tumor progression, and outcome for bladder cancer patients. Conversely, no such significance was found for nuclear expression of HuR. Previous studies have detected cytoplasmic accumulation in

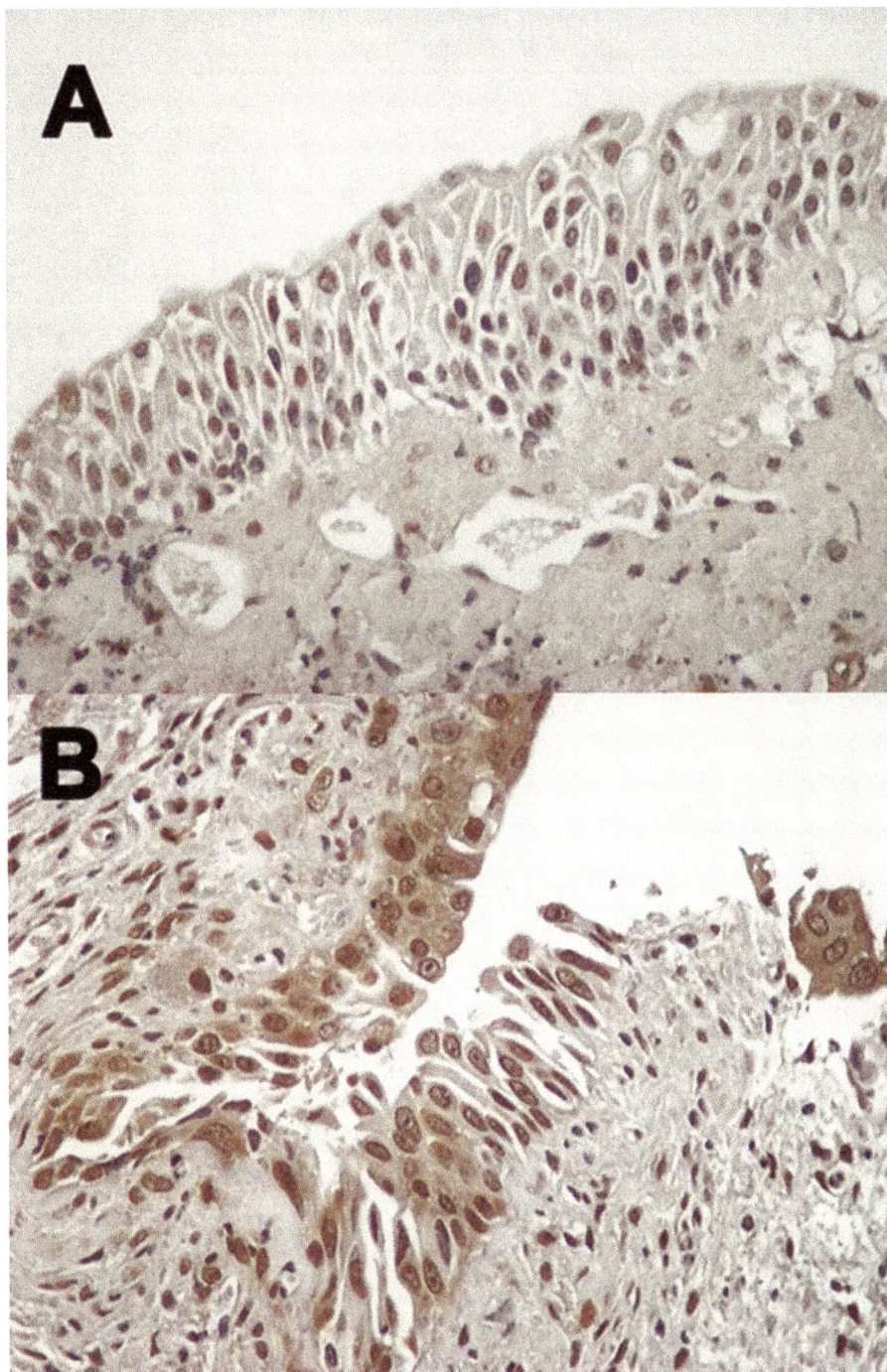

Figure 2. Representative examples of HuR immunoreactivity in normal cells (A) and cancer cells (B) of chemical-induced bladder cancer mouse model. (Magnification, x400). Staining pattern was close to human tissues.

several cancers, showing that nucleocytoplasmic translocation of HuR was essential for RNA stability [20,21]. Our results support a similar role in human bladder cancer tissues.

This is the first report on relationships between HuR expression and pathological features, recurrence, and survival in patients with urothelial carcinoma of the urinary bladder cancer. With regard to the pathological significance and prognostic roles of HuR, several previous studies have reported that over-expression is associated with high-grade malignancy, advanced stage, and poor survival in

patients with colon cancer [6], breast cancer [5], and renal cell carcinoma [7]. However, HuR expression does not appear to be associated with pathological status in patients with breast cancer, with high expression of HuR predicting a better prognosis [8]. Our results support former situation in patients with bladder cancer. As a mechanism underlying such pathological activities of HuR, regulation of angiogenesis has been suggested in various cancers [3,4]. Special attention was paid to the relationships between HuR expression, malignant potential and pathological

Table 1. Relationships between pathological features and HuR expression.

	N	HuR in nucleus (%) Negative	HuR in nucleus (%) Positive	HuR in cytoplasm (%) Negative	HuR in cytoplasm (%) Positive
pT stage					
Ta	33	12 (36.4)	21 (63.6)	31 (93.9)	2 (6.1)
T1	70	18 (25.7)	52 (74.3)	57 (81.4)	13 (18.6)
T2	11	2 (18.2)	9 (81.8)	2 (18.2)	9 (81.8)
T3	8	2 (18.2)	6 (75.0)	1 (12.5)	7 (87.5)
Low (Ta+1)	103	30 (29.1)	73 (70.9)	88 (85.4)	16 (14.6)
High(T2+3)	19	4 (21.1)	15 (78.9)	3 (15.8)	16 (84.1)
P value		0.471		<0.001	
Grade (G)					
G1	34	10 (29.4)	24 (70.6)	28 (82.4)	6 (17.6)
G2	43	10 (29.4)	33 (76.4)	38 (88.3)	5 (11.7)
G3	45	14 (31.1)	31 (68.9)	25 (55.6)	20 (44.4)
Low (G1+2)	77	20 (25.9)	57 (74.1)	66 (85.7)	11 (14.3)
High (G3)	45	14 (31.1)	31 (68.9)	25 (55.6)	20 (44.4)
P value		0.773		<0.001	

Table 2. Correlation with MVD, LVD and expressions of COX-2 and VEGF family.

	HuR in nucleus Negative	HuR in nucleus Positive	*P value*	HuR in cytoplasm Negative	HuR in cytoplasm Positive	*P Value*
COX-2 (%)	21.6 (8.5)	20.9 (9.3)	0.690	19.8 (8.9)	24.6 (8.7)	0.010
VEGF-A	33.6 (14.7)	33.9 (12.5)	0.919	32.2 (12.9)	38.5 (12.9)	0.021
VEGF-C	30.8 (15.5)	31.7 (16.3)	0.792	29.0 (14.6)	38.6 (17.8)	0.004
VEGF-D	31.0 (16.5)	32.1 (15.3)	0.737	30.6 (15.0)	35.4 (16.7)	0.134
MVD (/mm²)	69.9 (19.7)	67.8 (18.2)	0.599	65.9 (18.7)	75.8 (16.3)	0.010
LVD (/mm²)	25.1 (9.5)	27.8 (12.9)	0.271	25.6 (11.1)	31.1 (13.8)	0.023

COX: cyclooxygenase, VEGF: vascular endothelial growth factor, MVD: microvessel density, LVD: lymph-vessel density.

Furthermore, up-regulation of VEGF-A and -C expressions may be associated with such phenomenon in bladder cancer.

An additional important result in the present study was the fact that cytoplasmic HuR expression was a useful predictor of prognosis in bladder cancer patients who underwent TUR. In particular, expression was closely associated with postoperative metastasis. Many investigators have identified increased MVD and LVD as strong predictors of outcome in bladder cancer patients [13,23,24]. Based on these findings, we thought that such prognostic roles of MVD and LVD were reasonable. On the other hand, cytoplasmic expression of HuR was identified as a significant predictor of cause-specific survival in univariate analysis, but not as an independent predictor in multivariate analysis. We are not sure why such differences were encountered in this study. However, postoperative survival was influenced by numerous factors. We thus speculated that cytoplasmic HuR may play various roles in patient survival, while various other factors and molecules may have stronger effects in determining outcomes for patients with bladder cancer.

In this study, we showed that cytoplasmic HuR expressions in bladder cancer cells were higher than those in normal epithelial cells. Biological functions of HuR in human and mouse have been reported to be similar in previous report [25]. However, validation of specificity of HuR target is not still completely clear. Furthermore, newly and detailed pathological function of HuR in cancer cells are becoming more clearly in recent years [26].

features because stimulation of angiogenesis has been linked to tumor growth and progression in patients with several malignancies, including bladder cancer [13,22]. Finally, Our results showed the possibility that cytoplasmic expression of HuR was positively associated with malignant behavior and outcome in bladder cancer patients. In addition, there is a possibility that such malignant aggressiveness is associated with HuR-related angiogenesis.

One of the most interesting findings in this study was that cytoplasmic HuR expression correlated positively with lymphangiogenesis in bladder cancer tissues. To the best of our knowledge, this study is the first to report a relationship between HuR expression and lymphangiogenesis in patients with bladder cancer, although similar findings have been detected in lung cancer in previous reports [4]. In addition, interestingly, both that report and the present study showed that cytoplasmic HuR expression correlated with both angiogenesis and lymphangiogenesis. Given these results, we hypothesized that co-factors that can influence both angiogenesis and lymphangiogenesis may associate with such finding in cancer tissues.

Detailed regulatory mechanisms of angiogenesis and lymphangiogenesis by HuR in human cancer tissues are still not fully understood. Several molecules have been reported to be HuR-related, such as VEGF-A [10], VEGF-C, and COX-2 [7,9]. These factors are known to be associated with MVD and LVD in bladder cancer. However, the relationships between HuR expression and these angiogenesis- and lymphangiogenesis-related molecules in human bladder cancer tissues are still unclear. Our results showed that cytoplasmic HuR expression correlated positively with expressions of VEGF-A and -C, but not VEGF-D. We have previously reported that VEGF-A and -C were significantly associated with MVD and LVD in human bladder cancer tissues [13]. In addition, such significant relationships were not detected for nuclear HuR expression. Given these findings, we speculated that translocation from nucleus to cytoplasm is an important process in stimulating angiogenesis and lymphangiogenesis.

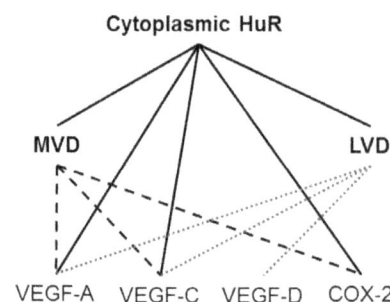

Figure 3. Schema of the relationships between cytoplasmic HuR expression and angiogenesis, lymphangiogenesis, and expressions of related molecules. MVD, microvessel density; LVD, lymphvessel density; VEGF, vascular endothelial growth factor; COX, cyclooxygenase.

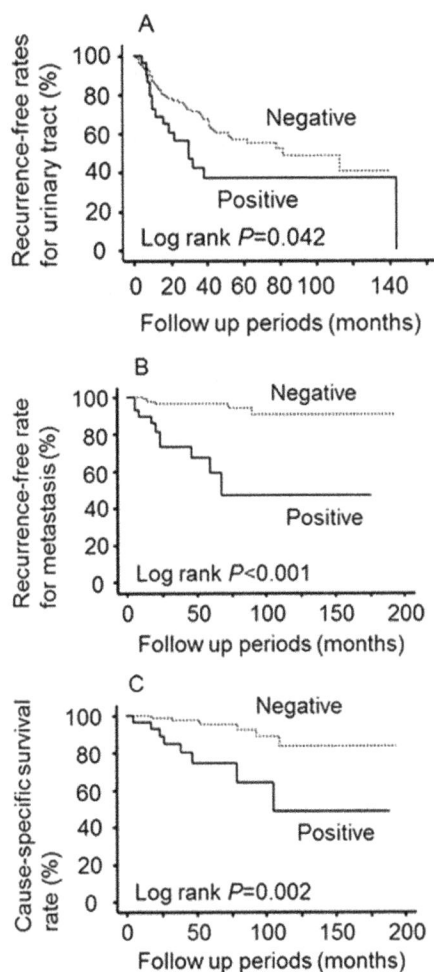

Figure 4. Kaplan-Meier curves for recurrence-free survival rates with urinary tract cancer (A), recurrence-free survival rates with metastasis (B), and cause-specific survival rates (C).

Table 3. Survival analyses for metastasis.

	Univariate analyses			Multivariate analyses		
	HR	95% CI	P value	HR	95% CI	P value
Grade						
High (Model A)	2.70	1.56–4.66	<0.001	1.47	0.49–4.40	0.489
(Model B)	–	–	–	1.15	0.38–3.51	0.805
pT stage						
High (A)	10.44	3.58–30.46	0.001	4.72	1.25–17.83	0.022
(B)	–	–	–	3.25	0.87–12.06	0.079
Adjuvant Tx						
Absence (A)	0.402	0.05–3.09	0.381	0.18	0.02–1.50	0.116
(B)	–	–	–	–	–	–
HuR in cytoplasm						
Positive (A)	9.60	3.19–28.88	<0.001	4.75	1.78–12.75	0.028
(B)	–	–	–	5.22	1.34–20.35	0.017

Tx: therapy, HR: hazard ratio, CI: confidential interval.
Model A: including cytoplasmic HuR expression, grade, pT stage, and adjuvant therapy.
Model B: including cytoplasmic HUR expression, grade, and pT stage, but not adjuvant TX.

ness and bladder cancer patient outcomes, whereas nuclear HUR expression was not. In addition, cytoplasmic HuR expression is associated with angiogenesis, lymphangiogenesis, and these-related molecules including VEGF-A, VEGF-C, and COX-2. Our results suggest that cytoplasmic HuR expression was useful as a predictive marker for metastasis after TUR in patients with bladder cancer. To obtain further mechanistic insight, further *in vivo* and *in vitro* studies in bladder cancer are necessary.

Acknowledgments

We are grateful to Mr. Takumi Shimogama and Mrs. Miho M. Kuninaka for their outstanding support.

Author Contributions

Conceived and designed the experiments: YM. Performed the experiments: YM SW YS KM. Analyzed the data: YM HS. Contributed reagents/materials/analysis tools: KO TM HS. Wrote the paper: YM YS KO SW TM HS.

Thus, further studies regarding molecular mechanism and cell biology experiments are necessary to understand more detailed pathological roles of HuR in bladder cancer.

In conclusion, our results showed that cytoplasmic HuR expression was significantly associated with malignant aggressive-

References

1. Hinman MN, Lou H (2008) Diverse molecular functions of Hu proteins. Cell Mol Life Sci 65: 3168–3181.
2. Cho SJ, Jung YS, Zhang J, Chen X (2012) The RNA-binding protein RNPC1 stabilizes the mRNA encoding the RNA-binding protein HuR and cooperates with HuR to suppress cell proliferation. J Biol Chem 287: 14535–14544.
3. Srikantan S, Gorospe M (2012) HuR function in disease. Front Biosci 17: 189–205.
4. Wang J, Wang B, Bi J, Zhang C (2010) Cytoplasmic HuR expression correlates with angiogenesis, lymphangiogenesis, and poor outcome in lung cancer. Med Oncol 28: S577–585.
5. Heinonen M, Fagerholm R, Aaltonen K, Kilpivaara O, Aittomäki K, et al. (2007) Prognostic role of HuR in hereditary breast cancer. Clin Cancer Res 13: 6959–6963.
6. Lim SJ, Lee SH, Joo SH, Song JY, Choi SI (2009) Cytoplasmic expression of HuR is related to cyclooxygenase 2 expression in colon cancer. Cancer Res Treat 13: 6959–6963.
7. Ronkainen H, Vaarala MH, Hirvikoski P, Ristimäki A (2011) HuR expression is a marker of poor prognosis in renal cell carcinoma. Tumor Biol 32: 481–487.
8. Yuan Z, Sanders AJ, Ye L, Wang Y, Jiang WG (2011) Prognostic value of human antigen R (HuR) in human breast cancer: high level predicts a favourable prognosis. Anticancer Res 31: 303–310.

9. Gately S, Li WW (2004) Multiple roles of COX-2 in tumor angiogenesis: a target for angiogenenic therapy. Semin Oncol 31: 2–11.
10. Sakuma T, Nakagawa T, Ido K, Takeuchi H, Sato K, et al. (2008) Expression of vascular endothelial growth factor-A and mRNA stability factor HuR in human meningiomas. J Neurooncol 88: 143–155.
11. Wang J, Zhao W, Guo Y, Zhang B, Xie Q, et al. (2009) The expression of RNA-binding protein HuR in non-small cell lung cancer correlated with vascular endothelial growth factor-C expression and lymph node metastasis. Oncology 76: 420–429.
12. Shariat SF, Matsumoto K, Kim J, Ayala GE, Zhou JH, et al. (2003) Correlation of cyclooxygenase-2 expression with molecular markers, pathological features and clinical outcome of transitional cell carcinoma of the bladder. J Urol 170: 985–989.
13. Miyata Y, Kanda S, Ohba K, Nomata K, Hayashida Y, et al. (2006) Lymphangiogenesis and angiogenesis in bladder cancer: prognostic implications and regulation by vascular endothelial growth factors-A, -C, and -D. Clin Cancer Res 12: 800–806.
14. Hinman MN, Lou H (2008) Diverse molecular functions of Hu proteins. Cell Mol Life Sci 65: 3168–3181.
15. Kim MY, Hur J, Jeong S (2009) Emerging roles of RNA and RNA-binding protein network in cancer cells. BMB Rep 42: 125–130.

16. Sagara Y, Miyata Y, Nomata K, Hayashi T, Kanetake H (2010) Green tea polyphenol suppresses tumor invasion and angiogenesis in N-butyl-(-4-hydroxybutyl) nitrosamine-induced bladder cancer. Cancer Epidemiol 34: 350–354.

17. Miyata Y, Koga S, Kanda S, Nishikido M, Hayashi T, et al (2003) Expression of cyclooxygenase-2 in renal cell carcinoma: correlation with tumor cell proliferation, apoptosis, angiogenesis, expression of matrix metalloproteinase-2, and survival. Clin Cancer Res 9: 1741–1749.

18. Iwata T, Miyata Y, Kanda S, Nishikido M, Hayashi T, et al. (2008) Lymphangiogenesis and angiogenesis in conventional renal cell carcinoma: association with vascular endothelial growth factors A to D immunohistochemistry. Urology 71: 749–754.

19. Costantino CL, Witkiewicz AK, Kuwano Y, Cozzitorto JA, Kennedy EP, et al. (2009) The role of HuR in gemcitabine efficacy in pancreatic cancer: HuR upregulates the expression of the gemcitabine metabolizing enzyme doxycytidine kinase. Cancer Res 69: 4567–4572.

20. Atasoy U, Watson J, Patel D, Keene JD (1998) ELAV protein HuA (HuR) can redistribute between nucleus and cytoplasm and is upregultaed during serum stimulation and T cell activation. J Cell Sci 111: 3145–3156.

21. Brennan CM, Steitz JA (2011) HuR and mRNA stability. Cell Mil Life Sci 58: 341–347.

22. Kadota K, Huang CL, Liu D, Ueno M, Kushida Y, et al. (2008) The clinical significance of lymphangiogenesis and angiogenesis in non-small cell lung cancer patients. Eur J Cancer 2008; 44: 1057–1067.Eur J Cancer 44: 1057–1067.

23. Afonso J, Santos LL, Amaro T, Lobo F, Longatto-Filho A (2009) The aggressiveness of urothelial carcinoma depends to a large extent on lymphovascular invasion–the prognostic contribution of related molecular markers. Histopathology 55: 514–524.

24. Ajili F, Kacem M, Tounsi H, Darouiche A, Enayfer E, et al. (2012) Prognostic Impact of Angiogenesis in Nonmuscle Invasive Bladder Cancer as Defined by Microvessel Density after Immunohistochemical Staining for CD34. Ultrastruct Pathol, in press.

25. Bergalet J, Fawal M, Lopez C, Desjobert C, Lamant L, Delsol G, et al. (2011) HuR mediated control of C/EBP beta mRNA stability and translation in ALK-positive anaplastic large cell lymphomas. Mol Cancer Res 9: 485–496.

26. Kim I, Kwak H, Lee HK, Hyun S, Jeong S (2012) β-catenin recognized a specific RNA motif in the cyclooxygenase-2 mRNA #'-UTR and interacts with HuR in colon cancer cells. Nucleic Acids Res 40: 6863–6872.

18

Complex Relationships between Occupation, Environment, DNA Adducts, Genetic Polymorphisms and Bladder Cancer in a Case-Control Study using a Structural Equation Modeling

Stefano Porru[1], **Sofia Pavanello**[2]*, **Angela Carta**[1], **Cecilia Arici**[1], **Claudio Simeone**[3], **Alberto Izzotti**[4], **Giuseppe Mastrangelo**[2]

1 Department of Medical-Surgical Specialties, Radiological Sciences and Public Health, Section of Public Health and Human Sciences, University of Brescia, Brescia, Italy, **2** Department of Cardiac, Thoracic, and Vascular Sciences, Unit of Occupational Medicine, University of Padova, Padova, Italy, **3** Department of Medical-Surgical Specialties, Radiological Sciences and Public Health, Section of Surgical Specialties, University of Brescia, Brescia, Italy, **4** Department of Health Sciences, University of Genoa, Italy/ Mutagenesis Unit, IRCCS Hospital-University San Martino Company – IST National Institute for Cancer Research, Genoa, Italy

Abstract

DNA adducts are considered an integrate measure of carcinogen exposure and the initial step of carcinogenesis. Their levels in more accessible peripheral blood lymphocytes (PBLs) mirror that in the bladder tissue. In this study we explore whether the formation of PBL DNA adducts may be associated with bladder cancer (BC) risk, and how this relationship is modulated by genetic polymorphisms, environmental and occupational risk factors for BC. These complex interrelationships, including direct and indirect effects of each variable, were appraised using the structural equation modeling (SEM) analysis. Within the framework of a hospital-based case/control study, study population included 199 BC cases and 213 non-cancer controls, all Caucasian males. Data were collected on lifetime smoking, coffee drinking, dietary habits and lifetime occupation, with particular reference to exposure to aromatic amines (AAs) and polycyclic aromatic hydrocarbons (PAHs). No indirect paths were found, disproving hypothesis on association between PBL DNA adducts and BC risk. DNA adducts were instead positively associated with occupational cumulative exposure to AAs (p = 0.028), whereas XRCC1 Arg 399 (p<0.006) was related with a decreased adduct levels, but with no impact on BC risk. Previous findings on increased BC risk by packyears (p<0.001), coffee (p<0.001), cumulative AAs exposure (p = 0.041) and *MnSOD* (p = 0.009) and a decreased risk by *MPO* (p< 0.008) were also confirmed by SEM analysis. Our results for the first time make evident an association between occupational cumulative exposure to AAs with DNA adducts and BC risk, strengthening the central role of AAs in bladder carcinogenesis. However the lack of an association between PBL DNA adducts and BC risk advises that these snapshot measurements are not representative of relevant exposures. This would envisage new scenarios for biomarker discovery and new challenges such as repeated measurements at different critical life stages.

Editor: Courtney G. Montgomery, Oklahoma Medical Research Foundation, United States of America

Funding: This work was funded by the Italian Ministry of University and Research and by the University of Brescia. The funders had no role in study design, data collection and analysis, decision to publish, or preparation of the manuscript.

Competing Interests: The authors have declared that no competing interests exist.

* E-mail: sofia.pavanello@unipd.it

Introduction

Tobacco smoking and occupational exposures to aromatic amines (AAs) and polycyclic aromatic hydrocarbons (PAHs) are the major risk factors for bladder cancer (BC) [1,2]. Moreover increasing evidence suggests a significant influence of genetic predisposition on BC incidence [3,4].

The formation of reactive metabolites of AAs and PAHs and their binding to DNA to give unrepaired/stable adducts, all modulated by genetic polymorphisms of metabolic and DNA repair enzymes, are considered critical events alongside the theoretical pathway that links exposure to BC [5]. "Bulky" DNA adduct measurement has been therefore considered an integrated marker of both exposure to aromatic compounds and ability to activate carcinogens and repair DNA damage [6,7].

Significantly higher levels of aromatic DNA adducts have been found in the bladder cancer biopsies from smokers [8,9]. Moreover persistent aromatic-DNA adducts causing mutations, including mutational "hot spots" in the bladder P53 gene, has provided a solid mechanistic view on how DNA adducts may drive bladder tumourigenesis [10]. Furthermore, some DNA modifications induced by aromatic compounds in the bladder are found to mirror those in the peripheral blood lymphocytes (PBLs) [11,12]. This has addressed the possibility of measuring such biomarker in accessible tissues which can be easily and non-invasively obtained from humans.

Many factors can however interfere in the theoretical pathway that links carcinogenic exposure to BC, such as multiple exposures (e.g., tobacco smoke, occupational exposure, fruit and vegetables consumption), their characterization (e.g., level, route, reliability) as well as the modulating role (increasing, protecting or having no effect) possibly played by polymorphic genes involved in metabolism and DNA repair [13]. To the best of our knowledge, only few studies have explored the hypothesis that PBLs DNA adduct levels can be associated to or predictive of BC risk. Results from three retrospective hospital based case-control showed that the risk indicator measuring the association between DNA adducts and BC was higher than 1.0 [14,15], not different from unity [17], or lower than 1.0 [16]. More precisely, DNA adducts were associated to the risk of BC but independently from smoking habits [14,15], while other authors [16] did not find any association between BC risk and bulky DNA adducts in never smokers. In the nested case-control prospective study, DNA adducts were not associated with BC risk [17]; overall, these conflicting results are hard to be explained from the biological viewpoint. Moreover, no study apparently estimated the complex interactions between DNA adducts, multiple genetic polymorphisms, occupational exposure to AAs and PAHs, and BC risk.

We previously assessed the interaction between occupational and environmental exposures with metabolic and DNA-repair polymorphisms on the risk of BC in retrospective hospital based case-control study [18–22].

The aim of this study was twofold: to investigate the extent to which PBL DNA adducts and BC risk were separately affected by genetic polymorphisms, environmental and occupational exposures; and to explore whether the formation of DNA adducts involved an additional increase in BC risk. These complex interrelationships were appraised using the analysis of structural equation modeling (SEM).

Subjects and Methods

Subjects

Study population, collection of data and statistical analysis are described in previous publications [18–22].

Briefly, the design was a hospital-based case-control study. The inclusion criteria were being male, aged between 20 and 80, resident in the Brescia province (Northern Italy). The cases were 201 newly diagnosed, histologically confirmed BC patients, admitted in the Urology Departments of the two main hospitals of Brescia from July 1997 to December 2000. The controls were 214 patients affected by various urological non-neoplastic diseases, frequency matched to cases by age (± 5 years), period and hospital of admission. A written informed consent was obtained from each recruited subject and the study was approved by the the Spedali Civili di Brescia Ethical Committee.

All subjects were administered a questionnaire during hospital admission to collect information on demographic variables and lifetime history of smoking, coffee and other liquid consumption, diet habits, occupations. Occupational exposures to PAHs and AAs were estimated according to methodology described in previous publication [22]. An index of cumulative exposure to AAs and PAHs, separately, was calculated as product ($i \times f \times l$) of length (l), intensity (i) and frequency (f) of exposure in each job, summing up as many products as were necessary to take into account all jobs done. Life-long consumption of cigarettes was calculated as packyears. The lifelong time-weighted average of cups/day of coffee was recoded as 0 (never drinkers), ≤ 3, 4, ≥ 5 cups/day. PAHs containing food, fruit, large leaf vegetables and other vegetables consumption was divided into four categories (less than once/month; less than once/week; 1–3 times/week; more than 3 times/week).

Genotyping of GSTM1, GSTT1, GSTP1, NAT1, NAT2, SULT1A1, XRCC1-3, XPD, CYP1A2, MPO, COMT, MnSOD

and NQO1 was assessed using Amplification Refractory Mutation System assay and using the GeneAmp PCR System 9700 (Applied Biosystems, Italy). PCR were followed by enzymatic digestion and PCR-RFLP analysis, as previously described [18–22].

All variables proved to be associated with BC risk at univariable logistic regression were forced in a multivariable unconditional logistic regression model and then chosen by backwards stepwise selection (with $p < 0.05$ as criterion). BC risk significantly increased with packyears, heavy coffee drinkers, MnSOD (Val/Val genotype), while decreased with large leaf vegetables consumption and MPO (G-463A homozygous variant). Cumulative exposure to AAs was not statistically significant but it was retained because being a substantial confounder [19,22].

DNA extraction from PBLs

Blood samples were collected from all the subjects during hospital admission and on the same day processed by centrifugation for obtaining peripheral blood lymphocytes (PBLs). The protocol for automated DNA extraction was performed according to Extragen kit (Extragen BC. by TALENT) following the manufacturer's instructions as previously described [20]. In particular 2.5 ml of buffy coats prepared from up to 10 ml of whole blood were processed for DNA extractions. A typical yield ranged from 150 to 400 μg DNA/extraction from a normal donor.

^{32}P-Post-labeling analysis of DNA adducts

Aliquots of 5 μg DNA were assayed for the presence of bulky-DNA adducts by ^{32}P-postlabeling after enrichment with Nuclease P1 as previously described [23,24]. Resolution of DNA adducts was performed by multidirectional thin-layer chromatography (TLC), using polyethyleneimine (PEI)-cellulose plates [25]. Briefly, 5 μg DNA were enzymatically digested to 3'-mononucleotides with 0,14 U/μg DNA of micrococcal nuclease and 1 mU/μg DNA of spleen phosphodiesterase for 3–4 hours at 37°C. After the enrichment procedure by Nuclease P1 digestion, DNA bases were labelled with 50 μCi of [gamma-^{32}P]ATP with a specific activity of 5000 Ci per mmol by using 2.5 units of T4 polynucleotide kinase. 20 μl of postlabeled sample were spotted on the origin of a premarked PEI cellulose sheet and run for the multidirectional TLC chromatography. Following chromatography, TLC sheets were dried and electronic autoradiography performed using a ^{32}P imager (InstanImager, Packard, MD, USA). A benzo(a)-pyrene diolepoxide-N2-dGp reference standard (National Cancer Institute Chemical Carcinogen Reference Standard Repository, Midwest Research Institute, Kansas City, Mo.) was used as a positive control in each labeling experiment. DNA adducts levels were measured as relative adduct level per 10^8 nucleotides.

Statistical analysis

In fitting SEM, packyears, coffee and vegetable consumption, *MnSOD*, *MPO*, cumulative AA exposure (variables associated with BC risk according to previous publications) plus *XRCC1* (see below) were used as exogenous variables (corresponding to predictors in regression based techniques). Both BC risk and adducts could be endogenous variables (corresponding to outcome variables), each affected by one or more exogenous variables (hypothesis 1). Alternatively, BC risk could be also influenced indirectly through the formation of DNA adducts (hypothesis 2). The two competing hypotheses were converted in two models of structural equations to find which model fitted best the observed data. SEM structural equations were fitted with "asymptotic distribution free" method because it did not make assumption on joint normality of all the variables and allowed using the variables (particularly adducts, see below) as given. The effect of each exogenous variable was expressed as standardized (or beta) coefficients that make comparisons easily by ignoring the independent variable's scale of units. SEM results were both tabulated and presented graphically. We used two SEM's goodness-of-fit statistics: (1) the chi square test for "model versus saturated" (the saturated model is the model that fits the covariances perfectly); and (2) the stability index obtained from the analysis of simultaneous equation systems.

The sample size required for SEM is dependent on model complexity, the estimation method used, and the distributional characteristics of observed variables [26]. The best option is to consider the model complexity (i.e., the number of exogenous variables) and the following rules of thumb: minimum ratio 5:1 [27,28]; recommended ratio 10:1 [26–28]; recommended ratio 15:1 for data with no normal distribution [29]. With eight exogenous variables used in the SEM model, we should have 120 ($= 15 \times 8$) subjects but they were actually 412 (see below) fulfilling the above requirements.

The analysis was carried out with the statistical package STATA 12.

Results

In the present study, complete individual data were available for 199 (out of 201) cases and 213 (out of 214) controls, totaling 412 (instead of 415) subjects.

Table 1 shows the main characteristics of cases and controls. Current and former smoking were more common (chi^2 test (2df) = 32.2377; p = 0.000) and coffee intake was higher (Wilcoxon rank-sum test z = −3.756; p = 0.0002) in cases than in controls. No significant differences between cases and controls were found for other demographic variables and putative risk factors of BC.

DNA adduct levels ranged from 0.3 to 70 adducts $\times 10^8$ nucleotides; the variable did not follow a normal distribution and any transformations failed to reduce its skewness (data not shown). Table 2 shows that mean, standard deviation, median, inter-quartile range and CV% of adduct levels were similar in cases and controls. A multivariable linear regression model with backwards stepwise selection gave XRCC1 as the only significant variable carrying protective effect (data not shown).

Table 3 shows three groups of SEM results.

1. Structural equations. It can be seen the beta coefficients (with "minus" sign indicating an inverse relationship), standard errors, z tests with p-values, and 95% confidence intervals for each of two structural equation models. The first model shows that cumulative occupational exposure to AAs (beta = 0.117; p = 0.028) is associated with increased DNA adduct levels, whereas XRCC1 Arg 399 (beta = −0.129; p<0.006) with decreased levels. We calculated the corresponding study-wise p-value as $(1-(1-alpha)^n)$, where "alpha" was 0.006 and "n" was 6. The result was 0,035464301 (well below the threshold of statistical significance), indicating that the error probability of 0.006 cannot be an effect of random fluctuations. The second model shows that cigarette smoking (packyears; beta = 0.256; p<0.001), coffee (beta = 0.166; p<0.001), cumulative occupational AAs exposure (beta = 0.084; p = 0.041) and MnSOD (beta = 0.119; p = 0.009) increased the BC risk whereas MPO (beta = −0.115; p<0.008) decreased it. No indirect paths were demonstrated (disproving hypothesis 2).

2. Variance explained by the above fitting was about 4% for DNA adducts and roughly 14% for the risk of BC.

3. Covariance between the two endogenous variables (BC risk and adducts) was not significant (p = 0.441, last row of table 1).

This finding demonstrated that these variables were not correlated to each other and that supported the hypothesis 2, i.e., DNA adducts did not affect BC risk in our population.

The value of chi square test for the discrepancy of the specified model versus saturated model was 0.00 with p-value equal to 1.00. The stability index was 0.00, indicating that SEM satisfies stability condition.

Using the graphical interface of SEM, the results shown in table 3 were displayed as path diagram in figure 1. In this figure, square boxes stand for variables, circles indicate variances, arrows specify the direction of causal flow, an arrowed route is a path, and the estimated beta coefficients appeared along the paths. The effect of one variable on another is called direct. There was no evidence of indirect effect (one variable affecting another variable which in turn affects a third), indicating that bladder cancer risk in our population was not further increased through formation of DNA adducts.

Discussion

DNA adducts as outcome

Since DNA adducts in PBLs are considered an integrate measure of carcinogen exposure, absorption, distribution, metabolism, and DNA repair, they have been referred to as biomarker of 'biologically effective dose' i.e. a measure of the amount of the carcinogen at the critical target [13]. Moreover carcinogen DNA adduct levels in more accessible circulating PBLs mirror those in the bladder tissue [11,12], which are considered an initial step in carcinogenesis.

However, in the present study, consistent with other literature findings, bulky DNA adducts detected by the nuclease P1 method of ^{32}P-post-labeling were not associated with an increased BC risk, probably because the adducts measured in PBLs at the time of BC diagnosis represent snapshots that are not necessarily representative of exposures relevant for BC risk that occurred in the past.

Adduct levels were instead associated with XRCC1399Arg carriers who presented a significant reduction in DNA adducts level, but with no effect on the risk of BC. Our results agree with previous studies reporting XRCC1399Arg associated with lower levels of bulky DNA adducts [30,31], due to higher DNA repair activity [32], and with two recent meta-analyses where XRCC1 Arg399Gln polymorphism was not related to BC risk [33,34].

In the present study, likewise the above reported studies [14,15,17], no relationship between DNA adduct levels and smoking was reported. Previous ^{32}P-postlabeling studies have reported inconsistent results on the association between the adduct levels in PBLs and tobacco smoking [35–39]. Discrepancies may depend on the marked interindividual variation in the metabolism of smoking carcinogens, which results in different DNA adduct levels for similar degrees of exposure [40]. Moreover, most of studies on the effect of smoking on PBLs bulky-DNA adduct levels did not reveal any significant differences [35,36,39], suggesting that adducts in PBLs from smokers may result from sources other than tobacco smoking.

We also found an association between cumulative occupational exposure to AAs and PBL adduct levels that was instead not reported by other authors most probably because information about occupational exposures was too limited to allow evaluation, even in the largest case-control study nested in EPIC cohort [17].

BC risk as outcome

We confirmed by SEM analysis the biological plausible protective effect of MPO A/A [21], and the risk effect of MnSOD

Table 1. Distribution of demographic characteristics, life habits, and occupational exposures in cases and controls.

	Cases (n = 199) Number (Percentage)	Controls (n = 213) Number (Percentage)
Age		
≤45	14 (7)	19 (9)
46–55	25 (13)	28 (13)
56–65	58 (29)	76 (36)
66–75	82 (41)	69 (32)
>75	20 (10)	21 (10)
Education		
0–5	106 (54)	111 (53)
6–8	60 (30)	47 (22)
9–13	25 (13)	41 (20)
≥14	7 (4)	11 (5)
Lifetime smoking		
Never	17 (9)	54 (25)
Light (≤26 packyears)	56 (28)	78 (37)
Heavy (>26 packyears)	126 (63)	81 (38)
Occupational cumulative exposure to PAHs		
Never	128 (64)	143 (67)
Ever	71 (36)	70 (33)
Occupational cumulative exposure to AAs		
Never	182 (91)	203 (95)
Ever	17 (9)	10 (5)
Coffee consumption (cups/day)		
Mean (± Standard Deviation)	2.33 (±2.30)	1.58 (±1.62)
5th–95th percentiles	0–8	0–6

Val/Val on BC [21,41]. The genetic polymorphism of enzymes involved in individual response to oxidative stress is likely involved in modulating the individual response to environmental exposures such as tobacco smoking, coffee drinks and AAs exposure [21]. In this study we also confirmed our previous results on the association between smoking habit and coffee drinking on BC risk, where the latter might be attributed to residual confounding by inadequate adjustment for cigarette smoking (which is over-represented among those who drink the most coffee/caffeine) [22]. As shown in table 3, the level of statistical significance of beta coefficients was particularly high for the association between BC risk and, on the other hand, packyears (beta = 0.256; p<0.001) and coffee (beta = 0.166; p<0.001); as well as for the association between decreased DNA adduct and *XRCC1 Arg 399* (beta = −0.129; p<0.006). Despite this, the proportion to which SEM fitting accounts for the dispersion of data (variance explained) was as low as 16% for BC risk, and 4% for DNA adducts. Therefore most variation of outcomes should be attributed to unknown predictors.

With regard to the relationship of occupational exposures to AAs and PAHs, DNA adducts and BC risk the literature is scanty and those few published studies have only found an exposure-independent association between adducts and BC risk. Our study precisely evaluated the occupational exposure history to AAs and PAHs, and noted a significant correlation between occupational exposure to AAs and BC, and adduct levels too. Therefore occupational exposure to AAs is confirmed as central risk factor for BC development. Finally the present work was carried out in the context of a biologically plausible and hypothesis-driven study design consistent with the available literature data.

Table 2. Summary statistics (mean, standard deviation, median, interquartile range, number of subjects) for "ln_adducts" in cases, controls, and total population.

	Mean	Std. Dev.	CV%	Median	Inter quartile range	N
Cases	0.82	1.20	146	0.57	2.00	185
Controls	0.77	1.09	142	0.46	1.73	180
Total	0.80	1.14	143	0.51	1.83	365

Table 3. SEM results: beta coefficients (with "minus" sign indicating inverse relationship), standard errors, z tests and the corresponding p-values, along with 95% confidence intervals for endogenous variables of structural equations; variances and covariance.

Endogenous variable	Exogenous variables	Beta Coef.	Std. Err.	z	P>|z|	95% CI Lower	Upper
Structural Equations							
Adducts	Packyears	0.064	0.048	1.35	0.177	−0.029	0.157
	Coffee	0.015	0.047	0.31	0.757	−0.078	0.107
	Occupational exposure to AAs	0.117	0.048	2.46	0.014	0.024	0.210
	XRCC1	−0.129	0.047	−2.75	0.006	−0.221	−0.037
	MPO	−0.024	0.039	−0.63	0.531	−0.100	0.052
	MnSOD	−0.053	0.045	−1.17	0.244	−0.142	0.036
Cancer Risk	Packyears	0.256	0.041	6.19	0.000	0.175	0.337
	Coffee	0.166	0.043	3.83	0.000	0.081	0.250
	AA	0.084	0.034	2.45	0.014	0.017	0.152
	XRCC1	−0.028	0.044	−0.65	0.519	−0.114	0.058
	MPO	−0.115	0.036	−3.21	0.001	−0.185	−0.045
	MnSOD	0.120	0.044	2.71	0.007	0.033	0.206
Variances							
Adducts		0.962	0.018			0.927	0.998
Cancer Risk		0.858	0.025			0.811	0.908
Covariance							
Adducts × Cancer Risk		−0.038	0.047	−0.80	0.421	−0.131	0.055

Packyears = Life-long consumption of cigarettes.
Coffee = Life-long time-weighted average of cups/day of coffee.
AA = Occupational cumulative exposure to aromatic amines.
XRCC1 = X-ray repair cross-complementing protein 1.
MPO = Myeloperoxidase (G-463A homozygous variant).
MnSOD = Manganese Superoxide Dismutase (Val/Val genotype).

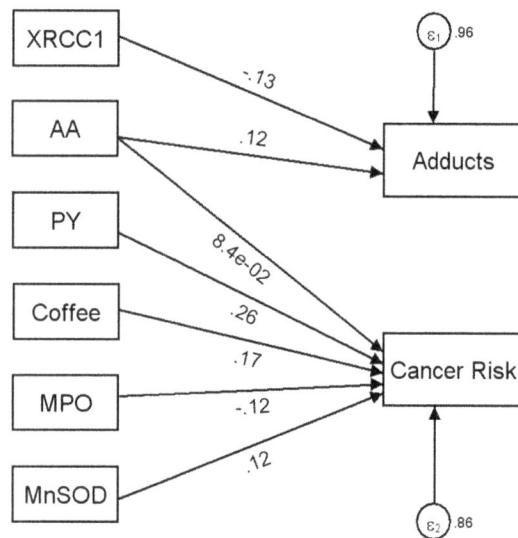

Figure 1. Path diagram of results shown in table 1. Variables (square boxes); variances (circles); causal flow (arrows); and paths (arrowed route). The estimated beta coefficients appeared along the paths. LEGEND: Packyears = Life-long consumption of cigarettes; Coffee = Life-long time-weighted average of cups/day of coffee; AA = Occupational cumulative exposure to aromatic amines; *XRCC1* = X-ray repair cross-complementing protein 1; *MPO* = Myeloperoxidase (G-463A homozygous variant); *MnSOD* = Manganese Superoxide Dismutase (Val/Val genotype).

In addition, the correlation we found between AAs exposure and BC risk is biologically plausible, because AAs are activated in liver and transported by blood proteins to the bladder where, under acidic conditions [42,43] or, enzymatically by O-acetylation of N-hydroxy arylamine (predominantly by the N- acetyltransfer-ase 1 (NAT1) isozyme), are further activated to the ultimate carcinogen [44]. This result also suggests that occupational exposure history collected by questionnaire through interview could be a reliable measurement of exposures to AAs in such studies.

Unlike AAs, cumulative exposure to PAHs was not associated with BC risk. Experimental evidence suggests that PAHs are slowly absorbed through most tissues. For instance, in the case of dermal exposure, considered the main route in the industry [45], absorption accounts for a small fraction of applied dose, and PAHs are enzymatically activated and degraded at this site of entry [46–48]. The concentration and persistence of PAHs in the lung is largely related with inhalation of PAHs containing dust [49,50]. The high propensity of PAHs to act as carcinogens at the sites of entry is supported by several experimental studies [51].

DNA adducts and BC risk

The results of literature on the association between DNA adducts and risk of BC are scanty and not consistent. A strong direct association between and the risk of BC and PBLs DNA adducts, measured at time of diagnosis and detected by means nuclease P1 and ^{32}P-postlabeling, was reported in two retrospec-tive hospital based case-control [14,15]. The association was however independent from smoking habits and was suggested to be dependent from other exposures (that the studies did not specify), and from *NAT2* as genetic factor. While, in a retrospective hospital based case-control among nonsmokers bulky DNA adducts were not associated with bladder cancer risk [16]. Lastly

PBLs DNA adducts (nuclease P1 and 32P-postlabeling) were not associated with the subsequent bladder cancer insurgence in a prospective nested case-control study [17]. The findings of this latter study are probably more reliable and meaningful than those of earlier investigations [14,15], because DNA adducts were measured years before the onset of disease, thus ruling out the possibility that the higher adduct levels were due to a condition associated with an already existing cancer.

We did not find any relation between DNA adducts and BC risk. However, we cannot exclude such relationship. In fact, a limitation of the present study is that adducts measured by nuclease P1 method of ^{32}P-postlabeling are non-specific because the responsible electrophilic substance cannot be identified. Moreover, DNA adducts measure at time of diagnosis may be not representative of cumulative doses of carcinogens that may cause cancer. Environmental and occupational exposures vary both qualitatively and quantitatively over time due to changes in lifestyle, place of residence, employment, etc., and the impact of a given exposure on the risk of cancer cannot be constant throughout the life of an individual [13]. This fact, combined with the awareness that the rate and speed of repair of various DNA adducts are different and their permanence mainly depends from life span of PBLs, from a few days to a few weeks, poses uncertainty on the significance of such short-term exposure biomarker in relation to the risk of cancer. Given the long latency of carcinogen-related malignancies – that is the time between the beginning of exposure and the onset of disease – the retrospective assessment of carcinogen exposures, especially via biomarkers, represents a challenge for both epidemiology and clinical medicine.

Perspectives (including SEM analysis)

New opportunities for biomonitoring of carcinogens may derive from measuring exposures from all sources both external and internal that occur throughout the lifespan. This approach named exposome by Wild [52] is represented by the set of chemicals derived from sources outside genetic control that include diet, pathogens, microbiome, smoking, psychological stress, drugs and pollution [53]. Indeed, these new technologies are opening new scenarios for biomarker discovery but new challenges as well, that include the need of repeated measurements of global sets of biomarkers to be collected at different critical life stages. Only in this way can the dynamics of exposures and early and late effects be captured.

In medicine and natural sciences a given outcome is often affected or influenced by more than one thing simultaneously. Multivariate techniques try to statistically account for these differences, adjusting an outcome measure Y to a 1 unit change in X, holding all other variables constant. However, it may be that other variables are not likely to remain constant: a change in X can produce a change in Z (direct effect) which in turn produces a change in Y (indirect effect). Both the direct and indirect effects of X on Y must be considered if we want to know what effect a change in X will have on Y. This can be done mathematically and statistically only using SEM. The procedure decomposes a correlation between two variables into its component parts: direct effects, indirect effects, common causes (X affects both Y and Z; this is spurious association) and correlated causes (X is a cause of Z and X is correlated with Y). The user is required to state, often using a path diagram, the way that he/she believes the variables are inter-related. Via some complex internal rules, SEM decides which model fits data better. This method is more suitable to analyze complex interrelationships because it tests causal relation-ships rather than mere correlations.

In our opinion, the statistical analysis with SEM is one strength of the present research. Other strengths of the study are the thorough and reliable collection of several personal, occupational and environmental variables, the multiple genetic polymorphisms and endpoints, the significant number of subjects, as compared to other similar studies with adduct analysis [14–17], the quality of DNA adduct analysis, the sample size required for calculation of SEM; here, the actual number of 412 cases was much higher than the maximum required sample size of 120 subjects estimated according to different assumptions (see above: statistical analysis).

Conclusions

Using the SEM analysis, a statistical technique that combines observed data and qualitative causal assumptions and tests whether and how variables are interrelated through a system of equations, we found that PBL DNA adducts was not associated with BC risk. This suggests that this measure at time of diagnosis may be not representative of dose of carcinogens that may cause cancer. However the new finding stemming from this study sustains that occupational cumulative exposure to AAs were instead associated with both DNA adducts and with BC risk. This agrees with the propensity of AAs to act as carcinogens away of the sites of entry after being transported by blood proteins to the bladder and confirm exposure to AAs, determined by blood DNA adduct, as central risk factor for BC development. Moreover *XRCC1399Arg* polymorphism has a role in repairing PBL DNA adducts but no impact on individual susceptibility to BC. Previous findings on the influence of smoking, coffee intake, *MPO A/A* and *MnSOD Val/Val* polymorphisms on BC risk were also confirmed by SEM analysis. A direct effect of these predictor variables was observed on each outcome variable. Our study envisages new scenarios, entailing the need of repeated DNA adduct measurements at different critical life stages and proper analytical techniques, for example during occupational exposure to AAs, as well as the appraisal of the complex relationship between gene and environment, by means of SEM analysis.

Author Contributions

Conceived and designed the experiments: SP SP GM. Performed the experiments: SP AC CA SP AI CS GM. Analyzed the data: SP AC CA SP AI CS GM. Contributed reagents/materials/analysis tools: SP AC CA SP AI CS GM. Wrote the paper: SP AC CA SP AI CS GM.

References

1. Pelucchi C, Bosetti C, Negri E, Malvezzi M, La Vecchia C (2006) Mechanisms of disease: the epidemiology of bladder cancer. Nat Clin Pract Urol 3: 327–340.
2. Bosetti C, Boffetta P, La Vecchia C (2007) Occupational exposures to polycyclic aromatic hydrocarbons, and respiratory and urinary tract cancers: a quantitative review to 2005. Ann Oncol 18: 431–446.
3. Burger M, Catto JW, Dalbagni G, Grossman HB, Herr H, et al. (2013) Epidemiology and risk factors of urothelial bladder cancer. Eur Urol 63: 234–241.
4. Chu H, Wang M, Zhang Z (2013) Bladder cancer epidemiology and genetic susceptibility. J Biomed Res 27: 170–178.
5. Pfeifer GP, Denissenko MF, Olivier M, Tretyakova N, Hecht SS, et al. (2002) Tobacco smoke carcinogens, DNA damage and p53 mutations in smoking-associated cancers. Oncogene 21: 7435–7451.
6. Pavanello S, Pulliero A, Clonfero E (2008) Influence of GSTM1 null and low repair XPC PAT+ on anti-B[a]PDE-DNA adduct in mononuclear white blood cells of subjects low exposed to PAHs through smoking and diet. Mutat Res 638: 195–204.
7. Loeb LA, Harris CC (2008) Advances in chemical carcinogenesis: a historical review and prospective. Cancer Res 68: 6863–6872.
8. Talaska G, Al-Juburi AZSS, Kadlubar FF (1991) Smoking related carcinogen–DNA adducts in biopsy samples of human urinary bladder: identification of N-(deoxyguanosin-8-yl)-4-aminobiphenyl as a major adduct. Proc Natl Acad Sci USA 88: 5350–5354.
9. Talaska G, Schamer M, Casetta G, Tizzani A, Vineis P (1994) Carcinogen-DNA adducts in bladder biopsies and urothelial cells: a risk assessment exercise. Cancer Lett 84: 93–97.
10. Yoon JI, Kim SI, Tommasi S, Besaratinia A (2012) Organ specificity of the bladder carcinogen 4-aminobiphenyl in inducing DNA damage and mutation in mice. Cancer Prev Res (Phila) 5: 299–308.
11. Zhou Q, Talaska G, Jaeger M, Bhatnagar VK, Hayes RB, et al. (1997) Benzidine-DNA adduct levels in human peripheral white blood cells significantly correlate with levels in exfoliated urothelial cells. Mutat Res 393: 199–205.
12. Airoldi L, Orsi F, Magagnotti C, Coda R, Randone D, et al. (2002) Determinants of 4-aminobiphenyl-DNA adducts in bladder cancer biopsies. Carcinogenesis 23: 861–866.
13. Wild CP (2009) Environmental exposure measurement in cancer epidemiology. Mutagenesis 24: 117–125.
14. Peluso M, Airoldi L, Armelle M, Martone T, Coda R, et al. (1998) White blood cell DNA adducts, smoking, and NAT2 and GSTM1 genotypes in bladder cancer: a case-control study. Cancer Epidemiol Biomarkers Prev 7: 341–346.
15. Peluso M, Airoldi L, Magagnotti C, Fiorini L, Munnia A, et al. (2000) White blood cell DNA adducts and fruit and vegetable consumption in bladder cancer. Carcinogenesis 21: 183–187.
16. Castaño-Vinyals G, Talaska G, Rothman N, Alguacil J, Garcia-Closas M, et al. (2007) Bulky DNA adduct formation and risk of bladder cancer. Cancer Epidemiol Biomarkers Prev 16: 2155–2159.
17. Peluso M, Munnia A, Hoek G, Krzyzanowski M, Veglia F, et al. (2005) DNA adducts and lung cancer risk: a prospective study. Cancer Res 65: 8042–8048.
18. Covolo L, Placidi D, Gelatti U, Carta A, Scotto Di Carlo A, et al. (2008) Bladder cancer, GSTs, NAT1, NAT2, SULT1A1, XRCC1, XRCC3, XPD genetic polymorphisms and coffee consumption: a case-control study. Eur J Epidemiol 23: 355–362.
19. Hung RJ, Boffetta P, Brennan P, Malaveille C, Hautefeuille A, et al. (2004) GST, NAT, SULT1A1, CYP1B1 genetic polymorphisms, interactions with environmental exposures and bladder cancer risk in a high-risk population. Int J Cancer 110: 598–604.
20. Shen M, Hung RJ, Brennan P, Malaveille C, Donato F, et al. (2003) Polymorphisms of the DNA repair genes XRCC1, XRCC3, XPD, interaction with environmental exposures, and bladder cancer risk in a case–control study in northern Italy. Cancer Epidemiol Biomarkers Prev 12: 1234–1240.
21. Hung RJ, Boffetta P, Brennan P, Malaveille C, Gelatti U, et al. (2004) Genetic polymorphisms of MPO, COMT, MnSOD, NQO1, interactions with environmental exposures and bladder cancer risk. Carcinogenesis 25: 973–978.
22. Pavanello S, Mastrangelo G, Placidi D, Campagna M, Pulliero A, et al. (2010) CYP1A2 polymorphisms, occupational and environmental exposures and risk of bladder cancer. Eur J Epidemiol 25: 491–500.
23. Pavanello S, Levis AG (1994) Human peripheral blood lymphocytes as a cell model to evaluate the genotoxic effect of coal tar treatment. Environ Health Perspect 102 Suppl 9: 95–99.
24. Izzotti A (1998) Detection of modified DNA nucleotides by postlabelling procedures. Toxicology Methods 8:175–205.
25. Gupta RC, Reddy MV, Randerath K (1982) 32P-postlabeling analysis of non-radioactive aromatic carcinogen—DNA adducts. Carcinogenesis 3: 1081–1092.
26. Kline R (2005) Principles and Practice of Structural Equation Modeling (2nd ed.). New York: The Guilford Press.
27. Bentler P, Chou C (1987) Practical issues in structural modeling. Sociological Methods and Research 16: 78–117.
28. Worthington R, Whittaker T (2006) Scale Development Research. A Content Analysis and Recommendations for Best Practices. The Counseling Psychologist 34: 806–838.
29. Hair J, Black W, Babin B, Anderson R, Tatham R (2006) Multivariate Data Analysis (6th ed.). New Jersey: Pearson Educational, Inc.
30. Matullo G, Palli D, Peluso M, Guarrera S, Carturan S, et al. (2001) XRCC1, XRCC3, XPD gene polymorphisms, smoking and (32)P-DNA adducts in a sample of healthy subjects. Carcinogenesis 22: 1437–445.
31. Ji G, Gu A, Zhou Y, Shi X, Xia Y, et al. (2010) Interactions between exposure to environmental polycyclic aromatic hydrocarbons and DNA repair gene polymorphisms on bulky DNA adducts in human sperm. PLoS One 5(10) pii: e13145.
32. Lunn RM, Langlois RG, Hsieh LL, Thompson CL, Bell DA (1999) XRCC1 polymorphisms: effects on aflatoxin B1-DNA adducts and glycophorin A variant frequency. Cancer Res 59: 2557–2561.
33. Fang Z, Chen F, Wang X, Yi S, Chen W, et al. (2013) XRCC1 Arg194Trp and Arg280His polymorphisms increase bladder cancer risk in asian population: evidence from a meta-analysis. PLoS One 8(5): e64001.
34. Zhuo W, Zhang L, Cai L, Zhu B, Chen Z (2013) XRCC1 Arg399Gln polymorphism and bladder cancer risk: updated meta-analyses based on 5767 cases and 6919 controls. Exp Biol Med (Maywood) 238: 66–76.
35. Phillips DH, Schoket B, Hewer A, Bailey E, Kostic S, et al. (1990) Influence of cigarette smoking on the levels of DNA adducts in human bronchial epithelium and white blood cells. Int J Cancer 46: 569–575.
36. Phillips DH, Hewer A, Grover PL (1986) Aromatic DNA adducts in human bone marrow and peripheral blood leukocytes. Carcinogenesis 7: 2071–2075.

37. Jahnke GA, Thompson CL, Walker MP, Gallagher JE, Lucier GW, et al. (1990) Multiple DNA adducts in lymphocytes of smokers and nonsmokers determined by 32-P-postlabelling analysis. Carcinogenesis 11: 205–211.

38. Savela K, Hemmink K (1991) DNA adducts in lymphocytes and granulocytes of smokers and nonsmokers detected by the 32-P-postlabelling assay. Carcinogenesis 12: 503–508.

39. Van Maanen JMS, Maas LM, Hageman G, Kleinjans JCS, Van Agen B (1994) DNA adduct and mutation analysis in white blood cell s of smokers and nonsmokers. Environ Mol Mutagen 24: 46–50.

40. Perera FP (1996) Molecular epidemiology: insights into cancer susceptibility, risk assessment, and prevention. J Natl Cancer Inst 88: 496–507.

41. Sutton A, Khoury H, Prip-Buus C, Cepanec C, Pessayre D, et al. (2003) The Ala16Val genetic dimorphism modulates the import of human manganese superoxide dismutase into rat liver mitochondria. Pharmacogenetics 13: 145–157.

42. Kadlubar FF (1991) Carcinogenic aromatic amine metabolism and DNA adduct detection in human. In: Emster L, editor. Xenobiotics and cancer. London: Taylor & Francis, Ltd. pp. 329–338.

43. Bartsch H, Malaveille C, Friesen M, Kadlubar FF, Vineis P (1993) Black (aircured) and blond (flue-cured) tobacco cancer risk. IV. Molecular dosimetrystudies implicates aromatic amines as bladder carcinogens. Eur J Cancer 29: 1199–1207.

44. Frederickson SM, Messing EM, Renikoff CA, Swaminathan S (1994) Relationship between in vivo acetylator phenotypes and cytosolic N-acetyltransferase and O-acetyltransferase activities in human uroepithelial cells. Cancer Epidemiol Biomark Prev 3: 25–32.

45. Jongeneelen FJ (1992) Biological exposure limit for occupational exposure to coal tar pitch volatiles at cokeovens. Int Arch Occup Environ Health 63: 511–516.

46. Kao J, Patterson FK, Hall J (1985) Skin penetration and metabolism of topically applied chemicals in six mammalian species, including man: an in vitro study with benzo[a]pyrene and testosterone. Toxicol Appl Pharmacol 81: 502–516.

47. Ng KM, Chu I, Bronaugh RL, Franklin CA, Somers DA (1992) Percutaneous absorption and metabolism of pyrene, benzo[a]pyrene, and di(2-ethylhexyl) phthalate: comparison of in vitro and in vivo results in the hairless guinea pig. Toxicol Appl Pharmacol 115: 216–223

48. VanRooij JG, De Roos JH, Bodelier-Bade MM, Jongeneelen FJ (1993) Absorption of polycyclic aromatic hydrocarbons through human skin: differences between anatomical sites and individuals. J Toxicol Environ Health 38:355–368.

49. Albert RE, Miller ML, Cody T, Andringa A, Shukla R, et al. (1991) Benzo[a]pyrene-induced skin damage and tumor promotion in the mouse. Carcinogenesis 12: 1273–1280.

50. Wolterbeek AP, Schoevers EJ, Rutten AA, Feron VJ (1995) A critical appraisal of intratracheal instillation of benzo[a]pyrene to Syrian golden hamsters as a model in respiratory tract carcinogenesis. Cancer Lett 89: 107–116.

51. IARC (2010) IARC monographs on the evaluation of carcinogenic risks to humans. Some non-heterocyclic polycyclic aromatic hydrocarbons and some related exposures. Volume 92. International Agency for Research on Cancer, Lyon, France39.

52. Wild CP (2012) The exposome: from concept to utility. Int J Epidemiol 41: 24–32.

53. Rappaport SM (2012) Biomarkers intersect with the exposome. Biomarkers 17(6):483–9.

19

Prognostic Relevance of Urinary Bladder Cancer Susceptibility Loci

Anne J. Grotenhuis[1], Aleksandra M. Dudek[2], Gerald W. Verhaegh[2], J. Alfred Witjes[2], Katja K. Aben[1,3], Saskia L. van der Marel[4], Sita H. Vermeulen[1,4], Lambertus A. Kiemeney[1,2]*

1 Department for Health Evidence, Radboud University Medical Center, Nijmegen, The Netherlands, 2 Department of Urology, Radboud University Medical Center, Nijmegen, The Netherlands, 3 Comprehensive Cancer Center The Netherlands, Utrecht, The Netherlands, 4 Department of Human Genetics, Radboud University Medical Center, Nijmegen, The Netherlands

Abstract

In the last few years, susceptibility loci have been identified for urinary bladder cancer (UBC) through candidate-gene and genome-wide association studies. Prognostic relevance of most of these loci is yet unknown. In this study, we used data of the Nijmegen Bladder Cancer Study (NBCS) to perform a comprehensive evaluation of the prognostic relevance of all confirmed UBC susceptibility loci. Detailed clinical data concerning diagnosis, stage, treatment, and disease course of a population-based series of 1,602 UBC patients were collected retrospectively based on a medical file survey. Kaplan-Meier survival analyses and Cox proportional hazard regression were performed, and log-rank tests calculated, to evaluate the association between 12 confirmed UBC susceptibility variants and recurrence and progression in non-muscle invasive bladder cancer (NMIBC) patients. Among muscle-invasive or metastatic bladder cancer (MIBC) patients, association of these variants with overall survival was tested. Subgroup analyses by tumor aggressiveness and smoking status were performed in NMIBC patients. In the overall NMIBC group (n = 1,269), a statistically significant association between rs9642880 at 8q24 and risk of progression was observed (GT vs. TT: HR = 1.08 (95% CI: 0.76–1.54), GG vs. TT: HR = 1.81 (95% CI: 1.23–2.66), P for trend = 2.6×10^{-3}). In subgroup analyses, several other variants showed suggestive, though non-significant, prognostic relevance for recurrence and progression in NMIBC and survival in MIBC. This study provides suggestive evidence that genetic loci involved in UBC etiology may influence disease prognosis. Elucidation of the causal variant(s) could further our understanding of the mechanism of disease, could point to new therapeutic targets, and might aid in improvement of prognostic tools.

Editor: Peter C Black, University of British Columbia, Canada

Funding: AG was supported by a research investment grant of the Radboud University Medical Centre. The funders had no role in study design, data collection and analysis, decision to publish, or preparation of the manuscript.

Competing Interests: The authors have declared that no competing interests exist.

* E-mail: Bart.Kiemeney@radboudumc.nl

Introduction

Urinary bladder cancer (UBC) is a heterogeneous disease with respect to its prognosis. The available prognostic tools that are based on clinicopathological variables, such as the European Organisation for Research and Treatment of Cancer (EORTC) risk tables and the Club Urológico Español de Tratamiento Oncológico (CUETO) scoring model, have insufficient discriminative ability to accurately predict the risk of disease recurrence and progression at the level of the individual patient. [1] The same holds for scores that include molecular markers. [2,3] Additional or better markers are clearly needed for personalized healthcare. There is growing evidence for a role of (germline) genetic polymorphisms in disease prognosis and treatment response. [4–7] Identification of such genetic variants may lead to improvement of disease outcome prediction in UBC patients. Discovery of such variants might also provide clues about the underlying mechanism of urothelial carcinogenesis and cancer progression, and thereby point the way to new therapeutic targets.

Sufficiently powered and well-designed studies into the prognostic and predictive value of germline genetic polymorphisms in UBC are rare. Chen *et al.* identified and (externally) validated the influence of genetic variation in the sonic hedgehog pathway (*i.e.,* rs1233560 in *SHH* (sonic hedgehog) and rs11685068 in *GLI2* (GLI family zinc finger 2)) on the risk of recurrence after transurethral resection of the tumor (TURT) in non-muscle invasive bladder cancer (NMIBC) patients. [8] The same research group discovered association of a polymorphism in one of the microRNA biogenesis genes (*i.e.,* rs197412 in *DDX20* (DEAD (Asp-Glu-Ala-Asp) box polypeptide 20)) with disease recurrence in the same UBC subgroup, which could be replicated in an additional NMIBC patient series. [9] The remainder of the published candidate-gene surveys for UBC prognosis is of small size and still awaits independent replications to exclude false-positive findings. [10–12] Genome-wide association studies (GWAS) into UBC prognosis are still lacking. For UBC *susceptibility*, the shift to an agnostic GWAS approach has led to the successful identification of several novel, established genetic polymorphisms. [13] For several cancer types, including colorectal, pancreatic, breast, lung, and prostate cancer, it has been shown that GWAS-identified susceptibility variants also have prognostic relevance. [14–20] Indeed, in one of our GWAS for UBC susceptibility, we found that the T allele of the identified risk variant rs798766 (*TACC3/FGFR3* (transforming, acidic coiled-coil containing protein 3/fibroblast growth factor receptor 3) locus) is associated with a higher risk of recurrence, specifically among patients with low-grade Ta tumors. [21] Here, we comprehensively evaluate the prognostic relevance of 12 variants at 11 (extensively) replicated UBC susceptibility loci. Our study indicates that there is overlap in genetic variants underlying UBC etiology and prognosis.

Materials and Methods

Ethics statement

The study was conducted according to the principles expressed in the declaration of Helsinki. All participants gave written informed consent and the study was approved by the Institutional Review Board of the Radboud university medical center, Nijmegen, the Netherlands.

Patient population

This study was performed in 1,602 patients with primary UBC from the Nijmegen Bladder Cancer Study (NBCS). The NBCS served as the Dutch discovery population in the UBC GWAS led by Radboud university medical center and deCODE Genetics (Reykjavik, Iceland). The NBCS has been described in detail before. [13] Patients with a previous or simultaneous (within three months) diagnosis of upper urinary tract cancer, based on information from the Netherlands Cancer Registry (NCR), were excluded. Detailed clinical data concerning diagnosis, stage, treatment, and disease course (tumor recurrence and progression) was collected retrospectively by a medical file survey. Based on stage and histological grade, all NMIBC patients were classified with regard to tumor aggressiveness (i.e., risk of progression). Subjects with low risk of progression were defined as those having TNM stage Ta in combination with WHO 1973 differentiation grade 1 or 2, WHO/ISUP 2004 low grade, or Malmström (modified Bergkvist) grade 1 or 2a. All other patients were classified as having tumors with high risk of progression (stage CIS ór T1 ór WHO 1973 grade 3, WHO/ISUP 2004 high grade, or Malmström (modified Bergkvist) grade 2b or 3). Self-reported data on smoking status was available based on a lifestyle questionnaire filled out by the participants at study inclusion.

Selection of variants and genotyping

The ten UBC susceptibility single-nucleotide polymorphisms (SNPs) that were identified through GWAS for UBC risk and replicated in at least one independent population, were selected for this study (see Table 1 for details). All of these SNPs were genotyped via the Illumina HumanCNV370-Duo BeadChip, except for rs2736098 that was genotyped by a single-SNP Centaurus (Nanogen) assay. [22] The genome-wide genotyping of SNPs in the NBCS, and related quality control (QC) procedures were described in detail before. [13] The concordance rate between (UBC susceptibility) SNP genotypes measured using the Illumina platform and those derived from a single-SNP Centaurus (Nanogen) assay was previously found to be >99.5%. [13,21,23]

In addition, deletion of the glutathione S-transferase mu 1 (GSTM1) gene (null genotype) and a tag SNP for the N-acetyltransferase 2 (NAT2) slow acetylation phenotype (rs1495741) [24], both with an established influence on UBC risk based on (meta-analysis of) candidate-gene studies, were included in this study (see Table 1). GSTM1 copy number variation (CNV) status was determined by an Applied Biosystems TaqMan Copy Number assay (Assay ID: Hs02575461_cn). The NAT2 tagSNP was genotyped through the Illumina HumanCNV370-Duo BeadChip.

As we realize that the 10 GWAS-identified genetic variants evaluated are not necessarily the causal variants, we also evaluated genetic variants in a 200 kb region centered on each of the susceptibility SNPs in relation to each of the prognostic endpoints. For this, we used genome-wide measured and imputed SNP data. Imputation was performed using the 1000 Genomes low-coverage pilot haplotypes (released June 2010, 120 chromosomes) and the HapMap3 haplotypes (released February 2009, 1920 chromosomes) as a combined reference panel. [13] We thereby automatically included the two UBC susceptibility variants (i.e., rs2978974 (8q24.3) and rs17863783 (2q37.1)) that were identified in previously published finemapping efforts. [25,26]

Outcome definition

In the NMIBC subgroup, the association of the 12 variants with the prognostic endpoints recurrence-free survival (RFS) and progression-free survival (PFS) was investigated. *Date of first recurrence* was defined as date of histological confirmation of a newly found bladder or prostatic urethra tumor following at least one tumor-negative follow-up cystoscopy or two surgical resection sessions for the primary tumor. *Date of first progression* was defined as date of first occurrence of grade progression, stage progression, local and/or distant metastasis, and/or cystectomy for therapy-resistant ('uncontrollable') disease. See Text S1 for a more detailed description of the prognostic endpoint definitions. NMIBC patients who were treated with an immediate radical cystectomy after primary diagnosis were considered not at risk of (intravesical) recurrence, and therefore excluded from further analyses. In case of no recurrence/progression, follow-up was censored at the last date of urological check-up. Only the first 5 years after the primary NMIBC diagnosis were considered in the analyses in order to focus on the most clinically relevant period for those prognostic endpoints, and also in order to reduce the effect of competing risks (especially for older patients). RFS and PFS were defined as the time period between date of the initial TURT and date of first event (recurrence or progression, respectively), date of censoring, or date of five-year follow-up, whichever came first.

In the subgroup of muscle-invasive ($\geq$T2) or metastatic bladder cancer (MIBC) patients, the association between the 12 variants and overall survival (OS) was evaluated. For this purpose, information on vital status was retrieved via the NCR through record linkage to the nationwide Dutch Municipal Personal Records Database. If patients were still alive at December 31st, 2011, follow-up was censored at this date. Again, follow-up time considered was restricted to the first five years after diagnosis. OS was defined as the time period between date of the initial TURT and date of death (of all causes), date of censoring, or date of five-year follow-up, whichever came first.

Statistical analysis

Kaplan-Meier survival and Cox proportional hazard regression analyses were performed, and log-rank tests calculated, to evaluate the association between the 12 variants and the above-mentioned prognostic endpoints. Multivariable Cox regression analysis was used to adjust the hazard ratio (HR) for the effect of treatment in NMIBC patients, and for extended/metastasized (i.e., primary stage T4(b) ór any T with N+/N$\geq$1 and/or M1) versus localized disease (i.e., primary stage T2-T4a with N0/NX and M0/MX) at diagnosis in MIBC patients. To evaluate subgroup-specific effects, a stratified analysis according to tumor aggressiveness of NMIBC (i.e., low vs. high risk of progression) and smoking status (i.e., never vs. ever cigarette smoking) was performed.

The association with disease prognosis was evaluated based on a genotypic model with the homozygous genotype of the most

Table 1. Extensively replicated germline UBC susceptibility loci.

Locus	Gene region	SNP	Risk allele[a]	Allelic OR[a]	Risk allele frequency[b]	Study type	Reference
8p22	NAT2	-	slow acetylator	1.4	0.56	Candidate-gene	[45]
1p13.3	GSTM1	-	null	1.5	0.51	Candidate-gene	[45]
8q24.21	MYC	rs9642880	T	1.22	0.45	GWAS	[23]
3q28	TP63	rs710521	A	1.19	0.73	GWAS	[23]
5p15.33	TERT	rs2736098	A	1.16	0.26	GWAS	[22]
5p15.33	CLPTM1L	rs401681	C	1.12	0.54	GWAS	[22]
8q24.3	PSCA	rs2294008	T	1.15	0.46	GWAS	[46]
4p16.3	TACC3-FGFR3	rs798766	T	1.24	0.19	GWAS	[21]
22q13.1	CBX6, APOBEC3A	rs1014971	T	1.14	0.62	GWAS	[47]
19q12	CCNE1	rs8102137	C	1.13	0.33	GWAS	[47]
2q37.1	UGT1A	rs11892031	A	1.19	0.92	GWAS	[47]
18q12.3	SLC14A1	rs1058396	G	1.14	0.50	GWAS	[13]

OR: odds ratio; *TP63*: tumor protein p63; *TERT*: telomerase reverse transcriptase; *CLPTM1L*: CLPTM1-like; *PSCA*: prostate stem cell antigen; *CBX6*: chromobox homolog 6; *APOBEC3A*: apolipoprotein B mRNA editing enzyme, catalytic polypeptide-like 3A; *CCNE1*: cyclin E1; *SLC14A1*: solute carrier family 14 (urea transporter), member 1
[a]for *NAT2* and *GSTM1* these do not refer to the risk allele but to the risk genotype;
[b]risk allele frequency among controls as published in candidate-gene study/GWAS paper

common (major) allele (based on our data) assigned as the reference category. For *GSTM1* we studied the association for patients with the null genotype compared to patients with at least one copy of the gene present, and for *NAT2* we evaluated the association of slow acetylators (rs1495741: AA) compared to intermediate/rapid acetylators (AG/GG). The Bonferroni correction was applied to adjust the statistical significance threshold for the 12 tested variants (alpha = $0.05/12 = 4 \times 10^{-3}$) (with P-values derived based on a (two-sided) trend test). At this alpha level and assuming a risk allele frequency of 0.20, our study had 80% power to detect a HR greater than 1.35 and 1.89 for recurrence (five-year risk: 50%), and a minimum HR of 1.57 and 2.36 for progression (five-year risk: 20%), according to a dominant and recessive mode of inheritance, respectively (IBM SPSS SamplePower release 3.01).

In addition to the single-SNP analyses, we evaluated the cumulative prognostic value of the UBC susceptibility variants by testing association with the genetic risk score, *i.e.*, total sum of the number of UBC risk alleles (0,1,2) for each SNP among individuals successfully genotyped for all 12 variants. For *NAT2* and *GSTM1*, we counted the risk genotype (0,1). Cumulative (additive) association with RFS and PFS among NMIBC patients was tested by including this genetic risk score as continuous (independent) variable in a Cox regression model (with adjustment for treatment type). Statistical analyses were performed using IBM SPSS Statistics for Windows 20 (IBM Corp., Armonk, NY, USA).

Association parameters for the imputed SNP variants surrounding the GWAS risk SNPs (according to an additive inheritance model) were obtained by Cox proportional hazards regression analyses performed with ProbABEL v0.1-3 from the GenABEL suite of programs. [27] The Cox proportional hazards model (*pacoxph* function) implemented in the ProbABEL-package makes use of the source code of the R package "survival" as implemented by T. Lumley. Regional association plots were drawn using LocusZoom software. [28]

Results

Non-muscle invasive bladder cancer (NMIBC)

Among the total study population of 1,602 UBC patients, 1,327 were diagnosed with NMIBC (stages Ta, T1, CIS). Thirty patients were excluded because they were previously or simultaneously diagnosed with cancer of the upper urinary tract. In addition, nine patients were excluded because the recurrence and progression status could not be validly assessed based on the medical file review. Finally, we excluded 19 NMIBC patients who had an immediate radical cystectomy (see Table S1 for patient and tumor characteristics). The median time between date of the initial TURT and date of the last urological check-up visit of the remaining 1,269 NMIBC patients was 5.3 (interquartile range (IQR): 3.7–8.7) years. Demographic and clinicopathological characteristics of both the NMIBC and MIBC group are shown in Table 2.

Association of UBC susceptibility loci with disease recurrence. Median time at risk for recurrence of the 1,269 included NMIBC patients was 2.9 years. During the first 5 years after the primary UBC diagnosis, 601 (Kaplan-Meier 5-year risk: 51.3%) NMIBC patients experienced disease recurrence. None of the 12 genetic variants examined showed a statistically significant association with RFS at the Bonferroni-adjusted or nominal significance level (P<0.05) (see Table 3).

Association of UBC susceptibility loci with disease progression. Median time at risk for progression of the 1,269 NMIBC patients was 4.9 years. 195 NMIBC patients (Kaplan-Meier 5-year risk: 17.2%) experienced disease progression during the first five years after the primary UBC diagnosis. One of the 12 genetic variants, *i.e.* rs9642880 at the *MYC* (v-myc avian myelocytomatosis viral oncogene homolog) locus showed a statistically significant association with the risk of disease progression (P for trend = 2.6×10^{-3}). The genotype-specific results suggest a recessive mode of action (GG vs. TT: HR = 1.81 (95% confidence interval (CI): 1.23–2.66)), with no evidence of a difference in progression risk between GT heterozygotes and TT homozygotes (see Table 3 and Figure 1). With a stricter progression definition, *i.e.*, transition from NMIBC (Ta/T1/CIS)

Table 2. Demographic and clinicopathological characteristics of included NMIBC and MIBC patients

N (%)		NMIBC	MIBC
		N = 1,269	N = 273
Male gender		1,065 (84)	196 (72)
Median age (range)		64 (25–92)	64 (27–93)
Smoking status	Never cigarette smoker	189 (15)	30 (11)
	Ever cigarette smoker	887 (70)	165 (60)
	Unknown	193 (15)	78 (29)
Tumor stage	0a	866 (68)	-
	0is	50 (4)	-
	I	336 (26)	-
	II	-	136 (50)
	III	-	50 (18)
	IV	-	87 (32)
	Unknown	17 (1.3)	-
Tumor grade	Low grade	775 (61)	15 (5.5)
	High grade	481 (38)	236 (86)
	Unknown	13 (1.0)	22 (8.1)
Tumor aggressiveness	Low risk of progression	703 (55)	-
	High risk of progression	552 (44)	-
	Unknown	14 (1.1)	-
Tumor histology	UCC	1,257 (99)	240 (88)
	SCC	-	11 (4.0)
	AC	1 (0.1)	9 (3.3)
	Other	2 (0.2)	11 (4.0)
	Unknown	9 (0.7)	2 (0.7)
Tumor size	<3 cm	181 (14)	15 (5.5)
	≥3 cm	93 (7.3)	39 (14)
	Unknown	995 (78)	219 (80)
Tumor focality	Solitary	699 (55)	179 (66)
	Multifocal	490 (39)	68 (25)
	Unknown	80 (6.3)	26 (9.5)
Initial treatment NMIBC	TURT only (± one immediate p.o. i.v. CT instillation)	552 (44)	-
	TURT + adjuvant i.v. CT	392 (31)	-
	TURT + adjuvant i.v. IT	248 (20)	-
	TURT + both adjuvant i.v. CT and IT	26 (2.1)	-
	Other	3 (0.2)	-
	Unknown	48 (3.8)	-
Initial treatment MIBC[a]	Curative intent	-	186 (68)
	Palliative intent	-	87 (32)

UCC: urothelial cell carcinoma; SCC: squamous cell carcinoma; AC: adenocarcinoma; p.o.: post-operative; i.v.: intravesical; CT: chemotherapy; IT: immunotherapy
[a]curative intent corresponds to treatment of tumors of stage T2-T4a with N0/NX and M0/MX; palliative intent corresponds to treatment of tumors of stage T4(b) or any T with N≥1/N+ and/or M1

to muscle-invasive disease (≥T2) (60 events within 5 years of diagnosis; Kaplan-Meier 5-year risk: 5.5%), the association of rs9642880 became even more pronounced and increased risk of progression was observed among both heterozygous and homozygous carriers of the G allele (GT vs TT: HR = 1.49 (95% CI: 0.72–3.08) and GG vs. TT: HR = 3.15 (95% CI: 1.50–6.61), P for trend = 1.32×10^{-3}). In addition, the stricter progression definition revealed nominal evidence for increased risk of progression among carriers of the rs710521 [G] allele (AG vs. AA: HR = 1.52 (95% CI: 0.89–2.61) and GG vs. AA: HR = 2.84 (95% CI: 1.24–6.51), P for trend = 0.01) in NMIBC patients. None of the other risk variants were nominally or statistically significantly associated with time to progression.

Subgroup analysis according to tumor aggressiveness. For several of the susceptibility loci, the etiologic link with bladder cancer was previously reported to be specific for (or most prominent among) the group with low or high risk of progression. Therefore, we also evaluated whether the

Table 3. Association of confirmed UBC susceptibility variants with NMIBC recurrence and progression

SNP/CNV	Genotype	Disease recurrence (N = 1,269)[a]			Disease progression (N = 1,269)[a]		
		N (n events)	HR (95% CI)	P trend	N (n events)	HR (95% CI)	P trend
rs9642880	TT	355 (180)	Ref.	0.98	355 (46)	Ref.	2.6×10^{-3}
	GT	637 (281)	0.84 (0.70–1.01)		637 (88)	1.08 (0.76–1.54)	
	GG	269 (135)	1.03 (0.82–1.28)		269 (59)	1.81 (1.23–2.66)	
rs710521	AA	732 (357)	Ref.	0.23	732 (107)	Ref.	0.25
	AG	468 (212)	0.88 (0.75–1.05)		468 (74)	1.09 (0.81–1.46)	
	GG	68 (31)	0.94 (0.65–1.36)		68 (14)	1.42 (0.82–2.49)	
rs2294008[b]	CC	323 (144)	Ref.	0.16	323 (50)	Ref.	0.97
	CT	699 (332)	1.09 (0.90–1.33)		699 (107)	0.97 (0.69–1.36)	
	TT	246 (125)	1.19 (0.94–1.51)		246 (38)	1.00 (0.65–1.52)	
rs798766	CC	747 (339)	Ref.	0.12	747 (118)	Ref.	0.40
	CT	452 (229)	1.17 (0.99–1.39)		452 (69)	0.96 (0.71–1.29)	
	TT	69 (33)	1.10 (0.77–1.57)		69 (8)	0.69 (0.34–1.42)	
rs401681	CC	436 (212)	Ref.	0.76	436 (73)	Ref.	0.35
	CT	633 (293)	0.89 (0.74–1.06)		633 (94)	0.87 (0.64–1.18)	
	TT	199 (96)	1.02 (0.80–1.29)		199 (28)	0.84 (0.54–1.30)	
rs2736098	GG	482 (211)	Ref.	0.36	482 (60)	Ref.	0.12
	AG	408 (198)	1.12 (0.92–1.36)		408 (64)	1.28 (0.90–1.82)	
	AA	100 (46)	1.08 (0.78–1.48)		100 (17)	1.39 (0.81–2.39)	
rs11892031[c]	AA	1063 (502)	Ref.	0.56	1063 (160)	Ref.	0.44
	AC	201 (95)	1.01 (0.81–1.26)		201 (34)	1.15 (0.79–1.66)	
	CC	5 (4)	2.43 (0.91–6.50)		5 (1)	1.36 (0.19–9.71)	
rs8102137	TT	535 (252)	Ref.	0.67	535 (77)	Ref.	0.20
	CT	580 (273)	0.98 (0.83–1.17)		580 (88)	1.05 (0.77–1.42)	
	CC	146 (71)	1.10 (0.84–1.43)		146 (28)	1.40 (0.91–2.15)	
rs1014971	AA	564 (273)	Ref.	0.46	564 (81)	Ref.	0.43
	AG	585 (274)	0.95 (0.80–1.12)		585 (95)	1.15 (0.86–1.55)	
	GG	119 (54)	0.92 (0.68–1.23)		119 (19)	1.12 (0.68–1.84)	
rs1058396	GG	381 (170)	Ref.	0.22	381 (55)	Ref.	0.36
	AG	625 (296)	1.05 (0.87–1.27)		625 (93)	1.03 (0.74–1.43)	
	AA	262 (135)	1.16 (0.92–1.45)		262 (47)	1.21 (0.82–1.79)	
rs1495741[d]	GG/AG	457 (207)	Ref.	0.25	457 (71)	Ref.	1.00
	AA	811 (394)	1.10 (0.93–1.31)		811 (124)	1.00 (0.75–1.34)	
GSTM1 deletion	+/+ and +/−	495 (226)	Ref.	0.16	495 (87)	Ref.	0.08
	−/−	680 (327)	1.13 (0.95–1.34)		680 (90)	0.77 (0.57–1.03)	

CNV: copy number variant; HR: hazard ratio; CI: confidence interval
[a]Presented effect estimates and statistical significance are based on univariable Cox proportional hazard regression;
[b]P for trend for independent rs2978974 SNP at the 8q24.3 locus is 0.75 and 0.83 in relation to NMIBC recurrence and progression, respectively;
[c]P for trend for causal risk variant (rs17863783) at the 2q37.1 locus is 0.36 and 0.85 in relation to NMIBC recurrence and progression, respectively;
[d]rs1495741: tag SNP for NAT2 acetylation status (GG = rapid, AG = intermediate, AA = slow)

association with disease recurrence and progression for the 12 genetic variants varies between these NMIBC subgroups. We adjusted for any remaining treatment variability within the two NMIBC subgroups. After restriction to NMIBC with known type of initial treatment, 672 were classified as 'at low risk of progression', and 534 as 'at high risk of progression', while for 12 cases aggressiveness could not be determined. Five-year risk of recurrence is 48% and 52% among low and high risk cases, respectively (indicating that tumor aggressiveness is not a good classifier for the risk of recurrence). With respect to progression, five-year risk varies between 9% among low risk and 26% among high risk cases. The stratified analysis did not reveal statistically significant associations in either of the subgroups, not for recurrence and not for progression; some suggestive findings of (borderline) nominal significance were found (see Table S2).

Effect modification by smoking status. Because of their involvement in the detoxification of xenobiotic and carcinogenic substances (including constituents of cigarette smoke, the main UBC risk factor), we also evaluated the association of NAT2 acetylation status, GSTM1 CNV, and of the rs11892031 SNP (in the UDP glucuronosyltransferase 1 family, polypeptide A complex locus (UGT1A) cluster) with NMIBC prognosis according to

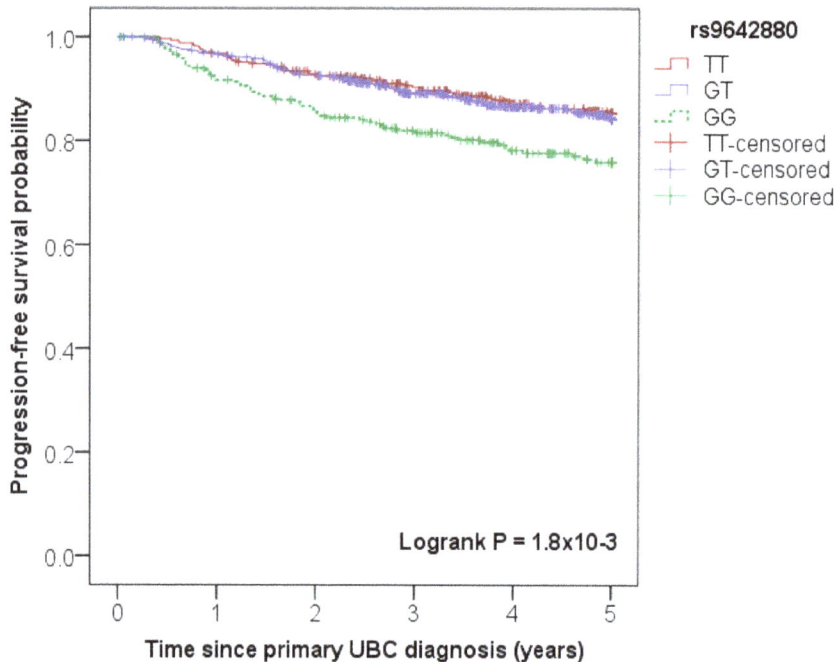

Figure 1. Association between rs9642880 (*MYC* locus) and progression-free survival in NMIBC patients. Kaplan-Meier survival plot showing association between rs9642880 genotype and progression-free survival (PFS) of non-muscle invasive bladder cancer (NMIBC) patients.

smoking status (see Table 4). Data on self-reported smoking status and type of initial treatment was available for 1,035 NMIBC patients (852 and 183 ever and never (cigarette) smokers, respectively). The analyses revealed some evidence for an elevated risk of disease recurrence in *NAT2* slow acetylators compared to patients with an intermediate or rapid acetylation status specifically among ever smokers (rs1495741 AA vs. AG/GG: $HR_{adj.}$ = 1.29 (1.04–1.61), P for trend = 0.02). Besides, among never smokers, *NAT2* slow acetylation status was found to correlate with a decreased risk of disease progression compared to intermediate/rapid acetylators ($HR_{adj.}$ = 0.42 (0.19–0.93), P for trend = 0.03). No evidence for effect modification by smoking status was found for the association between *GSTM1* CNV or rs11892031 and NMIBC prognosis.

Interestingly, an exploratory analysis for the other susceptibility loci indicated association of rs798766 at the 4p16.3 (*TACC3-FGFR3*) locus with the risk of disease recurrence specifically among never smoking NMIBC patients (never cigarette smokers: CT vs. CC: $HR_{adj.}$ = 2.71 (95% CI: 1.73–4.24) and TT vs. CC: $HR_{adj.}$ = 2.43 (95% CI: 0.73–8.05), P for trend = 2.7×10^{-5}; ever cigarette smokers: CT vs. CC: $HR_{adj.}$ = 1.07 (95% CI: 0.86–1.32) and TT vs. CC: $HR_{adj.}$ = 0.98 (95% CI: 0.63–1.52), P for trend = 0.75) (see Table 4 and Figure 2).

Prognostic analysis of genetic risk score. In addition to evaluation of the prognostic relevance of the UBC susceptibility variants at the single-SNP level, we assessed their cumulative (additive) effect on NMIBC prognosis by testing association with the overall number of UBC risk alleles (*i.e.*, the genetic risk score). After restriction to patients with complete genotype data for all 12 variants and known treatment type, 872 NMIBC patients (390 recurrence and 117 progression events) were included. The majority of ineligible patients for this analysis were due to a missing genotype for the rs2736098 SNP (N = 279: not included in Centaurus assay [22]) or the *GSTM1* CNV (N = 94; insufficient DNA amount or CNV analysis failed). This analysis indicated a

trend towards a slightly worse RFS ($HR_{adj.}$ = 1.05 (95% CI: 1.00–1.10, P for trend = 0.05) with each extra risk allele carried. This translates into a ~1,3-fold and 1,6-fold increased risk of recurrence among carriers of 5 and 10 risk alleles (compared to patients with zero UBC risk alleles), respectively. No association was observed between the genetic risk score and PFS among NMIBC patients ($HR_{adj.}$ = 0.99 (95% CI: 0.91–1.07), P for trend = 0.77).

Muscle-invasive and metastatic bladder cancer (MIBC)

The Nijmegen Bladder Cancer Study contains 275 MIBC patients. Two patients were excluded from the analysis because they were previously or simultaneously diagnosed with cancer of the upper urinary tract.

Association of UBC susceptibility loci with overall survival. Median time at risk for overall death of the 273 MIBC patients was 6.8 (IQR: 3.1–11)) years. During the first 5 years after the primary diagnosis, 81 of the MIBC patients (Kaplan-Meier 5-year risk: 29.9%) died. None of the 12 variants evaluated was found to be associated with OS at the Bonferroni-adjusted statistical significance level (see Table 5). *GSTM1* CNV showed a statistically significant association with OS at the nominal P<0.05: HR = 1.70 (95% CI: 1.04–2.79) for the patients with the null genotype versus all others. The association lost nominal significance however, after adjustment for the survival difference between patients with extended/metastasized and localized cancer (see Table 5). Because of the small sample size, no subgroup analyses were performed.

Regional association analysis

The evaluation of the association of (measured and imputed) genetic variants within a 200 kb region centered on each of the 10 GWAS-identified susceptibility SNPs did not reveal an association at the statistical significance threshold P<1×10^{-4} (on average ~500 variants in 200 kb region) for any of the genetic markers in

Table 4. Association of selected UBC susceptibility variants with NMIBC recurrence and progression by smoking status.

SNP/CNV	Genotype	Disease recurrence[a]						Disease progression[a]					
		Never (cigarette) smokers (N=183)			Ever (cigarette) smokers (N=852)			Never (cigarette) smokers (N=183)			Ever (cigarette) smokers (N=852)		
		N (n events)	HR (95% CI)	P trend	N (n events)	HR (95% CI)	P trend	N (n events)	HR (95% CI)	P trend	N (n events)	HR (95% CI)	P trend
rs1495741[b]	GG/AG	60 (23)	ref.	0.63	302 (119)	ref.	0.02	60 (13)	ref.	0.03	302 (34)	ref.	0.27
	AA	123 (58)	1.13 (0.69-1.83)		549 (258)	1.29 (1.04-1.61)		123 (13)	0.42 (0.19-0.93)		549 (78)	1.26 (0.84-1.89)	
GSTM1 del.	+/+ and +/−	74 (31)	ref.	0.25	335 (141)	ref.	0.42	74 (12)	ref.	0.86	335 (48)	ref.	0.29
	−/−	96 (44)	1.32 (0.83-2.11)		457 (203)	1.09 (0.88-1.36)		96 (12)	0.93 (0.42-2.09)		457 (50)	0.81 (0.54-1.20)	
rs11892031	AA	154 (68)	ref.	0.88	712 (316)	ref.	0.95	154 (23)	ref.	0.60	712 (91)	ref.	0.37
	AC	27 (12)	0.97 (0.52-1.80)		138 (59)	0.95 (0.72-1.26)		27 (3)	0.77 (0.23-2.58)		138 (21)	1.28 (0.79-2.07)	
	CC	2 (1)	1.88 (0.25-14)		2 (2)	2.08 (0.52-8.40)		2 (0)	C.E.		2 (0)	C.E.	
rs798766[c]	CC	119 (39)	ref.	2.7×10^{-5}	497 (216)	ref.	0.75	119 (11)	ref.	0.09	497 (68)	ref.	0.93
	CT	59 (39)	**2.71 (1.73-4.24)**		304 (139)	1.07 (0.86-1.32)		59 (14)	2.50 (1.14-5.52)		304 (38)	1.05 (0.70-1.56)	
	TT	5 (3)	**2.43 (0.73-8.05)**		50 (22)	0.98 (0.63-1.52)		5 (1)	1.14 (0.15-9.02)		50 (6)	0.86 (0.37-1.99)	

CNV: copy number variant; del. = deletion; C.E.: converging error; HR: hazard ratio; CI: confidence interval
[a]Presented effect estimates and statistical significance are based on multivariable Cox proportional hazard regression analyses with adjustment for treatment (TURT + both adjuvant i.v. CT and IT vs. CT and IT vs. TURT + adjuvant i.v. CT vs. TURT only (± one direct p.o. i.v. CT instillation)); IT vs. IT vs. TURT + adjuvant i.v. IT vs. TURT
[b]rs1495741: tag SNP for NAT2 acetylation status (GG = rapid, AG = intermediate, AA = slow);
[c]based on exploratory analysis

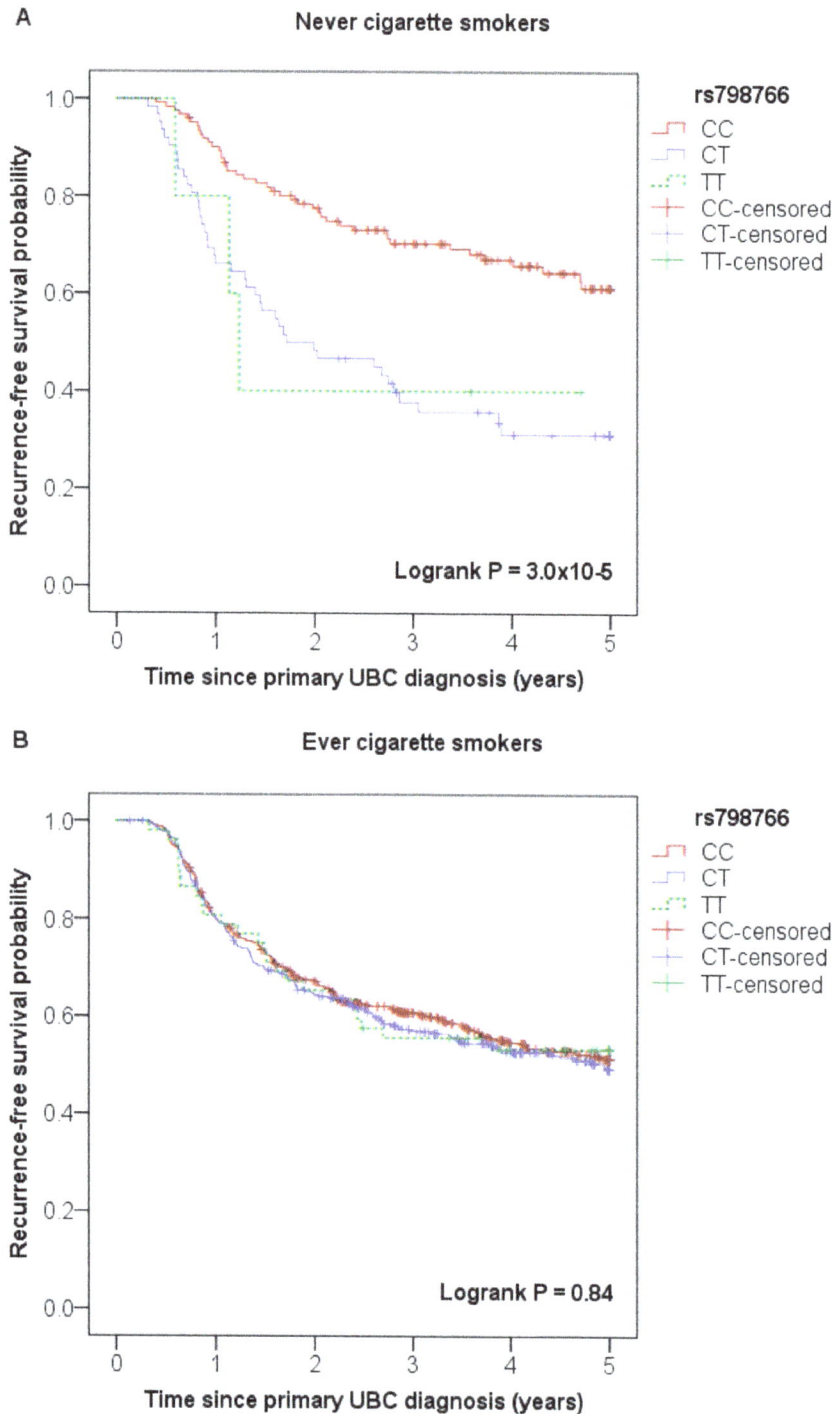

Figure 2. Association between rs798766 (*TACC3/FGFR3* locus) and recurrence-free survival in NMIBC patients by smoking status. Kaplan-Meier survival plots showing association between rs798766 genotype and recurrence-free survival (RFS) in **A**) never cigarette smokers (Logrank P = 3.0×10^{-5}) and **B**) ever cigarette smokers (Logrank P = 0.84) with non-muscle invasive bladder cancer (NMIBC).

relation to the endpoints RFS and PFS in the overall NMIBC subgroup (see Figure S1 and S2) and OS in the MIBC subgroup.

For the *MYC* locus, rs9642880 shows the second strongest association signal; rs10094872 shows a slightly stronger association signal with the risk of NMIBC progression (P = 1.8×10^{-3}; r^2 between the two SNPs based on 1000G Pilot 1 CEU data = 0.54). After adjusting for the effect of rs9642880, the association of rs10094872 lost strength in terms of the HR and statistical

significance (P = 0.25). The same holds for the association of rs9642880 (P = 0.37) conditional on the effect of rs10098472, indicating that both variants represent the same association signal.

Discussion

There is increasing evidence that the same genes or genetic variants could be implicated in both cancer predisposition, disease

Table 5. Association of confirmed UBC susceptibility variants with overall mortality among MIBC patients.

SNP/CNV	Genotype	N (n events)	Unadjusted (N = 273)		Adjusted[a] (N = 273)	
			HR (95% CI)	P trend	HR (95% CI)	P trend
rs9642880	TT	63 (18)	Ref.	0.69	Ref.	0.56
	GT	139 (39)	0.94 (0.54–1.64)		0.86 (0.49–1.50)	
	GG	70 (23)	1.12 (0.61–2.08)		1.18 (0.64–2.18)	
rs710521	AA	152 (50)	Ref.	0.16	Ref.	0.12
	AG	101 (27)	0.77 (0.48–1.23)		0.88 (0.55–1.41)	
	GG	20 (4)	0.59 (0.21–1.63)		0.52 (0.19–1.45)	
rs2294008[b]	CC	79 (18)	Ref.	0.22	Ref.	0.25
	CT	133 (43)	1.45 (0.84–2.52)		1.22 (0.70–2.13)	
	TT	61 (20)	1.48 (0.78–2.79)		1.45 (0.77–2.74)	
rs798766	CC	178 (49)	Ref.	0.21	Ref.	0.28
	CT	85 (27)	1.13 (0.71–1.80)		1.03 (0.65–1.65)	
	TT	10 (5)	2.14 (0.85–5.37)		2.41 (0.96–6.05)	
rs401681	CC	100 (24)	Ref.	0.13	Ref.	0.29
	CT	114 (36)	1.29 (0.77–2.17)		1.23 (0.73–2.06)	
	TT	59 (21)	1.56 (0.87–2.79)		1.39 (0.76–2.45)	
rs2736098	GG	99 (31)	Ref.	0.10	Ref.	0.35
	AG	80 (15)	0.54 (0.29–0.99)		0.64 (0.34–1.19)	
	AA	18 (4)	0.68 (0.24–1.93)		0.95 (0.33–2.72)	
rs11892031[c]	AA	243 (69)	Ref.	0.20	Ref.	0.20
	AC	30 (12)	1.50 (0.81–2.76)		1.49 (0.81–2.75)	
	CC	0 (0)	NA		NA	
rs8102137	TT	107 (34)	Ref.	0.49	Ref.	0.57
	CT	130 (38)	0.92 (0.58–1.45)		0.93 (0.59–1.48)	
	CC	36 (9)	0.77 (0.37–1.61)		0.81 (0.39–1.69)	
rs1014971	AA	123 (34)	Ref.	0.97	Ref.	0.92
	AG	124 (41)	1.20 (0.76–1.89)		1.05 (0.66–1.66)	
	GG	26 (6)	0.79 (0.33–1.89)		0.87 (0.37–2.08)	
rs1058396	GG	78 (28)	Ref.	0.29	Ref.	0.45
	AG	137 (37)	0.73 (0.44–1.19)		0.69 (0.42–1.13)	
	AA	58 (16)	0.75 (0.41–1.39)		0.85 (0.46–1.57)	
rs1495741[d]	GG/AG	92 (32)	Ref.	0.17	Ref.	0.09
	AA	181 (49)	0.73 (0.47–1.14)		0.68 (0.43–1.06)	
GSTM1 deletion	+/+ and +/−	104 (23)	Ref.	0.03	Ref.	0.09
	−/−	146 (51)	1.70 (1.04–2.79)		1.53 (0.93–2.51)	

CNV: copy number variant; HR: hazard ratio; CI: confidence interval;
[a]with adjustment for extended/metastasized (*i.e.*, primary stage T4(b) ór any T with N+/N≥1 and/or M1) *vs.* localized disease (*i.e.*, primary stage T2-T4a with N0/NX and M0/MX) in multivariable Cox proportional hazard regression analyses;
[b]P for trend (unadjusted) for independent rs2978974 SNP at the 8q24.3 locus is 0.16;
[c]P for trend (unadjusted) for causal risk variant (rs17863783) at the 2q37.1 locus is 0.92;
[d]rs1495741: tag SNP for *NAT2* acetylation status (GG = rapid, AG = intermediate, AA = slow)

prognosis, and treatment response. So far, this interrelatedness at the genetic level is particularly observed for genes involved in well-known oncogenic pathways such as xenobiotic metabolism, DNA repair, and cell cycle control. [29,30] In addition, several GWAS-identified cancer susceptibility loci (several with yet unknown mechanism) have been found to play a role in cancer prognosis. [14–21] This is the first comprehensive evaluation of the prognostic relevance of all confirmed UBC susceptibility loci.

Based on this study, for only one of the investigated UBC susceptibility loci an association with disease prognosis was identified which passed the multiple testing threshold. This main finding indicated an effect of the rs9642880 SNP at the *MYC* locus on PFS in the overall group of NMIBC patients. Patients with the rs9642880 GG genotype experienced an increased risk of disease progression compared to patients with the GT or TT genotype. Various etiological studies (including the initial GWAS) have indicated consistently that the risk of UBC is increased for carriers of the rs9642880[T] allele, which was most pronounced for low grade Ta tumors. [23,31–35] This etiologic link of rs9642880[T] with a less aggressive type of UBC could explain the decreased risk of progression in carriers of this allele. However, we do observe the decreased risk of progression in both the low and high risk of progression subgroups. This implies that within these risk strata rs9642880[T] confers an additional beneficial influence on the clinical disease course. Studies in other cancer types show an association for other (independent) SNPs in the 8q24 chromosomal region with disease aggressiveness and/or clinical outcome. [14,36–41] This strengthens the importance of unraveling the mystery of this 8q24 locus, a so-called gene desert, which seems to be involved in the susceptibility and clinical disease course of multiple cancer types. In addition to validation in an independent patient population, it requires further investigation whether the association that we found is mediated through a long-range, regulatory effect on the 30 kb upstream located *MYC* protooncogene, or through another biological mechanism. [42,43]

Previously, in one of the publications based on our GWAS for bladder cancer risk, we described association of the rs798766[T] allele (*TACC3/FGFR3* locus) with an increased risk of disease recurrence among low-stage low-grade NMIBC cases. [21] We do observe a similar trend in this paper (low risk of progression subgroup: CT vs. CC: $HR_{adj.}$ = 1.27 (95% CI: 1.00–1.61), and TT vs. CC: $HR_{adj.}$ = 1.18 (95% CI: 0.71–1.94), P for trend = 0.09). However the association is less pronounced and does not pass the significance threshold. This difference in effect estimates may be explained by the fact that this analysis and the previous GWAS analysis are based on only a partly overlapping patient series and use a slightly different recurrence definition. Also, in our current evaluation, we adjusted for the independent effect of treatment among the strata according to tumor aggressiveness. Based on an exploratory analysis, we found indications that the association between rs798766 and NMIBC recurrence might be mediated by smoking status, but this has to be confirmed by other studies.

For several other susceptibility loci, our study provides suggestive evidence for an association with UBC prognosis, especially in subgroup analyses, which could reflect the different molecular pathways that play a role in different disease subtypes. We presented the association results in this paper, but do not discuss them in further detail here as these findings first require replication in independent UBC patient series. Evaluation among the MIBC subgroup is hampered by the relatively small sample size. Future analyses should be performed in larger patient series that allow analyses in relevant subgroups with respect to disease stage and treatment.

Our prognostic evaluation based on a cumulative genetic risk score suggests that UBC risk loci might collectively influence NMIBC recurrence. This finding may be due to a cumulative effect of multiple small increases in recurrence risk conferred by several of the susceptibility variants.

Where classification of NMIBC patients into two risk strata with respect to tumor aggressiveness resulted in reasonable discrimination in the risk of progression in our cohort, it appeared to be a poor classifier for disease recurrence. Lack of data on tumor size and exact tumor number (two important recurrence predictors in the EORTC risk model but characteristics that are poorly documented in medical charts) for a large proportion of patients limited us in our possibilities to improve prognostic risk classification. Risk group stratification according to European Association of Urology (EAU) guidelines (*i.e.*, low, intermediate, high risk) resulted in too low event numbers to perform valid prognostic evaluation. [44] Consequently, the 'low risk of progression' subgroup contains a mix of low and intermediate risk cases, which could have diminished the power to detect subgroup-specific associations. However, we adjusted for remaining treatment variability among both risk strata, and thereby expect to have (indirectly) corrected for the correlated prognostic variables incorporated in the EORTC scoring system. In contrast to data underlying the EORTC prediction model, this study focused on primary bladder cancers (no prior recurrences), which most likely diminished variability in recurrence risk due to lack of cases at the higher end of the spectrum.

Major strengths of this study are the population-based nature, the relatively large sample size, and the medical file review of all patients. A weakness of the study is the prevalent sampling frame of part of the study cohort, which might have led to a relatively healthy study population with possible implications for the generalizability of our study findings to all UBC patients. We expect that this selection is negligible in NMIBC patients, especially with respect to the endpoint recurrence. The relatively high five-year OS in the MIBC subgroup (~70%) could reflect the effect of prevalent case sampling. The selection of patients with a less severe disease course could have resulted in some bias in the effect size measures.

With exception of our finding for the *MYC* locus, this study provides only suggestive evidence that genetic loci involved in UBC etiology have prognostic relevance. Replication studies in independent UBC series are necessary to confirm our findings, and should include evaluation among (disease) subgroups. Elucidation of the causal mechanism in functional analyses will further our understanding of the disease, might eventually point the way to potential new therapeutic targets, and could aid in further improvement of prognostic risk discrimination.

Note

After acceptance of this research paper, Figueroa *et al.* [48] reported on two new GWAS-identified UBC susceptibility loci. We included the association results of these two UBC risk variants (*i.e.*, rs10936599 (3q26.2) and rs907611 (11p15.5)) with disease prognosis in File S1. For both variants, we did not observe association with clinical outcome that passed the Bonferroni-adjusted statistical significance threshold, in both the NMIBC and MIBC subgroup.

Supporting Information

Figure S1 Regional association plots for NMIBC recurrence of 200 kb region centered on 10 GWAS-identified susceptibility SNPs. **A–J**) In the above plots, directly genotyped and imputed single-nucleotide polymorphisms (SNPs) distributed in a 200 kb region centered on each of the 10 respective GWAS-identified urinary bladder cancer (UBC) susceptibility SNPs are depicted by filled circles. For each SNP, the chromosomal location (NCBI Build 36/hg18) is shown on the x-axis and the significance level for association with non-muscle invasive bladder cancer (NMIBC) recurrence is indicated by a $-\log_{10}$ P-value on the left y-axis. In each plot, the GWAS-identified UBC susceptibility SNP at the respective locus is represented by a purple diamond. Local linkage disequilibrium (LD) structure is reflected by the plotted estimated recombination rates from 1000 Genomes Pilot June 2010 CEU (light blue line, right y-axis). The level of correlation (LD) of the UBC susceptibility SNP to other SNPs at the locus (pair wise r^2 values) are indicated by a color range from dark blue to red (see legend). SNPs with missing LD information are shown in grey. Below the graph, gene annotations are shown as horizontal dark blue lines. Regional association plots are shown for the **A**) 2q37.1 locus (rs11892031): most significant association for rs116323695 (P = 2.35E-02), **B**) 3q28 locus (rs710521): most significant association for rs3773928 (P = 2.03E-03), **C**) 4p16.3 locus (rs798766): most significant association for rs73081713 (P = 5.09E-03), **D**) 5p15.33 locus (rs2736098): most significant association for rs6420010 (P = 6.55E-03), **E**) 5p15.33 locus (rs401681): most significant association for rs116612249 (P = 8.29E-03), **F**) 8q24.3 locus (rs2294008): most significant association for rs118159558 (P = 2.33E-03), **G**) 8q24.21 locus (rs9642880): most significant association for rs80238840 (P = 7.65E-03), **H**) 18q12.3 locus (rs1058396): most significant association for rs8088466 (P = 7.72E-03), **I**) 19q12 locus (rs8102137): most significant association for rs117125197 (P = 6.16E-02), **J**) 22q13.1 locus (rs1014971): most significant association for rs7584 (P = 1.3E-02).

Figure S2 Regional association plots for NMIBC progression of 200 kb region centered on 10 GWAS-identified susceptibility SNPs. **A–J**) In the above plots, directly genotyped and imputed single-nucleotide polymorphisms (SNPs) distributed in a 200 kb region centered on each of the 10 respective GWAS-identified urinary bladder cancer (UBC) susceptibility SNPs are depicted by filled circles. For each SNP, the chromosomal location (NCBI Build 36/hg18) is shown on the x-axis and the significance level for association with non-muscle invasive bladder cancer (NMIBC) progression is indicated by a -$\log_{10}$ P-value on the left y-axis. In each plot, the GWAS-identified UBC susceptibility SNP at the respective locus is represented by a purple diamond. Local linkage disequilibrium (LD) structure is reflected by the plotted estimated recombination rates from 1000 Genomes Pilot June 2010 CEU (light blue line, right y-axis). The level of correlation (LD) of the UBC susceptibility SNP to other SNPs at the locus (pair wise r^2 values) are indicated by a color range from dark blue to red (see legend). SNPs with missing LD information are shown in grey. Below the graph, gene annotations are shown as horizontal dark blue lines. Regional association plots are shown for the **A**) 2q37.1 locus (rs11892031): most significant association for rs13009407 (P = 3.24E-03), **B**) 3q28 locus (rs710521): most significant association for rs76380205 (P = 5.07E-03), **C**) 4p16.3 locus (rs798766): most significant association for rs73081713

(P = 9.29E-03), **D**) 5p15.33 locus (rs2736098): most significant association for rs246993 (P = 2.49E-03), · **E**) 5p15.33 locus (rs401681): most significant association for rs246993 (P = 2.49E-03), **F**) 8q24.3 locus (rs2294008): most significant association for rs73716487 (P = 3.26E-04), **G**) 8q24.21 locus (rs9642880): most significant association for rs10094872 (P = 1.83E-03), **H**) 18q12.3 locus (rs1058396): most significant association for rs12454702 (P = 8.85E-03), **I**) 19q12 locus (rs8102137): most significant association for rs16963425 (P = 5.46E-02), **J**) 22q13.1 locus (rs1014971): most significant association for rs7289061 (P = 2.25E-04).

File S1 Association of two newly confirmed GWAS-identified UBC susceptibility variants with UBC prognosis.

Table S1 Descriptive characteristics of excluded NMIBC patients with immediate radical cystectomy (N = 19).

Table S2 Association of UBC susceptibility variants with NMIBC recurrence and progression by tumor aggressiveness.

Text S1 Detailed description of prognostic endpoint definitions.

Acknowledgments

We would like to thank all the participants in the study for their willingness to provide blood samples for genotyping. We thank our collaborators from deCODE Genetics in Reykjavik for all the genotyping.

Author Contributions

Conceived and designed the experiments: AG SV LK. Performed the experiments: AG AD GV JAW KA SvdM SV LK. Analyzed the data: AG. Wrote the paper: AG SV LK. Performed CNV genotyping: SvdM. Critically reviewed the manuscript: AD GV KA SvdM JAW.

References

1. Sylvester RJ (2011) How well can you actually predict which non-muscle-invasive bladder cancer patients will progress? Eur Urol 60: 431–433; discussion 433–434.
2. Tilki D, Burger M, Dalbagni G, Grossman HB, Hakenberg OW, et al. (2011) Urine markers for detection and surveillance of non-muscle-invasive bladder cancer. Eur Urol 60: 484–492.
3. van Rhijn BW (2012) Combining molecular and pathologic data to prognosticate non-muscle-invasive bladder cancer. Urol Oncol 30: 518–523.
4. Coate L, Cuffe S, Horgan A, Hung RJ, Christiani D, et al. (2010) Germline genetic variation, cancer outcome, and pharmacogenetics. J Clin Oncol 28: 4029–4037.
5. O'Donnell PH, Ratain MJ (2012) Germline pharmacogenomics in oncology: decoding the patient for targeting therapy. Mol Oncol 6: 251–259.
6. Wang L, McLeod HL, Weinshilboum RM (2011) Genomics and drug response. N Engl J Med 364: 1144–1153.
7. Wheeler HE, Maitland ML, Dolan ME, Cox NJ, Ratain MJ (2013) Cancer pharmacogenomics: strategies and challenges. Nat Rev Genet 14: 23–34.
8. Chen M, Hildebrandt MA, Clague J, Kamat AM, Picornell A, et al. (2010) Genetic variations in the sonic hedgehog pathway affect clinical outcomes in non-muscle-invasive bladder cancer. Cancer Prev Res (Phila) 3: 1235–1245.
9. Ke HL, Chen M, Ye Y, Hildebrandt MA, Wu WJ, et al. (2013) Genetic variations in micro-RNA biogenesis genes and clinical outcomes in non-muscle-invasive bladder cancer. Carcinogenesis 34: 1006–1011.
10. Chang DW, Gu J, Wu X (2012) Germline prognostic markers for urinary bladder cancer: obstacles and opportunities. Urol Oncol 30: 524–532.
11. Grotenhuis AJ, Vermeulen SH, Kiemeney LA (2010) Germline genetic markers for urinary bladder cancer risk, prognosis and treatment response. Future Oncol 6: 1433–1460.
12. Gu J, Wu X (2011) Genetic susceptibility to bladder cancer risk and outcome. Per Med 8: 365–374.
13. Rafnar T, Vermeulen SH, Sulem P, Thorleifsson G, Aben KK, et al. (2011) European genome-wide association study identifies SLC14A1 as a new urinary bladder cancer susceptibility gene. Hum Mol Genet 20: 4268–4281.
14. Dai J, Gu J, Huang M, Eng C, Kopetz ES, et al. (2012) GWAS-identified colorectal cancer susceptibility loci associated with clinical outcomes. Carcinogenesis 33: 1327–1331.
15. Fasching PA, Pharoah PD, Cox A, Nevanlinna H, Bojesen SE, et al. (2012) The role of genetic breast cancer susceptibility variants as prognostic factors. Hum Mol Genet 21: 3926–3939.
16. Gallagher DJ, Vijai J, Cronin AM, Bhatia J, Vickers AJ, et al. (2010) Susceptibility loci associated with prostate cancer progression and mortality. Clin Cancer Res 16: 2819–2832.
17. Rizzato C, Campa D, Giese N, Werner J, Rachakonda PS, et al. (2011) Pancreatic cancer susceptibility loci and their role in survival. PLoS One 6: e27921.
18. Shan J, Mahfoudh W, Dsouza SP, Hassen E, Bouaouina N, et al. (2012) Genome-Wide Association Studies (GWAS) breast cancer susceptibility loci in Arabs: susceptibility and prognostic implications in Tunisians. Breast Cancer Res Treat 135: 715–724.
19. Xing J, Myers RE, He X, Qu F, Zhou F, et al. (2011) GWAS-identified colorectal cancer susceptibility locus associates with disease prognosis. Eur J Cancer 47: 1699–1707.
20. Xun WW, Brennan P, Tjonneland A, Vogel U, Overvad K, et al. (2011) Single-nucleotide polymorphisms (5p15.33, 15q25.1, 6p22.1, 6q27 and 7p15.3) and lung cancer survival in the European Prospective Investigation into Cancer and Nutrition (EPIC). Mutagenesis 26: 657–666.
21. Kiemeney LA, Sulem P, Besenbacher S, Vermeulen SH, Sigurdsson A, et al. (2010) A sequence variant at 4p16.3 confers susceptibility to urinary bladder cancer. Nat Genet 42: 415–419.
22. Rafnar T, Sulem P, Stacey SN, Geller F, Gudmundsson J, et al. (2009) Sequence variants at the TERT-CLPTM1L locus associate with many cancer types. Nat Genet 41: 221–227.
23. Kiemeney LA, Thorlacius S, Sulem P, Geller F, Aben KK, et al. (2008) Sequence variant on 8q24 confers susceptibility to urinary bladder cancer. Nat Genet 40: 1307–1312.

24. Garcia-Closas M, Hein DW, Silverman D, Malats N, Yeager M, et al. (2011) A single nucleotide polymorphism tags variation in the arylamine N-acetyltransferase 2 phenotype in populations of European background. Pharmacogenet Genomics 21: 231–236.

25. Fu YP, Kohaar I, Rothman N, Earl J, Figueroa JD, et al. (2012) Common genetic variants in the PSCA gene influence gene expression and bladder cancer risk. Proc Natl Acad Sci U S A 109: 4974–4979.

26. Tang W, Fu YP, Figueroa JD, Malats N, Garcia-Closas M, et al. (2012) Mapping of the UGT1A locus identifies an uncommon coding variant that affects mRNA expression and protects from bladder cancer. Hum Mol Genet 21: 1918–1930.

27. Aulchenko YS, Struchalin MV, van Duijn CM (2010) ProbABEL package for genome-wide association analysis of imputed data. BMC Bioinformatics 11: 1–10.

28. Pruim RJ, Welch RP, Sanna S, Teslovich TM, Chines PS, et al. (2010) LocusZoom: Regional visualization of genome-wide association scan results. Bioinformatics 26: 2336–2337.

29. Savas S, Liu G (2009) Genetic variations as cancer prognostic markers: review and update. Hum Mutat 30: 1369–1377.

30. Spitz MR, Wu X, Mills G (2005) Integrative epidemiology: from risk assessment to outcome prediction. J Clin Oncol 23: 267–275.

31. Cortessis VK, Yuan JM, Van Den Berg D, Jiang X, Gago-Dominguez M, et al. (2010) Risk of urinary bladder cancer is associated with 8q24 variant rs9642880[T] in multiple racial/ethnic groups: results from the Los Angeles-Shanghai case-control study. Cancer Epidemiol Biomarkers Prev 19: 3150–3156.

32. Golka K, Hermes M, Selinski S, Blaszkewicz M, Bolt HM, et al. (2009) Susceptibility to urinary bladder cancer: relevance of rs9642880[T], GSTM1 0/0 and occupational exposure. Pharmacogenet Genomics 19: 903–906.

33. Ma Z, Hu Q, Chen Z, Tao S, Macnamara L, et al. (2013) Systematic evaluation of bladder cancer risk-associated single-nucleotide polymorphisms in a Chinese population. Mol Carcinog 52: 916–921.

34. Wang M, Wang M, Zhang W, Yuan L, Fu G, et al. (2009) Common genetic variants on 8q24 contribute to susceptibility to bladder cancer in a Chinese population. Carcinogenesis 30: 991–996.

35. Yates DR, Roupret M, Drouin SJ, Audouin M, Cancel-Tassin G, et al. (2013) Genetic polymorphisms on 8q24.1 and 4p16.3 are not linked with urothelial carcinoma of the bladder in contrast to their association with aggressive upper urinary tract tumours. World J Urol 31: 53–59.

36. Ahn J, Kibel AS, Park JY, Rebbeck TR, Rennert H, et al. (2011) Prostate cancer predisposition loci and risk of metastatic disease and prostate cancer recurrence. Clin Cancer Res 17: 1075–1081.

37. Bertucci F, Lagarde A, Ferrari A, Finetti P, Charafe-Jauffret E, et al. (2012) 8q24 Cancer risk allele associated with major metastatic risk in inflammatory breast cancer. PLoS One 7: e37943.

38. Hoskins JM, Ong PS, Keku TO, Galanko JA, Martin CF, et al. (2012) Association of eleven common, low-penetrance colorectal cancer susceptibility genetic variants at six risk loci with clinical outcome. PLoS One 7: e41954.

39. Suzuki M, Liu M, Kurosaki T, Suzuki M, Arai T, et al. (2011) Association of rs6983561 polymorphism at 8q24 with prostate cancer mortality in a Japanese population. Clin Genitourin Cancer 9: 46–52.

40. Takatsuno Y, Mimori K, Yamamoto K, Sato T, Niida A, et al. (2013) The rs6983267 SNP Is Associated with MYC Transcription Efficiency, Which Promotes Progression and Worsens Prognosis of Colorectal Cancer. Ann Surg Oncol 20: 1395–1402.

41. Zhang X, Chen Q, He C, Mao W, Zhang L, et al. (2012) Polymorphisms on 8q24 are associated with lung cancer risk and survival in Han Chinese. PLoS One 7: e41930.

42. Grisanzio C, Freedman ML (2010) Chromosome 8q24-Associated Cancers and MYC. Genes Cancer 1: 555–559.

43. Huppi K, Pitt JJ, Wahlberg BM, Caplen NJ (2012) The 8q24 gene desert: an oasis of non-coding transcriptional activity. Front Genet 3: 1–11.

44. Babjuk M, Burger M, Zigeuner R, Shariat SF, van Rhijn BW, et al. (2013) EAU Guidelines on Non-Muscle-invasive Urothelial Carcinoma of the Bladder: Update 2013. Eur Urol 64: 639–653.

45. Garcia-Closas M, Malats N, Silverman D, Dosemeci M, Kogevinas M, et al. (2005) NAT2 slow acetylation, GSTM1 null genotype, and risk of bladder cancer: results from the Spanish Bladder Cancer Study and meta-analyses. Lancet 366: 649–659.

46. Wu X, Ye Y, Kiemeney LA, Sulem P, Rafnar T, et al. (2009) Genetic variation in the prostate stem cell antigen gene PSCA confers susceptibility to urinary bladder cancer. Nat Genet 41: 991–995.

47. Rothman N, Garcia-Closas M, Chatterjee N, Malats N, Wu X, et al. (2010) A multi-stage genome-wide association study of bladder cancer identifies multiple susceptibility loci. Nat Genet 42: 978–984.

48. Figueroa JD, Ye Y, Siddiq A, Garcia-Closas M, Chatterjee N, et al. (2013) Genome-wide association study identifies multiple loci associated with bladder cancer risk. Hum Mol Genet doi:10.1093/hmg/ddt519.

20

Transcriptome Profiling of a Multiple Recurrent Muscle-Invasive Urothelial Carcinoma of the Bladder by Deep Sequencing

Shufang Zhang[1], Yanxuan Liu[2], Zhenxiang Liu[1], Chong Zhang[1], Hui Cao[1], Yongqing Ye[3], Shunlan Wang[1], Ying'ai Zhang[1], Sifang Xiao[1], Peng Yang[1], Jindong Li[1], Zhiming Bai[1]*

1 Affiliated Haikou Hospital, Xiangya School of Medicine Central South University, Haikou Municipal People's Hospital, Haikou, China, 2 Department of Genetic Disease, the First Affiliated Hospital of Xinxiang Medical University, Xinxiang, China, 3 Department of Shanghai Claison Bio-Technology, Shanghai, China

Abstract

Urothelial carcinoma of the bladder (UCB) is one of the commonly diagnosed cancers in the world. The UCB has the highest rate of recurrence of any malignancy. A genome-wide screening of transcriptome dysregulation between cancer and normal tissue would provide insight into the molecular basis of UCB recurrence and is a key step to discovering biomarkers for diagnosis and therapeutic targets. Compared with microarray technology, which is commonly used to identify expression level changes, the recently developed RNA-seq technique has the ability to detect other abnormal regulations in the cancer transcriptome, such as alternative splicing. In this study, we performed high-throughput transcriptome sequencing at ~50× coverage on a recurrent muscle-invasive cisplatin-resistance UCB tissue and the adjacent non-tumor tissue. The results revealed cancer-specific differentially expressed genes between the tumor and non-tumor tissue enriched in the cell adhesion molecules, focal adhesion and ECM-receptor interaction pathway. Five dysregulated genes, including CDH1, VEGFA, PTPRF, CLDN7, and MMP2 were confirmed by Real time qPCR in the sequencing samples and the additional eleven samples. Our data revealed that more than three hundred genes showed differential splicing patterns between tumor tissue and non-tumor tissue. Among these genes, we filtered 24 cancer-associated alternative splicing genes with differential exon usage. The findings from RNA-Seq were validated by Real time qPCR for CD44, PDGFA, NUMB, and LPHN2. This study provides a comprehensive survey of the UCB transcriptome, which provides better insight into the complexity of regulatory changes during recurrence and metastasis.

Editor: Georgios Gakis, Eberhard-Karls University, Germany

Funding: This work was supported by 2013 Hainan Provincial Natural Science Foundation (Grant number: 813256), Key Municipal Scientific Project of Haikou (Grant number: 2012-073), and Key Scientific Project of Hainan Province (Title: Preliminary screening of molecular markers in bladder cancer by high-throughput transcriptome sequencing). The funders had no role in study design, data collection and analysis, decision to publish, or preparation of the manuscript.

Competing Interests: The authors have declared that no competing interests exist. Yongqing Ye is employed by the Department of Shanghai Claison Bio-Technology, which was involved in helping the authors performthe sample collection. The authors have no other relationship with the Department of Shanghai Claison Bio-Technology relating to employment, consultancy, patents, products in development or marketed products.

* E-mail: hkbaizhiming@163.com

Introduction

The bladder cancer is the seventh most prevalent type of cancer worldwide. Global estimates suggest that in 2008, approximately 386,300 new bladder cancer cases were diagnosed and that 150,200 patients succumbed to the disease [1]. As the major subtype of bladder cancer, urothelial carcinoma of the bladder (UCB) is the fifth most expensive cancer to treat, accounting for $3.7 billion in direct costs in 2001 [2]. The costs are high because most patients survive long term, recurrence is frequent and lifelong surveillance is required. This disease occurs predominantly in men, yet it is increasing in incidence among women in a manner that cannot be entirely explained by increased tobacco use [3].

Approximately 80% of bladder cancers present as non-muscle invasive urothelial carcinoma, 70% of them will recur, and 10–20% of them will progress and invade the bladder muscle [4]. Of the patients initially presenting with muscle-invasive UCB, 50% will relapse with metastatic disease [5,6]. High-grade muscle-invasive disease represents a life-threatening condition and requires timely treatment [7,8].

Prior studies of genomic alterations have revealed that somatic changes, including point mutations [9,10], DNA rearrangements (reviewed in [6]) and copy number variations [11] [12], can result in mutations that drive the development of UCB. As a consequence of changes in the cancer genome, the reprogramming of the transcriptome leads to abnormal cellular behavior and thus directly contributes to cancer progression [13,14]. Studying the cancer transcriptome not only enables us to fill in the gap between driver mutations and cancer cell behavior, but also allows us to identify additional candidate cancer-related mutations and the molecular basis of gene regulation [14].

Alternative splicing (AS), the process by which splice sites are differentially utilized to produce different mRNA isoforms, is a key component in expanding a relatively limited number of genes into very complex proteomes in metazoans. Several evidences suggested that AS changes were associated with cancers [15,16,17]. The cancer-specific splice variants may potentially be used as diagnostic, prognostic, and predictive biomarkers as well as therapeutic targets [18].

The recent development of massively parallel sequencing (RNA-seq) provides a powerful approach to profile the transcriptome with greater efficiency and higher resolution [19]. The advantage of RNA-seq is that this technique makes feasible the study of the cancer transcriptome complexity, including alternative splicing, isoform usage, gene fusions and novel transcripts (reviewed in [20,21]. Despite the prevalence of using RNA-seq to study various cancer transcriptomes [20], the deep annotation of UCB gene expression profiling has not been performed.

In this study, we aimed to thoroughly annotate the transcriptomes of UCB tissue and adjacent non-tumor tissue from a single recurrent and cisplatin-resistance patient by RNA-seq. First, we found several dysregulated genes. Second, we performed the enrich analysis of Gene Ontology (GO) and pathway analysis of the dysregulated genes. Third, we investigated the differential splicing pattern between tumor and non-tumor tissue, and found out the cancer-associated genes with different exon skipping events. Finally, to validate our sequencing results, quantitative real-time PCR (qPCR) was used to confirm the difference of gene expression and the differential usage of splice variants in the sequencing patient and eleven additional patients.

Results

Analysis of RNA-Seq data

Two samples — UCB tissue (stage II, multiple recurrent and cisplatin-resistance) and distant non-tumor tissue — were collected from a Chinese male patient. Fig. S1 showed the pathological diagnostic images of the UCB tissue. All samples were subjected to massively parallel paired-end cDNA sequencing. In total, we obtained 32.0 million and 31.4 million read pairs from the UCB and non-tumor tissue, respectively. We used TopHat to align the reads to the UCSC (the University of California Santa) reference human genome Hg19. The uniquely aligned reads for the two samples ranged from 26.4 million to 28 million pairs. The proportion of reads that mapped to the Ensembl reference genes was ~78% for the both samples. The average coverage of our sequencing depth was approximately 50 times of human transcriptome (approximately 113 millon bp, based on the total length of the uniquely annotated exon region in the Ensembl database). In addition, only ~1% reads were mapped to rRNA, indicating that our libraries are properly constructed and faithfully represent the expression of genes with ploy (A). The details of the mapping results are listed in Table 1.

Analysis of differentially expressed genes

After mapping the RNA-Seq reads to the reference genome with TopHat, transcripts were assembled and their relative abundances were calculated using Cufflinks [22]. The Cufflinks use Cuffdiff algorithm to measure the gene expression and to identify the differentially expressed genes (DEGs). The normalized expression level of each gene was measured by Fragments Per Kilobase of exon per Million fragments mapped (FPKM). By requiring that the FPKM was greater than one, we detected 14,520 and 14,199 expressed genes in the tumor and non-tumor samples respectively, which included the majority of the annotated human reference genes (See Table S1 for details). The global gene expression profiles of two samples was correlated (Pearson correlation coefficient R = 0.77) (Fig. S2A). We totally detected 1879 significant DEGs (FDR<0.01, FDR: False Discovery Rate) between the two samples (Table S1). The "volcano plot" (Fig. S2B) and MA-plot (Fig. S2C) of the gene expression profiles show that the number of up- and down-regulated genes was nearly equal relative to the q-value and expression level, suggesting that the significance of the statistics test was not bias toward up- or down-regulated genes and the dysregulated genes is not biased toward highly or lowly expressed genes.

Function enrichment analysis of differentially expressed genes

To better understand the function of DEGs, we conducted an enrichment analysis of Gene Ontology (GO) for the dysregulated genes. We performed enrichment tests for significantly dysregulated genes that were detected in the UCB and non-tumor tissue using online tools from DAVID [23]. In total, the dysregulated genes in UCB were categorized into 22 GO terms of Biological Process (Table 2, p<0.05, corrected by Bonferroni correction). Most of terms were related to immune response, cell adhesion, response to wounding, extracellular structure organization, locomotion (chemotaxis and taxis), leukocyte activation, and so on.

A more informative analysis of functional annotation can be achieved by studying the enrichment of differentially expressed genes in a particular pathway. We used DAVID [23] to analyze which KEGG pathway was enriched with dysregulated genes in UCB. The pathways enriched with DEGs are listed in Table 3 (FDR<0.05). The cell adhesion molecules (CAMs) pathway was the most significant pathway (FDR = 2.67E-08). In addition, the focal adhesion, ECM (extracellular matrix)-receptor interaction pathway, and some disease pathway were also enriched.

To experimentally confirm the differentially expressed genes identified by RNA-seq, we performed the validation by quantitative real-time PCR (qRT-PCR). We chose five candidate genes

Table 1. Statistics of bladder cancer transcriptome mapping to human genome Hg19.

	Tumor	Non-tumor
Total reads	62,822,760 (100%)	63,977,860 (100%)
Uniquely Mapped Single Reads	3,143,012 (5.0%)	5,226,940 (8.2%)
Uniquely Mapped Paired Reads	52,859,962 (84.1%)	47,634,322 (74.5%)
Total Uniquely Mapped Reads	56,002,974 (89.1%)	52,861,262 (82.6%)
Uniquely Splice Junction Reads	10,935,040 (17.4%)	12,952,784 (20.2%)
Total Uniquely Mapped length (bp)	5,749,364,918(51x#)	5,462,298,875 (48x#)

#: Sequencing coverage on human transcriptome (approximately 113 million bps which was estimated as the total length of all unique exons according to Ensembl database).

Table 2. Gene Ontology terms of enriched differentially expressed genes in bladder cancer.

GO Term in Biological Process	Fold Enrichment[#]	Corrected p value[*]
GO:0006955~immune response	2.30	4.69E-18
GO:0007155~cell adhesion	2.15	1.84E-14
GO:0022610~biological adhesion	2.15	2.08E-14
GO:0009611~response to wounding	1.99	4.60E-07
GO:0006952~defense response	1.83	1.34E-05
GO:0006954~inflammatory response	2.13	8.59E-05
GO:0002684~positive regulation of immune system process	2.33	1.31E-04
GO:0050865~regulation of cell activation	2.53	4.71E-04
GO:0043062~extracellular structure organization	2.57	6.42E-04
GO:0016337~cell-cell adhesion	2.14	9.25E-04
GO:0050863~regulation of T cell activation	2.81	2.65E-03
GO:0030198~extracellular matrix organization	2.94	2.66E-03
GO:0006935~chemotaxis	2.48	3.60E-03
GO:0042330~taxis	2.48	3.60E-03
GO:0002694~regulation of leukocyte activation	2.39	8.66E-03
GO:0045321~leukocyte activation	2.11	9.44E-03
GO:0050867~positive regulation of cell activation	2.76	9.99E-03
GO:0051249~regulation of lymphocyte activation	2.45	1.46E-02
GO:0001775~cell activation	1.98	1.66E-02
GO:0050778~positive regulation of immune response	2.42	2.67E-02
GO:0046649~lymphocyte activation	2.17	3.37E-02
GO:0002252~immune effector process	2.45	4.33E-02

#: Fold Enrichment = (number of differentially expressed genes with the GO term/number of differentially expressed genes)/(number of expressed genes with the GO term/number of expressed genes)

*: p value corrected by method of Bonferroni, and only GO terms of the corrected p value less than 0.05 were shown.

(PTPRF, MMP2, VEGFA, CDH1 and CLDN7) that were detected differential expression by Cuffdiff (Table S2) and involved in Bladder cancer pathway, cell adhesion molecules (CAMs) pathway and focal adhesion pathway. We used GAPDH as an endogenous control in these reactions. The qRT-PCR results confirmed that all of these candidate genes expressed differently between UCB and non-tumor tissue, as shown in Fig. 1.

Table 3. KEGG pathways of enriched differentially expressed genes in bladder cancer.

KEGG pathway	Fold Enrichment[#]	FDR[*]
hsa04514:Cell adhesion molecules (CAMs)	3.02	2.67E-08
hsa05416:Viral myocarditis	2.81	1.63E-03
hsa04940:Type I diabetes mellitus	3.43	2.73E-03
hsa05340:Primary immunodeficiency	3.48	9.09E-03
hsa05330:Allograft rejection	3.39	1.16E-02
hsa04640:Hematopoietic cell lineage	2.32	1.74E-02
hsa05320:Autoimmune thyroid disease	2.82	1.84E-02
hsa05332:Graft-versus-host disease	3.12	2.25E-02
hsa05412:Arrhythmogenic right ventricular cardiomyopathy (ARVC)	2.33	3.30E-02
hsa04512:ECM-receptor interaction	2.24	3.52E-02
hsa04672:Intestinal immune network for IgA production	2.71	4.21E-02
hsa04510:Focal adhesion	1.71	4.36E-02

#: Fold Enrichment = (number of differentially expressed genes in the pathway/number of differentially expressed genes)/(number of expressed genes in the pathway/number of expressed genes)

*: False Discovery Rate provided by DAVID, only pathways of the FDR less than 0.05 were shown.

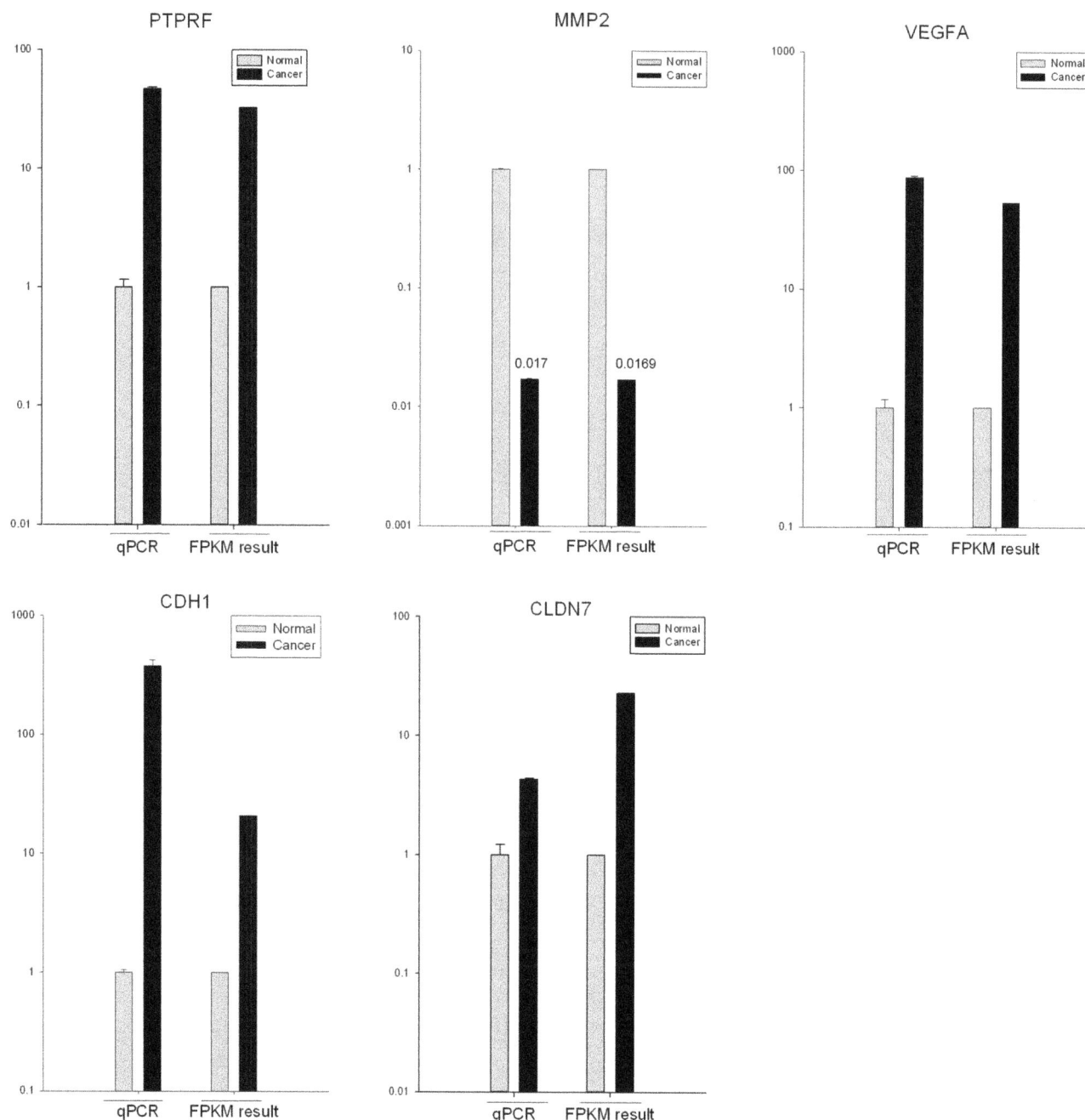

Figure 1. The differentially expressed genes detected by RNA-seq are confirmed by qRT-PCR. qRT-PCR was performed for five genes that are identified as differential expressed genes between UCB and non-tumor tissues. The expression level of each gene was normalized to the level in non-tumor tissue. A-E: PTPRF, MMP2, VEGFA, CDH1 and CLDN7.

To examine whether these genes were always dysregulated in the bladder cancer, we performed the qRT-PCR to test the expression changes for the five genes between the paired cancer and none-cancer tissue in eleven additional patients (which including 6 recurrent UCB patients and 5 newly diagnosed). The result showed that, CDH1, VEGFA, PTPRF and CLDN7 were up-regulated in six cancer samples, and MMP2 was down-regulated in ten cancer samples, suggested that these genes, especially MMP2, were dysregualted in most UCB samples (Table S3). And we also found that CDH1, VEGFA, PTPRF were up-regulated in 66.7% (4/6) recurrent patients but only 40% (2/5)

newly diagnosed patients (Fig. 2), suggesting the three genes might associated with the recurrence of UCB.

Alternative splicing events in bladder cancer

One gene locus can express multiple isoforms by alternative splicing (AS). The transcript diversity leads to plastic transcriptional networks in cancer, which are important to generate the unusual properties of cancer cells [17,24]. We thus perform genome-wide screening to identify the cancer-restricted alternative splicing events using software MISO (the Mixture of Isoforms) [25]. In total, we detected 25,695 and 23,769 alternative splicing

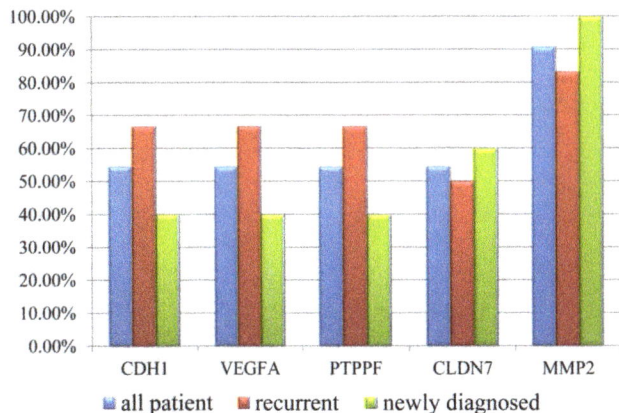

Figure 2. qRT-PCR validation of the differentially expressed genes in the additional patients. qRT-PCR was performed for five differentially expressed genes (CDH1, VEGFA, PTPRF, CLDN7 and MMP2) in the additional 11 patients (including 6 recurrent and drug-resistant UCB patients and 5 newly diagnosed patients). The histogram showed the proportion of validated patients in all cases (blue), the recurrent cases (red) and newly diagnosed (green).

events in the UCB and non-tumor tissue, respectively (Table 4). These events included seven different patterns: alternative 3′splice sites (A3SS), alternative 5′splice sites (A5SS), alternative first exons (AFE), mutually exclusive exons (MXE), retained introns (RI), skipped exons (SE) and tandem 3′UTRs (TUTR). Half of these events were exon skipping (Table 4).

We next detected the differential splicing events (DSEs) between UCB and non-tumor samples using MISO (Table S4 "raw"). We found 462 DSEs from 390 unique genes, and more than half of DSEs belong to skipped exon (Table 5). We defined the genes with DSEs as differential splicing genes (DSGs). To identify reliable DSGs associated with cancer, we further filtered the DSEs by a series steps (Materials and Methods) and obtained 43 reliable DSEs from 38 unique cancer-associated DSGs (Table S4 "cancer-associated"). Of these DSEs, 25 events from 24 DSGs belong to splicing pattern "skipped exon" (Table 6). As an example, Fig. 3 showed the coverage of reads of PDGFA in the differential exon usage. The ratio of junction-reads number for the exon inclusion versus the exon exclusion was obviously higher in the cancer tissue than that in the non-tumor tissue for both of the two genes. Since

Table 4. Statistics of alternative splicing events in bladder cancer.

Pattern of alternative splicing	Counts		Percentage	
	Tumor	Non-tumor	Tumor	Non-tumor
A3SS: Alternative 3′splice sites	3293	2950	12.8%	12.4%
A5SS: Alternative 5′splice sites	4185	3770	16.3%	15.9%
AFE: Alternative first exons	470	349	1.8%	1.5%
MXE: Mutually exclusive exons	681	657	2.7%	2.8%
RI: Retained introns	2666	2206	10.4%	9.3%
SE: Skipped exons	12697	11787	49.4%	49.6%
TUTR: Tandem 3′UTRs	1703	2050	6.6%	8.6%
TOTAL	25695	23769	100.0%	100.0%

the skipped exon is the most common way to generate protein products with alternative functions by truncating the functional domain in mammals [17], we focus on the analysis of differential splicing events of skipped exon in the future steps.

To experimentally confirm the skipped-exon DSGs identified by RNA-seq, the relative expression levels between skipped exons and their neighboring exon of selected genes were measured in the UCB and non-tumor sample by quantitative real-time PCR (qRT-PCR). We chose four candidate genes involved in KEGG pathways, including the CD44, GSK3B, PDGFA and NUMB, from above 24 differential splicing genes from MISO (the primers shown in Table S2). We used GAPDH as an endogenous control in these reactions. The result showed that except for GSK3B, another three genes, including CD44, PDGFA and NUMB, were validated (Fig. 4).

We next chose six differential splicing genes (CD44, PDGFA, NUMB, LPHN2, NIN, FAT1) to perform qRT-PCR validation in the eleven additional patients used in differentially expressed gene validation (Table S5). The result showed that CD44 (36%, 4/11), PDGFA (64%, 7/11), NUMB (64%, 7/11) and LPHN2 (73%, 8/11) showed exon increased exon inclusion in considerable number of UCB patients, but few patients showed the increased exon exclusion in gene NIN (18%, 2/11) and 9% (1/11). We also found that PDFGA showed increased exon inclusion in 83% (5/6) recurrent UCB samples, but only 40% (2/5) newly diagnosed samples (Fig. 5). And CD44 also showed higher proportion of exon inclusion in the recurrent samples (50%, 3/6) than that newly diagnosed (20%, 1/5). It suggested that the increased exon inclusion PDGFA (chr7:540068-540136) and CD44 (chr11:35231512-35231601) might associated with the recurrence of UCB.

Bioinformatics prediction of gene fusion events

We used two algorithms, deFuse [26] and TopHat-Fusion [27], to detect gene fusion based on the pair-ends reads in the two samples. Although various results were generated by deFuse and TopHat-Fusion (Table S6), however, none reliable fusion transcript was found by manually checking the reads mapping to the fusion sequence (Methods).

Discussion

Our study provides the first comprehensive insight into the transcriptome of a recurrent, drug-resistant and muscle-invasive urothelial carcinoma of the bladder with RNA-Seq. In total, approximately 60 million reads were generated per sample, which enabled us to quantify the gene expression abundance at a wide range [28]. The percentage of uniquely reads mapping, approximated uniform coverage in each gene (Fig. S3) and the number of expressed genes (FPKM>0) revealed that the data satisfied the quality standards of the RNA-seq and represented the majority of the transcriptome. We identified the levels of differentially expressed genes and alternative splicing patterns associated with cancer.

Differentially expressed genes in UCB

In this study, we sampled cancer and distant non-tumor tissue from a single individual to conduct transcriptome comparisons. To determine whether our findings were in agreement with previously reported results, we systematically compared the changes in the expression of specific UCB-related genes.

We found that the vascular endothelial growth factor A (VEGFA), a member of the PDGF/VEGF growth factor family that promotes angiogenesis through nitric oxide synthase, was

Table 5. Statistics of differential splicing genes in bladder cancer.

Pattern of alternative splicing	# of differential splicing events (percentage)	# of unique differential splicing genes (percentage)
A3SS: Alternative 3'splice sites	49(10.61%)	47(12.05%)
A5SS: Alternative 5'splice sites	52(11.26%)	46(11.79%)
AFE: Alternative first exons	14(3.03%)	10(2.56%)
MXE: Mutually exclusive exons	14(3.03%)	13(3.33%)
RI: Retained introns	101(21.86%)	95(24.36%)
SE: Skipped exons	232(50.22%)	203(52.05%)
TUTR: Tandem 3'UTRs	0(0.00%)	0(0.00%)
TOTAL	462(100.00%)	390(100.00%)

significantly up-regulated in UCB in cancer tissue compared to non-tumor tissue. Our result is coincident with the recent two studies using microarrays and digital gene expression profile, which both found the up-regulation of VEGFA in a large number of UCB patients [29,30], suggesting that VEGFA might be a commonly over-expressed gene in UCB.

We found that most of matrix metalloproteinases (MMPs), especially MMP2 and MMP9, is down-regulated in cancer tissues compared to non-tumor tissue. The MMPs activate basic and acidic fibroblast growth factors (bFGF and aFGF, respectively), which in turn restimulate the MMPs to promote endothelial cell migration [31]. MMPs also stimulate scatter factor (SF), which stimulates angiogenesis. High levels of MMP-2 and MMP-9 have

Table 6. Differential exon skipping events in cancer-associated genes.

Gene symbol	location of skipped exon	$\Psi1^{\&}$	$\Psi2^{\&}$	diff*	Bayes factor§	Gene description
MACF1	chr1:39946592–39946702	0.81	0.1	0.71	5.90E+275	microtubule-actin crosslinking factor 1
CTNND1	chr11:57583387–57583473	0.46	0.01	0.45	1.70E+244	catenin (cadherin-associated protein), delta 1
PDGFA	chr7:540068–540136	0.67	0.02	0.65	7.10E+219	platelet-derived growth factor alpha polypeptide
LPHN2	chr1:82452585–82452713	0.68	0.04	0.64	4.50E+216	latrophilin 2
ADD3	chr10:111892063–111892158	0.9	0.1	0.8	2.40E+184	adducin 3 (gamma)
CTNND1	chr11:57556509–57556627	0.17	0.92	−0.75	4.70E+140	catenin (cadherin-associated protein), delta 1
EIF4A2	chr3:186505197–186505373	0.9	0.48	0.42	1.50E+78	eukaryotic translation initiation factor 4A2
FAT1	chr4:187511522–187511557	0.08	0.46	−0.38	4.40E+73	FAT tumor suppressor homolog 1 (Drosophila)
CD151	chr11:834458–834591	0.19	0.49	−0.3	7.32E+37	CD151 molecule (Raph blood group)
NUMB	chr14:73745989–73746132	0.36	0.03	0.33	1.53E+34	numb homolog (Drosophila)
PACSIN2	chr22:43272894–43273016	0.67	0.97	−0.3	8.69E+28	protein kinase C and casein kinase substrate in neurons 2
FNBP4	chr11:47747289–47747388	0.77	0.24	0.53	5.61E+16	formin binding protein 4
TRIM37	chr17:57094657–57094785	0.41	0.91	−0.5	5.58E+15	tripartite motif containing 37
ACTB	chr7:5569166–5569364	0.78	0.33	0.45	1.00E+12	actin, beta
NIN	chr14:51223210–51225348	0.1	0.89	−0.79	1.00E+12	ninein (GSK3B interacting protein)
THSD1	chr13:52960163–52960321	0.33	0.91	−0.58	6.60E+09	thrombospondin, type I, domain containing 1
ELK1	chrX:47509320–47509425	0.75	0.38	0.37	3.03E+08	ELK1, member of ETS oncogene family
CD44	chr11:35231512–35231601	0.96	0.59	0.37	3.33E+07	CD44 molecule (Indian blood group)
GAS8	chr16:90102041–90102095	0.37	0.74	−0.37	2.20E+06	growth arrest-specific 8
TNC	chr9:117808689–117808961	0.43	0.85	−0.42	6.28E+05	tenascin C
GSK3B	chr3:119562102–119562200	0.95	0.42	0.53	5.30E+05	glycogen synthase kinase 3 beta
UBE2V1	chr20:48700666–48700791	0.64	0.97	−0.33	3.46E+04	ubiquitin-conjugating enzyme E2 variant 1
GTF2H1	chr11:18347494–18347700	0.04	0.38	−0.34	4.91E+03	general transcription factor IIH, polypeptide 1, 62kDa
ZMYND8	chr20:45841287–45841370	0.9	0.5	0.4	3.19E+03	zinc finger, MYND-type containing 8
CIRBP	chr19:1273493–1273714	0.49	0.88	−0.39	2.44E+03	cold inducible RNA binding protein

$^{\&}$: Ψ, percentage spliced in, denotes the fraction of mRNAs that represent the inclusion isoform; $\Psi1$: Ψ in cancer sample, $\Psi2$: Ψ in non-tumor sample.
*: The "diff" is provided by the MISO, and indicated the degree of splicing difference between samples. It was in [−1, 1]. The positive "diff" value means that the exon was skipped more in the non-tumor tissue than that in the cancer tissue, and the negative values means the exon skipped more in the cancer tissue.
§: The "bayes factor" provided by MISO indicate the significance of the splicing difference. It was in [0, +∞), and it was greater, then the difference was more significant.

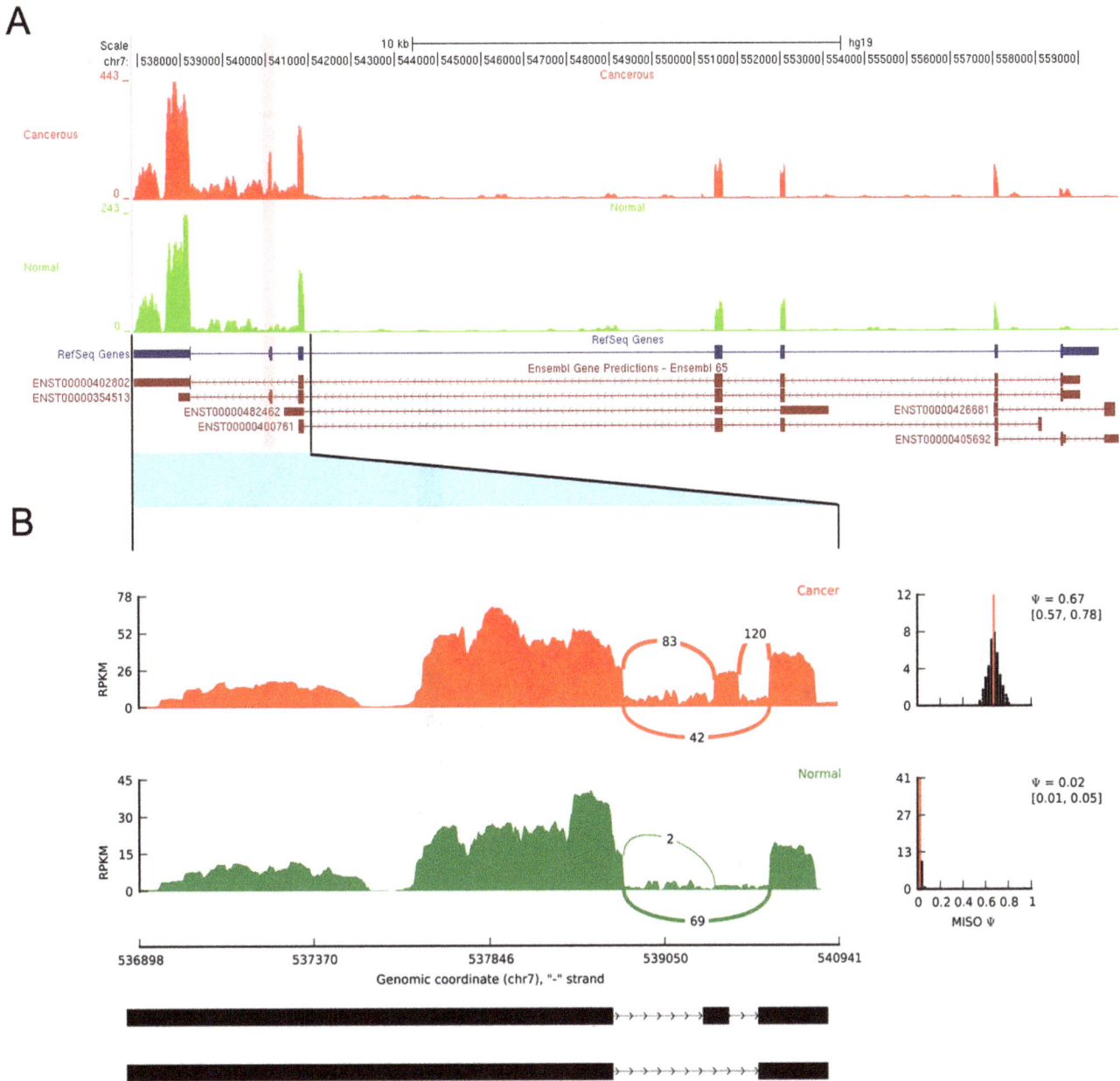

Figure 3. RNA-Seq read mapping to the reference gene PDGFA. A: RNA-Seq read mapping to the UCSC reference genome (hg19) of the gene PDGFA for UCB and non-tumor tissues in this study. The UCB tracks are shown in red and non-tumor tissue in green. The pink band indicated the location of skipped exon. B: The detail of junction reads mapping to the skipped exon and its neighboring exons. The Ψ ("percentage spliced in") indicates the ratio of reads supporting inclusion exon vs. total reads supporting both inclusion and exclusion exon. The Ψ posterior distributions [25] were shown in the right side.

been associated with increasing stage and grade of UCB [32,33], and MMP2 overexpression can predict poor relapse-free and disease-specific survival [34]. However, in the recent two studies, MMP2 was reported under-expression in UCB [29,30].

We also detected some biological markers in the diagnosis of recurrent bladder cancer was dysregulated in UCB, including KRT20 (Cytokeratin 20) [35], BIRC5 (Survivin) [36,37], CDH1 (E-cadherin) [38] and PSCA (Prostate Stem Cell Antigen-14) [39,40]. The investigation in DEGs showed that our findings from RNA-Seq agreed with previous reports.

In addition, several known driver factors that are frequently mutated in UCB, including ARPC5 (p16) [41] and FGF2 [42],

showed no change in expression in this study, suggesting that the genetic heterogeneity of UCB or the mutated products might be deleterious even if the expression level is unaffected.

The bladder cancer is characterized by chemoresistance although the mechanism is still not entirely known [43]. The UCB sample used in this study was diagnosed as the cisplatin resistance. We investigated the expression of the drug-resistant genes mentioned by Köberle et al., which listed the genes with cisplatin-based resistance in bladder cancer [44]. We found that genes associated with DNA repair and apoptosis pathway were dysregulated in UCB samples (Table S7), suggesting that the

A CD44

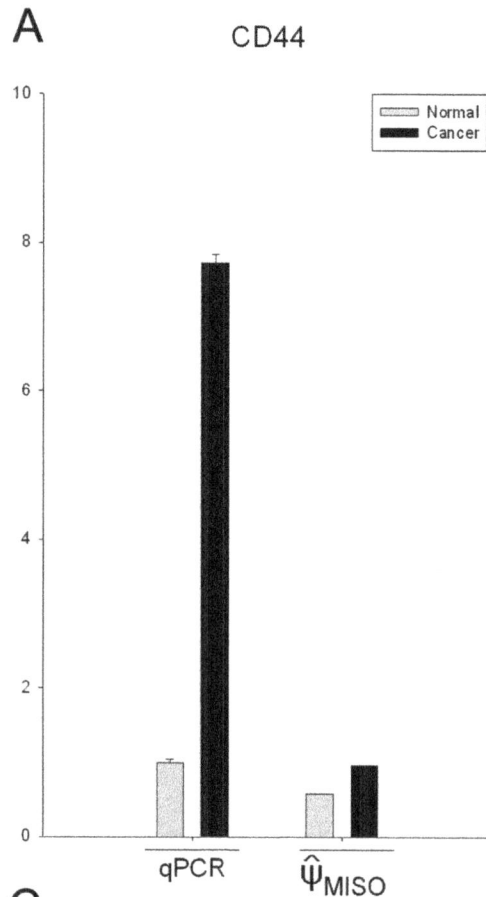

B PDGFA

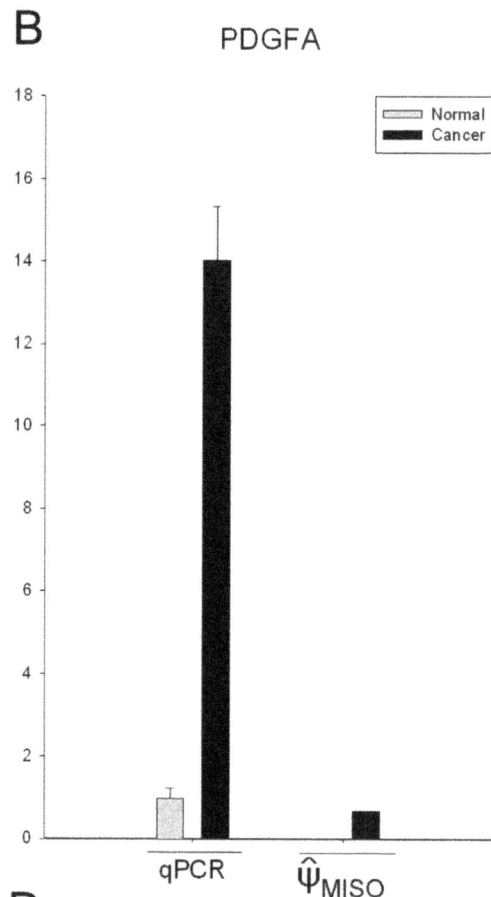

C NUMB

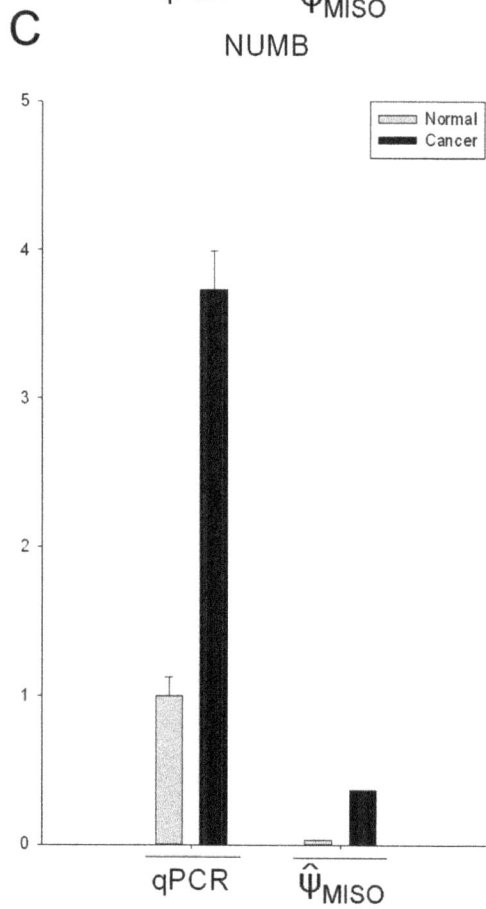

D GS3KB

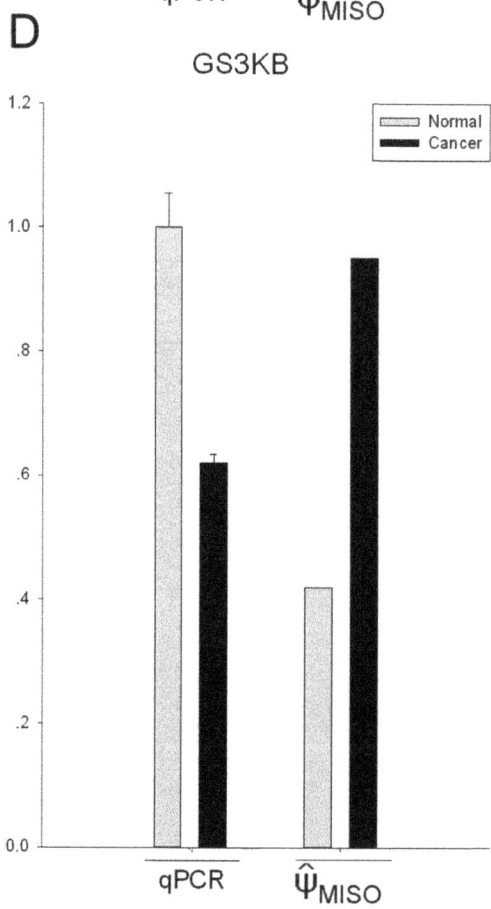

Figure 4. The qRT-PCR validation of differential splicing events detected by RNA-seq. qRT-PCR was performed for four genes that are identified as differential splicing genes between UCB and non-tumor tissues. The result of qRT-PCR is the relative expression level of the skipped exon and the neighboring constitutive exon. The expression level of each exon was normalized to the level in non-tumor tissue. The ΨMISO was the result of MISO, indicates the ratio of reads supporting inclusion exon vs. total reads supporting both inclusion and exclusion exon. A~D: CD44, PDGFA, NUMB and GSK3B.

chemoresistance of this cancer sample might be associated with the increased DNA repair and suppression of apoptosis.

In this study, the CAMs pathway is the most significant pathway enriched with DEGs, this result confirmed with the previous report that the CAMs is common pathway enriched with DEGs in carcinomas of the bladder, kidney and testis [30]. Aberration of the CAMs pathway and ECM receptors enables cancer cells to escape their primary tumor masses, invade adjacent tissues and colonize elsewhere [45,46]. Additionally, as demonstrated in our study, frequent deregulation of the cytokine-related pathways as well as the immune and inflammatory response processes is another common hallmark of human cancer [47]. For many solid tumors, cytokines, together with CAMs, play important roles in the induction of antitumor immune responses and tumor rejection in the tumor microenvironment where immune and malignant cells interact [48]. Moreover, recent emerging data suggested that cancer-related inflammation contributes to the proliferation and survival of tumor cells and linked this inflammation to the therapeutic response and prognosis of cancer patients [49].

Cancer-associated differential exon skipping events

Alternative regulation of gene expression can be achieved by transcriptional and post-transcriptional regulation. The first class of dysregulation of UCB at the transcriptional level has been well studied using microarray technology [50,51,52]. Quantifying the second class of regulatory change remains challenging despite the invention of the exon array [53]. RNA-seq technology enables the simultaneous study of these two different mechanisms [19,22,54,55]. In this study, we also investigated the second class of transcriptional dysregulation by analyzing the alternative splicing in UCB.

We performed the analysis by MISO, a probabilistic framework to quantitate the expression level of alternatively spliced genes

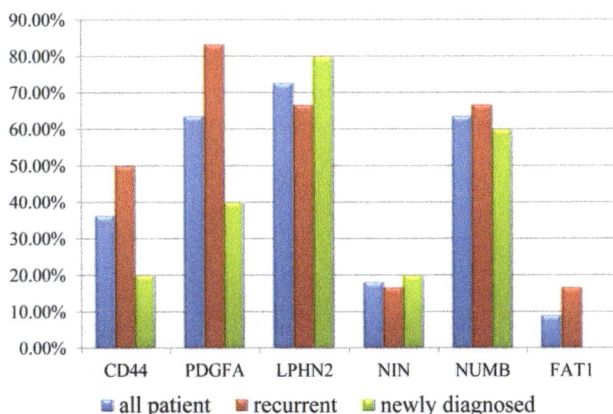

Figure 5. qRT-PCR validation of differential splicing events in the additional patients. qRT-PCR was performed for six differential splicing genes (CD44, PDGFA, NUMB, LPHN2, NIN and FAT1) in the additional 11 patients (including 6 recurrent and drug-resistant UCB patients and 5 newly diagnosed patients). The histogram showed the proportion of validated patients in all cases (blue), the recurrent cases (red) and newly diagnosed (green).

from RNA-Seq data, and identifies differentially regulated isoforms or exons across samples [25]. By adopting the more stringent cut-off and crossing with known cancer-associated genes, we find 24 highly reliable cancer-associated differential splicing genes.

Some splicing events have been reported to be related to bladder cancer using exon arrays, including CD44, CLSTN1 and CTNND1 [53]. CD44 is a transmembrane glycoprotein that participates in many cellular processes including regulation of cell division, survival, migration, and adhesion [56]. Its splice variant CD44E (exon v8-10 expressed) can serve as a prognostic predictor and indicator of disease extent in patients with urothelial cancer [57,58,59]. In our study, the variant exon v8, v9 and v10 expressed in the UCB tissue, but not in the non-tumor tissue (Fig. S4), suggesting that CD44E was cancer-specific. Our result supported the CD44E as a marker in the bladder cancer diagnose.

Some cancer-associated DSGs in our result were reported in the other cancers but not reported in the bladder cancer yet, such as PDGFA, MACF1, ADD3 and NUMB. PDGFA, a member of platelet-derived growth factor family, have two isoforms corresponding to a long (PDGFAA) and a short (PDGFAB) form due to alternative splicing of exon 6 [60]. In this study, the exon 6 was skipped in non-tumor tissue but not in the cancer tissue (Fig. 3), which means that the long isoform PDGFAA was mainly expressed in cancer tissues and the short isoform PDGFAB expressed in non-tumor tissue. PDGFAA has a basic carboxy-terminal tail encoded by exon 6, attaching it to the extracellular matrix whereas PDGFAB is freely diffusible in the extracellular fluid since it lacks this retention motif [61,62]. The role of the basic extension in PDGFAA and how it makes the long form functionally different from the short remain unknown. Expression of the long form of PDGFA was originally identified in tumor cells [60,63,64], and PDGFAA was cloned from a human glioma cell line [63]. The different expression of long isoforms of PDGFA was also reported in gliosarcomas of mouse [65] and liver cancer of rat [66]. A recent study showed that the long isoform of PDGFA overexpressed in the brain abnormalities and glioma-Like lesions in astrocytic cells in mice, and induced accumulation of immature cells in the mouse brain [65]. Further investigations are needed to understand the particular mechanism of the long isoform of PDGFA in UCB.

The AS events in MAFC1, ADD3 and NUMB were reported in the two recent researches in non-small cell lung cancer [67,68]. MAFC1 belongs to the plakin family of cytoskeletal linker proteins which form bridges between different cytoskeletal elements by specialized modular domains. Using exon array and qPCR validation, Misquitta-Ali et al. found that the exon number 8 (Ensembl exon id: ENSE00001770152) of MACF1 was expressed in non-small lung cancer and breast cancer but not in the pair-matched normal tissues [68]. Our study found this AS change between the UCB and the paired non-tumor tissue (Fig. S5), suggesting that the increased exon inclusion of exon 8 of MAFC1 might be common in these cancers. MACF1 has no direct relation with cancer, it has been reported to function in the Wnt signaling pathway and to be associated with a complex containing Axin, beta-catenin, glycogen synthase kinase 3 (GSK3B), and adenomatous polyposis coli (APC) [69], which have been linked to tumorigenesis [70,71]. Based on this, the increased inclusion of the alternative exon in MACF1 transcripts was proposed to contribute to altered Wnt signaling in the lung and colon cancers [68], and our result expands this supposition to the bladder cancer.

ADD3 (Gamma-adducin) is s a structural constituent of the spectrin-actin cytoskeleton that contains at least 16 exons, of which exon number 15 (ENSE00000986819) is a known cassette exon of 96 bp. Langer et al. reported that the long isoform of ADD3 with inclusion of exon number 15 was specifically expressed in the non-small cell lung cancer, but the cancer-special function of the isoform is unclear [67]. Our result showed the same AS event difference between in the UCB and non-tumor tissue (Fig. S6), suggesting that the long isoform of ADD3 might be also a cancer-specific transcript in bladder cancer.

NUMB plays a role in the determination of cell fates during development. The degradation of NUMB is induced in a proteasome-dependent manner by MDM2, is a membrane-bound protein that has been shown to associate with EPS15, LNX1, and NOTCH1. The increased inclusion exon 9 (ENSE00001689532) of NUMB transcripts is a highly widespread tumor-associated AS event, which was detected by exon arrays and validated by PCR in both of two independent laboratories [67,68]. The event was detected in 37 additional patients with lung, breast and colon cancer by Misquitta-Ali et al.[68], and in 5 of 6 patients in the study of Langer et al. [67]. In our study using RNA-Seq, the inclusion exon 9 of NUMB was also significantly increased in the UCB tissue (Fig. S7). Functional analysis in lung cancer showed that tumor-associated increases in NUMB exon 9 inclusion correlated with reduced levels of NUMB protein expression and activation of the Notch signaling pathway, an event that has been linked to tumorigenesis [68]. These findings suggested that the increased inclusion exon 9 of NUMB is supposed to be a candidate of marker in the diagnosis of multiple cancers including lung, breast, colon and bladder cancer.

There are also some differential splicing events which have not been reported to be associated with tumors, such as UCB increased exon inclusion of LPHN2 (chr1:82452585-82452713), EIF4A2 (chr3:186505197-186505373), FAT1 (chr4:187511522-187511557), exon exclusion of CD151 (chr11:834458-834591), and so on. The increased exon inclusion of LPHN2 was validated in 73% (8/11) UCB patients by qRT-PCR validation. The splicing events might be a novel alternative splicing changes associated with bladder cancer. Investigation of these events will help to understand the mechanism of tumor formation and progress. In addition, we tried to ask whether the drug-resistance was related to the differential alternative splicing due to the drug-resistance of this UCB tissue. We compared the drug-resistant genes listed in Table S7 with all DSEs we detected (listed in Table S4 "raw"). However, none of the drug-resistant genes showed the differential splicing events, suggesting that the drug-resistance might be majorly associated with the dysregulation in expression level but not in alternative splicing.

Materials and Methods

Patient Samples

Written informed consent from the patients were obtained, and this series of studies was reviewed and approved by Institutional Ethics Committees of Haikou Municipal People's Hospital (Haikou, China). Distant normaltissue of the urinary bladder and urothelial carcinoma of the bladder (UCB), were obtained from one 69-year-old Chinese male patient who initially suffered UCB in May 2010, and recurrently in October, November 2010 and June 2011, respectively. Partial cystectomies were performed

immediately following each detection. Samples used in this study were collected in the last surgery. H&E (hematoxylin and eosin stained) slides of frozen UBC tissue with patient-matched frozen normal tissue were examined by the pathologists of this study to ensure that the tumor tissues selected had high-density cancer foci and that the normal tissues were without tumor contamination. The tumor was consisted of pure transitional epithelium carcinoma, without any atypical glandular epithelial cells or squamous epithelial cells. Besides the histology, it was observed that the tumor invaded muscle (T2), no regional lymph nodes could not be assessed (N0) and no distant metastasis (M0). According TNM classification of carcinomas of the urinary bladder, the case should be defined as Stage II by the International agency of research on Cancer. Tumor chemosensitivity assay reported that the tumor was resistant to common used cisplatin-based chemotherapy drugs. Fig. S1 provides the histological image of the cancerous tissue. The percentage of tumor cells in the UCB tissue was 78% by counting the relative at a 400× magnification. The additional twenty-two paired cancer and non-cancer samples using in validation were collected from six recurrent and cisplatin-resistance UCB patients (stage II) and five newly diagnosed UCB patients (stage II). All samples were independently reviewed by an additional gynecologic pathologist. The treatment histories, including chemotherapy, of cases that represent recurrence were shown in Table S8.

Library preparation

Total RNA was extracted from non-tumor and cancerous bladder tissues with TRIzol according to the manufacturer's protocol (Invitrogen). For mRNA-seq sample preparation, the Illumina standard kit was used according to the TruSeq RNA SamplePrep Guide (Illumina). Briefly, 10 μg of total RNA from each sample was used for polyA mRNA selection using poly T oligo-conjugated magnetic beads by two rounds of purification, followed by thermal mRNA fragmentation. The fragmented mRNA was subjected to cDNA synthesis using reverse transcriptase (SuperScript II) and random primers. The cDNA was further converted into double-stranded cDNA, and after end repair (Klenow fragment, T4 polynucleotide kinase, T4 polymerase and 3-'A' add process [Klenow exo-fragment]), the product was ligated to Illumina Truseq adaptors. Size selection was performed using a 2% agarose gel, generating 380-bp cDNA libraries. Finally, the libraries were enriched using 15 cycles of PCR and purified with the QIAquick PCR purification kit (Qiagen). The enriched libraries were diluted with elution buffer to a final concentration of 10 nM.

Sequencing and quality filtering

Libraries from non-tumor tissue and cancerous bladder tissue were analyzed at a concentration of 11 pM on a single Genome Analyzer IIx (GAIIx) lane using 115-bp sequencing. Raw RNA-seq data were filtered by Fastx-tools (http://hannonlab.cshl.edu/fastx_toolkit/) according to the following criteria: 1) reads containing sequencing adaptors were removed; 2) nucleotides with a quality score lower than 20 were trimmed from the end of the sequence; 3) reads shorter than 50 were discarded; and 4) artificial reads were removed. After the filtering pipeline, a total of 21.5G bp of cleaned, paired-end reads were produced.

RNA-seq reads mapping

The clean reads were then aligned with the UCSC *H. sapiens* reference genome (build hg19) using TopHat v1.3.1[54], which initially removes a portion of the reads based on quality information accompanying each read and then maps the reads to the reference genome. The pre-built *H. sapiens* UCSC hg19 index was downloaded from the TopHat homepage and used as the reference genome. TopHat allows multiple alignments per read (up to 20 by default) and a maximum of two mismatches when mapping the reads to the reference. TopHat builds a database of potential splice junctions and confirms these by comparing the previously unmapped reads against the database of putative junctions. The default parameters for the TopHat method were used.

Transcript abundance estimation

The aligned read files were processed by Cufflinks v1.0.3 [22], which uses the normalized RNA-seq fragment counts to measure the relative abundances of the transcripts. The unit of measurement is Fragments Per Kilobase of exon per Million fragments mapped (FPKM). Confidence intervals for FPKM estimates were calculated using a Bayesian inference method [72]. The reference GTF annotation file used in Cufflinks was downloaded from the Ensembl database (Homo_sapiens.GRCh37.63.gtf [73]). The transcript abundance data has been submitted to the GEO database with accession ID GSE33782.

Detection of differentially expressed gene

The downloaded Ensembl GTF file was passed to Cuffdiff along with the original alignment (.SAM) files produced by TopHat. Cuffdiff re-estimates the abundance of the transcripts listed in the GTF file using alignments from the.SAM file and concurrently tests for differential expression. Only the comparisons with "q_value" less than 0.01 and test status marked as "OK" in the Cuffdiff output were regarded as showing differential expression.

Functional enrichment analysis of differentially expressed genes

The Database for Annotation, Visualization and Integrated Discovery (DAVID) v6.7 is a set of web-based functional annotation tools [23]. The unique lists of differentially expressed genes and all the expressed genes (FPKM>0 in any sample) were submitted to the web interface as the gene list and background, respectively. The cut-off of the False Discovery Rate (FDR) was set at 5%, and only the results from the GO FAT and KEGG pathways were selected as functional annotation categories for this analysis.

Detection of differential splicing events

The Mixture of Isoforms (MISO) analysis [25] was used to detect differentially regulated exons across samples. The MISO analysis was performed according to the tool's given workflow using paired-end reads (http://genes.mit.edu/burgelab/miso/docs/). The reads alignment files (.SAM) produced by TopHat and the pre-build human genome (Hg19) alternative events downloaded from the MISO reference manual page (http://genes.mit.edu/burgelab/miso/docs/#gff-event-annotation) were used as the input. To identify highly reliable cancer-associated DES events, we filtered the DES events by the flowing steps: 1) use the stringent cuff-offs to filter the result of MISO (the absolute value of diff >0.3 and bayes factor >1000, the default cut-off of MISO were 0.2 and 10); 2) keep the genes that are overlapped with the cancer-associated gene set, which were collected from the NCBI gene database (searched by "oncogene" and "tumor suppressor gene") and the Bushman Lab web (http://microb230.med.upenn.edu/protocols/cancergenes.html).

Visualization of mapped reads

The mapping results were visualized using the Integrative Genomics Viewer (IGV) available at http://www.broadinstitute.org/igv/. Views of other individual genes were generated by uploading coverage.wig files to the UCSC Genome browser.

Identifying and checking the gene fusions

All the filtered RNA-seq reads were mapped to the reference transcript sequences that were downloaded from the Ensembl database (Homo_sapiens.GRCh37.63.cdna.all.fa) using TopHat. The read pairs mapping to the same transcripts were removed, and the ends of remaining reads were truncated to maintain the 75-bp length using in-house Perl scripts. These fixed-length reads were passed to two software packages, deFuse (deFuse-0.4.2) [26] and TopHat-Fusion (TopHatFusion-0.1.0) [27], to find the candidate gene fusions. The bowtie-index used in the TopHat-Fusion was downloaded from the TopHat homepage (H. sapiens UCSC hg19). The parameters of the TopHat-Fusion used were obtained from the "Getting Started" (http://tophat-fusion.sourceforge.net/tutorial.html) tutorial. The deFuse parameters were the default settings, as described in the deFuse manual. The check of fusion transcripts was performed by mapping the reads to the identified fusion sequences. The count of unique reads spanned the fusion sites of the sequence should be greater than 5 and the reads was expected to be relatively uniformly distributed in the fusion sequences.

Differentially expressed gene validation

The differentially expressed genes were validated by Real-Time Quantitative Polymerase Chain Reaction (RT-qPCR) using a LightCycler 480 Instrument II (Roche). The PCR volume included 10 μl sample, 5 μl 2× SYBR Green Master Mix (TOYOBO), 1 μl cDNA template and 1 pmol/μl of each oligonucleotide. The RT-qPCR thermal profile was obtained using the following procedure: 95°C for 1 min, 40 cycles of 95°C for 10 sec, 60°C for 30 sec and 72°C for 10 sec, followed by 72°C for 5 min. The program was set to reveal the melting curve of each amplicon from 60°C to 95°C and obtain a read every 0.5°C. The primer sequences are listed in Table S2. All the RT-qPCR reactions were performed in triplicate to capture intra-assay variability.

The expression levels of each target gene in the tested experimental condition (cancerous bladder tissue) were compared to the control condition (non-tumor bladder tissue) according to Cook et al. [74]. The data were normalized using GAPDH, which had previously been identified as the best reference gene under different experimental conditions [75]. In the present analysis, GAPDH was confirmed to be stable and always showed variability less than ±1 cycle.

Differential splicing events validation

The primers (Table S2) were designed using Primer 5 software (PREMIER Biosoft International, Palo Alto, Calif.), and The PCR experiments were performed using a Veriti Thermal Cycler (ABI). The PCR volume used comprised 10 μl sample, 1 μl 10×PCR buffer, 1 μl cDNA template, 0.2 μl dNTP, 0.2 μl Taq Enzyme (Genscript), and 0.2 pmol/μl each oligonucleotide. PCR was performed using the following procedure: 95°C for 1 min, 40 cycles of 95°C for 15 sec, 55°C for 30 sec and 72°C for 15 sec, followed by 72°C for 5 min. We confirmed the presence of the fusion gene in cancerous colon tissue. GAPDH was used as the loading control. The PCR products of the fusion gene were cloned in the pGEM-T Easy Vector (Promega) and then sequenced with the T7 primer using a 3730 DNA Analyzer (ABI).

Data assessment

The raw sequencing data has been deposited to the NCBI Short Read Archive on accession number SRP009386.

Supporting Information

Figure S1   Histological image of a hematoxylin/eosin-stained section of the bladder cancer sample (original magnification ×400) (A) and distant non-tumor epithelial tissue of the urinary bladder and UCB tissues (B).

Figure S2   Differential expression analysis in the cancer and normal tissue. A: The scatter plot for global expression between samples; the Pearson correlation coefficient is shown; B: Volcano plots for all the genes to reveal the relation between expression fold-change and q value in DEG detecting. The red and blue dots indicate that up- and down-regulated DEGs were significant at q values less than 0.01. C: MA plots for all expressed genes to reveal the relation between expression level and fold-change. Each dots stands for one gene in comparison, the dotted line in grey indicates M = 0. Differentially expressed genes were plotted in red (up-regulated) and blue (down-regulated).

Figure S3   Homogeneity of reads coverage. The genes of which FPKM>1 and cDNA length≥300 bp were assigned as three groups according to gene expression (high: the top 25%, blue; middle: the middle 50%, red; and low: the bottom 25%, green). All cDNA were divided into 100 bins, the median of reads number in each bins was shown for each group. A: Reads coverage in normal tissue; B: Reads coverage in cancer tissue.

Figure S4   RNA-Seq read mapping to the reference gene CD44. A: RNA-Seq read mapping to the UCSC reference genome (hg19) of the gene PDGFA for UCB and normal tissues in this study. The UCB tracks are shown in red and normal tissue in green. The pink band indicated the location of skipped exon. B: The detail of junction reads mapping to the skipped exon and its neighboring exons. The Ψ ("percentage spliced in") indicates the ratio of reads supporting inclusion exon vs. total reads supporting both inclusion and exclusion exon. The Ψ posterior distributions were shown in the right side.

Figure S5   RNA-Seq read mapping to the reference gene MACF1. A: RNA-Seq read mapping to the UCSC reference genome (hg19) of the gene MACF1 for UCB and normal tissues in this study. The UCB tracks are shown in red and normal tissue in green. The pink band indicated the location of skipped exon. B:

The detail of junction reads mapping to the skipped exon and its neighboring exons.

Figure S6   RNA-Seq read mapping to the reference gene ADD3. A: RNA-Seq read mapping to the UCSC reference genome (hg19) of the gene ADD3 for UCB and normal tissues in this study. The UCB tracks are shown in red and normal tissue in green. The pink band indicated the location of skipped exon. B: The detail of junction reads mapping to the skipped exon and its neighboring exons.

Figure S7   RNA-Seq read mapping to the reference gene NUMB. A: RNA-Seq read mapping to the UCSC reference genome (hg19) of the gene NUMB for UCB and normal tissues in this study. The UCB tracks are shown in red and normal tissue in green. The pink band indicated the location of skipped exon. B: The detail of junction reads mapping to the skipped exon and its neighboring exons.

Table S1   Gene expression and differentially expressed genes.

Table S2   Primer sequences.

Table S3   qRT-PCR validation of five differentially expressed genes (fold change, cancer sample vs. non-cancer sample).

Table S4   Differential splicing events.

Table S5   qRT-PCR valication of six differential splicing genes.

Table S6   Gene fusions output by deFuse and TopHat-Fusion.

Table S7   Drug-resistant genes.

Table S8   The treatment history of cases that represent recurrence.

Author Contributions

Conceived and designed the experiments: ZB SZ. Performed the experiments: ZL CZ SW YZ SX. Analyzed the data: YL HC YY YZ. Contributed reagents/materials/analysis tools: YY PY JL. Wrote the paper: SZ ZB.

References

1. Jemal A, Siegel R, Ward E, Hao Y, Xu J, et al. (2008) Cancer statistics, 2008. CA Cancer J Clin 58: 71–96.
2. Botteman MF, Pashos CL, Redaelli A, Laskin B, Hauser R (2003) The health economics of bladder cancer: a comprehensive review of the published literature. Pharmacoeconomics 21: 1315–1330.
3. Hayne D, Arya M, Quinn MJ, Babb PJ, Beacock CJ, et al. (2004) Current trends in bladder cancer in England and Wales. J Urol 172: 1051–1055.
4. Knowles MA (2001) What we could do now: molecular pathology of bladder cancer. Molecular Pathology 54: 215–221.
5. Williams SG, Stein JP (2004) Molecular pathways in bladder cancer. Urological Research 32: 373–385.
6. Wolff EM, Liang G, Jones PA (2005) Mechanisms of Disease: genetic and epigenetic alterations that drive bladder cancer. Nat Clin Pract Urol 2: 502–510.
7. Chang SS, Hassan JM, Cookson MS, Wells N, Smith JA (2003) Delaying radical cystectomy for muscle invasive bladder cancer results in worse pathological stage. J Urol 170: 1085–1087.
8. Herr HW, Dotan Z, Donat SM, Bajorin DF (2007) Defining optimal therapy for muscle invasive bladder cancer. J Urol 177: 437–443.
9. Reddy EP, Reynolds RK, Santos E, Barbacid M (1982) A point mutation is responsible for the acquisition of transforming properties by the T24 human bladder carcinoma oncogene. Nature 300: 149–152.
10. Kompier LC, Lurkin I, van der Aa MNM, van Rhijn BWG, van der Kwast TH, et al. (2010) FGFR3, HRAS, KRAS, NRAS and PIK3CA Mutations in Bladder Cancer and Their Potential as Biomarkers for Surveillance and Therapy. PLoS ONE 5: e13821.

11. El-Rifai We, Kamel D, Larramendy ML, Shoman S, Gad Y, et al. (2000) DNA Copy Number Changes in Schistosoma-Associated and Non-Schistosoma-Associated Bladder Cancer. The American Journal of Pathology 156: 871–878.

12. Norskov MS, Frikke-Schmidt R, Bojesen SE, Nordestgaard BG, Loft S, et al. (2011) Copy number variation in glutathione-S-transferase T1 and M1 predicts incidence and 5-year survival from prostate and bladder cancer, and incidence of corpus uteri cancer in the general population. Pharmacogenomics J 11: 292–299.

13. Wong KM, Hudson TJ, McPherson JD (2011) Unraveling the genetics of cancer: genome sequencing and beyond. Annu Rev Genomics Hum Genet 12: 407–430.

14. Cancer Genome Atlas Research Network (2011) Integrated genomic analyses of ovarian carcinoma. Nature 474: 609–615.

15. Caceres JF, Kornblihtt AR (2002) Alternative splicing: multiple control mechanisms and involvement in human disease. Trends Genet 18: 186–193.

16. Cooper TA, Wan L, Dreyfuss G (2009) RNA and disease. Cell 136: 777–793.

17. Venables JP (2004) Aberrant and alternative splicing in cancer. Cancer Research 64: 7647–7654.

18. Pajares MJ, Ezponda T, Catena R, Calvo A, Pio R, et al. (2007) Alternative splicing: an emerging topic in molecular and clinical oncology. Lancet Oncol 8: 349–357.

19. Metzker ML (2010) Sequencing technologies — the next generation. Nat Rev Genet 11: 31–46.

20. Ozsolak F, Milos PM (2011) RNA sequencing: advances, challenges and opportunities. Nat Rev Genet 12: 87–98.

21. Wang Z, Gerstein M, Snyder M (2009) RNA-Seq: a revolutionary tool for transcriptomics. Nat Rev Genet 10: 57–63.

22. Trapnell C, Williams BA, Pertea G, Mortazavi A, Kwan G, et al. (2010) Transcript assembly and quantification by RNA-Seq reveals unannotated transcripts and isoform switching during cell differentiation. Nat Biotech 28: 511–515.

23. Huang da W, Sherman BT, Lempicki RA (2009) Systematic and integrative analysis of large gene lists using DAVID bioinformatics resources. Nat Protoc 4: 44–57.

24. David CJ, Manley JL (2010) Alternative pre-mRNA splicing regulation in cancer: pathways and programs unhinged. Genes Dev 24: 2343–2364.

25. Katz Y, Wang ET, Airoldi EM, Burge CB (2010) Analysis and design of RNA sequencing experiments for identifying isoform regulation. Nat Methods 7: 1009–1015.

26. McPherson A, Hormozdiari F, Zayed A, Giuliany R, Ha G, et al. (2011) deFuse: An Algorithm for Gene Fusion Discovery in Tumor RNA-Seq Data. PLoS Comput Biol 7: e1001138.

27. Kim D, Salzberg SL (2011) TopHat-Fusion: An algorithm for Discovery of Novel Fusion Transcripts. CSHL Biology of Genomes conference.

28. Mortazavi A, Williams BA, McCue K, Schaeffer L, Wold B (2008) Mapping and quantifying mammalian transcriptomes by RNA-Seq. Nat Methods 5: 621–628.

29. Zaravinos A, Lambrou GI, Boulalas I, Delakas D, Spandidos DA (2011) Identification of Common Differentially Expressed Genes in Urinary Bladder Cancer. PLoS ONE 6: e18135.

30. Li X, Chen J, Hu X, Huang Y, Li Z, et al. (2011) Comparative mRNA and microRNA Expression Profiling of Three Genitourinary Cancers Reveals Common Hallmarks and Cancer-Specific Molecular Events. PLoS ONE 6: e22570.

31. Mitra AP, Lin H, Datar RH, Cote RJ (2006) Molecular biology of bladder cancer: Prognostic and clinical implications. Clinical Genitourinary Cancer 5: 67–77.

32. Davies B, Waxman J, Wasan H, Abel P, Williams G, et al. (1993) Levels of matrix metalloproteases in bladder cancer correlate with tumor grade and invasion. Cancer Res 53: 5365–5369.

33. Gerhards S, Jung K, Koenig F, Daniltchenko D, Hauptmann S, et al. (2001) Excretion of matrix metalloproteinases 2 and 9 in urine is associated with a high stage and grade of bladder carcinoma. Urology 57: 675–679.

34. Vasala K, Pääkkö P, Turpeenniemi-Hujanen T (2003) Matrix metalloproteinase-2 immunoreactive protein as a prognostic marker in bladder cancer. Urology 62: 952–957.

35. Marín-Aguilera M, Mengual L, Ribal MJ, Ars E, Ríos J, et al. (2012) Utility of Urothelial mRNA Markers in Blood for Staging and Monitoring Bladder Cancer. Urology 79: 240.e249–240.e215.

36. Smith SD, Wheeler MA, Plescia J, Colberg JW, Weiss RM, et al. (2001) Urine detection of survivin and diagnosis of bladder cancer. JAMA 285: 324–328.

37. Swana HS, Grossman D, Anthony JN, Weiss RM, Altieri DC (1999) Tumor content of the antiapoptosis molecule survivin and recurrence of bladder cancer. N Engl J Med 341: 452–453.

38. Lipponen PK, Eskelinen MJ (1995) Reduced expression of E-cadherin is related to invasive disease and frequent recurrence in bladder cancer. Journal of Cancer Research and Clinical Oncology 121: 303–308.

39. Wu X, Ye Y, Kiemeney LA, Sulem P, Rafnar T, et al. (2009) Genetic variation in the prostate stem cell antigen gene PSCA confers susceptibility to urinary bladder cancer. Nat Genet 41: 991–995.

40. Elsamman E, Fukumori T, Kasai T, Nakatsuji H, Nishitani MA, et al. (2006) Prostate stem cell antigen predicts tumour recurrence in superficial transitional cell carcinoma of the urinary bladder. BJU Int 97: 1202–1207.

41. Korkolopoulou P, Christodoulou P, Lazaris A, Thomas-Tsagli E, Kapralos P, et al. (2001) Prognostic implications of aberrations in p16/pRb pathway in urothelial bladder carcinomas: a multivariate analysis including p53 expression and proliferation markers. Eur Urol 39: 167–177.

42. Bai Y, Mao QQ, Qin J, Zheng XY, Wang YB, et al. (2010) Resveratrol induces apoptosis and cell cycle arrest of human T24 bladder cancer cells in vitro and inhibits tumor growth in vivo. Cancer Sci 101: 488–493.

43. Drayton RM, Catto JWF (2012) Molecular mechanisms of cisplatin resistance in bladder cancer. Expert Review of Anticancer Therapy 12: 271–281.

44. Köberle B, Piee-Staffa A (2012) The Molecular Basis of Cisplatin Resistance in Bladder Cancer Cells.

45. Cavallaro U, Christofori G (2004) Cell adhesion and signalling by cadherins and Ig-CAMs in cancer. Nat Rev Cancer 4: 118–132.

46. Stetler-Stevenson WG, Aznavoorian S, Liotta LA (1993) Tumor Cell Interactions with the Extracellular Matrix During Invasion and Metastasis. Annual Review of Cell Biology 9: 541–573.

47. Yeh HJ, Ruit KG, Wang YX, Parks WC, Snider WD, et al. (1991) PDGF A-chain gene is expressed by mammalian neurons during development and in maturity. Cell 64: 209–216.

48. Emerich DF, Vasconcellos AV, Elliott RB, Skinner SJ, Borlongan CV (2004) The choroid plexus: function, pathology and therapeutic potential of its transplantation. Expert Opin Biol Ther 4: 1191–1201.

49. Crews L, Wyss-Coray T, Masliah E (2004) Insights into the pathogenesis of hydrocephalus from transgenic and experimental animal models. Brain Pathology 14: 312–316.

50. Zaravinos A, Lambrou GI, Volanis D, Delakas D, Spandidos DA (2011) Spotlight on Differentially Expressed Genes in Urinary Bladder Cancer. PLoS ONE 6: e18255.

51. Dong L, Bard AJ, Richards WG, Nitz MD, Theodorescu D, et al. (2009) A gene expression ratio-based diagnostic test for bladder cancer. Advances and Applications in Bioinformatics and Chemistry: 17.

52. Dyrskjøt L, Kruhøffer M, Thykjaer T, Marcussen N, Jensen JL, et al. (2004) Gene Expression in the Urinary Bladder. Cancer Research 64: 4040–4048.

53. Thorsen K, Sørensen KD, Brems-Eskildsen AS, Modin C, Gaustadnes M, et al. (2008) Alternative Splicing in Colon, Bladder, and Prostate Cancer Identified by Exon Array Analysis. Molecular & Cellular Proteomics 7: 1214–1224.

54. Trapnell C, Pachter L, Salzberg SL (2009) TopHat: discovering splice junctions with RNA-Seq. Bioinformatics 25: 1105–1111.

55. Garber M, Grabherr MG, Guttman M, Trapnell C (2011) Computational methods for transcriptome annotation and quantification using RNA-seq. Nat Meth 8: 469–477.

56. Götte M, Yip GW (2006) Heparanase, Hyaluronan, and CD44 in Cancers: A Breast Carcinoma Perspective. Cancer Research 66: 10233–10237.

57. Miyake H, Hara II, Arakawa S, Kamidono S (1999) Utility of Competitive Reverse Transcription-Polymerase Chain Reaction Analysis of Specific CD44 Variant RNA for Detecting Upper Urinary Tract Transitional-Cell Carcinoma. Mol Urol 3: 365–370.

58. Miyake H, Eto H, Arakawa S, Kamidono S, Hara I (2002) Over Expression of CD44V8-10 in Urinary Exfoliated Cells as an Independent Prognostic Predictor in Patients with Urothelial Cancer. The Journal of Urology 167: 1282–1287.

59. Miyake H, Hara I, Kamidono S, Eto H (2004) Multifocal Transitional Cell Carcinoma of the Bladder and Upper Urinary Tract: Molecular Screening of Clonal Origin by Characterizing CD44 Alternative Splicing Patterns. The Journal of Urology 172: 1127–1129.

60. Rorsman F, Bywater M, Knott TJ, Scott J, Betsholtz C (1988) Structural characterization of the human platelet-derived growth factor A-chain cDNA and gene: alternative exon usage predicts two different precursor proteins. Molecular and Cellular Biology 8: 571–577.

61. Heldin CH, Eriksson U, Ostman A (2002) New members of the platelet-derived growth factor family of mitogens. Archives of biochemistry and biophysics 398: 284–290.

62. Heldin CH, Westermark B (1999) Mechanism of Action and In Vivo Role of Platelet-Derived Growth Factor. Physiological Reviews 79: 1283–1316.

63. Betsholtz C, Johnsson A, Heldin CH, Westermark B, Lind P, et al. (1986) cDNA sequence and chromosomal localization of human platelet-derived growth factor A-chain and its expression in tumour cell lines. Nature 320: 695–699.

64. Collins T, Bonthron DT, Orkin SH (1987) Alternative RNA splicing affects function of encoded platelet-derived growth factor A chain. Nature 328: 621–624.

65. Nazarenko I, Hedrén A, Sjödin H, Orrego A, Andrae J, et al. (2011) Brain Abnormalities and Glioma-Like Lesions in Mice Overexpressing the Long Isoform of PDGF-A in Astrocytic Cells. PLoS ONE 6: e18303.

66. Cook JL, Giardina JF, Zhang Z, Re RN (2002) Intracellular Angiotensin II Increases the Long Isoform of PDGF mRNA in Rat Hepatoma Cells. Journal of Molecular and Cellular Cardiology 34: 1525–1537.

67. Langer W, Sohler F, Leder G, Beckmann G, Seidel H, et al. (2010) Exon Array Analysis using re-defined probe sets results in reliable identification of alternatively spliced genes in non-small cell lung cancer. BMC Genomics 11: 676.

68. Misquitta-Ali CM, Cheng E, O'Hanlon D, Liu N, McGlade CJ, et al. (2011) Global Profiling and Molecular Characterization of Alternative Splicing Events Misregulated in Lung Cancer. Molecular and Cellular Biology 31: 138–150.

69. Chen HJ, Lin CM, Lin CS, Perez-Olle R, Leung CL, et al. (2006) The role of microtubule actin cross-linking factor 1 (MACF1) in the Wnt signaling pathway. Genes Dev 20: 1933–1945.

70. Saadeddin A, Babaei-Jadidi R, Spencer-Dene B, Nateri AS (2009) The Links between Transcription, β-catenin/JNK Signaling, and Carcinogenesis. Molecular Cancer Research 7: 1189–1196.

71. Wang Y (2009) Wnt/Planar cell polarity signaling: A new paradigm for cancer therapy. Molecular Cancer Therapeutics 8: 2103–2109.

72. Jiang H, Wong WH (2009) Statistical inferences for isoform expression in RNA-Seq. Bioinformatics 25: 1026–1032.

73. Hubbard TJP, Aken BL, Ayling S, Ballester B, Beal K, et al. (2009) Ensembl 2009. Nucleic Acids Research 37: D690–D697.

74. Cook NL, Vink R, Donkin JJ, van den Heuvel C (2009) Validation of reference genes for normalization of real-time quantitative RT-PCR data in traumatic brain injury. J Neurosci Res 87: 34–41.

75. Barber RD, Harmer DW, Coleman RA, Clark BJ (2005) GAPDH as a housekeeping gene: analysis of GAPDH mRNA expression in a panel of 72 human tissues. Physiol Genomics 21: 389–395.

21

Incidental Prostate Cancer at the Time of Cystectomy: The Incidence and Clinicopathological Features in Chinese Patients

Jiahua Pan[9], Wei Xue[9], Jianjun Sha, Hu Yang, Fan Xu, Hanqing Xuan, Dong Li, Yiran Huang*

Department of Urology, Renji Hospital, Affiliated to Shanghai Jiao Tong University, School of Medicine, Shanghai, China

Abstract

Objectives: To evaluate the incidence and the clinicopathological features of incidental prostate cancer detected in radical cystoprostatectomy (RCP) specimens in Chinese men and to estimate the oncological risk of prostate apex-sparing surgery for such patients.

Methods: The clinical data and pathological feature of 504 patients who underwent RCP for bladder cancer from January 1999 to March 2013 were retrospectively reviewed. Whole mount serial section of the RCP specimens were cut transversely at 3–4 mm intervals and examined in same pathological institution.

Results: Thirty-four out of 504 patients (6.8%) had incidental prostate cancer with a mean age of 70.3 years. 12 cases (35.2%) were diagnosed as significant disease. 4 cases were found to have apex involvement of adenocarcinoma of the prostate while in 5 cases the prostate stroma invasion by urothelial carcinoma were identified (one involved prostate apex). The mean follow-up time was 46.4±33.8 months. Biochemical recurrence occurred in 3 patients but no prostate cancer-related death during the follow-up. There was no statistical significance in cancer specific survival between the clinically significant and insignificant cancer group.

Conclusions: The prevalence of incidental prostate cancer in RCP specimens in Chinese patients was remarkably lower than in western people. Most of the incidental prostate cancer was clinically insignificant and patient's prognosis was mainly related to the bladder cancer. Sparing the prostate apex was potentially associated with a 1.0% risk of leaving significant cancer of the prostate or urothelial carcinoma.

Editor: Peter C Black, University of British Columbia, Canada

Funding: The study was supported by National Natural Science Foundation of China (91129725) and Renji Medical Research Seed Project (RJZZ13-016). The funders had no role in study design, data collection and analysis, decision to publish, or preparation of the manuscript.

Competing Interests: The authors have declared that no competing interests exist.

* E-mail: viovilla@163.com

[9] These authors contributed equally to this work.

Introduction

Bladder cancer is the second most common genitourinary malignancy worldwide and the most frequently diagnosed genitourinary cancer in China [1,2]. It leads to significant morbidity and mortality. Up till now, RCP remains the golden standard for muscle invasive bladder cancer or recurrent superficial urothelial carcinoma at high risk [3]. Although the neobladder reconstruction and nerve-sparing technique offer a better quality of life for the patients, the recovery of erectile function and urinary continence after surgery are still far from satisfactory [4]. Therefore, the prostate apex-sparing or even the total prostate-sparing techniques have been developed to improve the postoperative urinary continence and sexual function [5,6]. However, the potential risk of prostate cancer residue and prostatic involvement with urothelial carcinoma become a major concern for these techniques.

The incidence of prostate cancer varies significant among different countries and ethnic groups. It is quite frequently diagnosed in North America and Europe but rare in Asians [7]. According to the latest reports, the incidence rate was only 12.10/100 000 in China and 12.70/100 000 in Japan [2,8–9]. More importantly, most of the prostate cancer diagnosed in the specimens from RCP for bladder cancer is considered as clinically insignificant disease [10–14]. However, in this issue, only few data of Chinese cohort are available with limited cases. In this study, we retrospectively reviewed 504 RCP cases for bladder cancer to investigate the incidence and clinicopathological features of incidental prostate cancer in RCP specimens in Chinese patients. To our knowledge, this study represents the largest series to date of incidental prostate cancer at RCP in China and even in Asia.

Materials and Methods

Cohort selection and pathological evaluation

The clinical data and pathological feature of 504 patients who underwent standard RCP for bladder cancer at our institution from January 1999 to March 2013 were retrospectively reviewed. As a tertiary referral center, these patients came from 31 out of 34 administrative zones of China. Patients with an abnormal result of digital rectal examination (DRE) or PSA suspicious of prostate cancer and finally confirmed by prostate biopsy before the surgery or patients having a history of prostate cancer were already excluded from the study. The study protocol was approved by the ethical committee of the faculty of medicine of Shanghai Jiao Tong University, School of Medicine. All patients enrolled in this study signed an informed consent before the surgery.

The preoperative assessment included DRE and upper urinary tract imaging such as intravenous urography (IVU), CT urography (CTU) or magnetic resonance urography (MRU). However, the PSA was only available in 296 cases before RCP. All the pathological examination was performed in the same institution. Whole mount serial section of the RCP specimens were cut transversely at 3–4 mm intervals. Besides the urothelial carcinoma of the urinary bladder, the location and tumor volume of the prostate cancer, prostate apex involvement, Gleason score, pathological staging and surgical margins were evaluated. Clinically significant prostate cancer was defined as a tumor volume$\geq$0.5 ml; Gleason 4 or 5 pattern, extracapsular extension, seminal vesicle invasion, lymph node metastasis or positive surgical margins [15].

Follow-up

The first postoperative PSA follow-up was scheduled at 3 months after the surgery, then every 3 months the first year, every 6 months the second year and annually thereafter. A biochemical recurrence was defined as an initial serum PSA of $\geq$0.2 ng/ml, with a second confirmatory level of PSA of >0.2 ng/ml [16].

Statistical Analysis

Proportions of the variables were analyzed using Chi-square test or Fisher's exact test while mean values were compared with one-way ANOVA test. The cancer specific survival was described using Kaplan-Meier curves. Survival differences were compared by the Log-rank test. Statistical significance was set at P<0.05 and all the P values were two-sided. The SPSS 18.0 was applied to perform the data analysis.

Results

Incidental prostate cancer

In this study, 34 out of 504 patients (34/504, 6.8%) who underwent RCP had incidentally diagnosed prostate cancer. The mean age was 70.3±8.9 years and the mean follow-up was 46.4±33.8 months. A preoperative PSA was available in 23 cases with incidental prostate cancer and their median PSA was 2.67±2.24 ng/ml. A tumor volume of more than 0.5 cm^3 was identified in 8 patients (8/34, 23.5%). 4 cases were found to have apex involvement of adenocarcinoma of the prostate while in 5 cases the prostate stroma invasion by urothelial carcinoma were identified (one involved the prostate apex). The detailed pathological staging and Gleason score were summarized in Table 1.

12 cases (12/34, 35.2%) were diagnosed as significant prostate cancer, while 22 (22/34, 64.8%) were clinically insignificant. The mean age of the patients with significant cancer and insignificant cancer was 66.83±6.83 years and 72.14±9.43 years, respectively. The preoperative PSA was available in 14 cases in insignificant cancer group with a median PSA of 2.0 ng/ml whereas available in 9 patients in significant cancer group with a median PSA of 3.7 ng/ml (P = 0.14). The positive surgical margin of prostate cancer was detected in 1 patient with significant disease. All the 4

cases with apex involvement of adenocarcinoma of the prostate were in significant cancer group and 3 of them had a preoperative PSA available. The median PSA of these 3 cases was 4.1 ng/ml. Although the prostate apex involvement was statistically higher in significant prostate cancer group, the biochemical recurrence rate was similar between the 2 groups during the follow-up. In addition, there was no statistical difference in pathological staging and the pelvic lymph node involvement of the bladder cancer between the 2 groups. The Clinical characteristics and pathologic feature of these 2 groups were listed in Table 2.

Prostatic stromal invasion by urothelial carcinoma

Prostatic stromal invasion is defined as the presence of invasive urothelial carcinoma nests or single cells penetrating through the basement membrane of prostatic ducts and acini. The prostate stroma invasion by bladder cancer were identified in 5 cases (one involved the prostate apex) in this cohort. 3 cases with prostate stroma invasion by urothelial carcinoma were in significant prostate cancer group while 2 in insignificant cancer group, respectively. (P = 0.32) When reviewing the pathological specimens, 4 out of these 5 cases were found to have high grade and multifocal urothelial carcinoma in urinary bladder and 3 of them had pelvic lymph node involvement.

Biochemical recurrence and cancer specific survival

After RCP, the PSA was below the limit of detection in all cases. During the follow-up, biochemical recurrence occurred in 3 patients (3/34, 8.8%) without prostate apex involvement and then treated with androgen deprivation therapy.

As for the survival, 10 patients (10/34, 32.4%) died of metastatic bladder cancer, 3 in clinically significant prostate cancer group (3/12, 25.0%) and 7 in clinically insignificant group (7/22, 31.8%), whereas 1 (1/22, 4.5%) died of myocardial infarction. There was no prostate cancer-related death in both groups during the follow-up. Concerning the cancer specific survival between the clinically significant and clinically insignificant cancer group, there was no statistical significance identified. (P = 0.51) (Figure 1)

Discussion

The frequency of incidental prostate cancer detected in RCP specimens is really variable all over the world. Abbas et al reported a 45% rate of incidental prostate cancer in a study of 40 cases [17]. Similar results were obtained by Montie et al, who found 33 of 84 men (33/84, 46%) undergoing cystoprostatectomy for bladder cancer had incidental prostate cancer [18]. However, the incidence rate was much lower in most of the Asian countries. According to the recent studies with 1207 cases from Asia, the prevalence of incidental prostate cancer was only about 10.9% [13,19–25]. It was extremely low in China, Japan and India. Nevertheless, the incidental prostate cancer seemed to be rather frequent in Korea, which was similar to that of western countries. Base on the findings form Joung et al, the prevalence was as high as 50% [20]. (The incidence of incidental prostate cancer in Asian countries was summarized in Table 3.)

Such a significant discrepancy of prostate cancer prevalence between China or some other Asian countries and western countries might relate to genetic backgrounds, lifestyles, socio-economical circumstances and dietary factors contributing to aggravate genomic susceptibility of prostate cancer. The varied geographic distribution across the world implies that the genetic background of prostate cancer might play a role in carcinogenesis. Carter et al reported that prostate cancer often occurred within a family [26]. In addition, males with a prostate cancer history in

Table 1. Patients demographic data of incidental prostate cancer

	Incidental prostate cancer (n = 34)
Age at RCP (Year)	70.3±8.9 (range 52–86)
Follow-up (Months)	46.4±33.8 (range 1–135)
Significant prostate cancer	12 (35.2)
Pathological stage of prostate cancer	
pT2a	19 (55.9)
pT2b	9 (26.5)
pT2c	2 (5.9)
pT3a	3 (8.8)
pT3b	1 (2.9)
Gleason Score	
3	1 (2.9)
4	4 (11.8)
5	4 (11.8)
6	18 (52.9)
7	5 (14.7)
8	1 (2.9)
9	1 (2.9)
Prostate cancer volume ≥0.5 ml	8 (23.5)
Prostate cancer positive surgical margin	1 (2.9)
Prostate apex involvement by incidental prostate cancer	4(11.8)
Prostate stroma invasion by urothelial carcinoma	5 (14.7)

relatives of the first and second orders are more susceptible to have the disease. The twins studies demonstrated that monozygotic twins have a significantly increased risk than dizygotes in both brothers [27–28]. However, even though African Americans are highly susceptible to prostate cancer in United States, their original African nations actually have remarkably lower incidence [29–31], which suggests other important factors also influence the incidence of prostate cancer. Meanwhile, the significant difference of the lifestyle and dietary habits might also relate to prostate cancer incidence. Recent study revealed that the risk of prostate cancer was inversely associated with total dietary fiber intake, insoluble and legume fiber intakes, which are the staple diet in many Asian countries [32]. What's more, as the most popular drink in China and Japan, green tea might also contribute to reduce the prostate cancer risk. A study of Green tea and cancer prevention from Cochrane database demonstrated a decreased risk of prostate cancer in men consuming higher quantities green tea or green tea extracts [33]. Kim et al has also approved that the polyphenon E, a green tea extract was an effective chemopreventive agent in preventing the progression of prostate cancer to metastasis in TRAMP mice model [34].

Up till now, only few reports with limited cases of incidental prostate cancer prevalence in Chinese population are available. We retrospectively reviewed the clinical data and pathological features of 34 out of 504 RCP cases to evaluate the incidence of incidental prostate cancer and the prostate apex involvement in Chinese people.

In this study, incidental prostate cancer was found in 6.8% of RCP specimens, of which 35.2% were considered clinically significant. Patients with an abnormal result of DRE and finally diagnosed with prostate cancer before the surgery had been already excluded from the study. However, a PSA test was not routinely conducted in bladder cancer patients in our institution according to the PSA best practice policy of the American Urological Association, because most of the patients with muscle-invasive bladder cancer have a limited life expectancy whereas most prostate cancer has a relatively long nature history [35]. Thus, a routine PSA screen before RCP for muscle-invasive bladder cancer may only have limited value.

As for the pathological features of the incidental prostate cancer, we found that most of them was pT2a (19/34, 55.9%), with a Gleason score≤6 (27/34, 79.4%) suggesting a more favorable prognosis, which was similar to results of Muzzucchelli et al [12]. There were 3 patients developed a biochemical recurrence after the surgery whereas no patients died of prostate cancer during the follow-up period of this study. As Delongchamps et al mentioned, in patients with concomitant prostate cancer, the poor survival rate was due to the majority of advanced bladder tumors and the outcome would be probably similar as the patients without coexisting prostate cancer [36]. Other authors also have found the same results [17,37–38]. In this case, another oncological problem would focus on whether incidental significant prostate cancer could affect the cancer specific survival of these patients. In this study, there are 12 cases with significant incidental prostate cancer and 22 cases with insignificant incidental prostate cancer. No statistic difference was found in mean age at cystoprostatectomy, in bladder cancer staging and in pelvic lymph node involvement rate by urothelial carcinoma between the groups. The Kaplan-Meier curves excluded a statistical difference in cancer specific survival rate between the 2 groups suggesting that the incidental significant prostate cancer also would not increase the risk of cancer specific mortality in patients with muscle-invasive bladder urothelial carcinoma.

Table 2. Clinical data and pathological feature of significant and insignificant incidental prostate cancer

	Significant prostate cancer(%)	Insignificant prostate cancer(%)	P
Number of Cases	12	22	
Mean Age at RCP (Year)	66.83±6.83 (range 54–77)	72.14±9.43 (range 52–86)	0.096
Preoperative PSA(ng/ml)	2.0	3.7	0.141
Prostate apex involvement by prostate cancer	4 (33.3)	0 (0)	0.011
Prostate stroma invasion by urothelial carcinoma	3 (25.0)	2 (9.1)	0.319
Biochemical recurrence	2 (15.4)	1 (4.5)	0.234
Prostate cancer staging			
pT2a	1 (7.7)	18 (81.8)	
pT2b	5 (41.7)	4 (18.2)	
pT2c	2 (15.4)	0 (0)	
pT3a	3 (25.0)	0 (0)	
pT3b	1(7.7)	0 (0)	
Gleason Score			
3	0 (0)	1 (4.5)	
4	0 (0)	4 (18.2)	
5	0 (0)	4 (18.2)	
6	5 (41.7)	13 (59.1)	
7	5 (41.7)	0 (0)	
8	1 (7.7)	0 (0)	
9	1 (7.7)	0 (0)	
Bladder cancer staging			
pT1	1(8.3)	2(9.1)	0.614
pT2	5(41.7)	13(59.1)	
pT3	3(25.0)	5(22.7)	
pT4	3(25.0)	2(9.1)	
Bladder cancer lymph node involvement			
N0	10(83.3)	18(81.8)	0.742
N1	2(16.7)	3(13.6)	
N2	0(0)	1(4.5)	

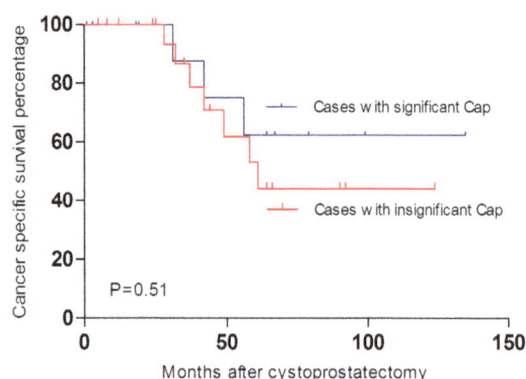

Figure 1. The Kaplan-Meier curves of cancer specific survival (including the urothelial carcinoma and the adenocarcinoma of the prostate) after radical cystoprostatectomy. The blue curve indicated the cancer specific survival of the cases with concomitant significant prostate cancer while the red curve showed the cancer specific survival of the cases with insignificant prostate cancer. There was no statistical significance identified between the 2 groups. (P = 0.51)

RCP has traditionally been considered as a golden standard for the treatment of muscle-invasive bladder cancer [3]. However, the risk of erectile dysfunction and urinary incontinence following this procedure is considerable and might delay the patients' acceptance of RCP, which can adversely affect the prognosis of these patients. Considering the important role of prostate apex for urinary continence and the erectile function, the apex-sparing approach has become a treatment of choice for muscle-invasive bladder cancer. Davila et al. found that erectile function could be significantly preserved by prostate apex-sparing cystectomy [39], meanwhile Colombo et al also proved that after prostate apex-sparing cystectomy with orthotopic urinary diversion, daytime and nighttime continence could be immediate and complete after catheter removal with normal erectile function clinically documented [40]. However, the cancer control must be taken seriously when considering the quality-of–life. In our series, 5 cases (5/34, 14.7%) were found to have prostate-apex involvement by adenocarcinoma of the prostate or urothelial carcinoma. Since the incidence rate of incidental prostate cancer was 6.8% in RCP specimens and the prostate-apex involvement rate was 14.7% (4 apical involvement by incidental prostate cancer and 1 apical involvement by urothelial carcinoma), sparing the prostate apex

Table 3. The incidence of incidental prostate cancer in Asian countries

Nations	Authors	Samples	PCa Cases (%)	Clinical significance
Japan	Yumura et al [19]	59	3 (5.1)	N/A
Japan	Kurahashi et al [13]	251	31 (12.3)	9
Korea	Joung et al [20]	36	18 (50.0)	5
India	Desai et al [21]	44	3 (6.8)	N/A
Saudi	Mosli et al [22]	93	14 (15.1)	N/A
Iran	Hosseini et al [23]	50	7 (14.0)	4
China	Liu et al [24]	49	4 (8.2)	1
China	Zhu et al [25]	92	3 (3.3)	1
Present study	Pan et al	504	34 (6.8)	12
Overall		1207	132 (10.9)	

would be potentially associated with a 1.0% risk of leaving significant cancer of the prostate or urothelial cancer, which was much lower than the estimated risk reported by Gakis et al from a Germany cohort [41].

On the other hand, the prostate stroma invasion by urothelial carcinoma was confirmed in 5 cases (5/34, 14.7%) and one of them had a prostate apex involvement, which was lower than most of the recent reports. In a large series from Pettus et al, 39 out of 122 patients (32%) were found to have prostatic urothelial carcinoma involvement with apical involvement in 18 specimens (15%) [42]. Shen et al also reported a 32% prostate involvement rate with urothelial carcinoma in RCP specimens for bladder cancer [43]. From these studies, we may find that bladder tumor stage, tumor grade, multifocality, tumor in bladder neck/trigone and presence of carcinoma in situ are important risk factors for prostate involvement. Patients with such risk factors are not appropriate candidates for prostate-apex sparing surgery.

Even though the probability of tumor residual in prostate apex is really low, the local recurrence could lead to serious problem in patients with orthotopic neobladder. Therefore, a positive preoperative prostate apical biopsy should preclude the apex-sparing RCP. However, since most incidentally detected prostate cancer are insignificant tumor with a tumor volume<0.5 ml, a negative biopsy cannot completely exclude apical involvement in these patients [44]. Currently no reliable preoperative factors are available to adequately identify whether patients with prostate cancer in the apex [45]. Meanwhile, considering the possibility of concomitant invasion of prostate apex by urothelial carcinoma, we believe the inclusion criteria for prostate apex-sparing surgery in Chinese patients should be limited as follows: young age (<60 years) and socially active, normal erectile function, normal DRE, pT2 solitary bladder cancer, no urothelial carcinoma in trigone, in bladder neck or in prostatic urethra and without carcinoma in situ. Hence, as the preoperative workup, an erectile function assessment before the surgery, a DRE, a serum PSA examination, a pelvic MRI and a cystoscopy with randomized biopsy should be absolutely essential in order to carefully evaluate these candidates.

Besides the apex-sparing radical cystoprostatectomy, there are other techniques such as prostate sparing cystectomy and bladder sparing strategies offering patients better quality of life when treating the muscle invasive bladder cancer. Theoretically, whole prostate sparing cystectomy might have more risk of leaving prostate cancer or urothelial carcinoma in prostate. A Canadian study revealed the overall rate of an underlying cancer within the prostate of cystoprostatectomy specimens was about 46% [46].

Mertens et al reported a 20-year single center experience of prostate sparing cystectomy for bladder cancer with a satisfactory oncological outcome [47]. The 2 and 5-year recurrence-free survival rates were 71.2% and 66.6% with complete daytime and nighttime continence in 96.2% and 81.9% of patients and erectile function intact in 89.7% of patients. Since the whole prostate was preserved, the patient selection should be very careful before the surgery. In their study, all patients underwent preoperative transurethral biopsy of the bladder neck and prostatic urethra and transrectal biopsies of prostate to rule out tumor in the bladder neck, prostatic urethra or prostate cancer. Meanwhile, the bladder sparing strategy is also a feasible procedure in well selected cases. Coen et al carried out a study of 325 cases with muscle invasive bladder cancer treated by transurethral resection and chemoradiation [48]. They established a nomogram including information on clinical T stage, presence of hydronephrosis, whether a visibly complete transurethral resection of bladder tumor was performed, age, sex, and tumor grade to predicting response to bladder-sparing therapy and oncological outcomes. Zapatero et al reported the long-term outcome of prospective bladder-sparing trimodality approach for invasive bladder cancer [49]. Five and 10-year cumulative overall survival were 60%–73% and the cancer-specific survival was 80%–82%. Of all surviving patients, 83% maintained their own bladder. However, these studies of bladder-sparing approach didn't report the erectile function of the patients after chemotherapy and radiotherapy while the chemoradiation could have great influence on it.

Limitation of our study was its retrospective nature. In this study, of all the 504 cases enrolled, the preoperative PSA was only available in 296 cases before radical cystoprostatectomy. For the rest of 208 cases without preoperative PSA, even no palpable nodule was found by DRE, the patients could have concomitant clinical prostate cancer which hadn't been discovered before the surgery. This might lead to a potential selection bias and influence the incidence of incidental prostate cancer in radical cystoprostatectomy specimens, although such an influence could be very limited because of the low incidence of clinical prostate cancer in China (12.10/100 000).A prospective randomized study with large case volumes should be carried out in the near future to evaluate the functional outcome and especially the oncological risk of prostate apex-sparing surgery for bladder urothelial carcinoma in Asia patients.

Conclusion

The prevalence of incidental prostate cancer in RCP specimens in Chinese patients was remarkably lower than in western people. Most of the incidental prostate cancer was clinically insignificant and the patient's prognosis was mainly related to the bladder cancer. Sparing the prostate apex was potentially associated with a 1.0% risk of leaving significant cancer of the prostate or urothelial carcinoma. Further prospective randomized study with large case volumes should be carried out to evaluate the functional outcome and especially the oncological risk of this technique in Asian patients.

Author Contributions

Conceived and designed the experiments: YH. Performed the experiments: JS WX YH HX. Analyzed the data: HY FX. Contributed reagents/materials/analysis tools: JP DL. Wrote the paper: JP WX.

References

1. Jemal A, Bray F, Center MM, Ferlay J, Ward E, et al (2011) Global cancer statistics. CA Cancer J Clin 61: 69–90.
2. Chen WQ, Zeng HM, Zheng RS, Zhang SW, He J (2012) Cancer incidence and mortality in china, 2007. Chin J Cancer Res 24(1):1–8.
3. Zietman AL, Shipley WU, Kaufman DS (2000) Organ-conserving approaches to muscle-invasive bladder cancer: future alternatives to radical cystectomy. Ann Med 32(1):34–42.
4. Novara G, Ficarra V, Minja A, De Marco V, Artibani W (2010) Functional results following vesical ileale Padovana (VIP) neobladder: midterm follow-up analysis with validated questionnaires. Eur Urol 57(6):1045–1051.
5. Wunderlich H, Wolf M, Reichelt O, Fröber R, Schubert J (2006) Radical cystectomy with ultrasound-guided partial prostatectomy for bladder cancer: a complication-preventing concept. Urology 68(3):554–559.
6. Davila HH, Weber T, Burday D, Thurman S, Carrion R, et al. (2007) Total or partial prostate sparing cystectomy for invasive bladder cancer: long-term implications on erectile function. BJU Int 100(5):1026–1029.
7. Gunderson K, Wang C Y and Wang R (2011) Global prostate cancer incidence and the migration, settlement, and admixture history of the Northern Europeans. Cancer Epidemiol 35(4): 320–327.
8. Katanoda K, Matsuda T, Matsuda A, Shibata A, Nishino Y, et al. (2013) An updated report of the trends in cancer incidence and mortality in Japan. Jpn J Clin Oncol 43(5):492–507.
9. Sim HG, Cheng C (2005) Changing demography of prostate cancer in Asia. Eur J Cancer 41(6):834–845.
10. Gakis G, Stenzl A, Renninger M (2013) Do we use the right criteria for determining the clinical significance of incidental prostate cancer at radical cystoprostatectomy? Scand J Urol 47(5):358–362.
11. Alsinnawi M, Loftus B, Flynn R, McDermott T, Grainger R, et al. (2012) The incidence and relevance of prostate cancer in radical cystoprostatectomy specimens. Int Urol Nephrol 44(6):1705–1710.
12. Mazzucchelli R, Montironi R, Morichetti D, Scarpelli M, Lopez-Beltran A, et al. (2010) Comparison between incidentally and clinically detected prostate cancer: implications for prostate cancer screening programs and focal therapy. Anal Quant Cytol Histol 32(3):151–154.
13. Kurahashi T, Miyake H, Furukawa J, Kumano M, Takenaka A, et al. (2010) Characterization of prostate cancer incidentally detected in radical cystoprostatectomy specimens from Japanese men with bladder cancer. Int Urol Nephrol 42(1):73–79.
14. Mazzucchelli R, Barbisan F, Scarpelli M, Lopez-Beltran A, van der Kwast TH, et al. (2009) Is incidentally detected prostate cancer in patients undergoing radical cystoprostatectomy clinically significant? Am J Clin Pathol 131(2):279–283.
15. Abdelhady M, Abusamra A, Pautler SE, Chin JL, Izawa JI (2007) Clinically significant prostate cancer found incidentally in radical cystoprostatectomy specimens. BJU Int 99(2):326–329.
16. Cookson MS, Aus G, Burnett AL, Canby-Hagino ED, D'Amico AV, et al. (2007) Variation in the definition of biochemical recurrence in patients treated for localized prostate cancer: the American Urological Association Prostate Guidelines for Localized Prostate Cancer Update Panel report and recommendations for a standard in the reporting of surgical outcomes. J Urol 177(2):540–545.
17. Abbas F, Hochberg D, Civantos F, Soloway M (1996) Incidental prostatic adenocarcinoma in patients undergoing radical cystoprostatectomy for bladder cancer. Eur Urol 30(3):322–326.
18. Montie JE, Wood DP Jr, Pontes JE, Boyett JM, Levin HS (1989) Adenocarcinoma of the prostate in cystoprostatectomy specimens removed for bladder cancer. Cancer 15;63(2):381–385.
19. Yumura Y, Oogo Y, Takase K, Kato Y, Hamano A, et al. (2006) Clinical analysis of double cancer involving bladder and prostate. Hinyokika kiyo 52: 255–258.
20. Joung JY, Yang SO, Seo HK, Kim TS, Han KS, et al. (2009) Incidental prostate cancer detected by cystoprostatectomy in Korean men. Urology 73(1):153–157.
21. Desai SB, Borges AM (2002) The prevalence of high-grade prostatic intraepithelial neoplasia in surgical resection specimens: an Indian experience. Cancer 94: 2350–2352.
22. Mosli HA, Abdel-Meguid TA, Al-Maghrabi JA, Kamal WK, Saadah HA, et al. (2009) The clinicopathologic patterns of prostatic diseases and prostate cancer in Saudi patients. Saudi Med J 30(11):1439–1443.
23. Hosseini SY, Danesh AK, Parvin M, Basiri A, Javadzadeh T, et al. (2007) Incidental prostatic adenocarcinoma in patients with PSA less than 4 ng/mL undergoing radical cystoprostatectomy for bladder cancer in Iranian men. Int Braz J Urol 33: 167–173.
24. Liu R, Shao GX, Qin RL, Fx K (1996) Coexistence of transitional cell carcinoma of bladder and adenocarcinoma of prostate (report of 5 cases). Chin J Urol 17: 738–739.
25. Zhu YP, Ye DW, Yao XD, Zhang SL, Dai B, et al. (2009) Prevalence of incidental prostate cancer in patients undergoing radical cystoprostatectomy: data from China and other Asian countries. Asian J Androl 11(1):104–108.
26. Carter BS, Steinberg GD, Beaty TH, Childs B, Walsh PC (1991) Familial risk factors for prostate cancer. Cancer Surv 11:5–13.
27. Ahlbom A, Lichtenstein P, Malmström H, Feychting M, Hemminki K, et al. (1997) Cancer in twins: genetic and nongenetic familial risk factors. J Natl Cancer Inst 89:287–293.
28. Schaid DJ, McDonnell SK, Blute ML, Thibodeau SN (1998) Evidence for autosomal dominant inheritance of prostate cancer. Am J Hum Genet 62:1425–1438.
29. Cussenot O, Valeri A (2001) Heterogeneity in genetic susceptibility to prostate cancer. Eur J Intern Med 12:11–16.
30. Ogunbiyi JO, Shittu OB (1999) Increased incidence of prostate cancer in Nigerians. J Natl Med Assoc 91:159–164.
31. Walker AR, Walker BF (2003) Puzzles in the causation and epidemiology of prostate cancer—a sombre outlook. S Afr Med J 93:773–774.
32. Deschasaux M, Pouchieu C, His M, Hercberg S, Latino-Martel P, et al. (2014) Dietary total and insoluble fiber intakes are inversely associated with prostate cancer risk. J Nutr 144(4):504–510.
33. Boehm K, Borrelli F, Ernst E, Habacher G, Hung SK, et al. (2009) Green tea (Camellia sinensis) for the prevention of cancer. Cochrane Database Syst Rev doi: 10.1002/14651858.CD005004.pub2
34. Kim S, Amankwah EK, Connors S, Park HY, Rincon M, et al. (2014) Safety and chemopreventive effect of Polyphenon E in preventing early and metastatic progression of prostate cancer in TRAMP mice. Cancer Prev Res (Phila) doi:10.1158/1940-6207.CAPR-13-0427-T
35. (2000) Prostate-specific antigen (PSA) best practice policy. American Urological Association. Oncology 14(2):267–272.
36. Delongchamps NB, Mao K, Theng H, Zerbib M, Debré B, et al. (2005) Outcome of patients with fortuitous prostate cancer after radical cystoprostatectomy for bladder cancer. Eur Urol 48:946–950.
37. Kouriefs C, Fazili T, Masood S, Naseem MS, Mufti GR (2005) Incidentally detected prostate cancer in cystoprostatectomy specimens. Urol Int 75:213–216.
38. Konski A, Rubin P, DiSantangnese PA, Mayer E, Keys H, et al. (1991) Simultaneous presentation of adenocarcinoma of prostate and transitional cell carcinoma of bladder. Urology 37:202–206.
39. Davila HH, Weber T, Burday D, Thurman S, Carrion R, et al. (2007) Total or partial prostate sparing cystectomy for invasive bladder cancer: long-term implications on erectile function. BJU Int 100(5):1026–1029.
40. Colombo R, Bertini R, Salonia A, Da Pozzo LF, Montorsi F, et al. (2001) Nerve and seminal sparing radical cystectomy with orthotopic urinary diversion for selected patients with superficial bladder cancer: An innovative surgical approach. J Urol 165:51–55.
41. Gakis G, Schilling D, Bedke J, Sievert KD, Stenzl A (2010) Incidental prostate cancer at radical cystoprostatectomy: implications for apex-sparing surgery. BJU Int 105(4):468–471.
42. Pettus JA, Al-Ahmadie H, Barocas DA (2006) Prostate involvement by urothelial and prostatic carcinomas in radical cystoprostatectomy specimens. Paper presented at: The 2006 Annual Meeting of the American Urological Association; May 20–25; Atlanta, GA.
43. Shen SS, Lerner SP, Muezzinoglu B, Truong LD, Amiel G, et al. (2006) Prostatic involvement by transitional cell carcinoma in patients with bladder cancer and its prognostic significance. Hum Pathol 37(6):726–734.
44. Moutzouris G, Barbatis C, Plastiras D, Mertziotis N, Katsifotis C, et al. (1999) Incidence and histological findings of unsuspected prostatic adenocarcinoma in radical cystoprostatectomy for transitional cell carcinoma of the bladder. Scand J Urol Nephrol 33(1):27–30.
45. Damiano R, Di Lorenzo G, Cantiello F, De Sio M, Perdonà S, et al. (2007) Clinicopathologic features of prostate adenocarcinoma incidentally discovered at the time of radical cystectomy: an evidence-based analysis. Eur Urol 52(3):648–657.

46. Sivalingam S, Drachenberg D (2013) The incidence of prostate cancer and urothelial cancer in the prostate in cystoprostatectomy specimens in a tertiary care Canadian centre. Can Urol Assoc J 7(1–2):35–38.

47. Mertens LS, Meijer RP, de Vries RR, Nieuwenhuijzen JA, van der Poel HG, et al. (2013) Prostate Sparing Cystectomy for Bladder Cancer: 20-Year Single Center Experience. J Urol doi: 10.1016/j.juro.2013.11.031.

48. Coen JJ, Paly JJ, Niemierko A, Kaufman DS, Heney NM, et al. (2013) Nomograms predicting response to therapy and outcomes after bladder-preserving trimodality therapy for muscle-invasive bladder cancer. Int J Radiat Oncol Biol Phys 1;86(2):311–316.

49. Zapatero A, Martin De Vidales C, Arellano R, Ibañez Y, Bocardo G, et al. (2012) Long-term results of two prospective bladder-sparing trimodality approaches for invasive bladder cancer: neoadjuvant chemotherapy and concurrent radio-chemotherapy. http://www.ncbi.nlm.nih.gov/pubmed/22999456Urology 80(5):1056–1062.

22

Investigating the Different Mechanisms of Genotoxic and Non-Genotoxic Carcinogens by a Gene Set Analysis

Won Jun Lee[1], Sang Cheol Kim[2]*, Seul Ji Lee[1], Jeongmi Lee[3], Jeong Hill Park[1], Kyung-Sang Yu[4], Johan Lim[5], Sung Won Kwon[1]*

1 College of Pharmacy and Research Institute of Pharmaceutical Sciences, Seoul National University, Seoul, Republic of Korea, 2 Samsung Genome Institute, Samsung Medical Center, Seoul, Republic of Korea, 3 School of Pharmacy, Sungkyunkwan University, Suwon, Republic of Korea, 4 Seoul National University College of Medicine and Hospital, Seoul, Republic of Korea, 5 Department of Statistics, Seoul National University, Seoul, Republic of Korea

Abstract

Based on the process of carcinogenesis, carcinogens are classified as either genotoxic or non-genotoxic. In contrast to non-genotoxic carcinogens, many genotoxic carcinogens have been reported to cause tumor in carcinogenic bioassays in animals. Thus evaluating the genotoxicity potential of chemicals is important to discriminate genotoxic from non-genotoxic carcinogens for health care and pharmaceutical industry safety. Additionally, investigating the difference between the mechanisms of genotoxic and non-genotoxic carcinogens could provide the foundation for a mechanism-based classification for unknown compounds. In this study, we investigated the gene expression of HepG2 cells treated with genotoxic or non-genotoxic carcinogens and compared their mechanisms of action. To enhance our understanding of the differences in the mechanisms of genotoxic and non-genotoxic carcinogens, we implemented a gene set analysis using 12 compounds for the training set (12, 24, 48 h) and validated significant gene sets using 22 compounds for the test set (24, 48 h). For a direct biological translation, we conducted a gene set analysis using Globaltest and selected significant gene sets. To validate the results, training and test compounds were predicted by the significant gene sets using a prediction analysis for microarrays (PAM). Finally, we obtained 6 gene sets, including sets enriched for genes involved in the adherens junction, bladder cancer, p53 signaling pathway, pathways in cancer, peroxisome and RNA degradation. Among the 6 gene sets, the bladder cancer and p53 signaling pathway sets were significant at 12, 24 and 48 h. We also found that the DDB2, RRM2B and GADD45A, genes related to the repair and damage prevention of DNA, were consistently up-regulated for genotoxic carcinogens. Our results suggest that a gene set analysis could provide a robust tool in the investigation of the different mechanisms of genotoxic and non-genotoxic carcinogens and construct a more detailed understanding of the perturbation of significant pathways.

Editor: Peiwen Fei, University of Hawaii Cancer Center, United States of America

Funding: This research was supported by Bio & Medical Technology Development Program of the National Research Foundation (NRF) funded by the Korean government (Ministry of Education, Science and Technology) (NRF- 2011-0019639), Basic Science Research Program through the NRF of Korea funded by the Ministry of Education, Science and Technology (NRF-2011-0023057) and NRF of Korea grant funded by the Korean government (MSIP)(NRF-2011-0030810). The funders had no role in study design, data collection and analysis, decision to publish, or preparation of the manuscript.

Competing Interests: The authors have declared that no competing interests exist.

* E-mail: swkwon@snu.ac.kr (SWK); sckim.sgi@gmail.com (SCK)

Introduction

Based on their mechanisms of action, chemical carcinogens are classified as genotoxic carcinogens (GTXs) or non-genotoxic carcinogens (NGTXs). GTXs covalently bind with DNA to form DNA adducts, which results in neoplastic initiation [1–3]. In *in vitro* and short-term *in vivo* assays, GTXs have been observed to damage DNA and generate chromosomal aberrations [1,2]. NGTXs, however, do not directly bind with DNA, instead, they cause neoplastic transformations through various mechanisms, including repression of the immune system and inducing oxidative stress [1,2]. Therefore, it is hypothesized that GTXs and NGTXs induce distinct gene expressions profiles, which may consequently be used to classify unknown compounds as either GTXs or NGTXs [4]. Unlike NGTXs, many GTXs also cause tumor in animal-based carcinogenic bioassays and environment exposures to chemical carcinogens have been reported to be major causal factors for cancer [5]. From the perspective of health care safety and the

pharmaceutical industry, determining the genotoxic potentials of chemicals to which humans are exposed is important to discriminate GTXs from NGTXs [5].

The potential genotoxicity of carcinogens is evaluated using *in vitro* tests, such as bacterial gene mutation test (Ames test), the mammalian micronuclei (MN) test, the chromosomal aberration (CA) test and the mouse lymphoma assay (MLA) [6]. To be classified as a genotoxic carcinogen, a chemical must exhibit *in vivo* genotoxicity in rodents. However, the *in vitro* results may not correspond with the results of *in vivo* evaluations, which result in numerous unnecessary animal experiments that are both costly and time consuming [7,8]. Thus, a more robust *in vitro* method is required.

Toxicogenomics, the application of gene expression profiling to toxicological investigations, provides novel approaches to address this problem, leading to deeper mechanistic insights. These approaches have been demonstrated to discriminate between GTXs and NGTXs [1,9]. To interpret gene expression profiling in a biologically meaningful way, individually identifying every gene with a statistically significant response is not sufficient [10]. Recently, the focus of studies has shifted from studying the effects of individual genes to studying the effects of a gene set, i.e., multiple functionally related genes [11,12]. A few studies including on by Kim HS *et al.* [10] have demonstrated the successful application of gene set analysis using gene expression data. In this study, we conducted gene set analysis to discriminate between genotoxic and non-genotoxic mechanisms for the first time.

To apply a gene set analysis, we used 12 compounds as the training set (12, 24, 48 h) and validated significant gene sets using 22 compounds for the test set (24, 48 h). Using a cut-off of $p<0.05$ for at least 1 time point, we selected 57 significant gene sets from 5 GTXs and 7 NGTXs in the training data. To validate the 57 gene sets, we utilized the prediction analysis for microarrays (PAM) and the accuracy of each gene set was calculated using the 24 and 48 h time points in both the training and test data. Compared with previous studies, our results suggest that this method of applying gene set analysis could be used to more clearly explain the differences between GTX and NGTX mechanisms.

Materials and Methods

Data collection

Raw gene expression profiling data were obtained from the Gene Expression Omnibus through accession number GSE28878. In a microarray experiment, HepG2 cells were treated with GTXs or NGTXs. The HepG2 cell culture medium was replaced with fresh medium containing either compound or with the corresponding control. HepG2 cells were treated with the training set compounds for 12, 24 and 48 h and the test set compounds for 24 and 48 h [5].

The liver plays an important role in the metabolism of many compounds and represents a major target organ in systemic toxicity, therefore, hepatic models are frequently used among the *in vitro* models [13]. As a preferred model of hepatic cell lines, the human liver cell line (HepG2) is widely employed in studies on the biotransformation of xenobiotic compounds because it does not carry the p53 mutation and enables cells to induce the DNA damage response pathway, arrest growth and activate apoptosis [13]. Many studies have revealed that HepG2 cells are suitable and applicable for genotoxic assays including the MN test and the comet assay [14].

The genotoxicity of the carcinogens was evaluated using *in vitro* genotoxicity assays (MN, CA, MLA) and *in vivo* genotoxicity assays (MN, CA). Carcinogens were classified as GTXs when they caused positive results in the genotoxicity assays and NGTXs if they caused negative results [5]. To observe a clear difference between GTXs and NGTXs, we selected 16 GTXs that showed consistent genotoxicity in both the *in vitro* and *in vivo* assays and 18 NGTXs that showed consistent non-genotoxicity in both *in vitro* and *in vivo* assays in GSE28878.

Table 1 displays the details for each of the selected compounds. We used 12 compounds for the training set and 22 compounds for the validation set. The training data included 12, 24 and 48 h time points that were used for expression profiling, and the validation data included 24 and 48 h time points.

Preprocessing

Human Genome U133 Plus 2.0 Gene Chip Arrays were used as the platform for the gene expression profile [5]. The data were normalized using a robust multi-array analysis (RMA) with the affy R package [15]. To convert the gene labels into Entrez IDs, we used the Database for Annotation, Visualization, and Integrated

Table 1. Thirty-four compounds were classified as part of the training sets and test sets.

Dataset		Compound	Time (h)
Training	GTX	Aflatoxin B1	12,24,48
		Benzo[a]pyrene	12,24,48
		2-Acetyl aminofluorene	12,24,48
		Dimethyl nitrosamine	12,24,48
		Mitomycin C	12,24,48
	NGTX	2,3,7,8-Tetrachloro	12,24,48
		dibenzo-p-dioxin	12,24,48
		Wy 14643	12,24,48
		Cyclosporine A	12,24,48
		Ampicillin trihydrate	12,24,48
		Di(2-ethylhexyl) phthalate	12,24,48
		d-Mannitol	12,24,48
		Diclofenac	12,24,48
Test	GTX	Azathioprine	24, 48
		4-Aminobiphenyl	24, 48
		Benzidine	24, 48
		Chlorambucil	24, 48
		1-Ethyl-1-nitrosourea	24, 48
		4,4'-Methylenebis(2chloroaniline)	24, 48
		2-Amino-3-methylimidazo[4,5-f] quinolone	24, 48
		Cyclophosphamide	24, 48
		Cisplatin	24, 48
		Furan	24, 48
		Diethylnitrosamine	24, 48
	NGTX	Caprolactam	24, 48
		Coumaphos	24, 48
		Diazinon	24, 48
		Acesulfame-K	24, 48
		Progesterone	24, 48
		1,1,1-Trichloro-2,2-di-(4chlorophenyl) ethane	24, 48
		Lindane	24, 48
		Nitrobenzene	24, 48
		Simazine	24, 48
		Tetrachloroethylene	24, 48
		Pentachlorophenol	24, 48

Training sets included 5 GTXs and 7 NGTXs, and the test sets included 11 GTXs and 11 NGTXs. The time points were 12, 24 and 48 h of exposure for the training set and 24 and 48 h of exposure for the test set.

Discovery (DAVID) software [16]. At each time point, fold changes were calculated for each compound through a comparison to a corresponding control.

To remove batch effects, we used the ComBat method in the sva R package. The ComBat method can be applied to high dimensional data matrices using an empirical Bayesian framework, and the ComBat output is a corrected expression profile [17]. Our training and test datasets were processed for each of the 3 different days. We found that our expression profile had severe batch effects that were removed by the ComBat method (Figure S1).

Selection and validation of significant gene sets

The aim of this gene set analysis was to search for gene set expression profiles related to GTXs or NGTXs [18]. We evaluated the differential gene expression patterns of gene sets derived from the Kyoto Encyclopedia of Genes and Genomes (KEGG) pathways and selected significant gene sets after exposure to 5 GTX and 7 NGTX.

For the gene set analysis, the Globaltest R package was used. Globaltest is a generalized linear model for predicting a response variable from the expression of gene sets [10,18]. The null hypothesis of Globaltest is that there are no associations between the response (GTXs vs. NGTXs) and expression of the gene sets [18]. P-values were calculated from the "gt" function in Globaltest. We found 57 gene sets with a p<0.05 for at least one of the 12, 24 and 48 h time points. Additionally, using the "comparative" function in Globaltest, we calculated comparative p-values as false discovery rate (FDR) for multiple-comparisons of KEGG pathways.

To determine whether the 57 gene sets were significant, a prediction analysis for microarrays (PAM) was conducted. The PAM classifies samples from gene expression data using the nearest shrunken centroid method [19]. The nearest shrunken centroid classification is a modified standard nearest centroid classification. Using the nearest shrunken centroid, samples were classified by the subsets of genes that best characterize each class. PAM has been employed by numerous studies to predict class from gene expression data [20–23].

Using the fold changes of each of the 57 selected gene sets, PAM was performed to develop prediction models from the training set. Using the 57 prediction models, 12 training and 22 test compounds were predicted to classify into GTXs or NGTXs at 24 and 48 h, respectively. To generate a predictive model, a balanced 10-fold cross validation was conducted for each gene set. Using the PAM results, accuracy, sensitivity and specificity, were calculated. We selected the final 6 gene sets using an accuracy of > 90% for the training set and an accuracy of > 70% for the test set.

Visualization

To visualize the 6 significant gene sets, we generated a gene plot using the Globaltest R package. The "Global Test Statistic" for each gene can be represented as the p-value from the component test in the Globaltest.

In the gene plot, we visualized the p-values of genes as bars. The gene with the lowest p-value contributed the most to the significance of the test result. The bars were colored to indicate a positive or a negative association of the gene expression with either GTXs or NGTXs. Thus, based on the comparison of GTXs with NGTXs, red bars indicate a gene that is up-regulated by a GTX and green bars indicate a gene that is down-regulated by a GTX. The threshold for statistical significance was set as p-value < 0.05. To further our understanding, we calculated the average fold change related to 5 GTXs and 7 NGTXs in training data and mapped the fold changes of individual gene to the KEGG pathway for each time point using pathview R package (http://bioconductor.org/packages/2.12/bioc/html/pathview.html). Pathview is used for data integration and visualization of pathways. This program maps a wide variety of biological data to a target pathway specified by user.

Principal component analysis (PCA) was performed using the R function, "prcomp" for the expression values of each of the 6 gene sets. Twelve compounds from the training data were distributed by 3D principal component analysis for each of the 3 time points.

To measure the classification performance, we used Kernel-based Orthogonal Projections to Latent Structures (K-OPLS)

[24,25]. Because the K-OPLS method has a unique ability to detect an unanticipated systemic variation, the results provide a robust model evaluation [24]. Additionally K-OPLS has been applied to model a variety of biological data [24,25]. Using the K-OPLS R package, we implemented 100-permutations and calculated the area under the curve (AUC).

Results and Discussion

Gene set analysis and classification

We conducted a gene set analysis to discriminate between GTXs and NGTXs and obtained a global test statistic. Because there were only a few gene sets that were significant at the p < 0.05 level, an unadjusted p-value below 0.05 was selected as the cut-off. There were 57 gene sets that satisfied p < 0.05 for at least one of the 12, 24 and 48 h time points (Table S1). We found that 12 gene sets were consistently activated at all 3 time points. The results also revealed that 29 gene sets were only activated at 12 h, 6 gene sets were activated only at 24 h and 5 gene sets were activated only at 48 h. We identified 3 gene sets that were activated both at 12 and 24 h but not 48 h. There were also 3 gene sets that were activated both at 12 and 48 h but not 24 h. We also found that 44, 24 and 20 gene sets were activated at 12, 24 and 48 h, respectively (Figure 1). This finding suggested that most gene sets were significantly activated at an earlier time point.

Using the 57 gene sets, 12 training and 22 test compounds were classified as GTXs or NGTXs and we determined the accuracy, sensitivity and specificity of the classification using PAM (Table S2). We calculated the accuracy, sensitivity and specificity as described in previous studies [26,27]. In the classification results, a positive or negative value indicated that the compound was classified as a GTX or NGTX, respectively. Thus, a true positives (TP) is an actual GTX that was predicted to be a GTX, and a false positive (FP) is an actual NGTX that was predicted to be a GTX. Similarly, a false negative (FN) is an actual GTX that was classified as a NGTX, and a true negative (TN) is an actual NGTX that was predicted to be an NGTX. From the TP, FP, FN and TN rates, we calculated the accuracy, sensitivity and specificity of the 12 training and 22 test compounds.

Compared with the test dataset, the accuracy of each gene set was higher for the training dataset. We selected 6 gene sets with >

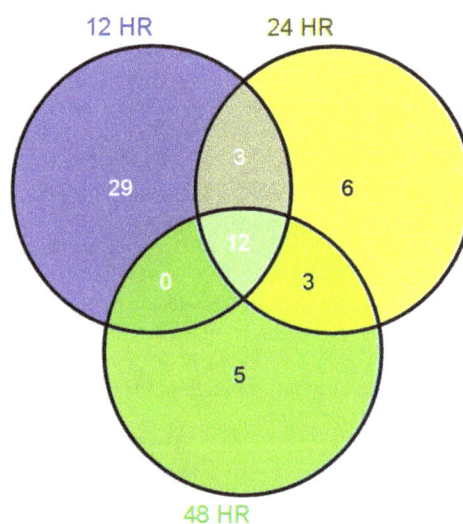

Figure 1. A Venn diagram displaying the 57 gene sets that met p < 0.05 for at least one of the 12, 24 or 48 h time points.

Table 2. To validate the 6 significant gene sets, PAM was conducted to classify the compounds using the fold changes of the 6 significant gene sets.

Gene Set Name	24 h Training accuracy (%)	sensitivity (%)	specificity (%)	24 h Test accuracy (%)	sensitivity (%)	specificity (%)	48 h Training accuracy (%)	sensitivity (%)	specificity (%)	48 h Test accuracy (%)	sensitivity (%)	specificity (%)
Adherens junction	92	80	100	73	55	91	100	100	100	73	45	100
Bladder cancer	92	80	100	73	45	100	92	80	100	77	55	100
p53 signaling pathway	92	80	100	73	45	100	92	80	100	73	45	100
Pathways in cancer	100	100	100	73	45	100	100	100	100	73	45	100
Peroxisome	100	100	100	77	64	91	92	100	86	77	82	73
RNA degradation	92	80	100	73	45	100	100	100	100	73	45	100
Mean	95	87	100	74	50	97	96	93	98	74	53	96

Accuracy, sensitivity and specificity were calculated for both the training dataset and the test dataset.

90% accuracy in the training set and $> 70\%$ accuracy in the test set (Table 2). These 6 gene sets included genes related to the adherens junction, bladder cancer, p53 signaling pathway, pathways in cancer, peroxisome and RNA degradation.

Among the 6 gene sets, we found that the bladder cancer and p53 signaling pathway gene sets were significant for all 3 time points, the other gene sets were significant only at 12 h (Table 3). Even after correcting the p-value for the FDR, the bladder cancer and p53 signaling pathway gene sets were still significant at all 3 time points. According to the FDR, more gene sets were significantly activated at 12 h than at 24 and 48 h (Table 3). Because all 6 gene sets were significantly activated at 12 h, investigations of the gene expression at earlier time points would be beneficial. Such an investigation may explain why the bladder cancer and p53 signaling pathway gene sets were significant at all three time points, whereas other gene sets were significant only at the early time point (Table S1).

The K-OPLS results indicated that 24 h of exposure to the training compounds resulted in a higher mean AUC than 48 h of exposure. Notably at 24 h, the p53 signaling pathway and bladder cancer gene sets exhibited robust performance with respect to classification, with an AUC of 0.907 and 0.861, respectively (Table 3).

Gene plot and PCA analysis

To further evaluate the significant gene sets including p53 signaling pathway and bladder cancer pathway, we investigated time-dependent expression in gene plot. A gene plot explains the contribution of each individual gene in the significant test, and therefore, we were able to identify genes that were differentially expressed in the gene set. For GTX treated HepG2 cells, the gene plot indicated that significantly up-regulated genes were more dominant than down-regulated genes. In the bladder cancer gene set, TP53, RASSF1, CDKN1A and PGF were significantly up-regulated after 12 h of GTX exposure. At 24 h, MDM2, PGF, CDKN1A and E2F1 were significantly up-regulated by GTXs. PGF, MDM2 and CDKN1A were up-regulated by GTXs at 48 h (Figure S2).

In the p53 signaling pathway gene set, 13 genes (DDB2, EI24, PIDD, TP53, TP73, CDK2, PPM1D, SESN1, RRM2, CASP9, CDKN1A, APAF1, BAX) were significantly up-regulated by GTXs at 12 h (Figure S2). Five of these genes (PIDD, BAX, PIGs, APAF-1, CASP9) are known to be involved in apoptosis, and three of these genes (DDB2, SENS1, RRM2) are associated with DNA repair. TP75 and PPM1D are related to the negative feedback of p53.

Table 3. P-values calculated from the Globaltest for each of the 3 time points in the training set.

Gene set Name	Training data 12 h	24 h	48 h
Adherens junction	0.035	0.111	0.338
Bladder cancer	0.010	0.008	0.015
p53 Signaling pathway	0.016	0.006	0.013
Pathways in cancer	0.039	0.056	0.277
Peroxisome	0.016	0.265	0.438
RNA degradation	0.008	0.205	0.207

We visualized the p53 signaling pathway as gene plots for the 24 and 48 h points, shown in Figure 2a and Figure 2b, respectively. In the p53 signaling pathway, we found 17 and 13 significant ($p < 0.05$) genes at 24 and 48 h, respectively; the number of significant genes decreased as exposure time increased from 24 to 48 h. In Figure 2a, it can be observed that 17 genes were significant (PIDD, DDB2, MDM2, BBC3, RRM2B, STEAP3, CCNB3, PPM1D, CDKN1A, RPRM, PTEN, BAX, EI24, GADD45A, ZMAT3, TP53I3, SESN1). In Figure 2b, it can be observed that 13 genes were significant (DDB2, CDKN1A, PPM1D, PIDD, TP53I3, EI24, MDM2, CCNG1, SESN3, PTEN, TP73, RRM2B, and SESN1).

We compared the significant genes in each functional group to understand the functional changes in the p53 signaling pathway. Figure 2a shows that four genes (PIDD, BBC3, BAX, EI24) were involved in apoptosis at 24 h, and three genes (DDB2, RRM2B, GADD45A) were associated with DNA repair at 24 h. MDM2 and PPM1D were related to the negative feedback of p53. Figure 2b shows that three genes (PIDD, TP53I3, EI24) were involved in apoptosis at 48 h, and three genes (DDB2, SESN3, RRM2B) were associated with DNA repair. MDM2, CCNG1 and PPM1D were related to the negative feedback of p53.

In both Figure 2a and Figure 2b, it can be observed that the identical number of DNA repair-related genes were consistently up-regulated; however, the number of apoptosis-related genes decreased from four (Figure 2a) to three (Figure 2b). The number of p53 negative feedback-related genes increased from two (Figure 2a) to three (Figure 2b).

The KEGG pathway and the fold-changes of individual genes, presented in the bottom of Figure 2, showed that several apoptosis-related genes (shown in Figure 2a) were up-regulated, but these up-regulated genes lost their expressions (Figure 2b). However, the fold-changes of the DNA repair-related genes shown in Figure 2a and Figure 2b were consistent.

By increasing the exposure time from 12 to 48 h, the number of significantly up-regulated genes related to apoptosis decreased from five to three, whereas the same number of DNA repair-related genes was consistently up-regulated for the GTX-treated HepG2 cells. Notably, TP53 is known to be involved in the suppression of tumors and was significantly up-regulated at 12 h; this significance was lost at 24 and 48 h. Instead, MDM2, a known negative regulator of the p53 tumor suppressor, was significantly up-regulated at 24 and 48 h.

At all 3 time points, the DNA damage-binding protein 2 (DDB2) was highly up-regulated in GTX- treated HepG2 cells. A recent study suggested that p53-triggered up-regulation of DDB2 is associated with a resistance to cell death that is induced by melanoma therapy in malignant melanoma cells [28]. Compared with the 12 h time point, the number of significantly up-regulated genes related to the negative feedback of p53 was increased at 48 h.

A PCA analysis revealed that the 12 compounds in the training set were appropriately classified into either GTXs or NGTXs for both the bladder cancer gene set and p53 signaling pathway gene set, particularly at 24 h (Figure 3). Additionally, 34 compounds in the training and test data were separated by the expression of the p53 signaling pathway and bladder cancer gene sets at 24 h (Figure S3).

Conclusions

To identify the differences between the GTX and NGTX biological mechanisms, we conducted a gene set analysis and validated significant gene sets. In previous studies, each gene was individually identified and classified using only statistical processes, and each of the individual classifiers was unrelated to biological mechanisms. However, information regarding biological processes is available for each gene in our study; thus, our method offers a

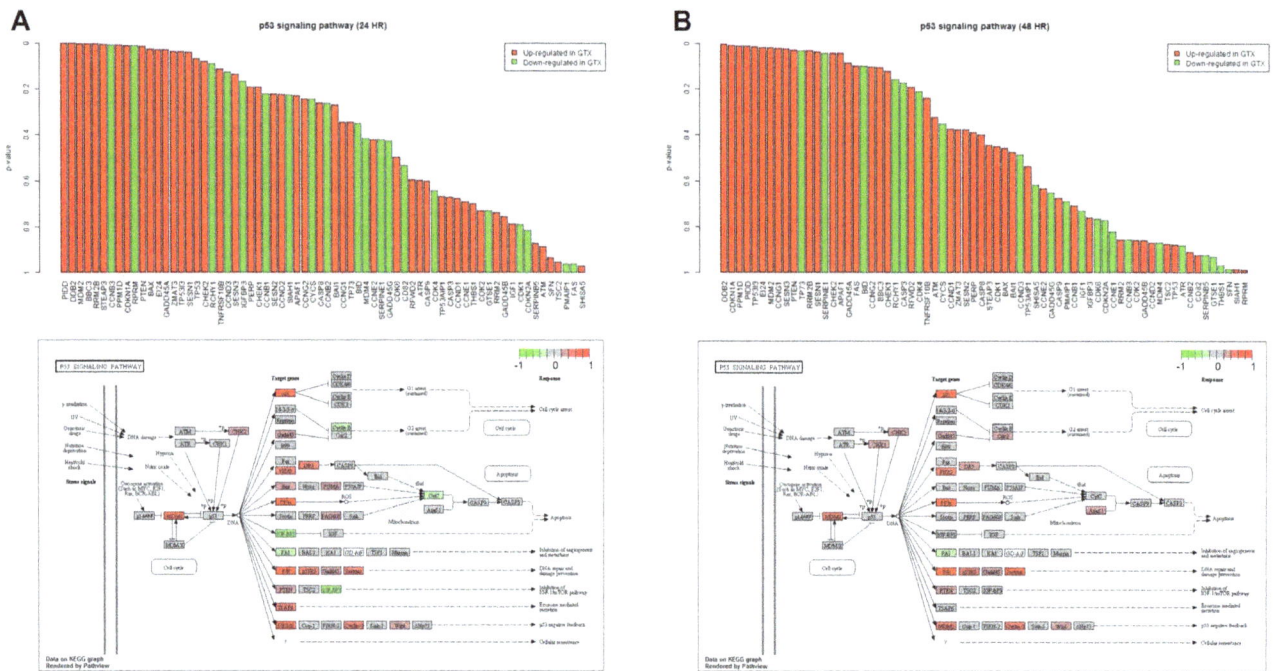

Figure 2. Gene plot (top) from Globaltest and KEGG pathway (bottom) showing the fold change of individual genes in the p53 signaling pathway. Red and green bars indicate up-regulated and down-regulated genes, respectively, after GTX exposure at A. 24 h or B. 48 h in comparison to NGTX exposure.

A

B

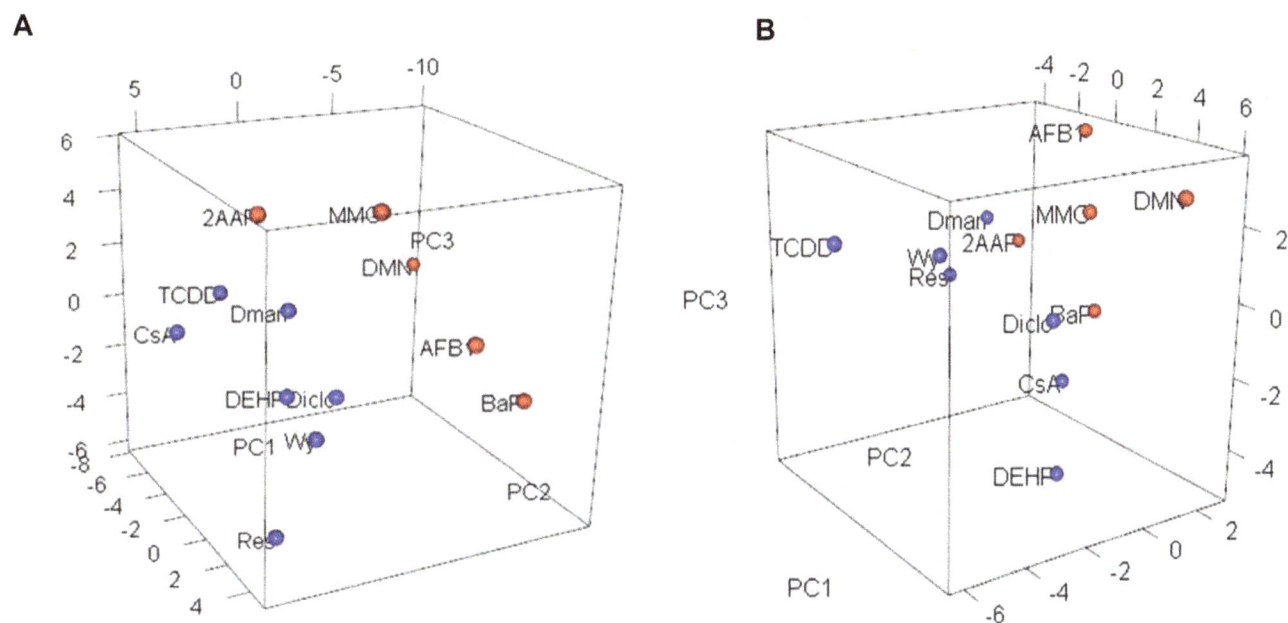

Figure 3. Principal component analysis revealed the distribution of 12 compounds in the training data. A. PCA results for gene expression in the p53 signaling pathway gene set at 24 h [red, 5 GTX; blue, 7 NGTX]. B. PCA results for gene expression in the bladder cancer gene set at 48 h [red, 5 GTX; blue, 7 NGTX].

simplified approach for explaining the different mechanisms of GTXs and NGTXs.

In a previous study, Magkoufopoulou *et al.* [5] suggested that their reported classifiers had a high classification accuracy at 24 h. Because they selected their classifiers from Ames-positive and Ames-negative compounds separately, the classifiers could be associated with different genotoxic properties. They also validated Ames-positive and Ames-negative compounds separately. This means that their classifiers may be limited in that they can only integrate information regarding Ames-positive and Ames-negative compounds. To evaluate genotoxicity using both *in vivo* results and Ames test results, we conducted gene sets analysis using 16 GTX that showed consistent genotoxicity in both the *in vitro* and *in vivo* assays and 18 NGTX that showed consistent non-genotoxicity in both *in vitro* and *in vivo* assays. The findings indicated that our gene sets could explain the genotoxic mechanism using both *in vivo* and Ames tests.

Our results revealed that at the 3 different time points, the expression of most gene sets was significantly activated at 12 h. Therefore, even if the previous study obtained their classifiers and validated them at 24 h, the expressions of genes at 12 h could provide more information on the mechanism of genotoxicity.

Although we identified gene sets that could discriminate between the GTXs and NGTXs biological processes, these gene sets could not explain why the compounds showed different results for the *in vivo* and *in vitro* assays. Additionally, in validation, the accuracy of test compounds was not as good as the training data. In conclusion, by employing gene set analysis, we found that the p53 signaling pathway and bladder cancer gene sets most accurately discriminated between GTXs and NGTXs. Additionally, our results suggested that gene expression at the early time point could provide more information regarding the initiation of carcinogenesis than that at a later time point. We further concluded that significantly expressed genes are involved in DNA repair, apoptosis and the negative feedback of p53.

Supporting Information

Figure S1 A. Clustering of the 12 h training data, which was influenced by 3 different groups [a, Series A; b, Series B; c, Series C]. **B.** After applying the ComBat method, the output revealed that batch effects from the different groups were removed.

Figure S2 Gene plot from Globaltest showed time-dependent expression of bladder cancer gene set. A. 12 h, **B.** 24 h, **C.** 48 h, **D.** Gene plot from Globaltest showing the p53 signaling pathway gene set at 12 h.

Figure S3 Thirty-four compounds including training and test data were separated using PCA. A. The expression of p53 signaling pathway was used in PCA at 24 h. **B.** The expression of bladder cancer was used in PCA at 24 h.

Table S1 Globaltest statistic of the 57 gene sets that satisfied p < 0.05 for at least one of the 12, 24 and 48 h time points.

Table S2 Using the 57 gene sets, 12 training and 22 test compounds were classified as GTXs or NGTXs and accuracy, sensitivity and specificity were obtained from the results of classification using PAM.

Table S3 In training dataset, FDR were calculated by function ''comparative'' of Globaltest. AUC generated by K-OPLS for measuring the performance of classification.

Author Contributions

Conceived and designed the experiments: WJL SCK JL SWK. Performed the experiments: WJL SCK SWK. Analyzed the data: WJL SJL JmL JHP

KSY. Contributed reagents/materials/analysis tools: JHP JL SWK. Wrote the paper: WJL SCK KSY SWK.

References

1. Ellinger-Ziegelbauer H, Stuart B, Wahle B, Bomann W, Ahr HJ (2005) Comparison of the expression profiles induced by genotoxic and nongenotoxic carcinogens in rat liver. Mutat Res 575: 61–84.
2. Williams GM (2001) Mechanisms of chemical carcinogenesis and application to human cancer risk assessment. Toxicology 166: 3–10.
3. Mathijs K, Brauers KJ, Jennen DG, Boorsma A, van Herwijnen MH, et al. (2009) Discrimination for genotoxic and nongenotoxic carcinogens by gene expression profiling in primary mouse hepatocytes improves with exposure time. Toxicol Sci 112: 374–384.
4. Watanabe T, Suzuki T, Natsume M, Nakajima M, Narumi K, et al. (2012) Discrimination of genotoxic and non-genotoxic hepatocarcinogens by statistical analysis based on gene expression profiling in the mouse liver as determined by quantitative real-time PCR. Mutat Res 747: 164–175.
5. Magkoufopoulou C, Claessen SM, Tsamou M, Jennen DG, Kleinjans JC, et al. (2012) A transcriptomics-based in vitro assay for predicting chemical genotoxicity in vivo. Carcinogenesis 33: 1421–1429.
6. Ames BN, Lee FD, Durston WE (1973) An improved bacterial test system for the detection and classification of mutagens and carcinogens. Proc Natl Acad Sci U S A 70: 782–786.
7. Kirkland D, Aardema M, Henderson L, Muller L (2005) Evaluation of the ability of a battery of three in vitro genotoxicity tests to discriminate rodent carcinogens and non-carcinogens I. Sensitivity, specificity and relative predictivity. Mutat Res 584: 1–256.
8. Gollapudi BB, Thybaud V, Kim JH, Holsapple M (2011) Strategies for the follow-up of positive results in the in vitro genotoxicity assays—an international collaborative initiative. Environ Mol Mutagen 52: 174–176.
9. van Delft JH, van Agen E, van Breda SG, Herwijnen MH, Staal YC, et al. (2004) Discrimination of genotoxic from non-genotoxic carcinogens by gene expression profiling. Carcinogenesis 25: 1265–1276.
10. Kim HS, Kim SC, Kim SJ, Park CH, Jeung HC, et al. (2012) Identification of a radiosensitivity signature using integrative metaanalysis of published microarray data for NCI-60 cancer cells. BMC Genomics 13: 348.
11. Al-Shahrour F, Diaz-Uriarte R, Dopazo J (2004) FatiGO: a web tool for finding significant associations of Gene Ontology terms with groups of genes. Bioinformatics 20: 578–580.
12. Beissbarth T, Speed TP (2004) GOstat: find statistically overrepresented Gene Ontologies within a group of genes. Bioinformatics 20: 1464–1465.
13. Jennen DG, Magkoufopoulou C, Ketelslegers HB, van Herwijnen MH, Kleinjans JC, et al. (2010) Comparison of HepG2 and HepaRG by whole-genome gene expression analysis for the purpose of chemical hazard identification. Toxicol Sci 115: 66–79.
14. Westerink WM, Stevenson JC, Horbach GJ, Schoonen WG (2010) The development of RAD51C, Cystatin A, p53 and Nrf2 luciferase-reporter assays in metabolically competent HepG2 cells for the assessment of mechanism-based genotoxicity and of oxidative stress in the early research phase of drug development. Mutat Res 696: 21–40.
15. Irizarry RA, Hobbs B, Collin F, Beazer-Barclay YD, Antonellis KJ, et al. (2003) Exploration, normalization, and summaries of high density oligonucleotide array probe level data. Biostatistics 4: 249–264.
16. Dennis G, Jr., Sherman BT, Hosack DA, Yang J, Gao W, et al. (2003) DAVID: Database for Annotation, Visualization, and Integrated Discovery. Genome Biol 4: P3.
17. Johnson WE, Li C, Rabinovic A (2007) Adjusting batch effects in microarray expression data using empirical Bayes methods. Biostatistics 8: 118–127.
18. Hulsegge I, Kommadath A, Smits MA (2009) Globaltest and GOEAST: two different approaches for Gene Ontology analysis. BMC Proc 3 Suppl 4: S10.
19. Tibshirani R, Hastie T, Narasimhan B, Chu G (2002) Diagnosis of multiple cancer types by shrunken centroids of gene expression. Proc Natl Acad Sci U S A 99: 6567–6572.
20. Bruin SC, Klijn C, Liefers GJ, Braaf LM, Joosse SA, et al. (2010) Specific genomic aberrations in primary colorectal cancer are associated with liver metastases. BMC Cancer 10: 662.
21. Lips EH, Laddach N, Savola SP, Vollebergh MA, Oonk AM, et al. (2011) Quantitative copy number analysis by Multiplex Ligation-dependent Probe Amplification (MLPA) of BRCA1-associated breast cancer regions identifies BRCAness. Breast Cancer Res 13: R107.
22. Oberthuer A, Warnat P, Kahlert Y, Westermann F, Spitz R, et al. (2007) Classification of neuroblastoma patients by published gene-expression markers reveals a low sensitivity for unfavorable courses of MYCN non-amplified disease. Cancer Lett 250: 250–267.
23. Chopra P, Lee J, Kang J, Lee S (2010) Improving cancer classification accuracy using gene pairs. PLoS One 5: e14305.
24. Bylesjo M, Rantalainen M, Nicholson JK, Holmes E, Trygg J (2008) K-OPLS package: kernel-based orthogonal projections to latent structures for prediction and interpretation in feature space. BMC Bioinformatics 9: 106.
25. Hilvo M, Denkert C, Lehtinen L, Muller B, Brockmoller S, et al. (2011) Novel theranostic opportunities offered by characterization of altered membrane lipid metabolism in breast cancer progression. Cancer Res 71: 3236–3245.
26. Altman DG, Bland JM (1994) Diagnostic tests. 1: Sensitivity and specificity. BMJ 308: 1552.
27. Swets JA (1988) Measuring the accuracy of diagnostic systems. Science 240: 1285–1293.
28. Barckhausen C, Roos WP, Naumann SC, Kaina B (2013) Malignant melanoma cells acquire resistance to DNA interstrand cross-linking chemotherapeutics by p53-triggered upregulation of DDB2/XPC-mediated DNA repair. Oncogene.

23

Role of Rip2 in Development of Tumor-Infiltrating MDSCs and Bladder Cancer Metastasis

Hanwei Zhang, Arnold I. Chin*

Department of Urology, Broad Stem Cell Research Center, Jonsson Comprehensive Cancer Center, University of California Los Angeles, Los Angeles, California, United States of America

Abstract

Tumor invasion and metastases represent a complex series of molecular events that portends a poor prognosis. The contribution of inflammatory pathways mediating this process is not well understood. Nod-like receptors (NLRs) of innate immunity function as intracellular sensors of pathogen motifs and danger molecules. We propose a role of NLRs in tumor surveillance and in programming tumor-infiltrating lymphocytes (TILs). In this study, we examined the downstream serine/threonine and tyrosine kinase Rip2 in a murine model of bladder cancer. In Rip2-deficient C57Bl6 mice, larger orthotopic MB49 tumors developed with more numerous and higher incidence of metastases compared to wild-type controls. As such, increased tumor infiltration of CD11b$^+$Gr1^{hi} myeloid-derived suppressor cells (MDSCs) with concomitant decrease in T cells and NK cells were observed in Rip2-deficient tumor bearing animals using orthotopic and subcutaneous tumor models. Rip2-deficient tumors showed enhanced epithelial-to-mesenchymal transition, with elevated expression of *zeb1, zeb2, twist,* and *snail* in the tumor microenvironment. We found that the absence of Rip2 plays an intrinsic role in fostering the development of granulocytic MDSCs by an autocrine and paracrine effect of granulocytic colony stimulating factor (G-CSF) expression. Our findings suggest that NLR pathways may be a novel modality to program TILs and influence tumor metastases.

Editor: Rajeev Samant, University of Alabama at Birmingham, United States of America

Funding: American Association of Cancer Research Career Development Award 10-20-14, Broad Stem Cell Research Center Scholars in Translational Medicine Program, STOP Cancer Research Career Development Award, Becton Dickinson Biosciences Research Grant (A.I. Chin) & Perkins Foundation. The funders had no role in study design, data collection and analysis, decision to publish, or preparation of the manuscript.

Competing Interests: The authors have declared that no competing interests exist.

* E-mail: aichin@ucla.edu

Introduction

The context of the immune tumor microenvironment can be predictive of tumor stage, cancer-specific survival, as well as response to chemotherapy [1–3]. In certain malignancies, the presence of infiltrating CD8$^+$ T lymphocytes correlates with improved outcomes, whereas infiltrating B cells, CD4$^+$ T lymphocytes, and negative regulators including myeloid-derived suppression cells (MDSCs) and T regulatory cells (Tregs) negatively correlate with survival [4]. These observations underscore the importance in defining pathways essential to programming the composition of tumor infiltrating lymphocytes (TILs), as selective modulation of the immune tumor microenvironment represents an emerging therapeutic modality.

Pattern recognition receptors such as the prototypic Toll-like receptor (TLR) family and intracellular nucleotide-binding oligomerization domain (NOD)-like receptor (NLR) family recognize conserved motifs on pathogens as well as endogenous molecules released by damaged cells [5]. Activation of these signaling pathways initiates innate and adaptive immune responses, and may promote tissue repair and regeneration. We previously implicated TLR3 in a murine model of prostate cancer tumor surveillance critical in programming the infiltration of T lymphocytes and NK cells, while suppressing Treg expansion [6]. In bladder cancer, the efficacy of immune modulation is highlighted by the use of intravesical Bacillus Calmette Guerin, which promotes an influx of macrophages and neutrophils within the tumor microenvironment mediated in part by TLR2 and 4 [7,8].

Receptor-interacting protein 2 (Rip2), a serine-threonine and tyrosine kinase downstream and common to Nod1 and Nod2, activates transcription factors such as NF-κB and MAP kinases through its kinase activity as well as through recruitment of E3 ubiquitin ligase [9–14]. Rip2-dependent pathways have emerged as critical in sensing diverse pathogens ranging from *Listeria monocytogenes, Staphylococcus aureus,* and *Legionella pneumophilia* to *Escherichia coli* as well as in mediating inflammatory disorders such as autoimmune encephalomyelitis [15–17]. In addition, polymorphisms of Nod2 have been linked with susceptibility to Crohn's disease, while polymorphisms of Rip2 have been linked with systemic lupus erythematosus [18,19]. The ability of NLRs to mediate tumor surveillance has not been investigated to date. Here, we postulate that Rip2 may mediate bladder cancer surveillance and explore its role using a murine orthotopic and subcutaneous bladder cancer model. We show that tumor bearing Rip2-deficient mice biases myeloid differentiation towards the MDSC lineage and plays an intrinsic role in the development of the CD11b$^+$Ly6G$^+$Ly6C^{lo} granulocytic MDSC population. Our findings are the first to implicate Rip2 and NLRs in tumor surveillance and their importance in programming the immune tumor microenvironment. The NLR pathway may represent a therapeutic opportunity in modulating cancer immunity to prevent tumor invasion and metastasis.

Materials and Methods

Ethics Statement

All animal work has been conducted in accordance with the Public Health Service Policy on Human Care and Use of Laboratory Animals and USDA Animal Welfare Act Regulations through an approved UCLA Institutional Animal Care and Use Committee protocol #2010-023-11C.

Mice

Rip2-deficient mice backcrossed to a C57Bl/6 background for 10 generations were genotyped as previously described [10]. Age-matched C57Bl/6 mice (Jackson Laboratories) were used as controls. Six- to 8-wk old female mice were used for the experiments. Mice were housed in pathogen-free conditions according to UCLA Animal Research Committee protocols.

Cell culture

MB49 cell lines (gift from Tim Ratliff) were derived from carcinogen-induced urothelial cell carcinomas in C57Bl6 mice and maintained at 37°C with 5% CO_2 in DMEM (Cellgro), supplemented with 10% FBS (Omega Scientific) and 1% penicillin and streptomycin [20].

Tumor models

For intravesical tumor implantation, female mice were sedated, catheterized with a 24 gauge catheter (BD Biosciences), and instilled with 10 µg of poly-L-lysine (Sigma) in 100 µl for 30 minutes before drainage and instillation of 2×10^6 MB49 cells in 100 µl for 60 minutes [21,22]. Mice were sacrificed 12 days following tumor inoculation, and the bladder and internal organs were examined. Bladder, lungs, and kidneys were fixed in formalin or embedded in OCT for staining by H&E or immunofluorescence [23]. Pulmonary and renal metastases were determined grossly and by light microscopy of H&E sections in a single representative coronal cross section. For subcutaneous tumor challenges, 5×10^5 MB49 cells were implanted subcutaneously in the flanks of mice with tumor growth monitored every other day. Following sacrifice of the mice 14 days following tumor inoculation, tumors were harvested, weighed, and dissociated for analysis.

Immunofluorescence and Immunohistochemistry

Immunofluorescence was performed on OCT-embedded frozen tissue sections. Sections were blocked with 10% goat serum and 10% BSA in PBS for 1 hour at RT, incubated with primary antibody overnight at 4°C, then washed and incubated with Al-448 or Al-466 goat anti-rat secondary antibody (Invitrogen) at 1:800 dilution. Immunohistochemistry was performed on formalin-fixed paraffin-embedded tumor sections. Sections were subject to heated antigen unmasking solution for 30 minutes, quenched in 0.3% hydrogen dioxide in PBS for 15 minutes, blocked with 10% goat serum and 10% BSA in PBS for 1 hour at RT, then incubated with primary antibody overnight at 4°C, incubated with biotinylated goat anti-rat secondary antibody at 1:800 dilution for 30 minutes at RT, and developed using the ABC kit (Vector Labs). Slides were counterstained with hematoxylin. Sections were mounted with Vectorshield and analyzed by fluorescence or light microscopy (Zeiss). Antibodies include CD11b (M1/70, R&D Systems), CD4 (RM4–5, Biolegend), CD8 (53.6–7, R&D Systems), CD49b (DX-5, Biolegend), Foxp3 (FJK-16s, eBioscience), Ly6G (RB6-BC5, eBioscience), Ly6C (AL-21, BD Biosciences), E-Cadherin (MAB7481, R&D Systems), N-cadherin (H-63, Santa

Cruz Biotechnology), and phospho-IκBα (Ser 32/36, #9246, Cell Signaling).

Cytokine array

An inflammatory cytokine array comparing serum from wild-type and Rip2-deficient mice implanted with intravesical MB49 cells was performed as described (ARY006, R&D Systems).

Flow cytometry analysis

Single-cell suspensions prepared from spleens, dissociated tumor cells, or differentiated bone marrow cells were analyzed by flow cytometry. Antibodies including CD4 (RM-4), CD8 (53–67), NK1.1 (pk-136), B220 (RA3-6B2), CD11b (M1/70), CD45.2 (104), Gr1 (RB6-8C5), Ly-6G (1A8), and Ly-6C (AL21) were obtained from BD Biosciences. Data acquisition was performed on a FACS LSRII (BD Biosciences) and analyzed using FlowJo.

Bone marrow-derived myeloid differentiation

BM-derived cells were obtained by flushing femurs and tibia from C57Bl/6 wild-type and RIP2$^{-/-}$ mice. Following lysis of red blood cells with ACK buffer, the remaining cells were cultured in DMEM supplemented with 10% FBS and 20% L929 cell-conditioned media. After incubation for 24 hours, non-adherent cells were harvested and plated at 2×10^5 cells/mL in DMEM supplemented with 10% fetal calf serum, 50 µM 2-mercaptoethanol, 10 mM HEPES, 1 mM sodium pyruvate, 1% penicillin and streptomycin, and supplemented using 20% L929 with 40 ng/mL G-CSF (Biolegend), 40 ng/mL GM-CSF (Invitrogen), or in combination. Cultures were incubated at 37°C with 5% CO_2 for 3 days. On Day 3, fresh medium with appropriate cytokines was added. On Day 4 cultured cells were harvested for FACS.

Isolation of tumor-infiltrating immune cells

Tumor tissue was minced in PBS with sterile scissors to approximately 1 mm pieces and digested in 0.25% collagenase IV in DMEM supplemented with 10% FBS at 37°C with 5% CO_2 for 3 hours [24]. Cell suspensions were filtered through a 70 µm cell strainer, subjected to ACK buffer for 5 minutes on ice, and then filtered through a 20 µM cell strainer for flow cytometry. Cells sorted using a FACS Aria (BD Biosciences) into CD45$^+$CD11b$^+$Gr1^{hi}, CD45$^+$CD11b$^+$GR1^{lo}, and CD45$^-$ fractions were collected for qPCR.

Quantitative RT-PCR

Total RNA extracted from sorted cells and fresh frozen bladder tumor as described (RNeasy Mini Kit, Qiagen) was used to synthesize cDNA using High Capacity cDNA Reverse Transcription Kits (Applied Biosystems). Relative gene expression was determined using SYBR Green PCR Master Mix (Applied Biosystems). A Bio-Rad iCycler was used to analyze the samples while the comparative threshold cycle method was used to calculate gene expression normalized to GAPDH as a gene reference. Primers sets for the following genes were used: Arginase-1, 5′-AGAGATACTTCCAACTGCCAGACT, 3′-ACTGGCCTTTGTTGATGTCCCTA; iNOS, 5′-GCTGGAAGCCACTGACACTTCG, 3′-CGAGATGGTCAGGGTCCCCT; IL-4, 5′- GTCATCCTGCTCTTCTTTC, 3′- ATGGCGTCCCTTCTCCTGT; IL-10, 5′-GCTCTTACTGACTGGCATGAG, 3′-CGCAGCTCTAGGAGCATGTG; IL-12 p40, 5′- TGGTTTGCCATCGTTTTGCTG, 3′- ACAGGTGAGGTTCACTGTTT; IFNγ, 5′- GGATGCATTCATGAGTATTGC, 3′- CCTTTTCCGCTTCCTGAGG; M-CSF, 5′-AGGACCTGTTGGAGTTCCCTC, 3′- TTTCGCCCTCA-

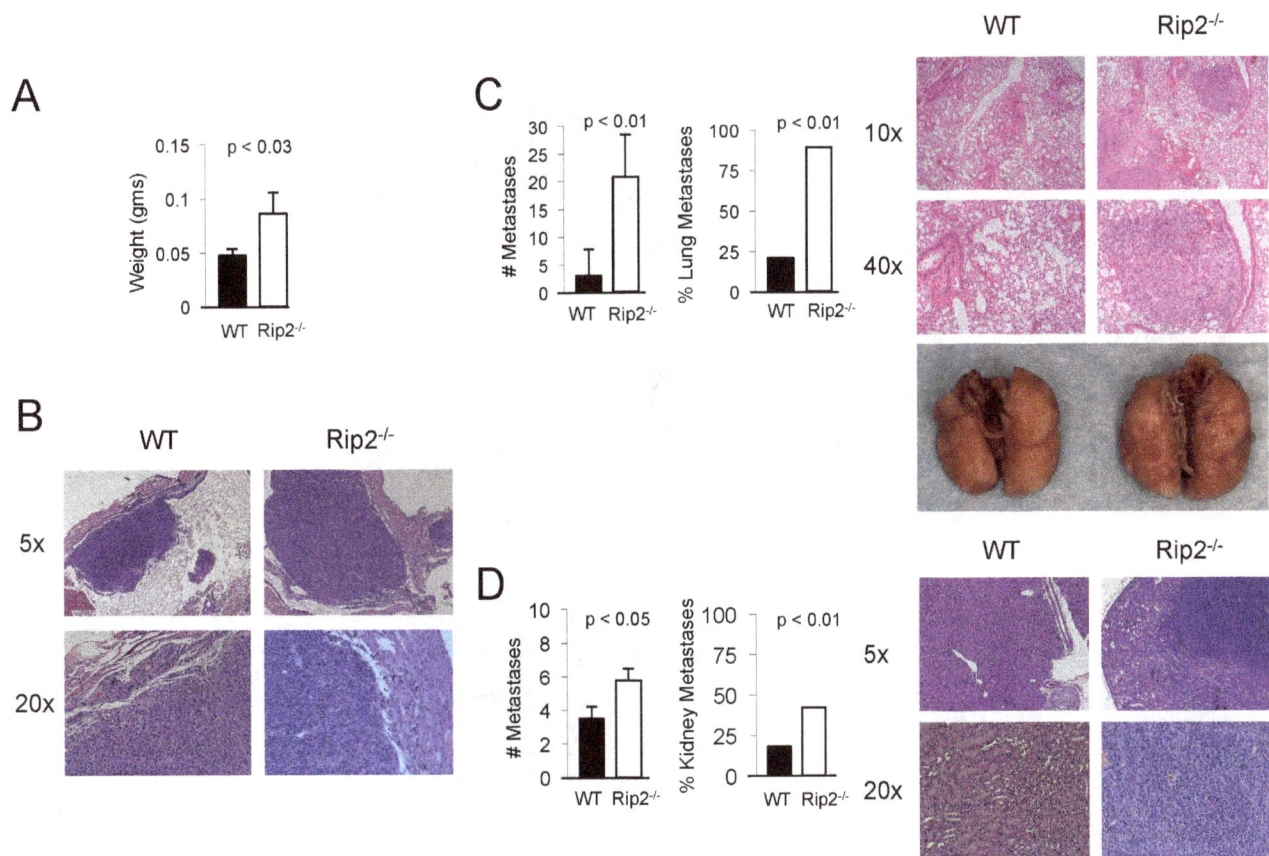

Figure 1. Increased tumor size and metastases in Rip2-deficient mice. Rip2$^{+/+}$ and Rip2$^{-/-}$ mice intravesically implanted with MB49 cells and sacrificed at 12 days were assessed for bladder tumor (A) weight, (B) histology with H&E staining at x5 and x20 magnification. C, Lungs were examined for metastasis by number of metastatic lesions per coronal cross section, % incidence, histology with H&E staining at x10 and x40 magnification, and gross examination. D, Kidneys were examined for metastasis by number of metastatic lesions per coronal cross section, % incidence, and histology with H&E staining at x5 and x20 magnification. Representative examples are shown. Columns, mean of 33 Rip2$^{+/+}$ and 19 Rip2$^{-/-}$ mice pooled from 5 independent experiments; bars, SEM. All p values were determined by two-tailed Student's t test, with statistically significance defined as p<0.05.

CACTTGATGA; G-CSF, 5′- CTCAACTTTCTGCCCA-GAGG, 3′- AGCTGGCTTAGGCACTGTGT; GM-CSF, 5′-GCCATCAAAGAAGCCCTGAA, 3′- GCGGGTCTGCACA-CATGTTA; Zeb1, 5′-AACGGAGATTTGTCTCCCAGT, 3′-CTGTCCAGCTTGCATCTTTTC; Zeb2, 5′-TAGCCGGTC-CAGAAGAAATG, 3′-GGCCATCTCTTTCCTCCAGT; Snail, 5′-GCGGAAGATCTTCAACTGCAAATATTGTAAC, 3′-GCAGTGGGAGCAGGAGAATGGCTTCTCAC; Twist, 5′-CGGGTCATGGCTAACGTG, 3′-CAGCTTGCCATCTTG-GAGTC; and GAPDH, 5′-GACCCCTTCATTGACCTCAAC, 3′-CTTCTCCATGGTGGTGAAGA.

Results

To investigate the role of Rip2 in tumor surveillance, we challenged wild-type and Rip2-deficient mice with syngeneic MB49 cells in an orthotopic bladder cancer model. We observed an almost two-fold increase in tumor weight in the absence of Rip2 (Fig 1A). Tumors harvested from mice of both genotypes demonstrated evidence of invasion into the detrusor muscle by H&E staining under light microscopy with larger tumors seen in Rip2-deficient animals (Fig 1B). Gross and histologic examination of internal organs revealed a greater number of metastasis in the lungs and kidneys of Rip2-deficient mice at an approximately three-fold and two-fold higher incidence respectively over wild-type controls (Fig 1C–D). No other gross metastases were observed including in the liver.

We have previously implicated Rip2 in development of Th1 and NK cells [10], while others reported a role in dendritic cell infiltration [17]. To investigate the role of Rip2 in the context of tumorigenesis, bladder tumor TILs were examined by immuno-fluorescence and immunohistochemistry. This revealed decreased infiltration of CD8$^+$ T lymphocytes, CD4$^+$ T lymphocytes, and NK cells in the absence of Rip2 as predicted. Examination of Foxp3$^+$ cells representative of T regulatory cells, showed an increasing trend in Rip2-deficient mice compared to wild-type mice although it did not reach statistical significance. Interestingly, tumors showed increased infiltration of CD11b$^+$ myeloid cells in Rip2-deficient compared to wild-type mice, while additional characterization of this myeloid population showed an expected increase in the macrophage marker F4/80 and in the Gr-1 subtype Ly6G, but not subtype Ly6C in tumors from Rip2-deficient mice (Fig 2).

To further examine the function of the tumor infiltrating populations, we subcutaneously implanted MB49 cells to generate larger tumors to facilitate subsequent sorting of cells. Similarly to orthotopic tumors, subcutaneous tumors developed in Rip2-deficient mice were of increased size compared to wild-type

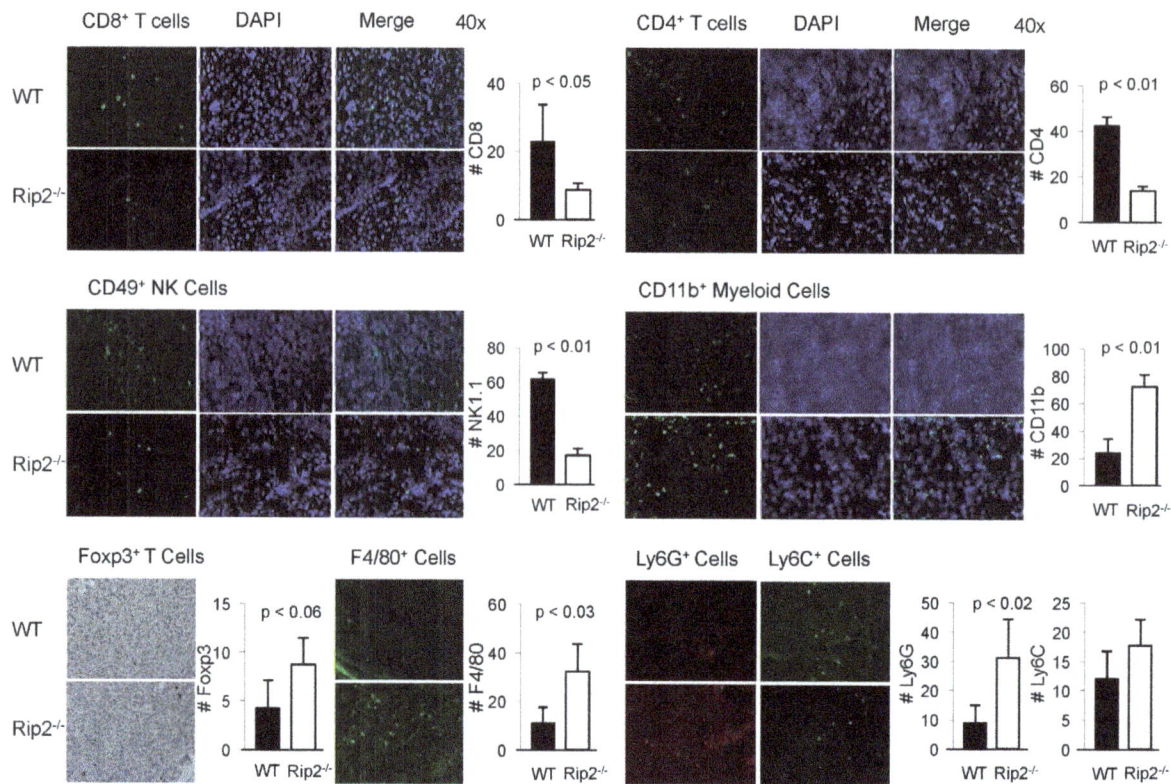

Figure 2. Loss of Rip2 alters composition of tumor infiltrating cells from Rip2-deficient mice. Infiltration of CD8, CD4, NK, CD11b, F4/80, Ly6G, and Ly6C expressing cells as indicated, were examined by immunofluorescence, and Foxp3 by immunohistochemistry in bladder tumors from Rip2$^{+/+}$ and Rip2$^{-/-}$ mice intravesically implanted with MB49 cells and sacrificed at 12 days. Left panels show specific antibody staining, middle panel shows DAPI staining, right panel shows merging of antibody and DAPI stains. Representative examples from each group of four to six mice in 4 independent experiments are shown at x40 magnification. Bar graphs enumerate mean number of cells per x40 field of 3 representative sections from groups of four mice; bars, SD. All p values were determined by two-tailed Student's t test, with statistically significance defined as $p<0.05$.

counterparts (Fig 3A). Dissociated tumors sorted for CD45^{+}NK1.1^{+} NK cells showed decreased numbers in Rip2-deficient compared to wild-type mice as expected (Fig 3B). The infiltrating numbers of CD4 and CD8 cells were too small to quantitate by flow cytometry (data not shown). Consistent with the previous orthotopic tumors, dissociated subcutaneous tumors sorted for surface markers CD11b^{+} and Gr1^{+} showed enriched numbers of CD11b^{+}Gr1^{hi} cells from Rip2-deficient compared to wild-type mice (Fig 3C). To further examine the functional characteristics of the CD11b^{+}Gr1^{hi} cells, we examined a panel of genes that represent a signature of MDSCs and myeloid subpopulations. Arginase-1 and iNOS mediate the T suppressive effects of MDSCs [25]. IFNγ supports the differentiation towards M1 cells, distinguished in turn by secretion of IL-12. IL-4 polarizes myeloid precursors towards a M2 phenotype, which is strongly associated with tumor associated MDSCs and express IL-10 to mediate their immune suppressive effects [26]. We show that Rip2-deficient CD11b^{+}Gr1^{hi} cells expressed higher levels of arginase-1 compared to cells from wild-type mice, with a similar trend in iNOS expression (Fig 3D). Consistently, increased IL-10 expression in Rip2-deficient CD11b^{+}Gr1^{hi} cells compared to cells from wild-type controls were observed, while no significant differences were seen in expression of IFNγ and IL-12, indicative of M2 polarization (Fig 3D). Levels of IL-4 were undetectable in the CD11b^{+}Gr1^{hi} cells (data not shown).

To examine the Rip-2-dependent systemic cues that may influence the development of the tumor microenvironment, cytokine levels were measured using an inflammatory cytokine

array comparing serum from wild-type and Rip2-deficient mice implanted with orthotopic MB49 bladder tumors. The levels of seven cytokines from the panel comprising 40 cytokines were found elevated in the absence of Rip2. The majority were associated with myeloid differentiation and chemotaxis, including G-CSF, M-CSF, IL-16, MCP-1, TREM-1, TIMP-1, and IL-1α with relative levels shown schematically [27–33] (Fig 4A). Splenocytes from tumor bearing mice were analyzed to assess the influence of these cytokine alterations, revealing no significant differences in the numbers of CD4^{+} and CD8^{+} T lymphocytes, B220^{+} B lymphocytes, and NK1.1^{+} cells, but increased development of CD11b^{+}Ly6G^{hi} cells in Rip2-deficient compared to wild-type mice, that represent the granulocytic MDSC population (Fig 4B). To further examine the bladder tumor microenvironment, we examined a panel of cytokines that influence the functional polarization of macrophages as well as differentiation of MDSCs in the intravesical bladder tumors [34]. Increased levels of IL-4, G-CSF, and GM-CSF were observed in bladder tumors from Rip2-deficient compared to wild-type mice, while no differences were detected in IFNγ and M-CSF expression, consistent with a tumor microenvironment fostering development of the tumor associated MDSCs (Fig 4C). To discriminate between cytokine production from tumor and surrounding stroma to the myeloid populations, we examined G-CSF expression in the CD45^{-} population representing tumor and stromal cells, and CD11b^{+}Gr1^{hi} population representing myeloid cells, and showed increased G-CSF in Rip2-deficient compared to wild-type

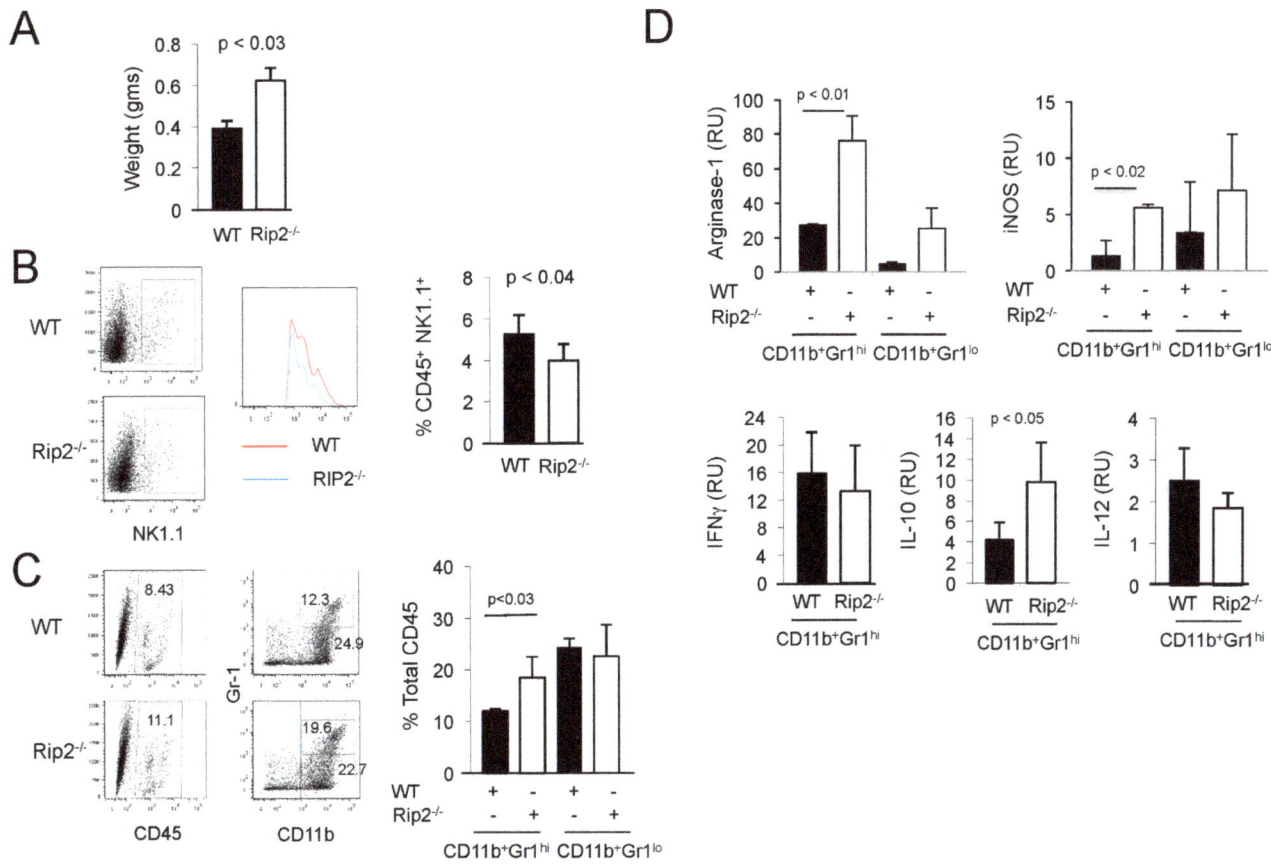

Figure 3. Increased tumor infiltrating granulocytic MDSCs in Rip2-deficient mice. Rip2$^{+/+}$ and Rip2$^{-/-}$ mice subcutaneously implanted with MB49 cells for 14 days were assessed for (A) tumor weight, and sorted by flow cytometry to examine (B) CD45$^+$NK1.1$^+$ cells, and (C) CD45$^+$CD11b$^+$Gr1^{hi} and CD45$^+$CD11b$^+$Gr1^{lo} cells. Column, mean of four mice; bars SD. Data are representative of two independent experiments. D, Sorted CD45$^+$CD11b$^+$Gr1^{hi} and CD45$^+$CD11b$^+$Gr1^{lo} cells in Rip2$^{+/+}$ and Rip2$^{-/-}$ mice were examined for expression of arginase-1 and iNOS by qPCR, while CD45$^+$CD11b$^+$Gr1^{hi} cells in Rip2$^{+/+}$ and Rip2$^{-/-}$ mice were examined for expression of IL10, IL-12, and IFNγ by qPCR. Column, mean of two mice; bars SD. Data are representative of three independent experiments. Representative examples are shown. All p values were determined by two-tailed Student's t test, with statistically significance defined as $p<0.05$.

CD11b$^+$Gr1^{hi} cells, suggesting an autocrine and paracrine regulation of MDSCs in absence of Rip2 (Fig 4D).

The MDSC population is comprised of immature myeloid cells and myeloid cell progenitors that can differentiate into mature macrophages, granulocytes, and dendritic cells. They are characterized by T lymphocyte suppressive ability and expression of arginase-1 and iNOS [25]. In the mouse, they can be further distinguished into granulocytic MDSCs by expression of surface markers CD11b$^+$Gr1^{hi} or CD11b$^+$Ly6G$^+$Ly6C^{lo} and monocytic MDSCs by expression of markers CD11b$^+$Gr1^{lo} or CD11b$^+$Ly6-G^{lo}Ly6C^{hi} [35]. To test the intrinsic role of Rip2 in myeloid development, naïve bone marrow from wild-type and Rip2-deficient mice were subject to *in vitro* differentiation using M-CSF, G-CSF, GM-CSF, or G-CSF and GM-CSF for 4 days and examined for expression of CD11b, Ly6G, and Ly6C. In the presence of G-CSF, GM-CSF, and G-CSF plus GM-CSF, the absence of Rip2 resulted in a bias towards the CD11b$^+$Ly6-G$^+$Ly6C^{lo} granulocytic MDSC population (Fig 5A). In BM-derived MDSCs differentiated using G-CSF or G-CSF and GM-CSF, increased arginase-1 and iNOS expression was uniformly observed in Rip2-deficient compared to wild-type cells, consistent with the increased development of MDSCs (Fig 5B).

MDSCs have been implicated in promoting EMT, a process critical in facilitating tumor invasion and subsequent tumor metastases [36]. A hallmark of EMT is a switch in surface adhesion markers with the loss of E-cadherin and expression of N-cadherin [37]. To investigate the influence of Rip2 in development of EMT, we examined expression of adhesion markers in intravesical tumors and observed decreased E-cadherin expression throughout the tumor with concomitant increased N-cadherin expression at the peripheral of the tumor in Rip2-deficient relative to wild-type mice (Fig 6A). NF-κB activation has been implicated in promoting EMT and thus we examined its activation in the absence of Rip2 [38]. Consistent with prior literature, we observed decreased canonical NF-κB activation exhibited by decreased p-IκB expression in Rip2-deficient tumors (Fig 6B), suggesting NF-κB independent mechanisms to account for EMT [39]. To investigate other mechanisms promoting EMT, a panel of transcription factors involved in EMT including *zeb-1*, *zeb-2*, *snail*, and *twist* were examined in tumor and stromal cells from dissociated subcutaneous tumors depleted of CD45, with the expression of *zeb-1*, *zeb-2*, and *snail* found increased in Rip2-deficient compared to wild-type tumor bearing mice, and increased expression of *twist* approaching statistical significance (Fig 6C). We also examined expression of these EMT inducing genes in lungs containing metastases from Rip2 wild-type and – deficient mice, revealing a similar trend with statistical significance for increased *twist* expression in absence of Rip2 (Fig 6D).

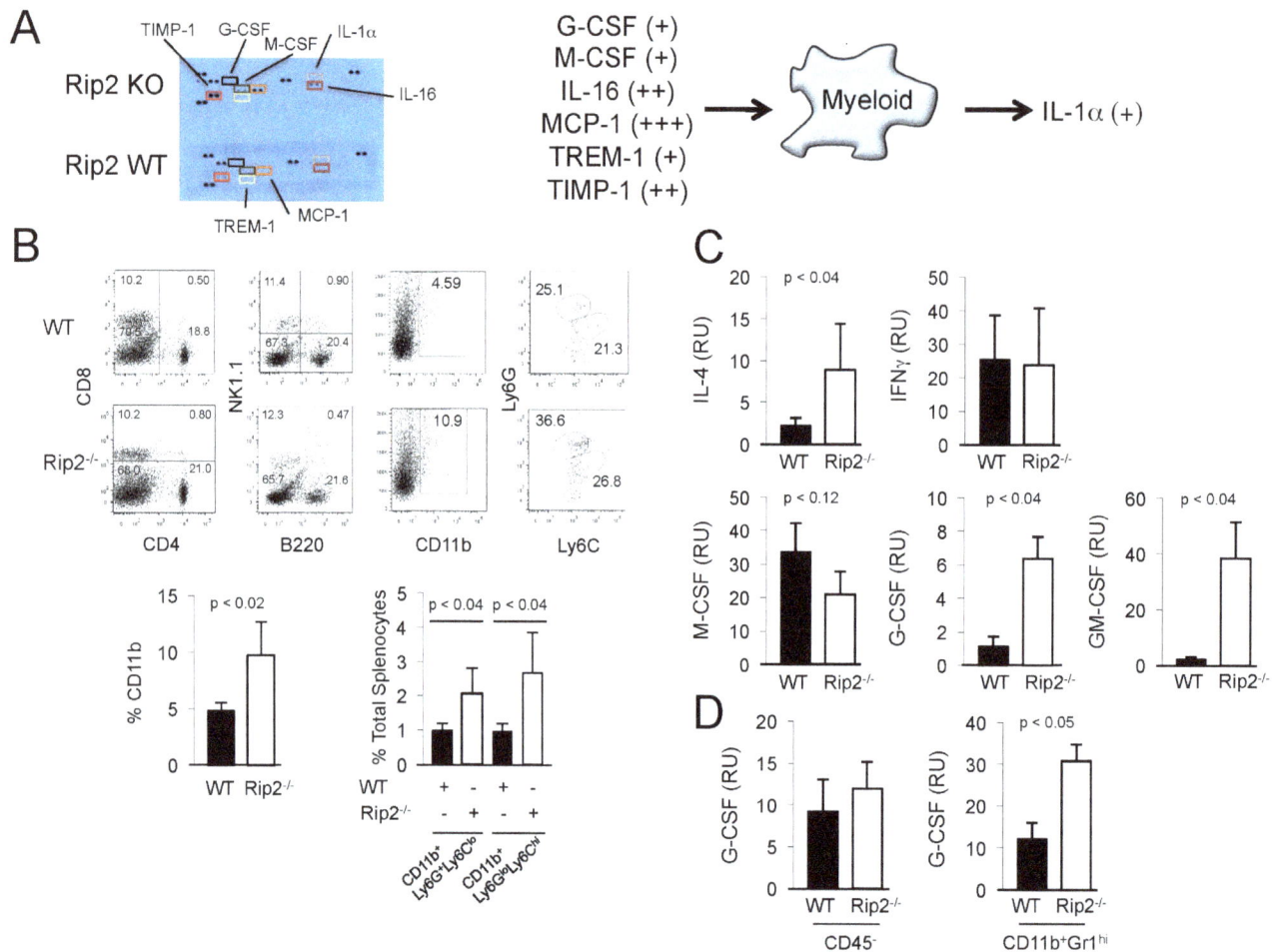

Figure 4. Biased development of granulocytic MDSCs in Rip2-deficient mice. A, Inflammatory cytokine expression in serum of $Rip2^{+/+}$ and $Rip2^{-/-}$ mice intravesically implanted with MB49 cells for 12 days was assessed by cytokine array analysis. Cytokines increased in $Rip2^{-/-}$ mice are depicted in the schematic as shown. (+) 2-5x, (++) 5-10x, (+++) >10x based on quantitation by ImageJ. Results are from duplicates and representative of two independent experiments. B, Splenocytes from $Rip2^{+/+}$ and $Rip2^{-/-}$ mice were examined for expression of CD4, CD8, B220, NK1.1, while $CD11b^+$ cells were examined for expression of Ly6G and Ly6C by flow cytometry as indicated. Column, mean of four mice; bars SD. Data are representative of two independent experiments. C, Total tumor from $Rip2^{+/+}$ and $Rip2^{-/-}$ mice intravesically implanted with MB49 cells and sacrificed at 12 days were examined for expression of IL4, IFNγ, M-CSF, G-CSF, and GM-CSF by qPCR. Column, mean of three mice; bars SD. D, Tumors from $Rip2^{+/+}$ and $Rip2^{-/-}$ mice subcutaneously implanted with MB49 cells for 14 days were fractioned to $CD45^-$ and $CD45^+CD11b^+Gr1^{hi}$ cells and examined for G-CSF expression by qPCR. Column, mean of three mice; bars SD. All p values were determined by two-tailed Student's t test, with statistically significance defined as p<0.05.

Discussion

The immune composition of the tumor microenvironment can be predictive of disease-free and overall survival. This has been shown in the context of $CD4^+$ T lymphocytes and CD1α dendritic cells in axillary lymph nodes correlating with disease-free survival in breast cancer patients [40], to tumor-infiltrating $CD3^+$ cells and $CD8^+$ T lymphocytes in colon [1] and bladder cancer respectively [2]. The balance of TILs may refine the predictive ability of the immune microenvironment, as $CD4^{lo}CD48^{lo}CD8^{hi}$ patients exhibited improved recurrence-free survival while the ratio of $CD8^+$ T cells to $CD68^+$ tumor associated macrophages predicted overall survival and response to neoadjuvant chemotherapy in breast cancer patients [3]. Anti-tumor immunity may be augmented by targeting negative regulators of T cell co-stimulation as evidenced by the development of anti-CTLA4 and anti-PD1 therapeutics, and may be extended to targeting Tregs and MDSCs [41]. This evidence suggests that active

programming of the tumor immune microenvironment may be a viable strategy to harness and bias immunity towards an anti-tumor response.

We have hypothesized that the ability of PRRs to sense contextual signals from pathogens to initiate an immune response is paralleled by the ability of DAMPs released by cellular damage in the tumor environment to shape tumor immunity. NLRs including Nod1 and Nod2 have been implicated in sensing various pathogens as well as cellular stresses [42]. The role of cytosolic PRRs, such as the NLR family in tumor surveillance is unclear. Recently, loss of Rip2 has been implicated in development of larger colorectal cancers in a murine model [43]. In this manuscript, we show that NLRs through Rip2 signaling can shape the tumor microenvironment towards tumor-infiltrating $CD8^+$ T lymphocytes, NK cells, and suppression of MDSCs. Similarly, in the absence of Rip2, larger orthotopic bladder tumors developed as well as increased tumor metastases in both the lung and kidneys.

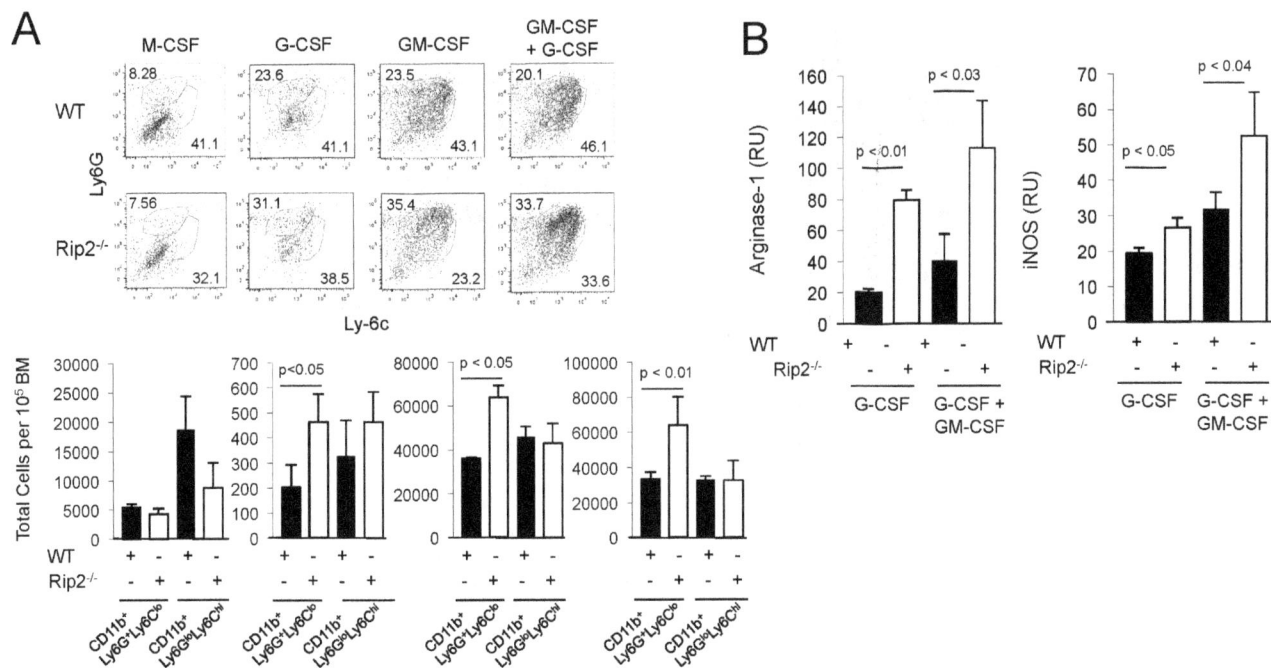

Figure 5. Intrinsic enhanced development of MDSC in absence of Rip2. A, Bone marrow from naïve Rip2$^{+/+}$ and Rip2$^{-/-}$ mice were differentiated by M-CSF, G-CSF, GM-CSF, and G-CSF plus GM-CSF as indicated for four days prior to flow cytometry to examine expression of Ly6G and Ly6C in CD11b$^+$ cells (ranging from 70–90%, not shown). CD11b$^+$LyG$^+$Ly6C^{lo} and CD11b$^+$LyG^{lo}Ly6C^{hi} populations for each group are shown as total cell counts per 10^5 starting BM cells. B, Expression of arginase-1 and iNOS by qPCR in G-CSF and G-CSF plus GM-CSF differentiated bone marrow from naïve Rip2$^{+/+}$ and Rip2$^{-/-}$ mice. Column, mean of three mice; bars SD. Data are representative of two independent experiments. Representative examples are shown. All p values were determined by two-tailed Student's t test, with statistically significance defined as $p<0.05$.

Rip2 was initially described based on sequence homology to its C-terminal CARD domain [44]. We developed Rip2-deficient animals and described a role in innate immunity implicating Rip2 downstream of Nod1, and adaptive immunity mediating IFNγ responses in Th1 and NK development [10]. Since then, the importance of Rip2 in NLR signaling and macrophage function has been validated and shown to play a critical role in innate immune signal transduction of Nod1 and Nod2 receptors [45]. In the absence of tumor growth, we found no significant differences in the development of all splenocytic lineages examined including CD11b$^+$Gr1$^+$ cells in Rip2-deficient compared to wild-type mice. However, in the presence of tumor growth we observed increased splenocytic CD11b$^+$Ly6G$^+$ cells representing granulocytic MDSCs in the absence of Rip2 [35].

We examined the systemic macroenvironment as well as local microenvironment levels of cytokines that were altered by the absence of Rip2 expression. Interestingly, elevated serum cytokines important in myeloid differentiation were found in Rip2-deficient tumor bearing animals, with increased levels of G-CSF and M-CSF, as well as MCP-1 and TREM-1. MCP-1 has been implicated in higher recurrence and worse bladder cancer prognosis by mediating tumor invasion, while TREM-1 has been implicated in activation of Kuffner cells in hepatocellular carcinoma [27,30]. Within the tumor microenvironment, in the absence of Rip2, we found a cytokine signature enriched in IL-4 and G-CSF, polarizing towards a M2 phenotype as reflected in increased production of IL-10 and arginase-1 [46]. M2 macrophages have been associated with tumor progression as well as MDSC development [47].

Examining the tumor infiltration population, we found not only increased proportion of CD11b$^+$Gr1^{hi} cells in Rip2-deficient animals, but also increased expression of arginase-1 and iNOS,

which leads to inhibition of T cells and NK cells, and suggests an intrinsic function of Rip2 in MDSC development. Rip2-deficient CD11b$^+$Gr1^{hi} MDSCs produced elevated levels of IL-10 which may further inhibit T cell activity by enhancing Tregs [48]. With the increased activation of Rip2-deficient MDSCs, we asked whether Rip2 plays an intrinsic role in the development of CD11b$^+$ subsets. Bone marrow-derived MDSCs using various cytokines showed increased development of CD11b$^+$Ly6G$^+$Ly6C^{lo} granulocytic MDSCs in the presence of G-CSF, GM-CSF, or their combination in Rip2-deficient compared to wild type cells, while there was no increased development of monocytic MDSC. The increased serum production of G-CSF as well as an intrinsic development of granulocytic MDSCs in vitro in response to G-CSF, suggests a mechanism for increased granulocytic MDSCs in the absence of Rip2.

Growing evidence has attributed MDSCs in cancer progression to immune suppression and modifying the microenvironment to foster tumor metastasis. Increased MDSCs have been described in cancer patients, including patients with bladder cancer [49,50]. Granulocytic MDSCs predominate in TIL populations and suppress CD8+T cells by producing reactive oxidative species (ROS), Arg1, and iNOS [25,35]. Recent studies support the role of granulocytic MDSCs to induce EMT in a melanoma model mediated by the chemokine receptor expressed on MDSCs, CXCR2 [36]. During metastasis, it is essential that cancer cells acquire a motile phenotype that allows for tumor invasion, extravasation into the blood stream or lymphatic channels for dissemination, followed by tumor implantation and growth. We noted increased tumor infiltrating MDSCs, decreased T lymphocytes and NK cells, and larger tumors with substantially higher numbers and rates of pulmonary metastases. With the observed increased metastasis in Rip2-deficient mice, we examined tumors

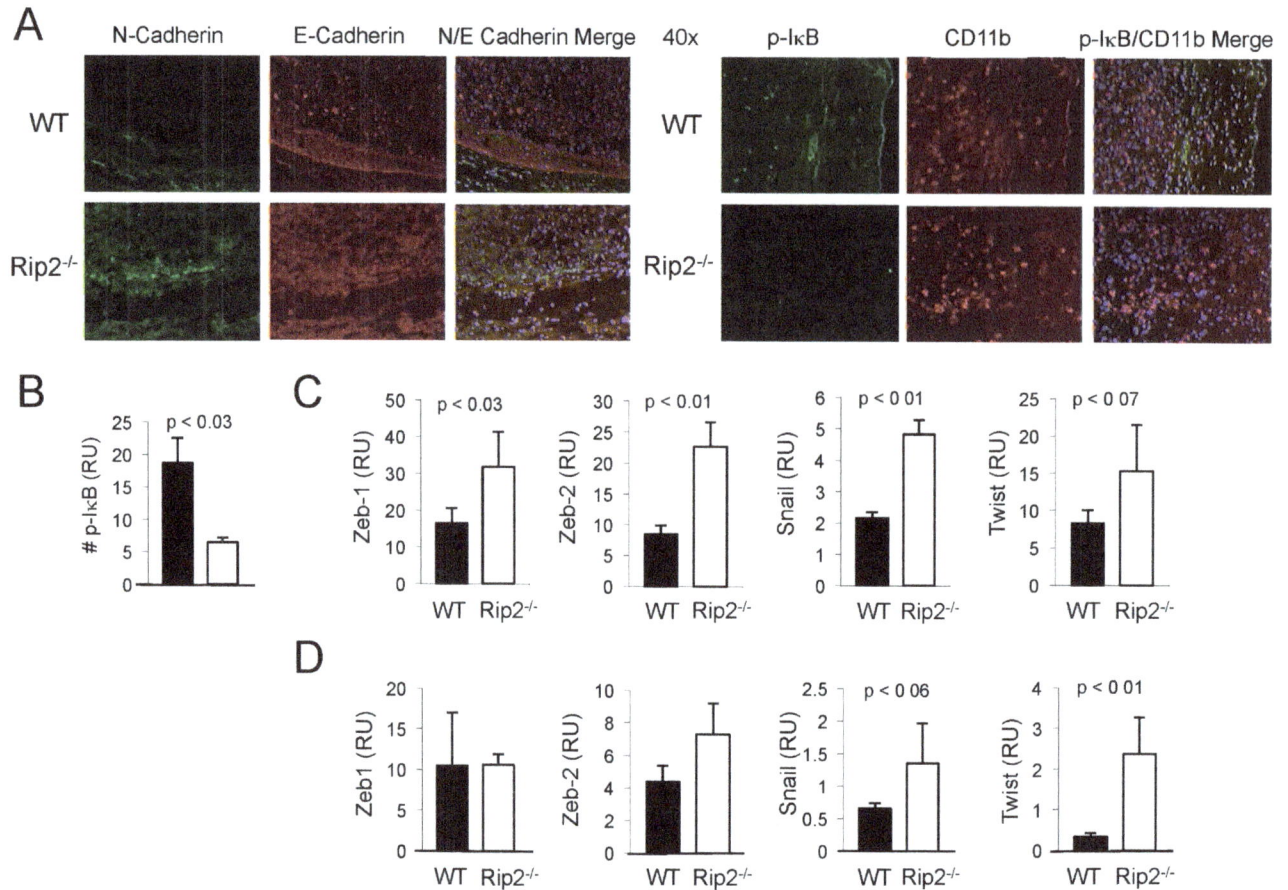

Figure 6. Enhanced epithelial-to-mesenchymal transition in tumors from Rip2-deficient mice. A, Rip2$^{+/+}$ and Rip2$^{-/-}$ mice intravesically implanted with MB49 cells for 12 days were assessed for E-cadherin and N-cadherin expression by immunofluorescence. Magnification of x40. Data are representative of two independent experiments. B, Bar graphs below enumerate mean number of cells per x40 field of 3 representative sections from groups of four mice; bars, SD. C, Expression of *zeb-1*, *zeb-2*, *snail*, and *twist* were examined from CD45$^-$ dissociated total tumor tissue by qPCR. Column, mean of four mice; bars SD. Data are representative of two independent experiments. D, Expression of *zeb-1*, *zeb-2*, *snail*, and *twist* were examined from dissociated lungs containing metastases by qPCR. Column, mean of four mice; bars SD. All *p* values were determined by two-tailed Student's *t* test, with statistically significance defined as p<0.05.

for features of EMT and demonstrated cadherin switching by loss of E-cadherin expression and gain of N-cadherin expression at the tumor periphery. We also showed increased tumoral expression of EMT transcription factors including *zeb-1*, *zeb-2*, and *snail*. NF-κB has been implicated in enhancing EMT, so the decreased activation in Rip2-deficient animals suggests an NF-κB-independent mechanism [38]. We found elevated levels of TIMP-1 in Rip2-deficient animals, which has been implicated in inducing expression of *slug*, *twist*, zeb1 and zeb2 [33]. A recent report describing down regulation of E-cadherin expression by Rip2 knockdown *in vitro* supports our findings [39]. These data support a local-regional shift in the tumor microenvironment enhanced by loss of Rip2 to facilitate EMT.

In humans, mutations in Nod2 are associated with Crohn's disease, while mutations in the Rip2 locus are linked with systemic lupus erythematosus [18,19]. These inflammatory diseases have been associated with susceptibility to cellular stress signals as well as pathogens in the gut flora. Our findings showing increased MDSCs in the absence of Rip2 appear seemingly contradictory. However, the development of MDSCs is not clear. Potentially, the activation of tumor associated MDSCs may be triggered in the context of endogenous ligands exposed during tumorigenesis. These contextual signals may differ from other endogenous or

pathogen-related signals that bias immune activation. Endogenous ligands expressed either from normal cells or specific to transformed cells that mediate these contextual signals for NLRs have yet to be identified and remain the subject of future investigations.

In the absence of Rip2, pathologic conditions such as the development of cancer, lead to microenvironment alterations and intrinsic activation of myeloid progenitors that expand the granulocytic MDSC population. These changes may influence EMT and development of metastases. Current therapeutic strategies have targeted negative T cell regulators. This includes utilizing anti-CTLA4 and anti-PD1 antibody therapies, or targeting MDSCs by inhibition of CSF-1R. The use of PRR modulation may be a novel strategy to program the TIL to favor anti-tumor immunity. This may be adopted on its own, or in conjunction with antigen-specific targeted therapy. The differences we have observed within the tumor microenvironment in our models of various PRR signaling mediator knockouts suggest that modulation of PRRs may need to be tailored to specific diseases and disease states. Our data suggest that TILs can by further shaped by activation of NLRs and function as immune modulators or adjuvant therapies.

In summary, we provide the initial evidence that intracellular NLRs represented by Rip2 can program the immune microenvironment and influence tumor invasion and metastasis in a bladder cancer model. We support a novel role of Rip2 in the development and recruitment of granulocytic MDSCs and highlight the contribution of MDSCs to the development of metastases in bladder cancer. Further study will be needed to clarify the contextual signals that trigger NLRs to mediate these functions. This study adds credence to our hypothesis that NLRs are critical sensors for the programming of the tumor immune microenvironment.

References

1. Galon J, Costes A, Sanchez-Cabo F, Kirilovsky A, Mlecnik B, et al. (2006) Type, density, and location of immune cells within human colorectal tumors predict clinical outcome. Science 313: 1960–1964.

2. Sharma P, Shen Y, Wen S, Yamada S, Jungbluth A, et al. (2007) CD8 tumor-infiltrating lymphocytes are predictive of survival in muscle-invasive urothelial carcinoma. Proc Natl Acad Sci U S A 104: 3967–3972.

3. DeNardo DG, Brennan DJ, Rexhepaj E, Ruffell B, Shiao SL, et al. (2011) Leukocyte complexity predicts breast cancer survival and functionally regulates response to chemotherapy. Cancer Discov 1: 54–67.

4. Fridman WH, Pagès F, Sautès-Fridman C, Galon J (2012) The immune contexture in human tumours: impact on clinical outcome. Nat Rev Cancer 12: 298–306.

5. Iwasaki A, Medzhitov R (2010) Regulation of adaptive immunity by the innate immune system. Science 327: 291–295.

6. Chin AI, Miyahira AK, Covarrubias A, Teague J, Guo B, et al. (2010) Toll-like receptor 3-mediated suppression of TRAMP prostate cancer shows the critical role of type I interferons in tumor immune surveillance. Cancer Res 70: 2595–2603.

7. Heldwein KA, Liang MD, Andresen TK, Thomas KE, Marty AM, et al. (2003) TLR2 and TLR4 serve distinct roles in the host immune response against Mycobacterium bovis BCG products. J Leukoc Biol 74: 277–286.

8. Simons MP, O'Donnell MA, Griffith TS (2008) Role of neutrophils in BCG immunotherapy for bladder cancer. Urol Oncol 26: 341–345.

9. Bertrand MJM, Lippens S, Staes A, Gilbert B, Roelandt R, et al. (2011) cIAP1/2 are direct E3 ligases conjugating diverse types of ubiquitin chains to receptor interacting proteins kinases 1 to 4 (RIP1-4). PLoS One 6: e22356.

10. Chin AI, Dempsey PW, Bruhn K, Miller JF, Xu Y, et al. (2002) Involvement of receptor-interacting protein 2 in innate and adaptive immune responses. Nature 416: 190–194.

11. Kobayashi K, Inohara N, Hernandez LD, Galán JE, Núñez G, et al. (2002) RICK/Rip2/CARDIAK mediates signalling for receptors of the innate and adaptive immune systems. Nature 416: 194–199.

12. Nembrini C, Kisielow J, Shamshiev AT, Tortola L, Coyle AJ, et al. (2009) The kinase activity of Rip2 determines its stability and consequently Nod1- and Nod2-mediated immune responses. J Biol Chem 284: 19183–19188.

13. Tigno-Aranjuez JT, Asara JM, Abbott DW (2010) Inhibition of RIP2's tyrosine kinase activity limits NOD2-driven cytokine responses. Genes Dev 24: 2666–2677.

14. Park J-H, Kim Y-G, McDonald C, Kanneganti T-D, Hasegawa M, et al. (2007) RICK/RIP2 mediates innate immune responses induced through Nod1 and Nod2 but not TLRs. J Immunol 178: 2380–2386.

15. Elinav E, Strowig T, Henao-Mejia J, Flavell R (2011) Regulation of the antimicrobial response by NLR proteins. Immunity 34: 665–679.

16. Biswas A, Liu Y-J, Hao L, Mizoguchi A, Salzman NH, et al. (2010) Induction and rescue of Nod2-dependent Th1-driven granulomatous inflammation of the ileum. Proc Natl Acad Sci U S A 107: 14739–14744.

17. Shaw PJ, Barr MJ, Lukens JR, McGargill M, Chi H, et al. (2011) Signaling via the RIP2 adaptor protein in central nervous system-infiltrating dendritic cells promotes inflammation and autoimmunity. Immunity 34: 75–84.

18. Abbott DW, Wilkins A, Asara JM, Cantley LC (2004) The Crohn's Disease Protein, NOD2, Requires RIP2 in Order to Induce Ubiquitinylation of a Novel Site on NEMO. Curr Biol 14: 2217–2227.

19. Li J, Tian J, Ma Y, Cen H, Leng R-X, et al. (2012) Association of RIP2 gene polymorphisms and systemic lupus erythematosus in a Chinese population. Mutagenesis 27: 319–322.

20. Hudson MA, Ritchey JK, Catalona WJ, Brown EJ, Ratliff TL (1990) Comparison of the Fibronectin-binding Ability and Antitumor Efficacy of Various Mycobacteria. Cancer Res 50: 3843–3847.

21. Shapiro A, Kelley DR, Oakley DM, Catalona WJ, Ratliff TL (1984) Technical Factors Affecting the Reproducibility of Intravesical Mouse Bladder Tumor Implantation during Therapy with Bacillus Calmette-Guérin. Cancer Res 44: 3051–3054.

22. Soloway MS (1977) Intravesical and systemic chemotherapy of urinary bladder cancer. Cancer Res 37: 2918–2929.

23. Jessen KA, Liu SY, Tepper CG, Karrim J, McGoldrick ET, et al. (2004) Molecular analysis of metastasis in a polyomavirus middle T mouse model: the role of osteopontin. Breast Cancer Res 6: 157–69.

24. Kortylewski M, Kujawski M, Wang T, Wei S, Zhang S, et al. (2005) Inhibiting Stat3 signaling in the hematopoietic system elicits multicomponent antitumor immunity. Nat Med 11: 1314–1321.

25. Sevko A, Umansky V (2013) Myeloid-derived suppressor cells interact with tumors in terms of myelopoiesis, tumorigenesis and immunosuppression: thick as thieves. J Cancer 4: 3–11.

26. Sinha P, Clements VK, Bunt SK, Albelda SM, Ostrand-Rosenberg S (2007) Cross-talk between myeloid-derived suppressor cells and macrophages subverts tumor immunity toward a type 2 response. J Immunol 179: 977–983.

27. Wu J, Li J, Salcedo R, Mivechi NF, Trinchieri G, et al. (2012) The proinflammatory myeloid cell receptor TREM-1 controls Kupffer cell activation and development of hepatocellular carcinoma. Cancer Res 72: 3977–3986.

28. Zanzinger K, Schellack C, Nausch N, Cerwenka A (2009) Regulation of triggering receptor expressed on myeloid cells 1 expression on mouse inflammatory monocytes. Immunology 128: 185–195.

29. Ben-Baruch A (2012) The Tumor-Promoting Flow of Cells Into, Within and Out of the Tumor Site: Regulation by the Inflammatory Axis of TNFα and Chemokines. Cancer Microenviron 5: 151–164.

30. Chiu H-Y, Sun K-H, Chen S-Y, Wang H-H, Lee M-Y, et al. (2012) Autocrine CCL2 promotes cell migration and invasion via PKC activation and tyrosine phosphorylation of paxillin in bladder cancer cells. Cytokine 59: 423–432.

31. Fridlender ZG, Sun J, Mishalian I, Singhal S, Cheng G, et al. (2012) Transcriptomic analysis comparing tumor-associated neutrophils with granulocytic myeloid-derived suppressor cells and normal neutrophils. PLoS One 7: e31524.

32. Glass WG, Sarisky RT, Vecchio AM Del (2006) Not-so-sweet sixteen: the role of IL-16 in infectious and immune-mediated inflammatory diseases. J Interferon Cytokine Res 26: 511–520.

33. Jung YS, Liu X-W, Chirco R, Warner RB, Fridman R, et al. (2012) TIMP-1 induces an EMT-like phenotypic conversion in MDCK cells independent of its MMP-inhibitory domain. PLoS One 7: e38773.

34. Waight J, Hu Q, Miller A, Liu S, Abrams S (2011) Tumor-derived G-CSF facilitates neoplastic growth through a branulocytic myeloid-derived suppressor cell-dependent mechanism. PLoS One 6.

35. Youn J-I, Nagaraj S, Collazo M, Gabrilovich DI (2008) Subsets of myeloid-derived suppressor cells in tumor-bearing mice. J Immunol 181: 5791–5802.

36. Toh B, Wang X, Keeble J, Sim WJ, Khoo K, et al. (2011) Mesenchymal transition and dissemination of cancer cells is driven by myeloid-derived suppressor cells infiltrating the primary tumor. PLoS Biol 9: e1001162.

37. Berx G, van Roy F (2009) Involvement of members of the cadherin superfamily in cancer. Cold Spring Harb Perspect Biol 1: a003120.

38. Chua HL, Bhat-Nakshatri P, Clare SE, Morimiya A, Badve S, et al. (2007) NF-kappaB represses E-cadherin expression and enhances epithelial to mesenchymal transition of mammary epithelial cells: potential involvement of ZEB-1 and ZEB-2. Oncogene 26: 711–724.

39. Wu S, Wang H, Nakamoto S, Imazeki F YO (2012) Knockdown of receptor-interacting serine/threonine protein kinase-2 (RIPK2) affects EMT-associated gene expression in human hepatoma cells. Anticancer Res 32: 3775–3783.

40. Kohrt HE, Nouri N, Nowels K, Johnson D, Holmes S, et al. (2005) Profile of immune cells in axillary lymph nodes predicts disease-free survival in breast cancer. PLoS Med 2: e284.

41. Ribas AA, Hersey PP, Midleton MR, Gogas HH, Flaherty KT, et al. (2013) New challenges in endpoints for drug development in advanced melanoma. Clin Cancer Res 18: 336–341.

42. Philpott DJ, Girardin SE (2010) Nod-like receptors: sentinels at host membranes. Curr Opin Immunol 22: 428–434.

43. Couturier-Maillard A, Secher T, Rehman A, Normand S, De Arcangelis A, et al. (2013) NOD2-mediated dysbiosis predisposes mice to transmissible colitis and colorectal cancer. J Clin Invest 123: 700–711.

44. Inohara N, del Peso L, Koseki T, Chen S, Núñez G (1998) RICK, a novel protein kinase containing a caspase recruitment domain, interacts with CLARP and regulates CD95-mediated apoptosis. J Biol Chem 273: 12296–12300.

Acknowledgments

We thank the UCLA Translational Pathology Core Laboratory for slide processing and the Broad Stem Cell Research Center Flow Cytometry Core.

Author Contributions

Conceived and designed the experiments: HZ AC. Performed the experiments: HZ AC. Analyzed the data: HZ AC. Contributed reagents/materials/analysis tools: HZ AC. Wrote the paper: HZ AC.

45. Magalhaes JG, Lee J, Geddes K, Rubino S, Philpott DJ, et al. (2011) Essential role of Rip2 in the modulation of innate and adaptive immunity triggered by Nod1 and Nod2 ligands. Eur J Immunol 41: 1445–1455.

46. Liu C, Li Y, Yu J, Feng L, Hou S, et al. (2013) Targeting the shift from M1 to M2 macrophages in experimental autoimmune encephalomyelitis mice treated with fasudil. PLoS One 8: e54841.

47. Yang W-C, Ma G, Chen S-H, Pan P-Y (2013) Polarization and reprogramming of myeloid-derived suppressor cells. J Mol Cell Biol 5: 207–209.

48. Chaudhry A, Samstein RM, Treuting P, Liang Y, Pils MC, et al. (2011) Interleukin-10 signaling in regulatory T cells is required for suppression of Th17 cell-mediated inflammation. Immunity 34: 566–578.

49. Brandau S, Trellakis S, Bruderek K, Schmaltz D, Stellar G, et al. (2011) Myeloid-derived suppressor cells in the peripheral blood of cancer patients contain a subset of immature neutrophils with impaired migratory properties. J Leukoc Biol 89: 311–317.

50. Eruslanov E, Neuberger M, Daurkin I, Perrin GQ, Algood C, et al. (2012) Circulating and tumor-infiltrating myeloid cell subsets in patients with bladder cancer. Int J Cancer 130: 1109–1119.

24

CKD-EPI and Cockcroft-Gault Equations Identify Similar Candidates for Neoadjuvant Chemotherapy in Muscle-Invasive Bladder Cancer

Sumanta K. Pal[1]*, Nora Ruel[2], Sergio Villegas[1], Mark Chang[1], Kara DeWalt[1], Timothy G. Wilson[3], Nicholas J. Vogelzang[4], Bertram E. Yuh[3]

1 Department of Medical Oncology and Experimental Therapeutics, City of Hope Comprehensive Cancer Center, Duarte, California, United States of America, **2** Division of Biostatistics, Department of Information Science, City of Hope Comprehensive Cancer Center, Duarte, California, United States of America, **3** Division of Urology, Department of Surgery, City of Hope Comprehensive Cancer Center, Duarte, California, United States of America, **4** US Oncology Research, Comprehensive Cancer Centers, Las Vegas, Nevada, United States of America

Abstract

Clinical guidelines suggest neoadjuvant cisplatin-based chemotherapy prior to cystectomy in the setting of muscle-invasive bladder cancer (MIBC). A creatinine clearance (CrCl) >60 mL/min is frequently used to characterize cisplatin-eligible patients, and use of the CKD-EPI equation to estimate CrCl has been advocated. From a prospectively maintained institutional database, patients with MIBC who received cystectomy were identified and clinicopathologic information was ascertained. CrCl prior to surgery was computed using three equations: (1) Cockcroft-Gault (CG), (2) CKD-EPI, and (3) MDRD. The primary objective was to determine if the CG and CKD-EPI equations identified a different proportion of patients who were cisplatin-eligible, based on an estimated CrCl of >60 mL/min. Cisplatin-eligibility was also assessed in subsets based on age, CCI score and race. Actuarial rates of neoadjuvant cisplatin-based chemotherapy use were also reported. Of 126 patients, 70% and 71% of patients were found to be cisplatin-eligible by the CKD-EPI and CG equations, respectively (P = 0.9). The MDRD did not result in significantly different characterization of cisplatin-eligibility as compared to the CKD-EPI and CG equations. In the subset of patients age >80, the CKD-EPI equation identified a much smaller proportion of cisplatin-eligible patients (25%) as compared to the CG equation (50%) or the MDRD equation (63%). Only 34 patients (27%) received neoadjuvant cisplatin-based chemotherapy. Of the 92 patients who did not receive neoadjuvant chemotherapy, 64% had a CrCl >60 mL/min by CG. In contrast to previous reports, the CKD-EPI equation does not appear to characterize a broader span of patients as cisplatin-eligible. Older patients (age >80) may less frequently be characterized as cisplatin-eligible by CKD-EPI. The discordance between actual rates of neoadjuvant chemotherapy use and rates of cisplatin eligibility suggest that other factors (e.g., patient and physician preference) may guide clinical decision-making.

Editor: Georgios Gakis, Eberhard-Karls University, Germany

Funding: This work was supported by NIH K12 2K12CA001727-16A1 (SKP). The funders had no role in study design, data collection and analysis, decision to publish, or preparation of the manuscript.

Competing Interests: The authors have declared that no competing interests exist.

* E-mail: spal@coh.org

Introduction

Several therapeutic options are available to patients with muscle-invasive bladder cancer (MIBC). For patients who opt to receive radical cystectomy, current guidelines strongly recommend consideration of neoadjuvant cisplatin-based chemotherapy.[1,2] These guidelines are predicated on randomized, phase III trials showing a survival benefit with this modality.[3,4] For instance, in Southwest Oncology Group (SWOG) 8710, a total of 307 patients with MIBC were randomized to receive either methotrexate, vinblastine, adriamycin and cisplatin (MVAC) followed by cystectomy or cystectomy alone.[4] Median survival was improved in those patients who received neoadjuvant MVAC (77 months *v* 46 months, P = 0.06). Alternatives to neoadjuvant MVAC include dose-dense MVAC (ddMVAC; supported by prospective phase II data), gemcitabine-cisplatin (GC; supported by retrospective series) and cisplatin/methotrexate/vinblastine (CMV; supported by a recently published phase III trial).[3,5,6] Meta-analytic data

pooled across multiple studies of neoadjuvant cisplatin-based trials suggest an absolute 5%.[7] From a theoretical perspective, the efficacy of neoadjuvant therapy may be based on (1) cytoreduction of primary tumor, resulting in more complete and successful surgery, or (2) elimination of micrometastatic disease burden.

Common to present neoadjuvant chemotherapy regimens for MIBC is the inclusion of cisplatin chemotherapy. Cisplatin has been used for the systemic management of bladder cancer for over three decades, and the nephrotoxicity associated with it has been well documented.[8,9] In light of this, clinical trials evaluating cisplatin-based regimens frequently include cutoffs for appropriate renal function. A common threshold in current day clinical trials is a creatinine clearance (CrCl) of 60 mL/min, below which patients are deemed ineligible.[10] These thresholds vary, with other groups utilizing thresholds of 45 and 55 mL/min to characterize eligibility for cisplatin-based studies.[11,12] Although it has been suggested that a measured CrCl is ideal, several studies allow for a calculated CrCl.

Methods for calculation of estimated CrCl vary. Although the Cockcroft-Gault equation has traditionally been employed, the reduced accuracy of this equation in certain populations (i.e., older adults) has long been recognized.[13] Alternatives to the Cockcroft-Gault equation include the Modified Diet in Renal Disease (MDRD) equation, developed from a training cohort of 1,070 patients, and validated in a cohort of 558 patients.[14] At the time this equation was conceived, it was thought to be more accurate than measured CrCl. More recently, in 2009, a new equation was introduced by the Chronic Kidney Disease Epidemiology (CKD-EPI) collaboration.[15] The eponymously titled CKD-EPI equation was suggested to offer a more precise assessment of glomerular filtration as compared to previous equations. Tsao *et al* have recently examined the Cockcroft-Gault and CKD-EPI equations in a series of 116 patients with bladder cancer treated at a single institution.[16] The authors reported that patients were 17% more likely to be deemed ineligible for cisplatin-based chemotherapy when using the Cockcroft-Gault equation as compared to the CKD-EPI equation, using a cutoff of 60 mL/min. In the current manuscript, we sought to validate these findings by comparing the two equations in an independent patient series. Our study captures a more extensive array of relevant clinical variables, such as comorbidity and actuarial use of chemotherapy, in a series of patients with muscle-invasive bladder cancer (MIBC) who received definitive management with cystectomy.

Patients and Methods

Patients

Patient data was obtained from an institutional bladder cancer database through the City of Hope Institutional Review Board approved protocol (IRB 12131). This database has been prospectively maintained from 1995 onwards with de-identified patient information. Prior to 2003, cases were primarily performed using a traditional open approach, whereas subsequent to 2003, cases were performed using robotic-assisted laparoscopic techniques. The database contains extensive clinical and demographic data, including age, race, gender, and Charlson comorbidity index (CCI). CCI is a system that assigns points for comorbidities and when added together can be used to predict mortality. Patients were included in the current study if they were noted to have muscle-invasive urothelial carcinoma of the bladder (other histologies, such as small cell and adenocarcinoma, were excluded). The nature and duration of neoadjuvant chemotherapy is also available within the database. Importantly, renal function and body-mass index (BMI) are recorded at the time of the initial patient encounter (i.e., prior to receipt of neoadjuvant chemotherapy and surgical intervention). These values were used to calculate CrCl using the subsequently defined methodology.

Calculation of CrCl

Standard methods were used to generate the estimates of CrCl using the Cockcroft-Gault, CKD-EPI, and MDRD equations. Specifically, the Cockcroft-Gault equation used was as follows:

$$CrCl = \frac{(140 - Age) \times Mass\ (kg) \times [0.85\ if\ female]}{72x \times SCr}$$

Notably, CrCl and SCr refer to CrCl and serum creatinine, respectively. The CDK-EPI equation used was as follows:

$$CrCl = 141 \times min\left(\frac{Scr}{k,1}\right)^{a} \times max\left(\frac{Scr}{k,1}\right)^{-1.209} \times$$

$$0.993^{Age} \times [1.018\ if\ female] \times [1.159\ if\ black]$$

The MDRD equation used was as follows:

$$CrCl = 186 \times SCr^{-1.154} \times Age^{-0.203} \times$$

$$[1.212\ if\ black] \times [0.742\ if\ female]$$

Statistical Analysis

Demographic, clinicopathologic information and clinical outcomes data were reported, with subgroups based on actuarial receipt of neoadjuvant cisplatin-based chemotherapy. The primary endpoint of this retrospective analysis was to determine if the Cockcroft-Gault and CKD-EPI equations identified different proportions of cisplatin-eligible patients amongst patients with MIBC who received cystectomy. Cisplatin eligibility was defined as a CrCl of 60 mL/min. Effect of calculation method on eligibility proportions was compared using a one way ANOVA test. Testing for differences in demographic or clinicopathologic variables between patient subgroups (Tables 1 and 2) was done using the chi-square test and student's t-test for categorical and continuous data, respectively. As a secondary endpoint, the proportion of patients deemed cisplatin-eligible by the MDRD equation was compared to the proportion derived from the CKD-EPI equation. Cisplatin-eligibility was also assessed in subsets based on age, CCI score and race.

Results

Patient Characteristics

A total of 126 patients were identified who had (1) a diagnosis of MIBC, (2) had received cystectomy at City of Hope, and (3) had sufficient data available to assess renal function by the three proposed methods. The majority of patients were male (83%). A total of 34 patients (27%) received neoadjuvant chemotherapy. Of these 34 patients, 29 patients (85%) had a CrCl >60 mL/min. Interestingly, amongst patients who did not receive chemotherapy (n = 92), the majority (64%) also had a CrCl >60 mL/min. As noted in Table 1, median age was higher in those patients with a CrCl ≤60 mL/min, and median body-mass index (BMI) was lower in these cohorts, as well. Few patients (<10%) were characterized as having clinical T3 or T4 disease.

Surgical Outcome and Pathologic Findings

As summarized in Table 2, Studer orthotopic neobladder, ileal conduit, and Indiana pouch urinary diversions were performed with similar frequency (40%, 35%, and 25% respectively). As it is our practice to avoid continent diversions in patients with reduced renal function, continent diversions (Indiana Pouch or Studer neobladder) were more frequent in patients with higher CrCl. Median operative time and estimated blood loss did not vary significantly amongst groups subdivided by chemotherapy receipt and Cockcroft-Gault calculated CrCl. Despite the fact that <10% of patients were characterized as having clinical T3/T4 disease prior to cystectomy, 31% were characterized as having pathologic T3 disease and 11% were characterized as having pathologic T4

Table 1. Demographic and clinicopathologic characteristics, as well as selected clinical outcomes, of patients with MIBC who received radical cystectomy.

	All Patients (n = 126)	(1) Chemo+ CG<=60 (n = 5)	(2) Chemo+ CG> 60 (n = 29)	(3) Chemo- CG< =60 (n = 33)	(4) Chemo- CG>60 (n = 59)	p-value
Gender, n (%)						
Female	21 (16.7%)	1 (20.0%)	2 (6.9%)	10 (27.8%)	8 (14.3%)	0.1
Male	105 (83.3%)	4 (80.0%)	27 (93.1%)	23 (69.7%)	51 (86.4%)	
Surgery Age, median (IQR)	71.5 (64–78)	77 (73–85)	65 (59–69)	79 (77–83)	69 (62–73)	<0.0001
BMI, median (IQR)	26.8 (24.1–30.9)	22.9 (21.0–29.0)	29.4 (26.7–33.3)	24.3 (23.4–25.9)	27.7 (24.7–32.2)	0.002
ASA, n (%)						
II	24 (19.0%)	2 (40.0%)	4 (13.8%)	3 (9.1%)	15 (25.4%)	0.2
III	80 (63.5%)	1 (20.0%)	21 (72.4%)	23 (69.7%)	35 (59.3%)	
IV	22 (17.5%)	2 (40.0%)	4 (13.8%)	7 (21.2%)	9 (15.3%)	
Total CCI, median (IQR)	5 (3–8)	6 (4–8)	5 (3–8)	8 (4–9)	4 (2–8)	0.2
Clinical T Stage, n (%)						
T2	117 (92.9%)	4 (80.0%)	26 (89.7%)	31 (93.9%)	56 (94.9%)	0.5
T3	6 (4.8%)	1 (20.0%)	2 (6.9%)	2 (6.1%)	1 (1.7%)	
T4	3 (2.4%)	0 (0.0%)	1 (3.4%)	0 (0.0%)	2 (3.4%)	

Subgroups are based on (1) receipt or non-receipt of neoadjuvant cisplatin-based chemotherapy and (2) CrCl (above or below 60) based on the Cockroft-Gault (CG) equation.

disease. The majority of patients with pathologic T3 and T4 disease had not received neoadjuvant chemotherapy, while the majority of patients with pathologic down-staging (i.e., findings of pathologic T0, Ta or T1 disease) had received this modality.

Cisplatin Eligibility

As previously noted, cisplatin eligibility was defined by a calculated CrCl of >60 mL/min. The primary objective of the study was to determine if the CKD-EPI equation identified a greater proportion of patients to be cisplatin-eligible as compared

Table 2. Surgical outcomes and pathologic findings of patients with MIBC who received radical cystectomy.

	All Patients (n = 126)	(1) Chemo+ CG<=60 (n = 5)	(2) Chemo+ CG>60 (n = 29)	(3) Chemo- CG<=60 (n = 33)	(4) Chemo- CG>60 (n = 59)	p-value
Diversion Type, n (%)						
Ileal Conduit	44 (34.9%)	3 (60.0%)	5 (17.2%)	17 (51.5%)	19 (32.2%)	0.005
Indiana Pouch	31 (24.6%)	1 (20.0%)	4 (13.8%)	10 (30.3%)	16 (27.1%)	
Studer neobladder	51 (40.5%)	1 (20.0%)	20 (69.0%)	6 (18.2%)	24 (40.7%)	
Surgery Length, hours median (IQR)	7.2 (6.3–8.4)	7.6 (7.3–8.1)	7.5 (6.6–8.3)	6.7 (5.9–7.8)	7.2 (6.4–8.8)	0.2
EBL, ml median (IQR)	400 (250–550)	500 (200–700)	350 (250–500)	350 (225–525)	400 (250–550)	0.4
Pathologic Stage, n (%)						
<T2	30 (23.8%)	1 (20.0%)	14 (48.3%)	2 (6.1%)	13 (22.0%)	0.03
T2	43 (34.1%)	1 (20.0%)	6 (20.7%)	12 (36.4%)	24 (40.7%)	
T3	39 (31.0%)	2 (40.0%)	6 (20.7%)	15 (45.4%)	16 (27.41%)	
T4	14 (11.1%)	1 (20.0%)	3 (10.3%)	4 (12.1%)	6 (10.2%)	
Pathologic Node Status, n (%)						
N0	89 (70.6%)	3 (60.0%)	17 (58.6%)	23 (69.7%)	46 (78.0%)	0.1
N1	11 (8.7%)	1 (20.0%)	5 (17.2%)	3 (9.1%)	2 (3.4%)	
N2	22 (17.5%)	0 (0.0%)	6 (20.7%)	6 (18.2%)	10 (16.9%)	
N3	1 (0.8%)	0 (0.0%)	0 (0.0%)	1 (3.0%)	0 (0.0%)	
NX	3 (2.4%)	1 (20.0%)	1 (3.4%)	0 (0.0%)	1 (178%)	
Length of Stay, days median (IQR)	9.5 (7–14)	10 (9–13)	9 (7–14)	11 (8–15)	9 (7–14)	0.4

Subgroups are based on (1) receipt or non-receipt of neoadjuvant cisplatin-based chemotherapy and (2) CrCl (above or below 60) based on the Cockroft-Gault (CG) equation.

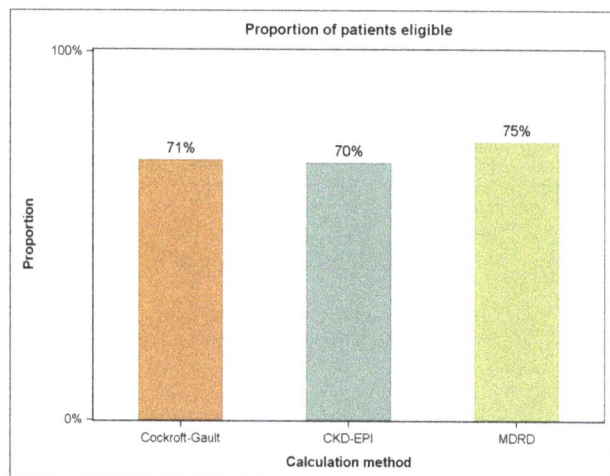

Figure 1. Proportion of patients defined as cisplatin-ineligible (i.e., creatinine clearance >60) based on the CKD-EPI equation, Cockroft-Gault equation, and MDRD equation (n = 126).

to the Cockcroft-Gault equation, to support previously published studies.[16] Ultimately, as noted in Figure 1, there was no difference in this proportion, with 70% and 71% of patients deemed cisplatin-eligible by the CKD-EPI and Cockcroft-Gault methods, respectively (P = 0.9). Similarly, the MDRD equation did not yield significant differences in cisplatin-eligibility.

Analyses were subsequently performed, assessing cisplatin eligibility using the same three equations in subsets divided by age, race and CCI score. No differences in the proportion of cisplatin-eligibility were seen in patients <60, 60–70 or 70–80 years of age (Figure 2a). However, in the subset of patients age >80 (n = 24), the CKD-EPI equation identified a much smaller proportion of cisplatin-eligible patients (25%) as compared to the Cockcroft-Gault equation (50%) or the MDRD equation (63%). By race, the three equations yielded few differences in cisplatin-eligibility amongst patients characterized as non-Hispanic white, Hispanic white, and other (Figure 2b). Notably, our study included only 1 black patient, limiting our ability to infer the concordance of the 3 equations in this racial group. No significant differences in cisplatin-eligibility were noted in subsets divided by CCI score, irrespective of the CrCl equation used (Figure 2c).

Discussion

In the current study, we could not replicate the results reported previously by Tsao et al.[16] Specifically, we did not find that the CKD-EPI equation was more likely to deem patients cisplatin-eligible as compared to the Cockcroft-Gault equation. On the contrary, our findings suggest that the CKD-EPI equation may be less likely to deem patients cisplatin-eligible in patients age >80. Similar findings were noted in the subset of patients defined as "other" race.

As also acknowledged by Tsao et al, reports such as these can only be characterized as hypothesis generating. However, we do take the added step of characterizing actuarial use of neoadjuvant chemotherapy in our cohort, which was comprised entirely of patients with MIBC (Tsao et al assessed a mixed cohort of patients with both localized and metastatic disease). As noted in Table 1, of 95 patients with a CrCl >60 mL/min by Cockcroft-Gault, only 31 patients (33%) received this modality. These data suggest that even if the CKD-EPI equation resulted in a modest increase in

estimated CrCl, many patients with satisfactory values would still not receive neoadjuvant chemotherapy. Other large series have produced similar findings. For instance, amongst 238 patients with MIBC receiving cystectomy at the University of Texas Southwestern Medical Center, it was noted that 97 patients (67%) had renal function adequate for cisplatin.[17] However, only 25 patients (17%) ultimately received neoadjuvant chemotherapy. A comparison of recipients and non-recipients of neoadjuvant chemotherapy with a CrCl >60 mL/min in our series shows little difference in baseline characteristics (e.g., BMI, CCI and clinical stage) between the groups. It is worth noting that there are other objective factors outside of CrCl that may impact use of neoadjuvant chemotherapy, such as neuropathy, hearing loss, performance status and comorbid conditions – certainly, these factors may limit use of neoadjuvant chemotherapy in a small proportion of patients. However, we envision that other subjective factors (patient preference, physician preference, etc.) may play a larger role in guiding the decision regarding neoadjuvant therapy.

Several limitations of the study should be noted. First, comparisons are offered between three equations frequently used to estimate CrCl. However, none of these equations represents a "gold standard" – ideally, comparisons would be made to measured CrCl. It has been suggested that the measured CrCl may be the optimal means by which to discern appropriately discern candidates for cisplatin therapy.[18] Although time consuming and perhaps more costly, the measured CrCl would likely offer the most precise estimate of renal function. An alternative to measured CrCl might be the addition of serum cystatin C to a standard laboratory panel; the combination of serum cystatin C to estimated GFR by CKD-EPI seemed to predict actual GFR with greater precision.[19] A second limitation is that the data presented herein is derived from a single institution. A larger sample derived from multiple institutions may provide a more realistic account of practice patterns for MIBC. As noted, only 17% of patients who were cisplatin-eligible (based on a Cockcroft-Gault estimated CrCl >60 mL/min) received neoadjuvant treatment. These numbers are lower than estimates of neoadjuvant chemotherapy use from the National Cancer Database published in 2007.[20] A third notable limitation is that we omit salient clinical endpoints from our analysis, such as disease-free survival (DFS) or overall survival (OS). We have previously published outcomes of patients receiving neoadjuvant CG and MVAC from our institutional series in a separate report.[21] Ultimately, it would be informative to know if misclassification of patients as cisplatin-ineligible has a detrimental effect on clinical outcome. However, as the data herein suggests, there are multiple factors that may ultimately dissuade use of neoadjuvant chemotherapy. Clearly, cisplatin "eligibility" based on renal function is not the only driver of neoadjuvant chemotherapy use. An additional limitation of our work is that the primary reason for non-receipt of neoadjuvant chemotherapy (e.g., patient preference, physician preference, renal function, etc.) was not consistently documented amongst our patients – collecting this data retrospectively would be challenging and subject to substantial biases. Finally, we have not reported receipt of adjuvant chemotherapy. The role of adjuvant chemotherapy is debatable, and many key trials of adjuvant treatment have been plagued by methodologic issues and problems with accrual that preclude useful results. Furthermore, given that we are a tertiary care center, many patients receive their preoperative and operative treatment at our site but return to a local practitioner for further care. As such, our capture of receipt of adjuvant therapy may be incomplete.

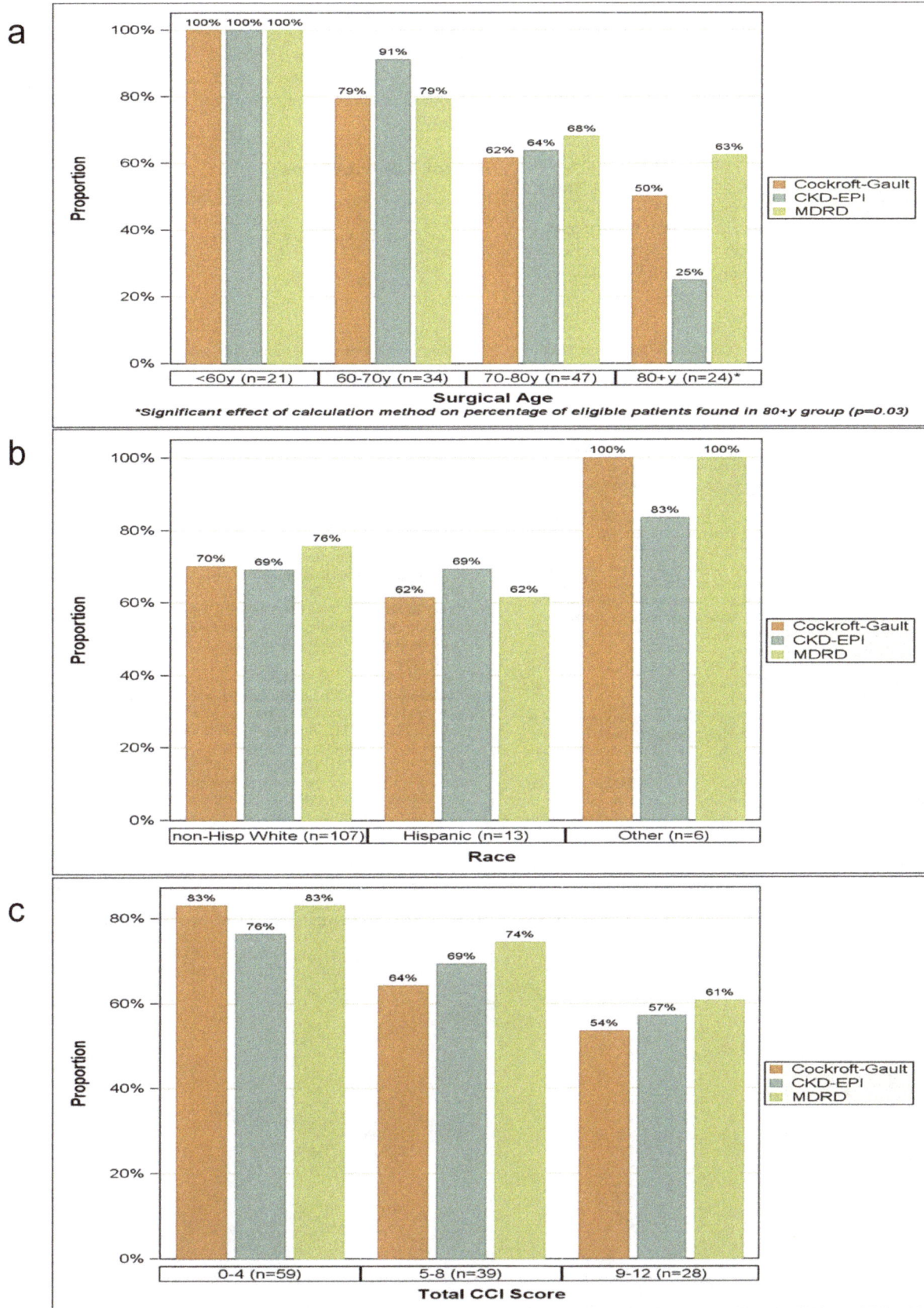

Figure 2. Proportion of patients defined as cisplatin-eligible (i.e., creatinine clearance >60) based on the CKD-EPI equation, Cockroft-Gault equation, and MDRD equation in subsets based on age (a), race (b) and comorbidity (c).

Galsky *et al* have proposed a consensus definition to identify patients with metastatic urothelial carcinoma "unfit" for cisplatin chemotherapy.[10,22] The definition is based in part on renal function, either measured or estimated. If estimated, a suggestion is made that the CKD-EPI equation be used, referencing a pooled analysis comparing the MDRD and CKD-EPI in non-oncology populations.[15] Although our study has the previously noted limitations, we reflect on the relative merits of the Cockroft-Gault, MDRD and CKD-EPI equations in a population solely comprised of patients with MIBC. Based on our data, it may be premature to substitute the CKD-EPI equation for the Cockroft-Gault equation in forthcoming trials in bladder cancer evaluating cisplatin-based neoadjuvant chemotherapy. To err on the side of caution, these studies may default to using measured CrCl to determine eligibility. Although a trial specifically dedicated evaluating the aforementioned equations is unlikely to occur, a prospective comparison of these equations could easily be embedded in any forthcoming study assessing neoadjuvant cisplatin-based chemotherapy.

Author Contributions

Conceived and designed the experiments: SKP NR SV MC KD TW NV BY. Analyzed the data: SKP NR SV MC KD TW NV BY. Wrote the paper: SKP NR SV MC KD TW NV BY.

References

1. NCCN Clinical Practice Guidelines in Oncology, version 1.2013: Bladder Cancer (Available at http://www.nccn.org; last accessed January 10, 2013.)
2. Sternberg CN, Bellmunt J, Sonpavde G, Siefker-Radtke AO, Stadler WM, et al. (2013) ICUD-EAU International Consultation on Bladder Cancer 2012: Chemotherapy for urothelial carcinoma-neoadjuvant and adjuvant settings. Eur Urol 63: 58–66.
3. Griffiths G, Hall R, Sylvester R, Raghavan D, Parmar MK (2011) International phase III trial assessing neoadjuvant cisplatin, methotrexate, and vinblastine chemotherapy for muscle-invasive bladder cancer: long-term results of the BA06 30894 trial. J Clin Oncol 29: 2171–2177.
4. Grossman HB, Natale RB, Tangen CM, Speights VO, Vogelzang NJ, et al. (2003) Neoadjuvant chemotherapy plus cystectomy compared with cystectomy alone for locally advanced bladder cancer. N Engl J Med 349: 859–866.
5. Qu AQ, Jacobus SJ, Signoretti S, Stack EC, Krajewski KM, et al. (2013) Phase II study of neoadjuvant dose-dense methotrexate, vinblastine, doxorubicin, and cisplatin (ddMVAC) chemotherapy in patients with muscle-invasive urothelial cancer (MI-UC): Pathologic and radiologic response, serum tumor markers, and DNA excision repair pathway biomarkers in relation to disease-free survival (DFS). ASCO Meeting Abstracts 31: 4530.
6. Yuh BE, Ruel N, Wilson TG, Vogelzang N, Pal SK (2012) Pooled Analysis of Clinical Outcomes with Neoadjuvant Cisplatin and Gemcitabine Chemotherapy for Muscle-Invasive Bladder Cancer. J Urol.
7. (2005) Neoadjuvant chemotherapy in invasive bladder cancer: update of a systematic review and meta-analysis of individual patient data advanced bladder cancer (ABC) meta-analysis collaboration. Eur Urol 48: 202–205; discussion 205–206.
8. Rossof AH, Talley RW, Stephens R, Thigpen T, Samson MK, et al. (1979) Phase II evaluation of cis-dichlorodiammineplatinum(II) in advanced malignancies of the genitourinary and gynecologic organs: a Southwest Oncology Group Study. Cancer Treat Rep 63: 1557–1564.
9. Ostrow S, Egorin MJ, Hahn D, Markus S, Leroy A, et al. (1980) Cis-Dichlorodiammine platinum and adriamycin therapy for advanced gynecological and genitourinary neoplasms. Cancer 46: 1715–1721.
10. Galsky MD, Hahn NM, Rosenberg J, Sonpavde G, Hutson T, et al. (2011) A consensus definition of patients with metastatic urothelial carcinoma who are unfit for cisplatin-based chemotherapy. Lancet Oncol 12: 211–214.
11. Siefker-Radtke AO, Dinney CP, Shen Y, Williams DL, Kamat AM, et al. (2012) A phase 2 clinical trial of sequential neoadjuvant chemotherapy with ifosfamide, doxorubicin, and gemcitabine followed by cisplatin, gemcitabine, and ifosfamide in locally advanced urothelial cancer: Final results. Cancer.
12. Bellmunt J, Guillem V, Paz-Ares L, Gonzalez-Larriba JL, Carles J, et al. (2000) Phase I-II study of paclitaxel, cisplatin, and gemcitabine in advanced transitional-cell carcinoma of the urothelium. Spanish Oncology Genitourinary Group. J Clin Oncol 18: 3247–3255.
13. Goldberg TH, Finkelstein MS (1987) Difficulties in estimating glomerular filtration rate in the elderly. Arch Intern Med 147: 1430–1433.
14. Levey AS, Bosch JP, Lewis JB, Greene T, Rogers N, et al. (1999) A More Accurate Method To Estimate Glomerular Filtration Rate from Serum Creatinine: A New Prediction Equation. Annals of Internal Medicine 130: 461–470.
15. Levey AS, Stevens LA, Schmid CH, Zhang YL, Castro AF, 3rd, et al. (2009) A new equation to estimate glomerular filtration rate. Ann Intern Med 150: 604–612.
16. Tsao CK, Moshier E, Seng SM, Godbold J, Grossman S, et al. (2012) Impact of the CKD-EPI equation for estimating renal function on eligibility for cisplatin-based chemotherapy in patients with urothelial cancer. Clin Genitourin Cancer 10: 15–20.
17. Raj GV, Karavadia S, Schlomer B, Arriaga Y, Lotan Y, et al. (2011) Contemporary use of perioperative cisplatin-based chemotherapy in patients with muscle-invasive bladder cancer. Cancer 117: 276–282.
18. Pal SK, Milowsky MI, Plimack ER (2013) Optimizing systemic therapy for bladder cancer. J Natl Compr Canc Netw 11: 793–804.
19. Inker LA, Schmid CH, Tighiouart H, Eckfeldt JH, Feldman HI, et al. (2012) Estimating Glomerular Filtration Rate from Serum Creatinine and Cystatin C. New England Journal of Medicine 367: 20–29.
20. Fedeli U, Fedewa SA, Ward EM (2011) Treatment of muscle invasive bladder cancer: evidence from the National Cancer Database, 2003 to 2007. J Urol 185: 72–78.
21. Pal SK, Ruel NH, Wilson TG, Yuh BE (2012) Retrospective analysis of clinical outcomes with neoadjuvant cisplatin-based regimens for muscle-invasive bladder cancer. Clin Genitourin Cancer 10: 246–250.
22. Galsky MD, Hahn NM, Rosenberg J, Sonpavde G, Hutson T, et al. (2011) Treatment of patients with metastatic urothelial cancer "unfit" for Cisplatin-based chemotherapy. J Clin Oncol 29: 2432–2438.

25

Galactodendritic Phthalocyanine Targets Carbohydrate-Binding Proteins Enhancing Photodynamic Therapy

Patrícia M. R. Pereira[1,2]**, Sandrina Silva**[1]**, José A. S. Cavaleiro**[1]**, Carlos A. F. Ribeiro**[2]**, João P. C. Tomé**[1,3]***,
Rosa Fernandes[2,4,5]*

1 QOPNA and Department of Chemistry, University of Aveiro, Aveiro, Portugal, **2** Laboratory of Pharmacology and Experimental Therapeutics, Institute for Biomedical Imaging and Life Sciences (IBILI), Faculty of Medicine, University of Coimbra, Azinhaga de Santa Comba, Coimbra, Portugal, **3** Department of Organic Chemistry, Ghent University, Gent, Belgium, **4** Center of Investigation in Environment, Genetics and Oncobiology, Coimbra, Portugal, **5** Center of Ophthalmology and Vision Sciences, IBILI, Faculty of Medicine, University of Coimbra, Coimbra, Portugal

Abstract

Photosensitizers (PSs) are of crucial importance in the effectiveness of photodynamic therapy (PDT) for cancer. Due to their high reactive oxygen species production and strong absorption in the wavelength range between 650 and 850 nm, where tissue light penetration is rather high, phthalocyanines (Pcs) have been studied as PSs of excellence. In this work, we report the evaluation of a phthalocyanine surrounded by a carbohydrate shell of sixteen galactose units distributed in a dendritic manner (PcGal$_{16}$) as a new and efficient third generation PSs for PDT against two bladder cancer cell lines, HT-1376 and UM-UC-3. Here, we define the role of galacto-dendritic units in promoting the uptake of a Pc through interaction with GLUT1 and galectin-1. The photoactivation of PcGal$_{16}$ induces cell death by generating oxidative stress. Although PDT with PcGal$_{16}$ induces an increase on the activity of antioxidant enzymes immediately after PDT, bladder cancer cells are unable to recover from the PDT-induced damage effects for at least 72 h after treatment. PcGal$_{16}$ co-localization with galectin-1 and GLUT1 and/or generation of oxidative stress after PcGal$_{16}$ photoactivation induces changes in the levels of these proteins. Knockdown of galectin-1 and GLUT1, via small interfering RNA (siRNA), in bladder cancer cells decreases intracellular uptake and phototoxicity of PcGal$_{16}$. The results reported herein show PcGal$_{16}$ as a promising therapeutic agent for the treatment of bladder cancer, which is the fifth most common type of cancer with the highest rate of recurrence of any cancer.

Editor: Michael Hamblin, MGH, MMS, United States of America

Funding: The synthesis of the photosensitizer was supported by the grant PTDC/CTM/101538/2008 (FCT- Fundação para a Ciência e a Tecnologia, Portugal). Thanks are due to FCT and Fundo Europeu de Desenvolvimento Regional (FEDER) for funding IBILI (Pest-C/SAU/UI3282/2011 and Pest-C/SAU/UI3282/2013) and QOPNA (PEst-C/QUI/UI0062/2013) research units. Thanks are due to ACIMAGO (ref. 12/12). The funders had no role in study design, data collection and analysis, decision to publish, or preparation of the manuscript.

Competing Interests: The authors have declared that no competing interests exist.

* E-mail: jtome@ua.pt (JT); rcfernandes@fmed.uc.pt (RF)

Introduction

Conventional photodynamic therapy (PDT) combines a non-toxic photosensitizer (PS), light irradiation at a specific wavelength and tissue molecular oxygen to produce cytotoxic reactive oxygen species (ROS) [1,2]. The molecular mechanisms underlying PDT are not clearly understood. However, it has been described that the generation of ROS will trigger signalling pathways that ultimately destroy the targeted tissue. Cell death in PDT may occur by apoptotic and by non-apoptotic mechanisms (*e.g.* necrosis), or even by a combination of the two mechanisms [2]. Additionally, studies suggest that cell death pathway induced after PDT depends on the PS and its intracellular localization, the PDT dose and the cell metabolic potential (*e.g.* its intrinsic antioxidant capacity) [2]. To enhance the specific deliver/target of PSs in cancer cells, third generation PSs have been synthesized, by conjugating them with biochemical motifs [3–5]. Among new third generation PSs, the advances in the past years concerning glycobiology have spurred the development of carbohydrate-based molecules for cancer treatment by PDT [3,4,6–14].

Carbohydrates have a strong potential as PS-delivery systems, because they are biocompatible molecules with a rapid cellular uptake and specific recognition by lectin proteins, which play an important role in several biochemical signalling pathways implicated in cancer metastasis, cell growth and inflammation [15,16]. The exact interaction mechanism of PS-carbohydrate conjugates with cancer cells is still unknown. However, it is expected that the specific (non-covalent) binding of carbohydrates with lectins [16], promotes the accumulation of the glyco-conjugate inside cells by the endocytic pathway. In addition, the expression of certain carbohydrate-binding lectins (*e.g.* galectins) is higher in cancer cells than in non-tumoral cells [17].

Among carbohydrates, the biocompatibility of galactose molecules and their specific recognition by galectins overexpressed in cancer cells (*e.g.* galectin-1 and galectin-3 [18]) have led to the development of galacto-conjugated PSs. Besides galectins, galactose carbohydrates can bind to GLUT1 (a well-known glucose transporter [19–21]). The steriospecificity of GLUT1 (recognizing both D-glucose and D-galactose) has been reported [19–21]. Galactose is a C4 epimer of glucose that can bind the glucose-binding site of GLUT1. There is strong evidence in literature that conjugation of carbohydrates (monosaccharides such as glucose and galactose, disaccharides such as lactose) with porphyrinoids [6,8,9,22–30] can improve the accumulation of PSs in cancer cells and, consequently, their photoactivity. Furthermore, it has been reported a marked contrast in terms of adsorption on the cells between galactose and glucose conjugated PSs. The former presented a selective uptake by rat hepatoma RLC-116 cells [29].

Recently, the emerging role of dendrimers (with well-defined nano-scaled structures) in biological systems has highlighted their potential benefits for the preparation of new anticancer drugs [31–33]. Regarding dendritic units of specific carbohydrates, it is well-known their multivalent interactions with lectins, promoting a synergistic increase in binding affinity [31]. The photodynamic efficiency of porphyrins conjugated with glycodendrimers has been reported in the literature [12,34–37]. However, the *in vitro* PDT studies with the corresponding phthalocyanines (Pcs) are scarce.

Recently, we have reported the synthesis of a new Pc decorated with sixteen molecules of galactose (in a dendritic manner, $PcGal_{16}$, Figure S1) [34]. $PcGal_{16}$ demonstrated strong absorbance in the red spectral region (600–800 nm), fluorescence emission bands at 734 and 805 nm, solubility in a phosphate buffered saline (PBS) solution and interaction with human serum albumin [34]. Additionally, $PcGal_{16}$ demonstrated photostability and ability to generate ROS after photoactivation. The present study was undertaken to validate the *in vitro* photodynamic efficacy of this $PcGal_{16}$ from the standpoint of its uptake by bladder cancer cells (HT-1376 and UM-UC-3, derived from transitional cell carcinoma) to interaction with carbohydrate-binding proteins; induction of phototoxicity, ROS production and activity of antioxidant enzymes after PDT. Our findings show that $PcGal_{16}$ has a strong photodynamic efficiency in an *in vitro* system of bladder cancer.

Materials and Methods

Synthesis of galacto-dendrimer phthalocyanine ($PcGal_{16}$)

$PcGal_{16}$ was synthesized as previously described [34]. Zinc 1,2,3,4,8,9,10,11,15,16,17,18,22,23,24,25-hexadeca-fluoro-phthalocyaninato zinc(II) (PcF_{16}) was obtained from Sigma. Stock solutions of PSs were prepared at a concentration of 2 mM in dimethyl sulfoxide (DMSO; Sigma-Aldrich, St Louis, MO, USA). Working solutions of $PcGal_{16}$ 0.5–9 µM were freshly prepared in sterile phosphate-buffered saline (PBS) keeping the concentration of DMSO always lower than 0.45% (v/v).

Cells culture and treatments

Human bladder cancer cell lines UM-UC-3 and HT-1376 derived from high-grade transitional cell carcinoma (from the American Type Culture Collection, ATCC, Manassas, VA, USA) were cultured in Eagle's Minimum Essential Medium (EMEM; ATCC) supplemented with 10% (v/v) of fetal bovine serum (Life Technologies, Carlsbad, CA, USA), 100 U/mL penicillin, 100 µg/mL streptomycin and 0.25 µg/mL amphotericin B (Sigma).

UM-UC-3 and HT-1376 cells were seeded at a density of 3×10^4 and 4×10^5 cells/well in 96- and 6-well culture plates (Orange Scientific, Braine-l'Alleud, Belgium), respectively. Twenty-four hours after plating, cells were incubated with the desired concentrations of PSs in the dark for the indicated period of time.

Photodynamic irradiation was carried out in fresh culture medium, devoid of PS, covering UM-UC-3 and HT-1376 cell monolayers and exposing them to red light (620–750 nm) delivered by an illumination system (LC-122 LumaCare, London). The light was delivered for 10 min or 40 min at a fluence rate of 2.5 mW/cm^2 or 10 mW/cm^2, as measured with an energy meter (Coherent FieldMaxII-Top) combined with a Coherent Power-Sens PS19Q energy sensor [34]. Sham-irradiated cells, used as

controls, consisted in cells kept in the dark for the same durations and under the same environmental conditions as the irradiated cells. In all treatments, triplicate wells were established under each experimental condition, and each experiment was repeated at least three times.

Cellular uptake of $PcGal_{16}$

After incubation with $PcGal_{16}$ in the dark, UM-UC-3 and HT-1376 cells were immediately washed with PBS buffer and lysed in 1% m/v sodium dodecyl sulfate (SDS; Sigma) in PBS buffer at pH 7.0. $PcGal_{16}$ intracellular concentration was determined by spectrofluorimetry using an IVIS Lumina XR equipment (Caliper Life Sciences, Hopkinton MA) with excitation and emission wavelengths set at 675 nm and Cy 5.5 (695–770 nm), respectively, and the results were normalized for protein concentration (determined by bicinchoninic acid reagent; Pierce, Rockford, IL, USA).

For microscopic evaluation, UM-UC-3 and HT-1376 bladder cancer cells were grown for 24 h on glass coverslips coated with poly-L-lysine (Sigma). The cells were incubated with 5 µM $PcGal_{16}$ for 2 h, at 37°C. After incubation, cells were fixed with 4% paraformaldehyde (PFA; Merck, Darmstadt, Germany) for 10 min at room temperature. The samples were then rinsed in PBS, and mounted in VectaSHIELD mounting medium containing 4',6-diamidino-2-phenylindole (DAPI; Vector Laboratories, CA, Burlingame) for visualization under a confocal microscope (LSM 510, Carl Zeiss, Gottingen, Germany). For detection of $PcGal_{16}$, the specimen was excited at 633 nm and its emitted light was collected between 653–750 nm. For DAPI detection, specimen was excited at 405 nm and its emitted light was collected between 430–500 nm.

Cell metabolic activity and membrane integrity

Trypan Blue dye exclusion. Cell membrane integrity after $PcGal_{16}$ incubation in the dark, irradiation, or both was determined by the trypan blue dye (Biowhittaker, Walkersville, MD, USA) exclusion test 24, 48 and 72 h after each treatment. Cells with intact membrane were counted on a Neubauer chamber after trypsinization and the cell viability of treated cells was normalized to that of the untreated cells.

MTT assay. Cell metabolic activity after $PcGal_{16}$ incubation in the dark, irradiation, or both was determined 24, 48 and 72 h after treatments by measuring the ability of bladder cancer cells to reduce 3-[4,5-dimethylthiazol-2-yl]-2,5-diphenyl-tetrazolium bromide (MTT, Sigma), to a colored formazan using a microplate reader (Synergy HT, Biotek, Winooski, VT, USA). The data were expressed in percentage of control (*i.e.* optical density of formazan from cells not exposed to $PcGal_{16}$).

IC_{50} values (*i.e.* concentration of $PcGal_{16}$ required to reduce cell viability by 50% as compared to the control cells) were calculated using non-linear regression analysis to fit dose-response curves in GraphPad Prism 5.0 software (La Jolla, CA, USA).

Detection of intracellular Reactive Oxygen Species (ROS) generation

Immediately after irradiation or sham-irradiation, cancer cells were washed twice with PBS and incubated with either 2 or 5 µM 2',7'-dichlorodihydrofluorescein diacetate (H_2DCFDA; Invitrogen Life Technologies, Carlsbad, CA, USA) for an additional 1 h period, at 37°C, protected from light. After incubation, cells were washed with PBS and lysed in 1% (m/v) SDS solution in PBS (pH 7.0). DCF fluorescence was determined using a microtiter plate reader (Synergy HT) with the excitation and emission filters set at 485/20 nm and 528/20 nm, respectively. Protein concentration was determined using the Pierce BCA Protein Assay Kit.

The ROS levels were also qualitatively evaluated by fluorescence microscopy. After PDT treatments, UM-UC-3 and HT-1376 human bladder cancer cells grown on coverslips were incubated with 5 µM of H_2DCFDA in PBS buffer (in dark conditions). After washing steps and fixation in 4% (m/v) PFA, coverslips were mounted using VectaSHIELD mounting medium and the slides were visualized under a confocal microscope (LSM 710, Carl Zeiss).

Redox quenching studies

Immediately after $PcGal_{16}$ uptake, photodynamic treatment was performed with cell monolayers covered with culture medium containing 50 nM of redox quenchers sodium azide, L-histidine and L-cysteine obtained from Sigma. The effect of quenchers on cell viability was evaluated 24 h after PDT by the MTT viability assay.

TUNEL assay

Cell death was detected by terminal deoxynucleotidyltransferasedUTP nick end-labeling (TUNEL) assay, using the DeadEnd Fluorometric TUNEL System (Promega, Madison, WI, USA), according to the manufacturer's instructions. Briefly, 24 and 72 h after PDT treatment, bladder cancer cells were fixed in 4% (m/v) PFA and permeabilized with 0.2% v/v Triton X-100 in PBS solution. Cells were stained with TdT reaction cocktail for 60 min at 37°C. The nuclei were stained with DAPI and the cells were analyzed under a fluorescence microscope (Leica DFC350 FX, Leica Microsystems, Bannockburn, IL, USA). Tunel-positive DAPI-stained cells were counted in 10 randomly selected fields from three independent experiments. Percentage of dead cells was expressed as ratio of TUNEL-positive cell numbers to DAPI-stained cell numbers.

Antioxidant enzyme activities

Cell homogenates were obtained immediately after PDT and centrifuged at 10,000 g for 10 min at 4°C. The supernatants were used for measurements of glutathione peroxidase (GPox), glutathione reductase (GR), glutathione S-transferase (GST), superoxide dismutase (SOD) and catalase (CAT) activities in 96-well plates using a Biotek Synergy HT spectrophotometer (Biotek). The activity was expressed as nmol of substrate oxidized per minute per mg of protein (mU/mg).

GPox activity was determined at 30°C, measuring the NADPH (Merck) oxidation at 340 nm. Supernatants were mixed with 1 mM of glutathione-reduced form (GSH; Sigma), 0.5 U/mL GR (Sigma), 0.18 mM NaDPH, 1 mM EDTA (Sigma) and 0.7 mM *tert*-butyl hydroperoxide (t-BOOH; Sigma) in 50 mM imidazole (Sigma) at pH 7.4. The activity was calculated using the NADPH extinction coefficient of 0.62 m^2/mmoL.

GR activity in cell supernatants was determined at 30°C by measuring the rate of NADPH oxidation at 340 nm in the presence of 3 mM glutathione-oxidised form (Sigma), 0.12 mM NADPH, and 2.5 mM EDTA, in 50 mM Hepes (pH 7.4). The activity was calculated using the NADPH extinction coefficient of 0.62 m^2/mmoL.

GST activity was determined at 30°C by monitoring the formation of GSH conjugate with 1-chloro-2,4-dinitrobenzene (CDNB; Sigma) at 340 nm in the presence of 1 mM GSH and 1 mM CDNB in 50 mM Hepes (pH 7.4). The activity was calculated using the conjugate extinction coefficient of 0.96 m^2/mmoL.

SOD activity was determined at 25°C measuring the cytochrome c (Merck) reduction at 550 nm. The supernatants were mixed with 40 µM cytochrome c solution (0.05 M potassium phosphate, 0.5 mM EDTA, pH 7.8) containing 80 µM xanthine (Merck). To initiate the reaction, 2 U/mL xanthine oxidase (Merck) was added. The increase in cytochrome c absorbance at 550 nm was recorded. SOD activity was calculated considering that one unit of SOD activity represents the inhibition of 50% in the rate of increase in absorbance at 550 nm when compared with control (sample without SOD under the conditions of the assay).

CAT activity was determined at 25°C by monitoring the rate of hydrogen peroxide (0.04% w/w) decomposition in 0.05 M potassium phosphate, pH 7.0. One unit of catalase activity was defined by the enzyme quantity that produced an absorbance reduction of 0.43 per minute at 240 nm in this system.

Transfection assays

Galectin-1 or GLUT1 was depleted in human bladder cancer cells using a pool of three target-specific 20–25 nt siRNA (Santa Cruz Biotechnology, Inc., Santa Cruz, CA, USA). UM-UC-3 and HT-1376 bladder cancer cells were transfected in 6- or 96-well culture plates, at 60–80% confluence, with galectin-1 and GLUT1, respectively. Cells were also transfected with a scrambled siRNA in parallel as controls.

For each transfection, cells were treated for 5 h with 2.4 µM of siRNA in transfection medium (Santa Cruz) containing 0.5 µL/cm^2 of transfection reagent (Santa Cruz). After incubation, complete media was added and the cells were incubated for 24 or 48 h. Galectin-1 or GLUT1 downregulation was evaluated 24 h or 48 h post-transfection by Western blotting. The uptake and PDT experiments were performed 24 h or 48 h post-transfection with GLUT1 hsiRNA or galectin-1 hsiRNA, respectively.

Western blot

After PDT treatment, UM-UC-3 and HT 1376 cells were washed twice with ice-cold PBS and harvested in RIPA buffer (150 mM NaCl, 50 mM Tris-HCl, pH 7.5, 5 mM ethylene glycol tetraacetic acid (EGTA), 1% Triton X-100, 0.5% sodium deoxycholate (DOC), 0.1% SDS, 2 mM phenylmethanesulfonyl (PMSF), 2 mM iodoacetamide (IAD),) and 1× protease inhibitor cocktail (Roche, Indianapolis, IN, USA)). After centrifugation at 16,000 g for 10 min at 4°C, supernatants were used for protein quantification using the Pierce BCA Protein Assay Kit, followed by denaturation of the sample with Laemmli buffer. For the Western Blotting analysis, 60 µg proteins were loaded per lane on sodium dodecyl sulphate-polyacrilamide gels (SDS-PAGE). Following electrophoresis and transfer to PVDF membranes (Bio-Rad, Hercules, CA, USA), the blots were incubated in 5% (m/v) nonfat milk in TBS-T (20 mM Tris, 150 mM NaCl, Tween 0.2%, pH 7.6) and probed with rabbit anti-galectin-1 1:1,000 (Abcam, Cambridge, UK), rabbit anti-GLUT1 1:1,000 (Chemicon, Boston, MA, USA) and mouse anti β-actin 1:20,000 (Sigma) antibodies. After washing, the membranes were probed with secondary anti-rabbit or anti-mouse IgG-HRP-linked antibodies (1:10,000; Bio-Rad). Immunoreactive bands were detected by enhanced chemiluminiscence (ECL) substrate using an imaging system (VersaDoc 4000 MP, Bio-Rad) followed by densitometric analysis.

Immunofluorescence

UM-UC-3 and HT-1376 human bladder cancer cells were grown on coverslips as previously described [20,21]. After treatment, cells were washed with PBS and fixed in 4% PFA. Cells were then permeabilized with 1% Triton X-100 in PBS (pH 7.4) and blocked with 5% bovine serum albumin in PBS buffer, before incubation with primary antibodies rabbit anti-galectin-1 1:100 (Abcam) and rabbit anti-GLUT1 1:250 (Chemicon). The cells were then rinsed with PBS buffer and incubated with DAPI and secondary fluorescent antibodies. After washing, samples were imaged using a confocal microscope (LSM 710, Carl Zeiss).

Statistical analysis

The results are presented as mean ± standard deviation (S.D.) with n indicating the number of experiments. Statistical significance among two conditions was assessed using the nonparametric Mann-Whitney test. Statistical significance among three conditions was assessed by the nonparametric Kruskal-Wallis test. Statistical significance among several conditions was assessed with the Friedman test. P-value was considered at the 5% level of significance to deduce inference of the significance of the data. All graphs and statistics were prepared using the GraphPad Prism 5.0 software.

Results

PcGal$_{16}$ accumulates in cancer cells and is non-toxic in darkness

To study the cellular uptake of PcGal$_{16}$, HT-1376 and UM-UC-3 bladder cancer cells have been incubated with increasing concentrations (0.5, 2.5, 5 and 9 μM) of PcGal$_{16}$ in PBS for up to 4 h. PcGal$_{16}$ intracellular accumulation was determined by quantitative spectrofluorimetry and fluorescence microscopy. As shown in Figure 1A, the uptake of PcGal$_{16}$ was both concentration- and time- dependent, reaching a plateau in less than 2 h. Addition of 5 μM PcGal$_{16}$ to HT-1376 and UM-UC-3 cells resulted in an intracellular concentration of 3531±125.9 and 2973±119.1 nmol PcGal$_{16}$ per mg of protein, respectively, after 2 h of incubation (Figure 1A). This spectrofluorimetric data was confirmed by confocal microscopy showing that cells treated with PcGal$_{16}$ exhibit strong fluorescence, with occasional bright spots in the perinuclear region (Figure 1B). PcF$_{16}$, the non-conjugated Pc (Figure S1), was used as control. No significant intracellular accumulation was observed when the cells were incubated with 0.5–9 μM PcF$_{16}$ (data not shown), showing that the uptake of the PcGal$_{16}$ by cancer cells is enhanced relatively to unconjugated PcF$_{16}$. After confirmation of PcGal$_{16}$ uptake by bladder cancer cells, its cytotoxic effect in darkness was assessed by the MTT colorimetric assay (Figure S2). No dark toxicity was observed in untreated cells (up to 4 h) in the presence of 0.45% or less DMSO in the incubation medium. Moreover, PcGal$_{16}$ showed no significant cytotoxicity at concentrations up to 9 μM up to 72 h after treatment (Figure S2).

PcGal$_{16}$ induces cytotoxicity after photodynamic activation

To test the effect of light irradiation (red light at 620–750 nm delivered at 2.5 mW/cm^2 for 40 min, i.e. 6 J/cm^2) after PcGal$_{16}$ uptake on cell viability, MTT was performed 24 h after treatment (Figure 2). No cytotoxicity was observed in the untreated sham-irradiated cells (Figure 2A) or untreated irradiated cells in the presence of 0.45% (v/v) or less DMSO in PBS (data not shown). However, when HT-1376 and UM-UC-3 cells were incubated with PcGal$_{16}$ and then irradiated, there was an increased phototoxicity in a concentration- and uptake time-dependent manner (Figure 2A). Data showed that PcGal$_{16}$ exerted a higher phototoxicity on UM-UC-3 cells compared to HT-1376 cells (Figure 2A). Moreover, the percentage of cell death in treated cells

compared to untreated cells was significantly influenced by the dose of light (Figure 2B). The phototoxicity was higher in cells irradiated at 6 J/cm^2 than in cells irradiated at 1.5 J/cm^2 (cells irradiated with light at 2.5 mW/cm^2 for 40 min or 10 min, respectively). On the other hand, irradiation of cells with light at 10 mW/cm^2 for 10 min (i.e. 6 J/cm^2) resulted in induction of cell death in untreated control cells. In subsequent experiments, we then performed cells irradiation with light at 2.5 mW/cm^2 for 40 min. Based on the uptake results (Figure 1A) and MTT data before (Figure S2) and after PcGal$_{16}$ photoactivation (Figures 2A and 2B), we estimate the lowest concentration of PcGal$_{16}$ and the lowest dose of light necessary to achieve high phototoxicity for both bladder cancer cell lines. When cells were incubated with 5 μM PcGal$_{16}$ for 2 h and then irradiated with light at 6 J/cm^2 (cells irradiated for 40 min with light at 2.5 mW/cm^2), we observed a significant increase in phototoxicity of HT-1376 and UM-UC-3 cells. The cells were also incubated with 5 μM of PcF$_{16}$ during 2 h and then irradiated. As shown in Figures S2 and 2, the phototoxicity was higher for PcGal$_{16}$ than for non-conjugated PcF$_{16}$. Based on the critical role of ROS in causing cell death after PDT and considering the different PDT-induced phototoxicity observed in UM-UC-3 and HT-1376 cells, the intracellular production of ROS was evaluated immediately after PDT in the cells previously incubated with 5 μM PcGal$_{16}$ for 2 h. The application of PcGal$_{16}$ in combination with PDT led to a high significant augmentation of ROS in both bladder cancer cell lines compared with the control (Figures 2C and 2D). The ROS levels (DCF fluorescence fold increase per mg of protein) in HT-1376 and UM-UC-3 cells were 50.52±12.77 and 74.88±11.49, respectively, when 5 μM H$_2$DCFDA was used for ROS detection (Figure 2D).

To assess the contribution of ROS in PcGal$_{16}$-mediated cell death, quenchers of ROS (histidine, sodium azide [38] and cysteine [39]) were added at non-toxic concentrations to the incubation medium when the cells were irradiated. Cell viability evaluated 24 h after treatment was dependent on the used scavenger and cell type (Figure 2E). For the cell line UM-UC-3, all quenchers at the employed concentration partially decrease the PcGal$_{16}$–PDT-induced phototoxicity. For the cell line HT-1376, none of the quenchers used in these experiments were able to reduce the phototoxicity induced by photoactivated PcGal$_{16}$.

To assess whether PDT has a long-term phototoxic effect, we evaluated cell viability for up to 72 h after PDT treatment. In both cell lines, the results obtained with the MTT colorimetric assay (cell metabolic activity) were correlated with the loss of cell membrane integrity (trypan blue staining) (Figures 3A and 3B). Overall, UM-UC-3 and HT-1376 bladder cancer cells were unable to recover from the PDT-induced damage effects 48 or 72 h after treatment, for PcGal$_{16}$ concentrations above 5 μM. TUNEL data revealed that there is an induction of cell death in a time-dependent manner in the cells irradiated after incubation with PcGal$_{16}$ (Figure 3C). Twenty-four hours after PDT with PcGal$_{16}$, the percentage of TUNEL positive cells in UM-UC-3 cell line was 1.8 higher than that of the HT-1376 cells, but after 72 h there was almost the same percentage of TUNEL-positive cells in both cell lines. The concentrations of PcGal$_{16}$ necessary to inhibit the metabolic activity of UM-UC-3 and HT-1376 bladder cancer cells in 50% can be estimated from Figure 3A. These values, named as "photocytotoxic concentrations" (IC$_{50}$) are reported in Table 1. Data show that 24 h after PDT, IC$_{50}$ value is lower for UM-UC-3 when compared with HT-1376 cells and similar for these cell lines 72 h after PDT.

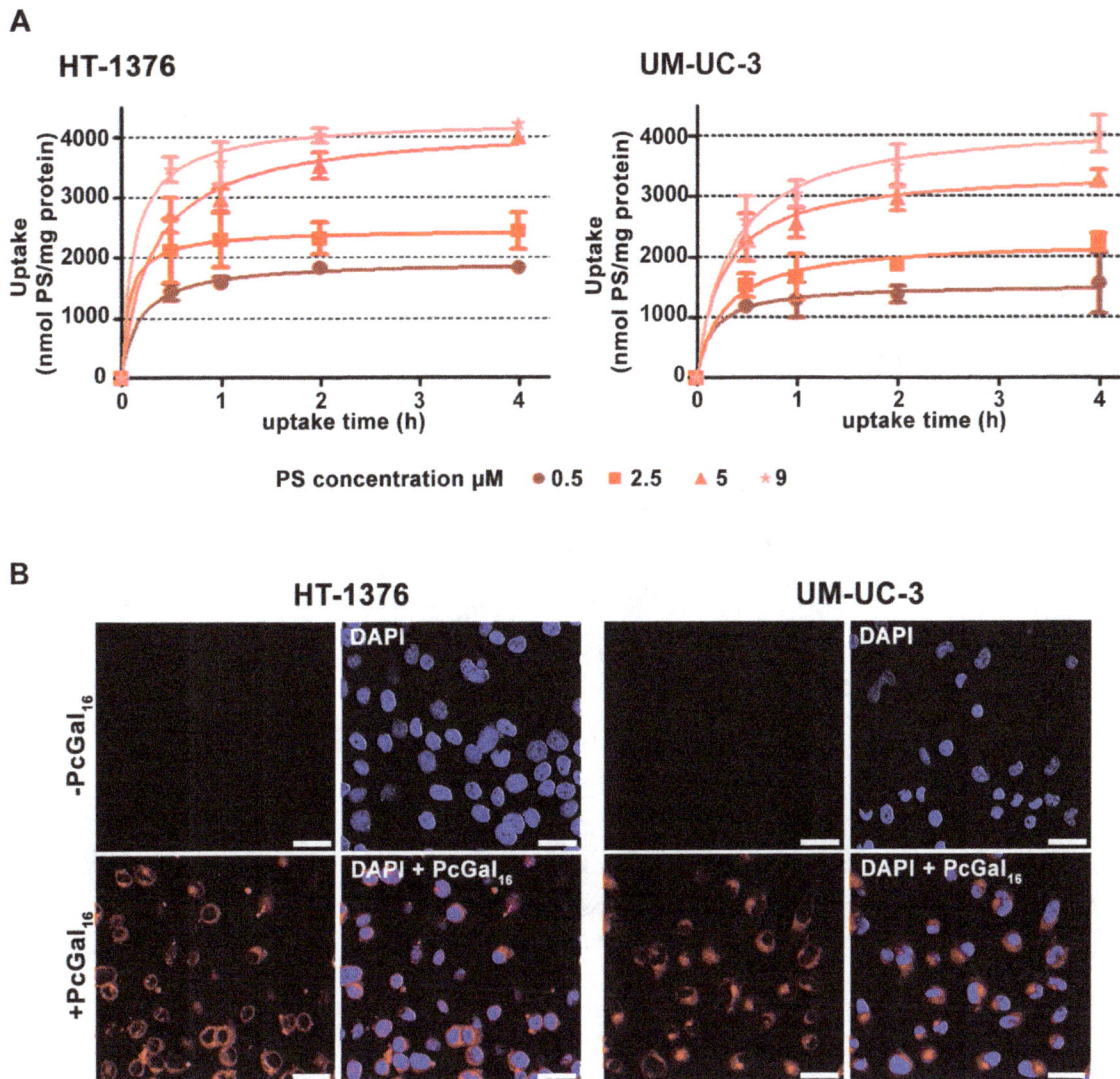

Figure 1. PcGal$_{16}$ accumulates in UM-UC-3 and HT-1376 human bladder cancer cells. Intracellular uptake of PcGal$_{16}$ by HT-1376 and UM-UC-3 bladder cancer cells (panel A). The concentration of PcGal$_{16}$ was determined by fluorescence spectroscopy and the results were normalized to protein quantity. Data are the mean ± S.D. of at least three independent experiments performed in triplicates. Representative fluorescence images (panel B) of bladder cancer cells incubated with PcGal$_{16}$ (red) in darkness and cell nucleus stained with DAPI (blue). *Scale bars* 20 μm.

PcGal$_{16}$ induces antioxidant enzyme response after photodynamic therapy

Considering the different levels of ROS produced in the two bladder cancer cell lines after PDT with PcGal$_{16}$, we investigated (immediately after PDT) the involvement of specific antioxidant enzymes [40] in the detoxification of ROS and/or resulting toxic products. For that, the activities of the three major antioxidant enzymes, SOD, CAT, and GPox were determined by spectroscopy [41]. SOD catalyses the dismutation of superoxide radical anions into hydrogen peroxide and molecular oxygen. Hydrogen peroxide is then removed by CAT when it is present at high concentrations or by GPox when present at low concentrations. Knowing about the indirect antioxidant function [40] of GR in the replenishment of gluthathione levels in reduced form (GSH) and of GST in the elimination of reactive compounds through their conjugation with GSH, their activities were also determined.

In UM-UC-3 control cells, the activities of GR, SOD and CAT were 1.5-fold, 1.9-fold and 1.5-fold higher, respectively, than in HT-1376 control cells (Table 2). There was no significant difference in the activities of GST and GPox between the control cells of the two cell lines. After PDT with PcGal$_{16}$, there was a 1.3-fold, 3.1-fold and 1.5-fold increase in the activities of GR, SOD and CAT in UM-UC-3 cells. In HT-1376 cells, there was a 2.2-fold, 4.6-fold and 4.8-fold increase in GR, SOD and CAT activities and a 2-fold decrease in the activity of GST after PDT with PcGal$_{16}$. Treatment of HT-1376 resulted in a 2.3-fold increased of CAT activity as compared to UM-UC-3-treated cells. The ability of HT-1376 cells to produce an antioxidant adaptive response, activating the antioxidant enzymes GR, SOD and CAT can explain the higher resistance observed 24 h after PDT with PcGal$_{16}$ as compared with UM-UC-3 cells.

Knockdown of galectin-1 and GLUT1 decreases the uptake and phototoxicity of PcGal$_{16}$

We investigated whether the presence of the dendritic galactose units around the core of Pc molecule could facilitate the

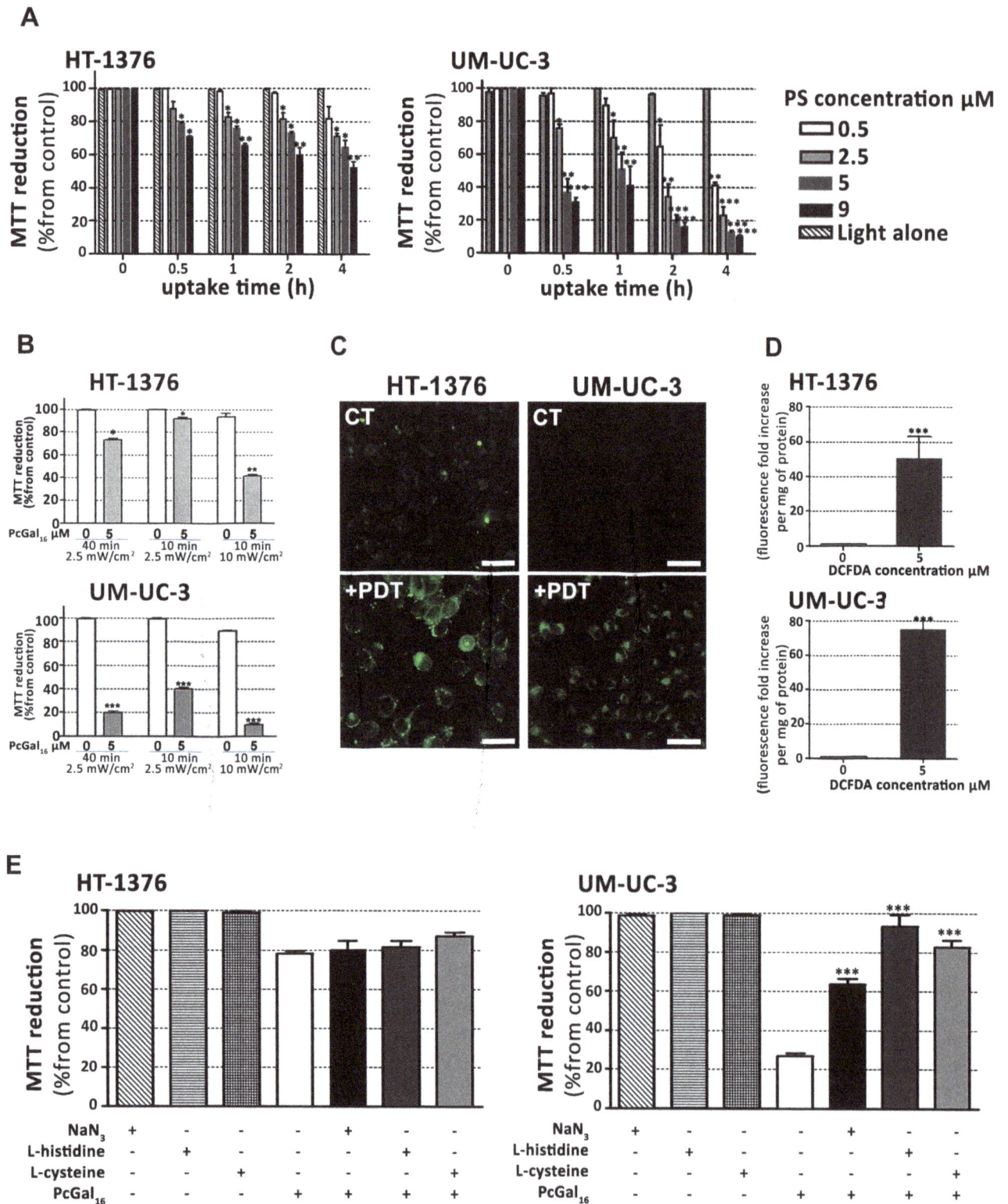

Figure 2. PcGal$_{16}$ generates ROS and produces toxicity after PDT. Photocytotoxic effects after PcGal$_{16}$-PDT in HT-1376 and UM-UC-3 cells evaluated 24 h after PDT using the MTT assay (panel A). The percentage of toxicity was calculated relatively to control cells (cells incubated with PBS and irradiated). Data are the mean ± S.D. of at least three independent experiments performed in triplicates. *($p<0.05$), **($p<0.001$), ***($p<0.0001$) significantly different from control cells. Irradiation dose-dependent cell death in response to PDT with PcGal$_{16}$ (panel B). Cytotoxicity was assessed 24 h after treatment using the MTT assay. The percentage of cytotoxicity was calculated relatively to control cells (untreated cells). Data are the mean value ± S.D. of at least three independent experiments performed in triplicates. *($p<0.05$), **($p<0.001$), ***($p<0.0001$) significantly different from control cells. Representative fluorescence images (panel C) and quantification (panel D) of DCF fluorescence increase (as a measure of ROS production) in HT-1376 and UM-UC-3 cells, after PDT with PcGal$_{16}$. *Scale bars* 20 μm. Data are the mean ± S.D. of at least three independent experiments performed in triplicates. *($p<0.05$), ***($p<0.0001$) significantly different from control cells Photocytotoxicity after PDT with PcGal$_{16}$ in

the presence of 50 nM of ROS quenchers (sodium azide, histidine and cysteine) in HT-1376 and UM-UC-3 cells (panel E). Cytotoxicity was assessed 24 h after treatment using the MTT assay. The percentage of cytotoxicity was calculated relatively to control cells (untreated cells). Data are the mean value $\pm$ S.D. of at least three independent experiments performed in triplicates. ***($p < 0.0001$) significantly different from MTT reduction (%) after PcGal$_{16}$-PDT.

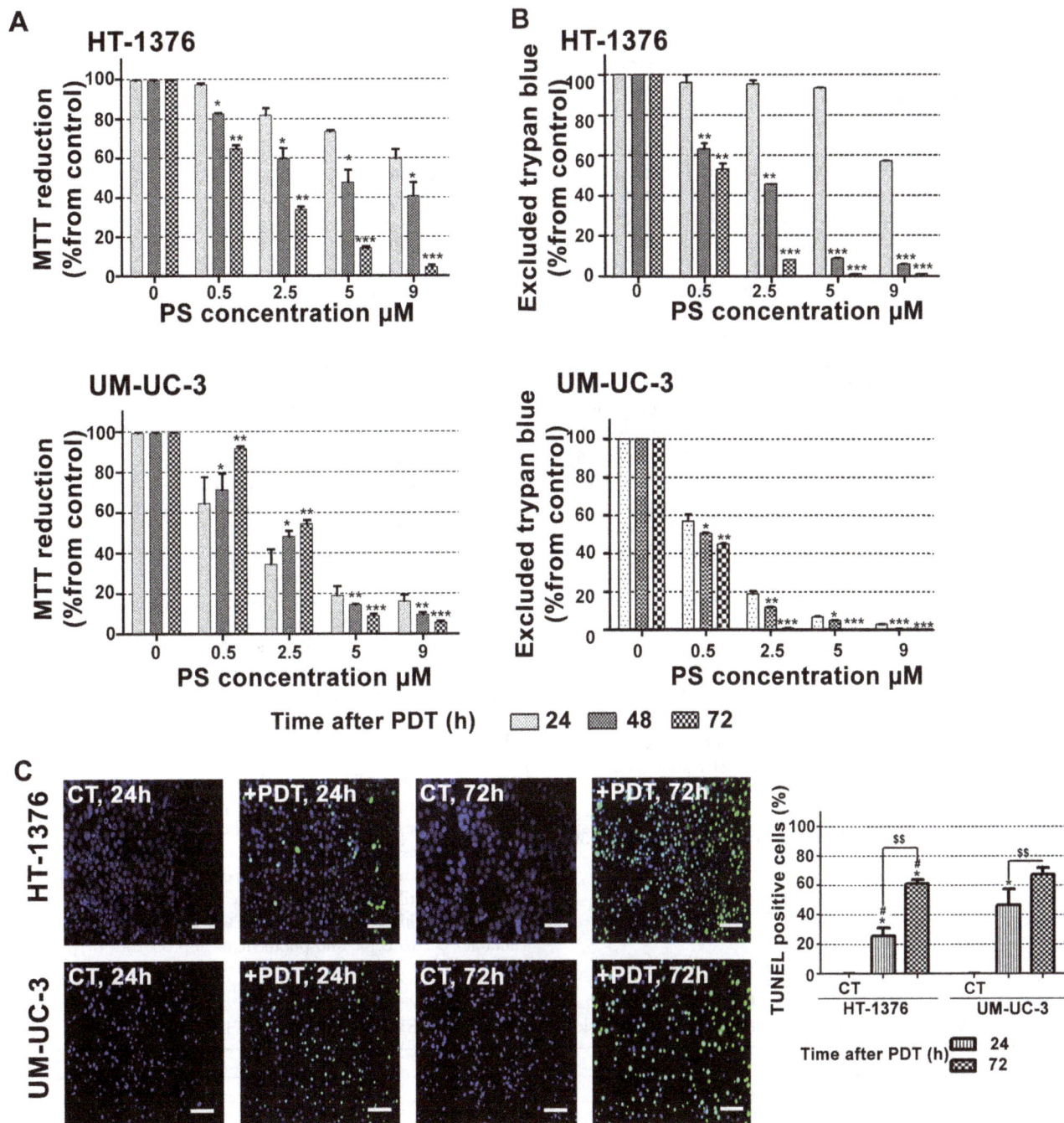

Figure 3. PDT with PcGal$_{16}$ has a long-term phototoxicity effect. Cytotoxicity was assessed 24, 48, and 72 h after PcGal$_{16}$-PDT using the MTT (panel A) and trypan blue staining (panel B) assays. The percentage of cytotoxicity was calculated relatively to control cells (cells incubated with PBS in darkness and then irradiated) at the respective uptake time. Data are the mean value $\pm$ S.D. of at least three independent experiments performed in triplicates. *($p < 0.05$), **($p < 0.001$), ***($p < 0.0001$) significantly different from MTT reduction (%) or excluded trypan blue (%) at 24 h after PDT for the respective concentration. Representative fluorescence images revealing cell death in HT-1376 and UM-UC-3 cells after PDT with PcGal$_{16}$ by TUNEL staining 24 and 72 h after treatment (panel C). DAPI was used for nuclei staining (blue) and TUNEL staining was used to visualize dead cells (green). *Scale bars* 20 μm. Quantification of TUNEL-positive cells 24 and 72 h after PDT with PcGal$_{16}$. *($p < 0.05$) significantly. different from control cells. $^{\$\$}$($p < 0.001$) significantly different from TUNEL-positive cells 24 h after PDT. $^{\#}$($p < 0.05$) significantly different from TUNEL-positive UM-UC-3 cells at the respective time after PDT.

Table 1. Values for photocytotoxic concentration (IC$_{50}$, µM) of photoactivated PcGal$_{16}$ on human bladder cancer cell lines, HT-1376 and UM-UC-3.

	HT-1376 cell line			UM-UC-3 cell line		
Hours after PDT	24	48	72	24	48	72
IC$_{50}$ (µM), CI$_{95\%}$	-	3.3 [0.6;10.7]	2.5 [2.2;2.9]	2.1 [0.9;5.0]	2.8 [2.4; 3.2]	2.6 [2.6;2.7]

IC$_{50}$ is the incubation concentration that inhibits the proliferation of cultures in 50%, after cells' incubation with **PcGal$_{16}$** and irradiation. IC$_{50}$ values were calculated using the MTT dose response curves (24, 48, and 72 h after PDT), obtained for cells incubated with **PcGal$_{16}$** at various concentrations for 2 h. CI$_{95\%}$: 95% Confidence interval.

interaction of this PS with specific domains in the plasma membrane of cancer cells. We hypothesized that domains enriched in carbohydrate-binding proteins [42] could facilitate the interaction with PcGal$_{16}$, enhancing somehow its cellular uptake, and therefore its photodynamic potential.

Galectin [18] and glucose [19] proteins are expressed in high levels in cancer cells and both have affinity for galactose molecules. Therefore, we have evaluated the protein levels of galectin-1 and GLUT 1 in UM-UC-3 and HT-1376 cells, by Western Blotting and immunofluorescence (Figures 4 and 5).

The galectin-1 protein levels were higher in UM-UC-3 than in HT-1376 control cells (Figure 4A). To determine whether galectin-1 plays a role in the uptake of PcGal$_{16}$ by cancer cells, siRNA was used to knockdown galectin-1 within UM-UC-3 bladder cancer cells. The treatment of UM-UC-3 cells with a pool of three target-specific siRNAs maximally suppressed galectin-1 by ≈50% at 24 h and 48 h post-transfection (Figure 4B), without affecting the expression of the housekeeping protein β-actin. The transfected cells were then treated with PcGal$_{16}$ 48 h post-transfection. As shown in Figures 4C and 4D, transfected cells displayed a markedly decreased uptake and phototoxicity of PcGal$_{16}$. The GLUT1 protein levels were higher in HT-1376 than in UM-UC-3 control cells (Figure 5A). Therefore, HT-1376 bladder cancer cells were also treated with a pool of three target-specific GLUT1 siRNAs. Application of GLUT1 siRNA suppressed GLUT1 by ≈50% and ≈90% at 24 h and 48 h post-transfection, respectively (Figure 5B). Treatment of HT-1376 cells with PcGal$_{16}$ twenty-four hours post-transfection, resulted in a substantial decrease in the uptake and phototoxicity (Figures 5C and D).

PcGal$_{16}$ decreases the galectin-1 and GLUT1 protein levels

To further explore the role of galectin-1 and GLUT1 in the photodynamic effect induced by PcGal$_{16}$, we determined the levels of these proteins before and after PDT. Both incubation of cancer cells with PcGal$_{16}$ (i.e. incubation of cancer cells with PcGal$_{16}$ in darkness) and PDT with PcGal$_{16}$ induced a decrease in galectin-1 as observed by Western Blotting and immunofluorescence (Figures 4E, 4F and 4G). The decrease observed in galectin-1 was higher in UM-UC-3 cells as compared to HT-1376 cells and it was more evident after PDT. Using confocal fluorescence microscopy, we observed co-localization of PcGal$_{16}$ with galectin-1 inside bladder cancer cells (Figure 4G).

Similar to what was observed for galectin-1, there was also a decrease in GLUT1 (Figures 5E, 5F and 5G) both after PcGal$_{16}$ uptake and after PDT treatment in HT-1376 cancer cells. Furthermore, in these cancer cells it was higher after PDT than after PcGal$_{16}$ uptake in darkness. In UM-UC-3 cells, PcGal$_{16}$ was not able to reduce GLUT1 protein levels (Figure 5F). In both bladder cancer cell lines there was co-localization of PcGal$_{16}$ with GLUT1 (Figure 5G). Overall, these findings clearly indicate show the critical involvement of the carbohydrate-binding proteins in the potential of PcGal$_{16}$ as a therapeutic agent.

Discussion

Third-generation PSs such as Pc coupled to carbohydrates are interesting for PDT, because they can be recognized by glycoprotein-based membrane proteins that are overexpressed in tumors [6]. Besides the enhancement of cellular recognition, the presence of dendritic galactose molecules improves Pc solubility and biocompatibility [34]. We have recently reported the synthesis of a new Pc with dendrimers of galactose sugar (PcGal$_{16}$) that has valuable spectroscopic and photochemical properties [34]. In this

Table 2. Values of activity (mU/mg of protein) of antioxidant enzymes superoxide dismutase (SOD), catalase (CAT), glutathione peroxidase (GPox), glutathione reductase (GR) and glutathione S-transferase (GST) determined after PDT.

Cell line	PcGal$_{16}$-PDT	Enzyme activity (mU/mg of protein)				
		GST	GPox	GR	SOD	CAT
UM-UC-3	–	44.0±1.4	232.4±23.6	252.3±13.9§	56.0±13.1§	36.31±1.3§
	+	39.7±2.7	243.6±12.0	316.1±11.3$^{\#}$	173.6±4.8$^{\#}$	52.89±2.7$^{\#}$
HT-1376	–	50.4±2.4	236.1±9.9	163.4±1.9	29.56±1.9	24.85±2.2
	+	24.6±0.5§,*	252.3±18.2	356.9±30.6§	134.7±4.3§,*	119.8±3.3§,*

§(p<0.05): significantly different from HT-1376 control cells;
$^{\#}$(p<0.05): significantly different from UM-UC-3 control cells;
*(p<0.05): significantly different from UM-UC-3 treated cells.

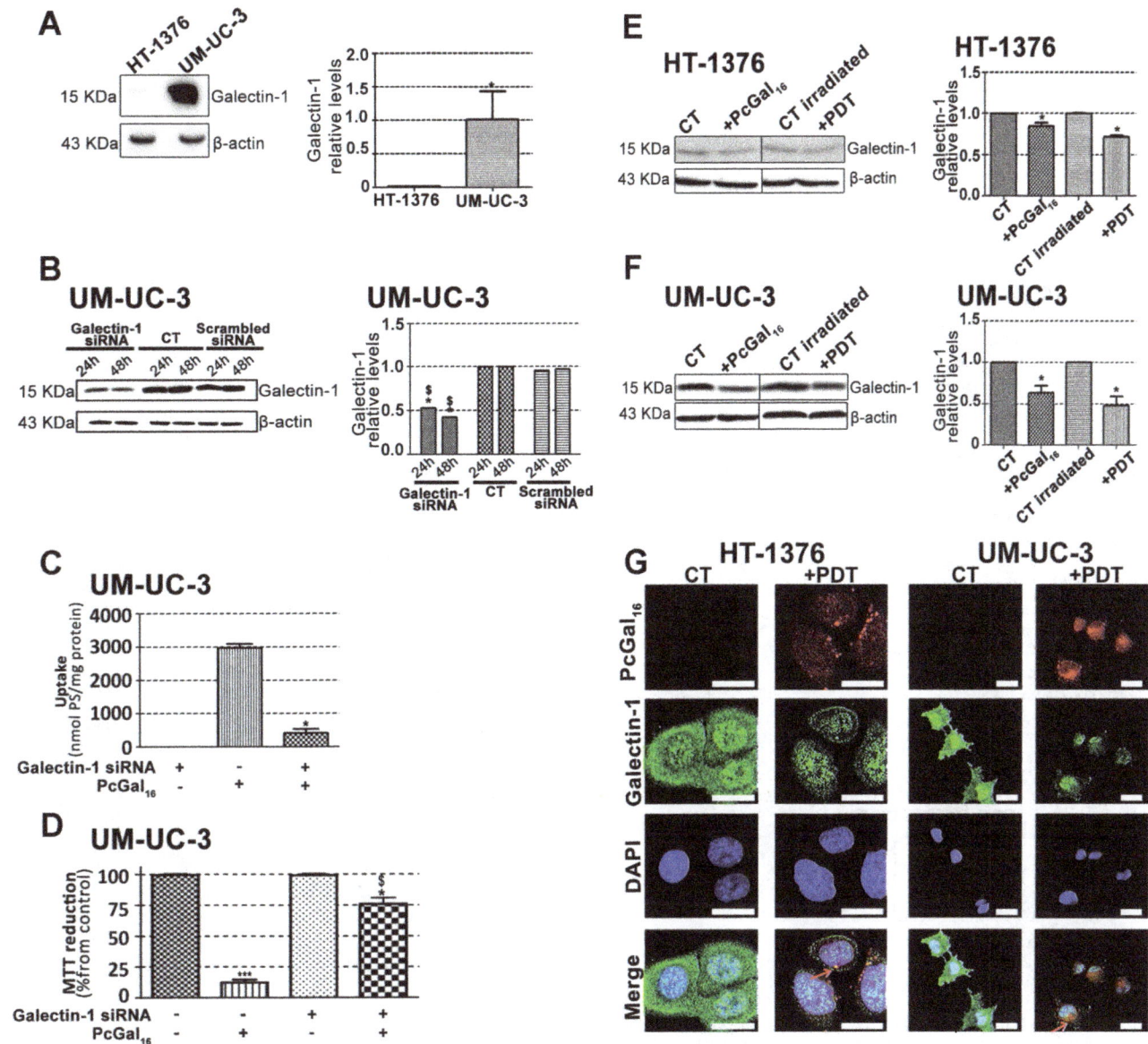

Figure 4. Knockdown of galectin-1 decreases de uptake and phototoxicity of PcGal₁₆. Western blotting analysis and quantification of galectin-1 protein levels in HT-1376 and UM-UC-3 cells (panel A), in HT-1376 cells (panel E) or UM-UC-3 cells (panel F) after uptake with PcGal$_{16}$ in darkness and after PDT. β-actin was blotted as loading control. Quantitative analysis of galectin-1 (normalized to β-actin) expressed as a ratio of the levels found in HT-1376 cells. *($p<0.05$) significantly different from HT-1376 cells. Quantitative analysis of galectin-1 (normalized to β-actin) expressed as a ratio of the levels found in untreated HT-1376 or UM-UC-3 cells (panel E, F). Data represents mean ± S.D. of five independent experiments. *($p<0.05$) significantly different from untreated HT-1376 or UM-UC-3 cells. Knockdown of galectin-1 in UM-UC-3 bladder cancer cells as determined by Western blotting 24 and 48 h post-transfection (panel B). Quantitative analysis of galectin-1 (normalized to β-actin) expressed as a ratio of the levels found in non-transfected control cells. Data represents mean ± S.D. of five independent experiments. *($p<0.05$), $^\$$($p<0.05$) significantly different from non-transfected control cells or cells treated with scrambled siRNA, respectively. Intracellular uptake of PcGal$_{16}$ by UM-UC-3 bladder cancer cells transfected with galectin-1 siRNA (panel C). The cells were incubated with PcGal$_{16}$ 48 h post-transfection with galectin-1 siRNA. Data are the mean ± S.D. of at least three independent experiments performed in triplicates. *($p<0.05$) significantly different from non-transfected control cells. Photocytotoxic effects after PcGal$_{16}$-PDT in UM-UC-3 cells transfected with galectin-1 siRNA (panel D). Phototoxicity was evaluated 72 h after PDT. Data are the mean ± S.D. of at least three independent experiments performed in triplicates. *($p<0.05$), ***($p<0.0001$) significantly different from control cells. $^\$$($p<0.05$), significantly different from PDT with PcGal$_{16}$ in non-transfected cells. Representative fluorescence images (panel G) of galectin-1 protein (green) in cancer cells before and after incubation with PcGal$_{16}$ (red), with DAPI staining the nucleus (blue). *Scale bars* 20 μm.

study, we showed that PcGal$_{16}$ is a nontoxic compound *per se*, and has high photocytotoxic efficiency in two bladder cancer cell lines, which is paralleled with its high ability to produce ROS and to induce oxidative stress (Figure 6).

The high intracellular uptake of the glycoconjugated PS, PcGal$_{16}$, can be explained by the presence of carbohydrate cellular transporters or receptors present at the cell surface. Although the PcGal$_{16}$ uptake was quite similar in the two bladder cancer cell lines, the expression of carbohydrate-binding proteins GLUT1 and galectin-1 is different amongst them. Besides its role in the import and export of glucose [19], the isoform of glucose transporter GLUT1 also transports D-galactose [19] having lower

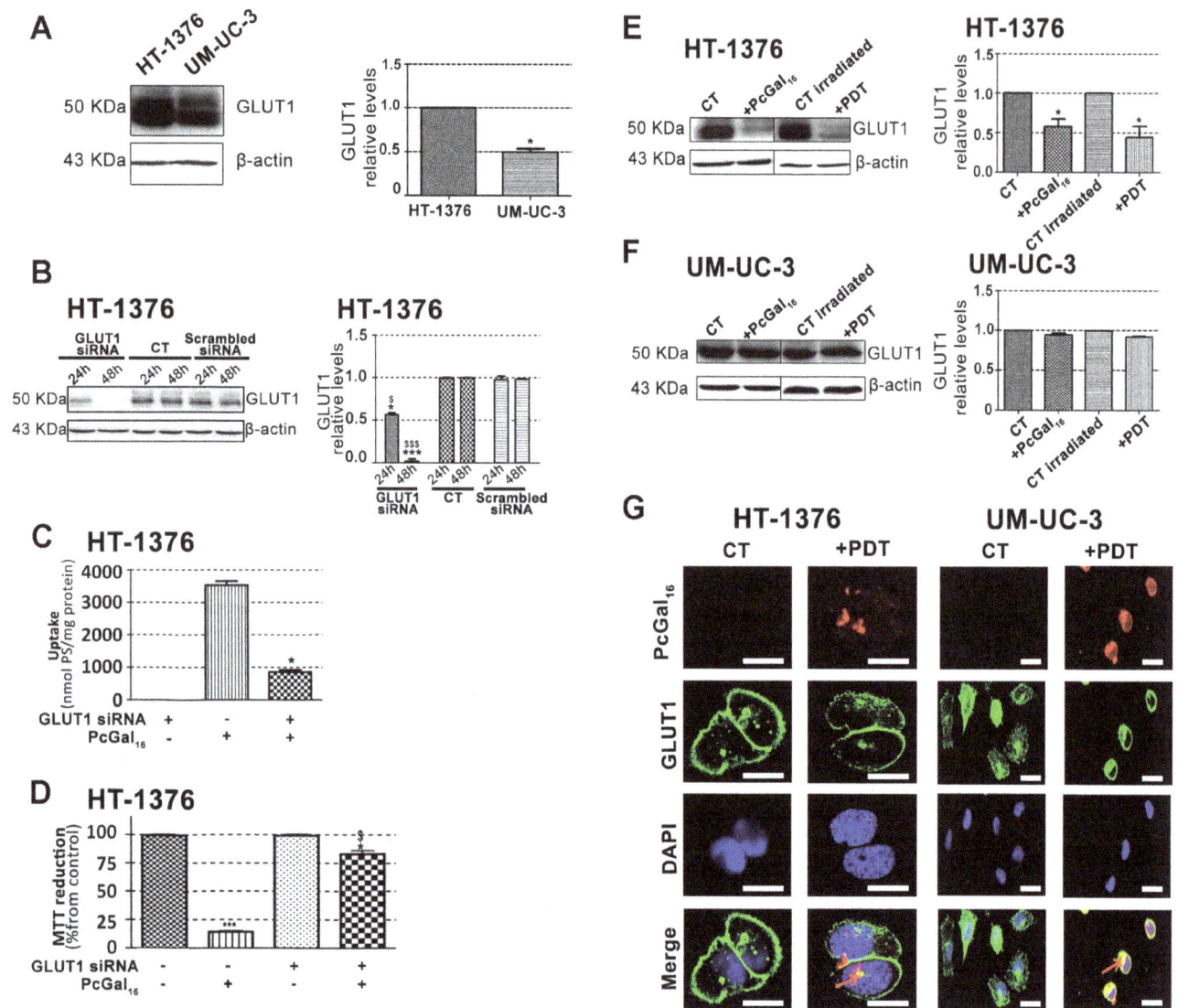

Figure 5. Knockdown of GLUT1 decreases de uptake and phototoxicity of PcGal₁₆. Western blotting analysis and quantification of GLUT1 protein levels in HT-1376 and UM-UC-3 cells (panel A), in HT-1376 cells (panel E) or UM-UC-3 cells (panel F) after uptake with PcGal₁₆ in darkness and after PDT. β-actin was blotted as loading control. Quantitative analysis of GLUT1 (normalized to β-actin) expressed as a ratio of the levels found in HT-1376 cells (panel A). *($p<0.05$) significantly different from HT-1376 cells. Quantitative analysis of GLUT1 (normalized to β-actin) expressed as a ratio of the levels found in untreated HT-1376 or UM-UC-3 cells (panel E, F). Data represents mean ± S.D. of five independent experiments. *($p<0.05$) significantly different from untreated HT-1376 cells. Knockdown of GLUT1 in HT-1376 bladder cancer cells as determined by Western blotting 24 and 48 h post-transfection (panel B). Quantitative analysis of GLUT1 (normalized to β-actin) expressed as a ratio of the levels found in non-transfected control cells. Data represents mean ± S.D. of five independent experiments. *($p<0.05$), ***($p<0.0001$) significantly different from non-transfected control cells. $($p<0.05$), $$$($p<0.0001$) significantly different from cells treated with scrambled siRNA. Intracellular uptake of PcGal₁₆ by HT-1376 bladder cancer cells transfected with GLUT1 siRNA (panel C). The cells were incubated with PcGal₁₆ 24 h post-transfection. Data are the mean ± S.D. of at least three independent experiments performed in triplicates. *($p<0.05$) significantly different from non-transfected control cells. Photocytotoxic effects after PcGal₁₆-PDT in UM-UC-3 cells transfected with galectin-1 siRNA (panel D). Phototoxicity was evaluated 72 h after PDT. Data are the mean ± S.D. of at least three independent experiments performed in triplicates. *($p<0.05$), ***($p<0.0001$) significantly different from control cells. *($p<0.05$), significantly different from PDT with PcGal₁₆ in non-transfected cells. Representative fluorescence images (panel G) of GLUT1 protein (green) in HT-1376 and UM-UC-3 cells before and after incubation with PcGal₁₆ (red), with DAPI staining the nucleus (blue). *Scale bars* 20 μm.

affinity for it than for D-glucose. Studies have been suggested that the hydroxyl groups in C1, C3 and C4 positions of D-galactose are hydrogen bond acceptors for GLUT1 sugar uptake site [43]. Like other galectins, galectin-1 has a carbohydrate-recognition domain (CRD) able to recognize and bind β-galactose [17]. Our assays demonstrated that galectin-1 and GLUT1 are both expressed by UM-UC-3 and HT-1376 cells. However, HT-1376 cells present higher GLUT1 levels compared with UM-UC-3 cells, and the

contrary was observed for galectin-1. Although a similar PcGal₁₆ uptake was observed in the two bladder cancer cell lines, both GLUT1 and galectin-1 may contribute for its specificity modulating the intracellular uptake. Knockdown of galectin-1 and GLUT1 in UM-UC-3 and HT-1376 cells, respectively, was associated with a marked decrease of PcGal₁₆ uptake and phototoxicity. Together, these data demonstrated that galectin-1

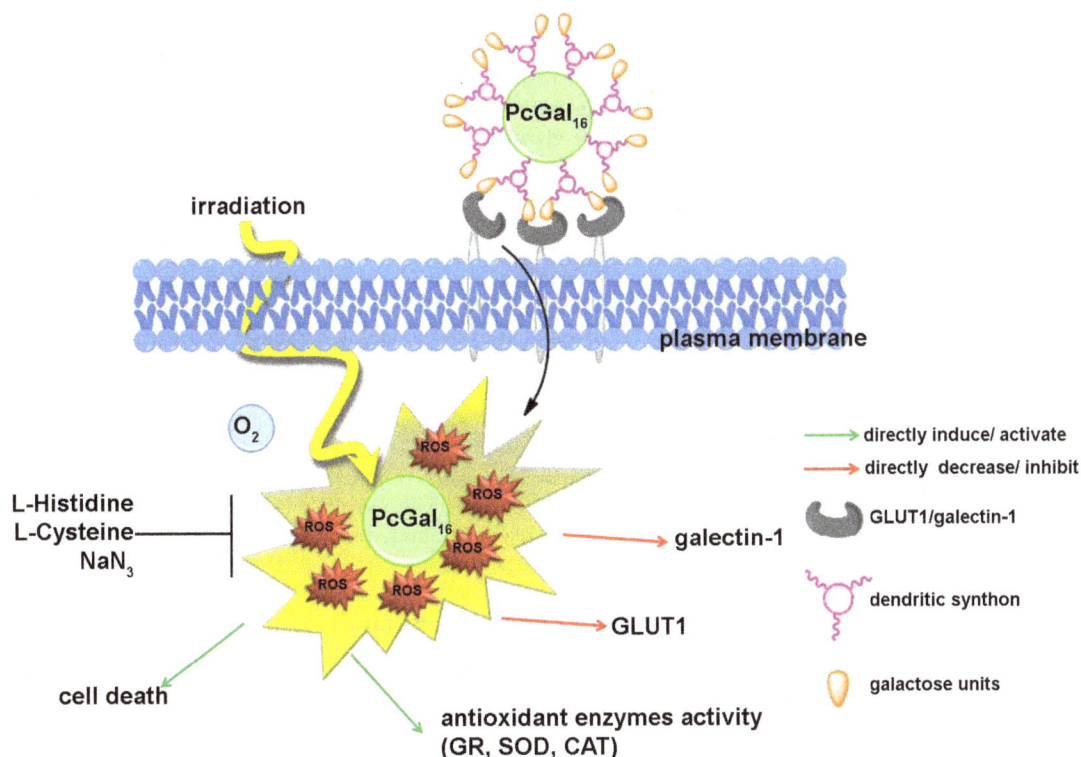

Figure 6. Hypothetic illustration of phototoxicity of PcGal₁₆ in human bladder cancer cells. The uptake of PcGal₁₆ by bladder cancer cells is modulated by the presence of carbohydrate-binding proteins present at the cell surface (*i.e.* GLUT1 and galectin-1). PcGal₁₆ is a nontoxic compound *per se*, and has high photocytotoxic efficiency against bladder cancer cell lines. Treatment with ROS quenchers demonstrated that cell death in bladder cancer cells is mediated by the production of ROS after PDT. Immediately after PDT with PcGal₁₆ there is an increase on the activity of antioxidant enzymes (SOD, CAT and GR antioxidant enzymes). The photoactivated PcGal₁₆ co-localizes with galectin-1 and GLUT1 and reduces their levels.

and GLUT1 contribute for the efficacy of PDT mediated by PcGal₁₆.

Interestingly, although the similar uptake of PcGal₁₆ by UM-UC-3 and HT-1376 cells, the phototoxicity induced 24 h after PDT was higher in UM-UC-3 cells than in HT-1376 cells. Such lack of association between uptake and phototoxicity has been described [44,45]. We investigated whether the higher phototoxicity observed in UM-UC-3 cells was due to higher production of ROS and/or higher oxidative damage compared with that in HT-1376 cells. As expected, the ability of PcGal₁₆ to produce ROS was higher in UM-UC-3 than in HT-1376 cells.

In PDT, it has been described that ROS can be generated by two photochemical reactions [46,47]. In type-II photochemical reactions, the excited PS in its triplet state can transfer its energy to molecular oxygen leading to the formation of singlet oxygen. Type-I photochemical reactions happen when an excited PS reacts with a biological substrate forming radicals and radical ions. Treatment with ROS quenchers demonstrated that in UM-UC-3 cells, singlet oxygen should have a high effect since cell death was highly reduced with quenchers of singlet oxygen (sodium azide and histidine). Further studies are needed to gain insight into the contribution of specific ROS in PcGal₁₆-mediated cell death after PDT.

Interestingly, we observed that PDT with PcGal₁₆ has a long-term phototoxic effect in both cancer cell lines. Cytotoxicity assays (MTT, trypan blue and TUNEL assays) performed 72 h after PDT demonstrated that UM-UC-3 cells were not able to recover. Moreover, in HT-1376 cells there was a marked induction of cell

death occurring from 24 to 72 h after PDT with PcGal₁₆. The three distinct cytotoxic methods used in the present work are widely applied in the study of cell death: MTT (indicator of metabolic activity), trypan blue staining (indicator of membrane integrity loss occurring in necrosis or in late stages of apoptosis) and TUNEL assay (indicator of DNA fragmentation, a key factor of apoptosis). Cell death in PDT may occur by apoptosis or necrosis, or even by a combination of the two mechanisms [2]. A more specific and comprehensive study is needed to understand the specific cell death pathways induced after PDT with PcGal₁₆ in the bladder cancer cells used in this study. The different cell death obtained 24 h after PDT in UM-UC-3 and HT-1376 cells can be partially explained by the different amount of ROS present in both cells lines after irradiation. In addition, the resistance exhibited by HT-1376 cells could be due to the presence of efficient protective mechanisms, at least in the first stages after photodynamic treatment. Cytoprotective mechanisms initiated by cancer cells after PDT are well-known [47]. The increase of antioxidant molecules (*e.g.* gluthathione, vitamin C and vitamin E) [48] and the induction of genes encoding proteins involved in apoptosis or in the repair of lesions [49] are two of the well-known cytoprotective mechanisms induced after PDT. Another one is based on the equilibrium between photo-oxidative impairment of cells by ROS *versus* elimination of ROS by the activity of cellular antioxidant enzymes. Recent studies have shown that PDT caused increased-antioxidant enzymes activity and expression [50]. Thus, PDT efficacy can be influenced by the antioxidant response of the enzymes SOD, the GSH system and CAT.

Our data demonstrated that after PDT with PcGal$_{16}$ there was an increase in the activity of SOD, CAT and GR antioxidant enzymes in both cell lines, being higher in HT-1376 than in UM-UC-3 cells. This higher antioxidant defense of HT-1376 cells against ROS can explain the results obtained 24 h after treatment. However, it is hypothesized that this was not maintained for 72 h after PDT since for this time point there was a massive cell death. This not only suggests that in this cell line there is a temporal relationship between ROS levels and cell death, but shows that antioxidant enzymes activity is of greater importance in protecting HT-1376 cells for at least 24 h after PDT with PcGal$_{16}$. Regarding the activity of antioxidant enzymes, in HT-1376 cells it was also observed a decrease in the activity of GST, which is an enzyme implicated in cells defense against oxidation products. This enzyme has been described as protecting cells from DNA desintegration and drug toxicity [51]. GST isoforms are overexpressed in multidrug resistant tumors having an important role in tumors drug resistance by direct detoxification or inhibition of the MAP kinase pathway [51]. Thus, the higher cell death observed in HT-1376 cells 72 h after treatment can be also related with the activity of GST. A decrease in the activity of GST can be associated with DNA fragmentation and cell death 72 h after treatment.

Understanding the role of galactose moieties in the recognition of the PS by cancer cells may allow the investigation and development of more focused therapeutic strategies. Thus, we investigated whether PcGal$_{16}$ could be directly recognized by specific carbohydrate-binding proteins present at the plasma membrane. Consistently, the photoactivated PcGal$_{16}$ was shown to co-localize and reduce the levels of the plasma membrane proteins galectin-1 and GLUT1. Moreover, the immunofluorescence and Western Blotting studies demonstrated that, although its non-dark toxicity, PcGal$_{16}$ decreases the levels of galectin-1 and GLUT1 proteins. A plausible explanation for the decreased levels of the galactose binding proteins, galectin-1 and GLUT1, after incubation with PcGal$_{16}$ can be the masking of the epitope, which can block antibody-epitope binding due to changes in protein conformation or, eventually, endocytosis of these proteins and subsequent degradation. Thus, the changes observed in the levels of galectin-1 and GLUT1 could be induced directly by the binding of PcGal$_{16}$ to the carbohydrate-binding proteins and/or indirectly by the generation of ROS after PDT with PcGal$_{16}$.

Although significant progress has been made in research related with the role of galectins in cancer, the information underlying the molecular mechanisms that control the expression of these proteins in tumour cells is scarce. The interaction of PSs with galectins (namely galectin-1 and galectin-3) has been studied by spectroscopic studies [52] and molecular modeling analysis [6,27]; however, they have not been validated by in vitro studies. As far as we know, there are no in vitro reports indicating whether PSs can modulate the expression of carbohydrate-binding proteins such as galectin-1 and GLUT1. Knowing that galectin-1 expression is correlated with cell metastatic potential [18,53] and contributes to tumor progression and resistance after conventional cancer therapeutic modalities [18], the ability of PcGal$_{16}$ to reduce the

levels of galectin-1 after its uptake and/or photoactivation prompted us to envisage PcGal$_{16}$ as a potential candidate for cancer treatment.

Knowing that the overexpression of GLUTs is involved in tumor glycolysis - one of the biochemical "hallmarks" of cancer - the efficiency of PcGal$_{16}$ as an efficient anti-cancer PS is also evidenced by its ability to reduce GLUT1. GLUT1 is an attractive target to consider in the development of new PSs because it is lower expressed in normal-epithelial tissues or benign epithelial cell tumors when compared with human cancer cells [54]. The function of GLUT1 in the tumorogenesis process has been demonstrated by in vitro and in vivo studies, where the overexpression of GLUT1 antisense resulted in the inhibition of HL60 leukaemia cells proliferation and MKN-45 derived xenografs, respectively [55,56]. Based on the results of the current study, we envisage PcGal$_{16}$ as a promising therapeutic agent for the treatment of bladder cancer. Further studies are warranted to investigate the selectivity and photototoxicity of this PS in an in vivo model of bladder cancer, to contribute to a possible impact on clinical practice.

Supporting Information

Figure S1 Chemical structures of free phthalocyanine PcF$_{16}$ and galacto-dendrimer phthalocyanine PcGal$_{16}$.

Figure S2 PcGal$_{16}$ is non-toxic in darkness, PcF$_{16}$ is non-toxic in darkness and after PDT. Non-dark toxicity of various concentrations of PcGal$_{16}$ in HT-1376 and UM-UC-3 cells (panel A). Non-dark toxicity was assessed using the MTT colorimetric assay 24, 48, and 72 h after treat HT-1376 and UM-UC-3 cells (panel B). Toxicity of PcF$_{16}$ at 5 μM in darkness and after PDT (panel C) in HT-1376 and UM-UC-3 cells. The toxicity was assessed using the MTT colorimetric assay 24 h after treat HT-1376 and UM-UC-3 cells. Data are the mean $\pm$ S.D. of at least three independent experiments performed in triplicates.

Acknowledgments

We grateful appreciate the help of Dr. Célia Gomes (IBILI-FMUC, Portugal) with the spectrofluorometric measurements in IVIS Lumina XR equipment.

We thank Dr. Filomena Botelho (IBILI-FMUC, Portugal) for the generous supply of HT-1376 human bladder cancer cells.

P. Pereira and S. Silva acknowledge fellowships from FCT (SFRH/BD/85941/2012 and SFRH/BPD/64812/2009, respectively).

We appreciate the help of Dr. Célia Gomes (IBILI-FMUC, Portugal) with the spectrofluorometric measurements in IVIS Lumina XR equipment.

Author Contributions

Conceived and designed the experiments: PP RF JT. Performed the experiments: PP SS. Analyzed the data: PP RF JT. Contributed reagents/materials/analysis tools: PP SS. Wrote the paper: PP RF JT CFR JC.

References

1. Allison RR, Sibata CH (2010) Oncologic photodynamic therapy photosensitizers: a clinical review. Photodiagnosis Photodyn Ther 7:61–75.
2. Almeida RD, Manadas BJ, Carvalho AP, Duarte CB (2004) Intracellular signaling mechanisms in photodynamic therapy. Biochim Biophys Acta 1704:59–86.
3. Soares ARM, Tome JPC, Neves MGPMS, Tome AC, Cavaleiro JAS, et al. (2009) Synthesis of water-soluble phthalocyanines bearing four or eight D-galactose units, Carbohyd Res 334:507–510.
4. Silva JN, Silva AMG, Tome JPC, Ribeiro AO, Domingues MRM, et al. (2008) Photophysical properties of a photocytotoxic fluorinated chlorinconjugated to four β-cyclodextrins. Photochem Photobiol Sci 7:834–843.
5. Pereira PMR, Carvalho JJ, Silva S, Cavaleiro JAS, Schneider RJ, et al. (2014) Porphyrin conjugated with serum albumins and monoclonal antibodies boosts efficiency in targeted destruction of human bladder cancer cells, Org Biomol Chem 12:1804–1811.

6. Zheng G, Graham A, Shibata M, Missert JR, Oseroff AR, et al. (2001) Synthesis of beta-galactose-conjugated chlorins derived by enyne metathesis as galectin-specific photosensitizers for photodynamic therapy. J Org Chem 66:8709–8716.

7. Soares ARM, Neves MGPMS, Tome AC, Iglesias-de la Cruz MC, Zamarron A, et al. (2012) Glycophthalocyanines as Photosensitizers for Triggering Mitotic: Catastrophe and Apoptosis On Cancer Cells. Chem Res Toxicol 25:940–951.

8. Daly R, Vaz G, Davies AM, Senge MO, Scanlan EM (2012) Synthesis and biological evaluation of a library of glycoporphyrin compounds. Chemistry 18:14671–14679.

9. Vedachalam S, Choi BH, Pasunooti KK, Ching KM, Lee K, et al. (2011) Glycosylated porphyrin derivatives and their photodynamic activity in cancer cells. MedChemComm 2:371–377.

10. Ernst B, Magnani JL (2009) From carbohydrate leads to glycomimetic drugs. Nat Rev Drug Discov 8:661–677.

11. Lourenço LMO, Tome JPC, Domingues MRM, Domingues P, Costa PJ, et al. (2009) Synthesis and differentiation of alpha- and beta-glycoporphyrin stereoisomers by electrospray tandem mass spectrometry. Rapid Commun Mass Spectrom 23:3478–3483.

12. Figueira F, Pereira PMR, Silva S, Cavaleiro JAS, Tome JPC (2014) Porphyrins and Phthalocyanines decorated with dendrimers: Synthesis and biomedical applications. Curr Org Synth In press.

13. Gary-Bobo M, Vaillant O, Maynadier M, Basile I, Gallud A, et al. (2013) Targeting multiplicity: the key factor for anti-cancer nanoparticles. Curr Med Chem 20:1946–1955.

14. Lourenço LMO, Neves MGPMS, Cavaleiro JAS, Tome JPC (2014) Synthetic approaches to glycophthalocyanines. Tetrahedron In press.

15. David A (2010) Carbohydrate-based Biomedical Copolymers for Targeted Delivery of Anticancer Drugs. Isr J Chem 50:204–219.

16. Sharon N, Lis H (1989) Lectins as cell recognition molecules. Science 246:227–234.

17. Liu FT, Rabinovich GA (2005) Galectins as modulators of tumour progression. Nat Rev Cancer 5:29–41.

18. Cindolo L, Benvenuto G, Salvatore P, Pero R, Salvatore G, et al. (1999) Galectin-1 and galectin-3 expression in human bladder transitional-cell carcinomas. Int J Cancer 84:39–43.

19. Carruthers A, DeZutter J, Ganguly A, Devaskar SU (2009) Will the original glucose transporter isoform please stand up! Am J Physiol Endocrinol Metab 297:E836–E848.

20. Fernandes R, Carvalho AL, Kumagai A, Seica R, Hosoya K, et al. (2004) Downregulation of retinal GLUT1 in diabetes by ubiquitinylation. Mol Vis 10:618–628.

21. Fernandes R, Hosoya K, Pereira P (2011) Reactive oxygen species downregulate glucose transport system in retinal endothelial cells. Am J Physiol-Cell Ph 300: C927–C936.

22. Silva AMG, Tome AC, Neves MGPMS, Cavaleiro JAS, Perrone D, et al. (2005) Porphyrins in 1,3-dipolar cycloadditions with sugar azomethine ylides. Synthesis of pyrrolidinoporphyrin glycoconjugates. Synlett 0857–0859.

23. Choi CF, Huang JD, Lo PC, Fong WP, Ng DKP (2008) Glycosylated zinc(II) phthalocyanines as efficient photosensitisers for photodynamic therapy. Synthesis, photophysical properties and in vitro photodynamic activity. Org Biomol Chem 6:2173–2181.

24. Iqbal Z, Hanack M, Ziegler T (2009) Synthesis of an octasubstituted galactose zinc(II) phthalocyanine. Tetrahedron Lett 50:873–875.

25. Lee PPS, Lo PC, Chan EYM, Fong WP, Ko WH, et al. (2005) Synthesis and in vitro photodynamic activity of novel galactose-containing phthalocyanines. Tetrahedron Lett 46:1551–1554.

26. Park YK, Bold B, Cui BC, Bai JQ, Lee WK, et al. (2008) Binding affinities of carbohydrate-conjugated chlorins for galectin-3. B Korean Chem Soc 29:130–134.

27. Pandey SK, Zheng X, Morgan J, Missert JR, Liu TH, et al. (2007) Purpurinimide carbohydrate conjugates: effect of the position of the carbohydrate moiety in photosensitizing efficacy. Mol Pharm 4:448–464.

28. Singh S, Aggarwal A, Thompson S, Tome JPC, Zhu X, et al. (2010) Synthesis and photophysical properties of thioglycosylated- chlorins, isobacteriochlorins and bacteriochlorins for bioimaging and diagnostics. Bioconjugate Chem 21:2136–2146.

29. Fujimoto K, Miyata T, Aoyama Y (2000) Saccharide-directed cell recognition and molecular delivery using macrocyclic saccharide clusters: Masking of hydrophobicity to enhance the saccharide specificity. J Am Chem Soc 122:3558–3559.

30. Ribeiro AO, Tome JPC, Neves MGPMS, Tome AC, Cavaleiro JAS, et al. (2006) [1,2,3,4-tetrakis(alpha/beta-D-galactopyranos-6-yl)-phthalocyaninato]-zinc(II): a water-soluble phthalocyanine. Tetrahedron Lett 47:9177–9180.

31. Gillies ER, Frechet JMJ (2005) Dendrimers and dendritic polymers in drug delivery. Drug Discov Today 10:35–43.

32. Wolinsky JB, Grinstaff MW (2008) Therapeutic and diagnostic applications of dendrimers for cancer treatment. Adv Drug Deliv Rev 60:1037–1055.

33. Klajnert B, Rozanek M, Bryszewska M (2012) Dendrimers in photodynamic therapy. Curr Med Chem 19:4903–4912.

34. Silva S, Pereira PMR, Silva P, Paz FA, Faustino MA, et al. (2012) Porphyrin and phthalocyanine glycodendritic conjugates: synthesis, photophysical and photochemical properties. Chem Commun 48:3608–3610.

35. Ballardini R, Colonna B, Gandolfi MT, Kalovidouris SA, Orzel L, et al. (2003) Porphyrin-containing glycodendrimers. Eur J Org Chem 2:288–294.

36. Wang ZJ, Chauvin B, Maillard P, Hammerer F, Carez D, et al. (2012) Glycodendrimeric phenylporphyrins as new candidates for retinoblastoma PDT: Blood carriers and photodynamic activity in cells. J Photochem Photobiol B 115:16–24.

37. Ballut S, Makky A, Loock B, Michel JP, Maillard P, et al. (2009) New strategy for targeting of photosensitizers. Synthesis of glycodendrimeric phenylporphyrins, incorporation into a liposome membrane and interaction with a specific lectin. Chem Comm 2:224–226.

38. Bancirova M (2011) Sodium azide as a specific quencher of singlet oxygen during chemiluminescent detection by luminol and Cypridina luciferin analogues. Luminescence 26:685–688.

39. Aruoma OI, Halliwell B, Hoey BM, Butler J (1989) The antioxidant action of N-acetylcysteine: its reaction with hydrogen peroxide, hydroxyl radical, superoxide, and hypochlorous acid. Free Radic Biol Med 6:593–597.

40. Sies H (1993) Strategies of antioxidant defense. Eur J Biochem 215:213–219.

41. Weydert CJ, Cullen JJ (2010) Measurement of superoxide dismutase, catalase and glutathione peroxidase in cultured cells and tissue. Nat Protoc 5:51–66.

42. Lotan R, Raz A (1988) Lectins in cancer cells. Ann N Y Acad Sci 551:385–398.

43. Barnett JEG, Holman GD, Chalkley RA, Munday KA (1975) Evidence for two asymmetric conformational states in the human erythrocyte sugar-transport system. Biochem J 145:417–429.

44. Hirohara S, Obata M, Ogata S, Ohtsuki C, Higashida S, et al. (2005) Cellular uptake and photocytotoxicity of glycoconjugated chlorins in HeLa cells. J Photoch Photobio B 78:7–15.

45. Laville I, Pigaglio S, Blais JC, Doz F, Loock B, et al. (2006) Photodynamic efficiency of diethylene glycol-linked glycoconjugated porphyrins in human retinoblastoma cells. J Med Chem 49:2558–2567.

46. Plaetzer K, Krammer B, Berlanda J, Berr F, Kiesslich T (2009) Photophysics and photochemistry of photodynamic therapy: fundamental aspects. Laser Med Sci 24:259–268.

47. Buytaert E, Dewaele M, Agostinis P (2007) Molecular effectors of multiple cell death pathways initiated by photodynamic therapy. Biochimica et biophysica acta 1776:86–107.

48. Sattler UGA, Mueller-Klieser W (2009) The anti-oxidant capacity of tumour glycolysis. International journal of radiation biology 85:963–971.

49. Oleinick NL, Morris RL, Belichenko I (2002) The role of apoptosis in response to photodynamic therapy: what, where, why, and how. Photochemical & photobiological sciences : Official journal of the European Photochemistry Association and the European Society for Photobiology 1:1–21.

50. Saczko J, Kulbacka J, Chwilkowska A, Pola A, Lugowski M, et al. (2007) Cytosolic superoxide dismutase activity after photodynamic therapy, intracellular distribution of Photofrin II and hypericin, and P-glycoprotein localization in human colon adenocarcinoma. Folia Histochem Cyto 45:93–98.

51. Townsend DM, Tew KD (2003) The role of glutathione-S-transferase in anti-cancer drug resistance. Oncogene 22:7369–7375.

52. Bogoeva VP, Varriale A, John CM, D'Auria S (2010) Human galectin-3 interacts with two anticancer drugs. Proteomics 10:1946–1953.

53. Chiariotti L, Berlingieri MT, De Rosa P, Battaglia C, Berger N, et al. (1992) Increased expression of the negative growth factor, galactoside-binding protein, gene in transformed thyroid cells and in human thyroid carcinomas. Oncogene 7:2507–2511.

54. Younes M, Lechago LV, Somoano JR, Mosharaf M, Lechago J (1996) Wide expression of the human erythrocyte glucose transporter Glut1 in human cancers. Cancer Res 56:1164–1167.

55. Chan JYW, Kong SK, Choy YM, Lee CY, Fung KP (1999) Inhibition of glucose transporter gene expression by antisense nucleic acids in HL-60 leukemia cells. Life Sci 65:63–70.

56. Noguchi Y, Saito A, Miyagi Y, Yamanaka S, Marat D, et al. (2000) Suppression of facilitative glucose transporter 1 mRNA can suppress tumor growth. Cancer Letters 154:175–182.

26

Genetic Variation in the *TP53* Pathway and Bladder Cancer Risk

Silvia Pineda[1], **Roger L. Milne**[1], **M. Luz Calle**[2], **Nathaniel Rothman**[3], **Evangelina López de Maturana**[1], **Jesús Herranz**[1], **Manolis Kogevinas**[4,5], **Stephen J. Chanock**[3], **Adonina Tardón**[6], **Mirari Márquez**[1], **Lin T. Guey**[1], **Montserrat García-Closas**[3], **Josep Lloreta**[5,7], **Erin Baum**[1], **Anna González-Neira**[1], **Alfredo Carrato**[8,9], **Arcadi Navarro**[10,11,12,13], **Debra T. Silverman**[3], **Francisco X. Real**[1,10], **Núria Malats**[1]*

1 Spanish National Cancer Research Center (CNIO), Madrid, Spain, **2** Systems Biology Department, University of Vic, Vic, Spain, **3** Division of Cancer Epidemiology and Genetics, National Cancer Institute, Department of Health and Human Services, Bethesda, Maryland, United States of America, **4** Centre for Research in Environmental Epidemiology (CREAL), Barcelona, Spain, **5** Institut Municipal d'Investigació Mèdica – Hospital del Mar, Barcelona, Spain, **6** Department of Preventive Medicine, Universidad de Oviedo, Oviedo, Spain, **7** Departament de Patologia, Hospital del Mar – IMAS, Barcelona, Spain, **8** Servicio de Oncología, Hospital Universitario de Elche, Elche, Spain, **9** Servicio de Oncología, Hospital Universitario Ramon y Cajal, Madrid, Spain, **10** Departament de Ciències Experimentals i de la Salut, Universitat Pompeu Fabra, Barcelona, Spain, **11** Institut de Biologia Evolutiva (UPF-CSIC), Barcelona, Spain, **12** Institució Catalana de Recerca i Estudis Avançats (ICREA), Barcelona, Spain, **13** Instituto Nacional de Bioinformática, Barcelona, Spain

Abstract

Introduction: Germline variants in *TP63* have been consistently associated with several tumors, including bladder cancer, indicating the importance of *TP53* pathway in cancer genetic susceptibility. However, variants in other related genes, including *TP53* rs1042522 (Arg72Pro), still present controversial results. We carried out an in depth assessment of associations between common germline variants in the *TP53* pathway and bladder cancer risk.

Material and Methods: We investigated 184 tagSNPs from 18 genes in 1,058 cases and 1,138 controls from the Spanish Bladder Cancer/EPICURO Study. Cases were newly-diagnosed bladder cancer patients during 1998–2001. Hospital controls were age-gender, and area matched to cases. SNPs were genotyped in blood DNA using Illumina Golden Gate and TaqMan assays. Cases were subphenotyped according to stage/grade and tumor p53 expression. We applied classical tests to assess individual SNP associations and the Least Absolute Shrinkage and Selection Operator (LASSO)-penalized logistic regression analysis to assess multiple SNPs simultaneously.

Results: Based on classical analyses, SNPs in *BAK1* (1), *IGF1R* (5), *P53AIP1* (1), *PMAIP1* (2), *SERINPB5* (3), *TP63* (3), and *TP73* (1) showed significant associations at p-value≤0.05. However, no evidence of association, either with overall risk or with specific disease subtypes, was observed after correction for multiple testing (p-value≥0.8). LASSO selected the SNP rs6567355 in *SERPINB5* with 83% of reproducibility. This SNP provided an OR = 1.21, 95%CI 1.05–1.38, p-value = 0.006, and a corrected p-value = 0.5 when controlling for over-estimation.

Discussion: We found no strong evidence that common variants in the *TP53* pathway are associated with bladder cancer susceptibility. Our study suggests that it is unlikely that *TP53* Arg72Pro is implicated in the UCB in white Europeans. *SERPINB5* and *TP63* variation deserve further exploration in extended studies.

Editor: Masaru Katoh, National Cancer Center, Japan

Funding: This work was supported by the Fondo de Investigación Sanitaria, Spain (grant numbers 00/0745, PI051436, PI061614, G03/174); Red Temática de Investigación Cooperativa en Cáncer (grant number RD06/0020-RTICC), Spain; Marató TV3 (grant number 050830); European Commission (grant numbers EU-FP7-HEALTH-F2-2008-201663-UROMOL; US National Institutes of Health (grant number USA-NIH-RO1-CA089715); and the Intramural Research Program of the Division of Cancer Epidemiology and Genetics, National Cancer Institute at the National Institutes of Health, USA; Consolíder ONCOBIO (Ministerio de Economía y Competitividad, Madrid, Spain). The funders had no role in study design, data collection and analysis, decision to publish, or preparation of the manuscript.

* E-mail: nmalats@cnio.es

Introduction

In more developed countries, urothelial carcinoma of the bladder (UCB) is the fourth most common cancer in men and the seventeenth in women, the overall male:female ratio being 3:1. This ratio is greater (6:1) in Spain, where the disease presents one of the highest incidence rates among men (51 per 100,000 man-year) [1]. Tobacco smoking and occupational exposure to aromatic amines have been established as the strongest risk factors, among others [2]. While no high-penetrance allele/gene has been identified to date as associated with UCB, there is well-established evidence that UCB risk is influenced by common genetic variants [3,4].

Previous studies characterizing UCB are consistent with the existence of, at least, two disease subtypes based on their morphological and genetic features. The first subtype includes low-risk, papillary, non-muscle invasive tumors (NMIT, 60–65% of all UCB) and the second type includes both high-risk NMIT (15–20% of all UCB) and muscle invasive tumors (MIT, 20%–30% of all UCB). Supporting these morphological subtypes, differential genetic pathways were described and were associated with distinct UCB evolution. Somatic mutations in *FGFR3* are more frequent in low-risk NMIT, while mutations in *TP53* and *RB* are mainly involved in high-risk NMIT and MIT [5,6]; mutations in *PIK3CA* and *HRAS* occur similarly in the two tumor subtypes. Interestingly, an exploratory analysis has shown that some germline genetic variants might be differentially associated with the risk of developing distinct UCB subphenotypes defined according to tumor stage (T) and grade (G) [7].

TP53 is the most important human tumor suppressor gene and its implications in UCB have been extensively studied [8]. *TP53* is located in17p13, a region that is frequently deleted in human cancers, and it encodes the p53 protein. p53 is a transcription factor controlling cell proliferation, cell cycle, cell survival, and genomic integrity and - therefore - it regulates a large number of genes. Under normal cellular conditions, p53 is rapidly degraded due to the activity of *MDM2*, a negative p53 regulator that is also a p53 target gene. Upon DNA damage or other stresses, p53 is stabilized and regulates the expression of many genes involved in cell cycle arrest, apoptosis, and DNA repair among others. Somatic alterations in *TP53*/p53 are one of the most frequent alterations associated with UCB, especially with the more aggressive tumors [9].

Germline *TP53* mutations predispose to a wide spectrum of early-onset cancers and cause Li-Fraumeni and related syndromes [10,11]. These mutations are usually single-base substitutions. Over 200 germline single nucleotide polymorphisms (SNPs) in *TP53* have been identified at present [12]. SNP rs1042522 (Arg72Pro) has been assessed in association with several cancers, among them UCB. However, the results of these studies are inconsistent [13,14,15,16,17,18]. In contrast, an association between SNP rs710521 in *TP63*, a *TP53* family member, and risk of UCB has been convincingly replicated, pointing to the involvement of *TP53* pathway members in UCB susceptibility [4].

The aim of this study was to comprehensively investigate whether germline SNPs in genes involved in the *TP53* pathway are associated with risk of UCB. To this end, a total of 184 tagSNPs in 18 key genes were assessed using data from the Spanish Bladder Cancer/EPICURO study.

Materials and Methods

Study Subjects

The Spanish Bladder Cancer/EPICURO Study is a case-control study carried out in 18 hospitals from five areas in Spain and described elsewhere [2,4,7]. Briefly, cases were patients diagnosed with primary UCB at age 21–80 years between 1998 and 2001. All participants were of self-reported white European ancestry. Diagnostic slides from each patient were reviewed by a panel of expert pathologists to confirm the diagnosis and to ensure that uniform classification criteria were applied based on the 1999 World Health Organization and International Society of Urological Pathology systems [19].

Controls were patients admitted to participating hospitals for conditions thought to be unrelated to the UCB risk factors. The main reasons for hospital admission were: hernia (37%), other abdominal surgery (11%), fracture (23%), other orthopaedic

problem (7%), hydrocoele (12%), circulatory disorder (4%), dermatological disorder (2%), ophthalmological disorder (1%), and other diseases (3%). Controls were individually matched to the cases on age within 5-year categories, gender, ethnic origin and region of residence.

Information on sociodemographics, smoking habits, occupational and environmental exposures, and past medical and familial history of cancer was collected by trained study monitors who conducted a comprehensive computer- assisted personal interview with the study participants during their hospital stay. Of 1,457 eligible cases and 1,465 controls, 1,219 (84%) and 1,271 (87%), were interviewed, respectively.

All subjects gave written informed consent to participate in the study, which was approved by the ethics committees of the participating centers.

Genotyping

A total of 184 tagSNPs from 18 genes participating in the *TP53* pathway were selected using the Select Your SNPs (SYSNPs) program [20]. SYSNP used information from dbSNP b25, hg17 and HapMap Release #21. Haploview's Tagger algorithm (v3.32) was applied with default parameter values. The tool considers all available information for each SNP and implements algorithms that provide the status of each SNP as a tagSNP, a captured SNP or a non-captured SNP. According to this information tagSNPs were selected. The following groups of genes were considered: 1) *TP53* family members (*TP53*, *TP63* and *TP73*) and 2) genes known to be targets of p53 or regulators of p53 function [*BAK1*, *BAX*, *BBC3*, *BIRC5*, *CDKN1A*, *FAS*, *GADD45A*, *IGF1R*, *MDM2*, *PCNA*, *PMAIP1*, *SERPINB5*, *SFN* (Stratifin, 14-3-3sigma), *TP53AIP1*], and 3) c-*MYC*, a major oncogene involved in a broad range of human cancers that regulates p53 pro-apoptotic activity (See Table S1 in File S1). SNPs were genotyped using Illumina Golden Gate and TaqMan (Applied Biosystems) assays at the Spanish Core Genotyping Facility at the CNIO (CEGEN- CNIO). Genotyping was successful for 1,058 cases and 1,138 controls. We calculated the coverage for each gene using Haploview 4.2 by selecting the SNPs within a gene with a MAF≥0.05 from the 1000 genomes project, as reference, and obtained the number of SNPs captured with the SNPs genotyped at r2≥0.8 within each gene.

Statistical Analysis

Departure from Hardy-Weinberg equilibrium was assessed in controls using Pearson's chi-squared test. Missing genotypes were imputed for the multi-SNP model using the BEAGLE 3.0 method [21]. Associations between UCB and the SNPs considered were assessed using two approaches: classical logistic and polytomous regression analyses applied to each SNP individually, and the Least Absolute Shrinkage and Selection Operator (LASSO)-penalized logistic regression to assess all SNPs simultaneously. All models were adjusted for age at diagnosis (cases) or interview (controls), gender, region, and smoking status. Smoking status was coded in four categories (never: <100 cigarettes in their lifetime; occasional: at least one per day for ≥6 months; former: if they had smoked regularly, but stopped at least 1 year before the study inclusion date; and current: if they had smoked regularly within a year of the inclusion date [2].

With the "classical" statistical approaches we assessed SNP main effects for the whole disease and for different subtypes of UCB, as well as SNP*SNP and SNP*smoking interactions. Disease subtypes were defined in two ways. First, according to established criteria based on tumor stage (T) and grade (G) as low-risk NMIT (TaG1 and TaG2), high-risk NMIT (TaG3, T1G2, T1G3, and Tis), and MIT (T2, T3, and T4); and second, according to the

Table 1. Demographics and smoking status of patients included in the study.

	Cases (n = 1058)	Controls (n = 1138)	[1]p-value
Gender			
Male	920 (87%)	991 (87%)	
Female	138 (13%)	147 (13%)	0.9
Age			
<55	149 (14%)	181 (16%)	
55–64	222 (21%)	278 (24%)	
65–69	241 (23%)	263 (23%)	
70–74	225 (21%)	222 (20%)	
75+	221 (21%)	194 (17%)	0.06
Region			
1-Barcelona	214 (20%)	233 (21%)	
2-Valles	173 (16%)	181 (16%)	
3-Elche	83 (8%)	80 (7%)	
4-Tenerife	195 (19%)	207 (18%)	
5-Asturias	393 (37%)	437 (38%)	0.9
Smoking			
Never	147 (14%)	334 (29%)	
Occasional	43 (4%)	81 (7%)	
Former	409 (38%)	429 (38%)	
Current	454 (43%)	283 (25%)	<0.001
Missing	5 (1%)	11 (1%)	

[1]p-value from Pearson's χ^2 test for association.

tumor expression of p53 determined using DO7 antibody. We applied the histoscore as $z = \sum_{i=1}^{3} i * pos\%cells_i$, where $pos\%cells_i$ was the percentage of cells with intensity $i (i = 1,2,3)$. We then classified cases as having low or high p53 expression relative to the median histoscore.

To assess overall main effects, the four modes of inheritance were considered: co-dominant, dominant, recessive, and additive. The statistical significance of associations was determined using the Likelihood Ratio Test (LRT). We evaluated associations between individual SNPs and subtypes of UCB using polytomous logistic regression. Heterogeneity by disease subtype was tested by a LRT comparing this model to that with the ln(OR) restricted to be equal across subtypes. We also evaluated all two-way interactions between SNPs by a LRT comparing logistic regression models with the two SNPs (additive model) and covariates described above, with and without a single interaction term for multiplicative, per-allele effects. Interactions between each SNP and cigarette use (never vs. ever) were assessed using a similar method. Multiple testing was accounted for by applying a permutation test with 1,000 replicates. We applied Quanto (http://hydra.usc.edu/gxe/) to assess statistical power considering the available sample size.

We also assessed combined SNP effects using LASSO. The method has been described in detail by [22]. Briefly, the log-likelihood function applied in classical logistic regression

$$L_n(\beta) \sum_{i=1}^{n} [y_i \log \pi(X'_i\beta) + (1-y_i)\log(1-\pi(X'_i\beta))], \quad (1)$$

where n is the number of observations, is reconstructed incorporating a penalty so that

$$g(\beta; \lambda) = L_n(\beta) + \lambda \sum_{j=1}^{p} |\beta_j|, \quad (2)$$

where p is the number of SNPs and λ is the lasso penalty. The Newton-Raphson algorithm is applied to equation (2) to estimate β's in an iterative way.

The LASSO method is based on the idea of removing irrelevant predictor variables ($\beta = 0$) via the penalty parameter, thereby selecting only the most relevant SNPs as the subset of markers most associated with the disease. The application of the penalty parameter also avoids overfitting due to both high-dimensionality and collinearity between covariates. We only considered additive genetic mode of inheritance.

This technique gives biased estimators to reduce their variance. Because of this, the implemented package in R does not provide estimates p-values for the regression beta coefficients, since standard errors are not meaningful under a biased estimator. We therefore evaluated the results by first applying the LASSO using a 5-fold cross-validation (CV) method [23] to choose the optimal λ as that giving the minimum Akaike information criterion (AIC); we then selected the subset of SNPs that were most informative with that λ. We assessed the robustness of each SNP selected in the optimal model by calculating the reproducibility as the proportion of times each SNP was selected to be in the multivariate model from 1,000 bootstrap subsamples [24].

To evaluate the association with UCB risk of that subset of SNPs, we tested them by the LRT in a multivariate regression

Table 2. SNPs in TP53 and bladder cancer risk.

SNP	Cases			Controls			Additive model			Co-dominant model						P-trend	Repr. (%)
	AA	Aa	aa	AA	Aa	aa	OR	95% CI	p-value	OR(Aa)	95% CI	p-value	OR(aa)	95% CI	p-value		
rs1042522[1]	588	372	72	628	388	84	1.04	0.91-1.20	0.5	1.10	0.91-1.33	0.3	0.97	0.68-1.37	0.8	0.5	24%
rs12951053	915	109	3	972	122	5	0.98	0.75-1.27	0.9	1.04	0.79-1.39	0.7	0.64	0.14-2.88	0.5	0.8	35%
rs1625895	761	241	28	793	266	26	1.04	0.88-1.24	0.6	0.99	0.80-1.21	0.9	1.28	0.73-2.26	0.4	0.7	13%
rs2287497	835	183	9	869	207	11	0.95	0.77-1.17	0.7	0.97	0.77-1.22	0.8	0.70	0.28-1.74	0.4	0.7	48%
rs2909430	749	251	28	800	272	27	1.03	0.87-1.23	0.7	1.04	0.85-1.27	0.7	1.23	0.70-2.16	0.5	0.7	36%
rs8073498	425	467	132	435	521	128	0.99	0.87-1.13	0.9	0.94	0.78-1.13	0.5	1.01	0.75-1.34	0.9	0.8	44%
rs8079544	923	103	2	993	102	4	1.05	0.79-1.39	0.7	1.10	0.81-1.48	0.5	0.42	0.07-2.33	0.3	0.5	40%

Repr. (%),percentage reproducibility assessing the robustness of each SNP by LASSO.
AA, Aa and aa represent common-homozygotes, heterozygotes and rare-allele homozygotes, respectively.
OR, odds ratio; CI, confidence interval; OR(Aa) and OR(aa) were estimated relative to genotype AA.
[1]Arg72Pro polymorphism.
All models were adjusted for age, gender, region and cigarette smoking status.

model with all the SNPs in comparison to the null model. To correct for the over-estimation due the pre-selection of the best SNPs, we performed a permutation test with 10,000 replicates.

STATA 10 was used to run the classical logistic and multinomial regression analyses. All other statistical analyses were run in R (http://www.R-project.org), using the penalized library [25] for LASSO penalized logistic regression.

Results

Table 1 shows the distribution of the study subjects included in the analysis: 1,058 cases and 1,138 controls. Most individuals (87%) were male and cases were more likely to be current smokers than controls (43% vs. 25%, respectively, p-value<0.001).

No evidence of departure from Hardy-Weinberg equilibrium was observed for any SNPs after consideration of multiple testing (unadjusted p-value$>10^{-4}$). Polymorphisms in TP53 were not individually associated with UCB risk, even at a nominal, uncorrected 5% significance level (uncorrected p-value>0.4). The percentage of reproducibility from the LASSO model using 1,000 bootstrap subsamples was <50%, indicating a poor robustness of the models. Results for the additive and co-dominant models are summarized in Table 2.

Using classical logistic regression, SNPs in BAK1 (1), IGF1R (5), P53AIP1 (1), PMAIP1 (2), SERPINB5 (3), TP63 (3), and TP73 (1) showed significant results, at a non-corrected p-value≤0.05, with overall UCB risk (Table 3). However, no evidence of association with risk was observed for any individual SNPs after correcting for multiple testing (permutation test p-value>0.8). This was also the case for the associations with the established disease subtypes defined according to stage/grade or by p53 expression (Figure 1). Of note, SNPs rs3758483 and rs983751 in FAS were differentially and inversely associated with MIT and high p53 expressing tumors in uncorrected analyses (Tables S2 and S3 in File S1). We also observed no evidence of SNP*SNP interactions or interactions between SNPs and smoking status (data not shown).

When all 184 SNPs were simultaneously assessed using LASSO, the method selected rs6567355 in SERPINB5 with a reproducibility = 83%. This SNP provided an OR = 1.21, 95%CI 1.05–1.38, p-value = 0.006 in the main effect logistic regression model and a corrected p-value = 0.5 when controlling for over-estimation (Table 3). While not selected by LASSO in the last model under the stringent criteria applied, IGF1R-rs1058696 (OR = 0.63, 95%CI 0.44–0.90, p-value = 0.010) and TP63-rs13321831 (OR = 1.36, 95%CI 1.06–1.73, p-value = 0.014) showed a percentage of reproducibility >80%.

Discussion

We genotyped common variants in genes in the TP53 pathway in 1,058 cases and 1,138 controls of white European ancestry and found no strong evidence of association with risk of UCB overall, or with subtypes of the disease defined by stage and grade or by p53 expression.

A key gene in the pathway is TP53, and the most commonly studied variant in this particular gene is Arg72Pro (rs1042522). Its implication in susceptibility to various cancers has been reported in Asian populations, but not in white Europeans. A meta-analysis of 49 cervical cancer studies contributing a total of 7,946 cases and 7,888 controls found that the Arg allele was associated with an increased risk of cervix cancer [14]. However, another meta-analysis of 39 studies (26,041 cases and 29,679 controls) found weak evidence for an association of the same variant with reduced breast cancer risk [18]. Regarding gastric cancer, a combined analysis of 6,859 cases and 9,277 controls from 28 studies found a

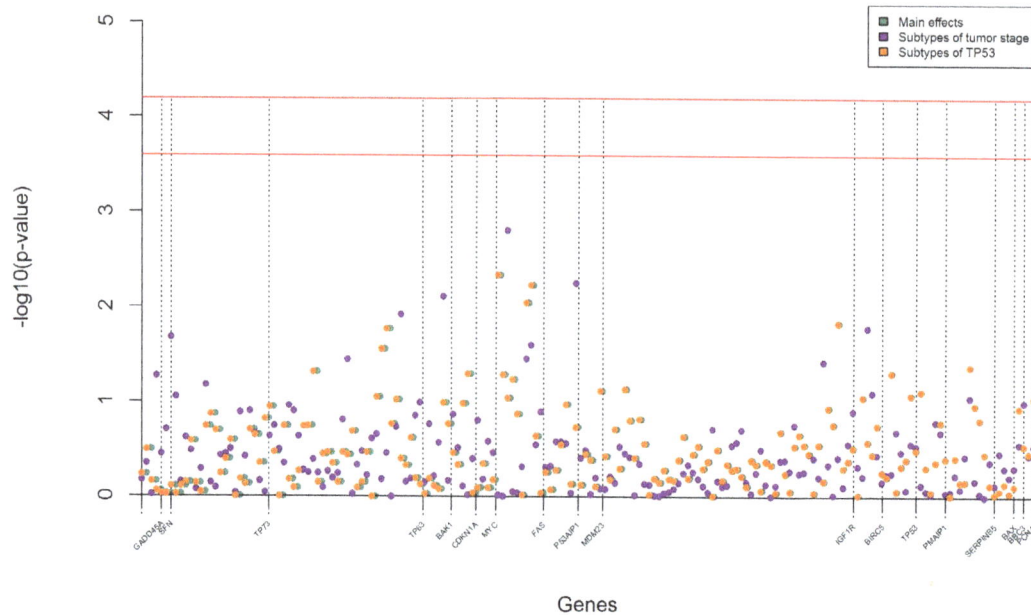

Figure 1. Main effect *p-values* for bladder cancer risk (overall and for each subphenotype) for each tag-SNP under the additive mode of inheritance. A SNP *p-value* above the red line is considered as associated with the phenotype after multiple testing correction by Bonferroni (4.2 for main effects and 3.6 for subtypes). All models are adjusted for age, gender, region and cigarette smoking status.

stronger inverse association only among Asians [26]. For lung cancer, a marginally significant increased risk was in a combined analysis of data with 15,647 cases and 14,391 controls from 36 studies, though the association seemed to be also confined to the Asian population [27].

The association between *TP53* Arg72Pro and UCB risk has been assessed by two meta-analyses. Overall, no association was observed by Jiang et al. when comparing 1,601 cases and 1,948 controls from 10 studies, although a marginally significant association was seen among Asians (OR = 0.77, 95%CI 0.59–1.00, for ArgArg/ArgPro vs. ProPro) [13]. Discordant results have been recently reported combining data from 14 studies contributing with 2,176 cases and 2,798 controls (OR = 1.268, 95%CI 1.003–1.602, for ArgArg/ArgPro vs. ProPro among the Asian population) [17]. A large number of studies overlap between the two meta-analyses. The lack of information on gene-gene and gene-environment interactions, as well as on the concomitant effect of *TP53* somatic mutations may explain the discordant results [28].

The findings from our study confirm the lack of association of Arg72Pro in *TP53* with risk of UCB in white Europeans (OR = 0.98, 95%CI 0.77–1.26, for ArgPro vs. ArgArg and OR = 0.91, 95%CI 0.75–1.09, for ProPro vs. ArgArg, p-value = 0.5 for overall effects) [13,17]. However, we cannot rule out that lack of statistical power may hamper identification of a small effect association: even with its large sample size, the present study sample size could detect an OR≥1.3 per-allele for this SNP with 90% statistical power and at a significance level of 5%.

Regarding other SNPs in *TP53*, Lin et al reported an association with rs9895829 and rs1788227 (p-value = 0.003 and 0.027, respectively) in a smaller study with 201 cases and 311 controls in an Asian population [29]. We did not genotype these SNPs, though they are in high LD with two SNPs considered here: rs8079544 (LD = 1.0) and rs12951053 (LD = 0.7), respectively. Nonetheless, none of the assessed additional SNPs in *TP53* appeared to be associated with UCB risk. The partial coverage of

the gene with the assessed SNPs (38%) does not allow us to dismiss the role of *TP53* in UCB susceptibility.

TP63 is another key member of the studied pathway. One SNP (rs710521) located in this gene has been reported to be associated with risk of UCB by a GWAS (per-allele OR = 1.19, 95%CI 1.12–1.27, p-value = 1.15×10^{-7}) [30]. This association was convincingly replicated in a combined analysis of data from different studies (allele-specific OR = 1.18, 95%CI 1.12–1.24, p-value = 1.8×10^{-10}), including ours, for which it was genotyped as part of a separate initiative [4]. Of note, this particular SNP did not show significant results in our study (OR = 0.95, 95%CI 0.83–1.10, p-value = 0.5), a fact that can be explained by the different geographical location related exposures of the participating studies, being UCB an environmental driven disease [31]. The present study assessed 32 SNPs in *TP63*, providing 24% of the gene coverage. Three of them showed uncorrected significant results in the overall UCB association analysis with a percentage of reproducibility >70% from LASSO. These results warrant an extended UCB study on this region.

Regarding other SNPs in the selected genes, we did not find any strong evidence of association after correcting for multiple testing (permutation test p-value≥0.8 for overall main effects and p-value≥0.3 for subtype effects). The top (uncorrected) significant SNPs were located in *BAK1*, *IGF1R*, *P53AIP1*, *PMAIP1*, *SERPINB5*, and *TP73*. Common variants in these genes have not previously been reported as associated with UCB risk, though an altered expression of *BAK1* and *IGF1R* has been described in bladder tumors.

Many complex diseases, such as UCB, are likely due to the combined effects of multiple loci [32] and most traditional association studies assessing main effects for one SNP at a time are underpowered to detect small effects [33]. Therefore, the implication of common genetic variants may be better assessed by a method that both selects a far-reduced set of potentially associated SNPs and tests for association globally. This has been a challenge due to the high-dimensionality and collinearity

Table 3. Significant SNPs at α = 0.05 in the logistic regression main effect models.

GENE	SNP	Cases			Controls			MAF(a)	pHWE	Risk of bladder cancer			MOI	Repr. (%)
		AA	Aa	aa	AA	Aa	Aa			OR	95% CI	p-value		
BAK1	rs11757379	654	330	42	642	390	54	0.23	0.67	0.86	0.74–0.99	0.047	Add.	33%
IGF1R	rs1058696	968	56	2	998	90	0	0.04	-	0.63	0.44–0.90	0.010	Dom.	81%
IGF1R	rs12591122	758	244	25	824	250	14	0.13	0.34	2.23	1.11–4.51	0.025	Rec.	66%
IGF1R	rs4966015	722	283	21	771	276	41	0.16	0.01	0.44	0.25–0.77	0.004	Rec.	43%
IGF1R	rs702497	633	342	50	645	366	73	0.24	0.04	0.69	0.50–0.94	0.019	Rec.	73%
IGF1R	rs7166348	618	365	45	670	355	62	0.22	0.11	0.67	0.44–1.00	0.050	Rec.	33%
P53AIP1	rs2604235	431	484	109	463	473	149	0.36	0.11	0.74	0.56–0.97	0.029	Rec.	30%
PMAIP1	rs1942919	270	547	207	353	509	224	0.44	0.11	1.27	1.05–1.55	0.015	Dom.	33%
PMAIP1	rs7240884	449	476	100	477	471	138	0.34	0.20	0.75	0.56–0.99	0.047	Rec.	25%
SERPINB5	rs1509476	532	413	82	614	405	69	0.25	0.87	1.20	1.04–1.38	0.012	Add.	14%
SERPINB5	rs1509478	378	490	159	450	493	139	0.36	0.84	1.18	1.04–1.34	0.011	Add.	51%
SERPINB5	rs6567355	466	442	114	552	435	93	0.29	0.60	1.21	1.05–1.38	0.006	Add.	83%
TP63	rs12489753	863	159	5	934	146	7	0.07	0.65	1.31	1.02–1.69	0.035	Dom.	71%
TP63	rs13321831	847	172	8	927	155	6	0.08	1.00	1.36	1.06–1.73	0.014	Dom.	83%
TP63	rs6779677	328	476	224	347	547	194	0.43	0.42	1.29	1.04–1.61	0.022	Rec.	76%
TP73	rs3765731	554	385	86	544	446	96	0.29	0.77	0.85	0.71–1.00	0.050	Dom	71%

MAF(a), minor allele frequency); pHWE, p-value from the Hardy Weinberg equilibrium test; MOI, Mode of Inheritance.
Repr. (%), percentage reproducibility assessing the robustness of each SNP by LASSO.
All models are adjusted for age, gender, region and smoking status.
Odd ratio and 95%CI under the model of inheritance that provided the lowest p-value, and percentage reproducibility from LASSO under the additive mode of inheritance.

between SNPs. Nevertheless, penalized techniques can deal with these problems and they are starting to emerge in genetic association studies. Wu et al used penalized logistic regression in a genome-wide association study applied to coeliac disease data and Zhou et al extended this work to the assessment of association for common and rare variants applied to family cancer registry data [34] [35]. In the present study, we applied the LASSO algorithm to account for the combination effects of the SNPs in the TP53 pathway and UCB risk. Under the criteria applied, this method selected one SNP (rs6567355) that showed a non-corrected p-value = 0.006 for the additive mode of inheritance with a percentage of reproducibility = 83%. This is a frequent G> A SNP (MAF = 0.29) located in the intron region of *SERPINB5*. As mentioned before, no evidences of previous association between this SNP and any disease have been reported at present. *SERPINB5* is a tumor suppressor (Table S1 in File S1). The expression levels of this gene has been correlated with those of *DBC1* (Deleted in bladder cancer 1) in UCB specimens, suggesting its involvement in the urokinase-plasminogen pathway [36]. *SERPINB5* would deserve of further exploration in extended studies, as well.

A limitation of our study is the incomplete tagging of the selected genes due to the use of an earlier HapMap release to select tag SNPs, prior to the availability of data from the 1000 genomes project. The median coverage of the 18 genes considered in the pathway is, according to the updated HapMap releases, 44%, ranging from 21% to 86%. Therefore, we cannot rule out completely the implication of common variation in these genes in UCB susceptibility.

For common SNPs (MAF>0.05), our study is powered (90%) to detect ORs≥1.4 at a significance level of 0.05, assuming an additive mode of inheritance. Therefore, the study is not conclusive with OR<1.4. While this study represents one of the largest assessments conducted till present, much larger studies will be required to rule out smaller main effects associated with common variants in the genes of this pathway. This is even more important when subphenotype analyses are considered. We also found no evidence of SNP-SNP interactions (permutation test p-value≥0.3) and SNP-smoking interactions (permutation test p-value≥0.07), although the power was even more limited to detect these. According to the candidate pathway, the studied SNPs were selected as tags; therefore, they were not correlated showing a low LD. This fact, let us overcome a potential limitation affecting the percentage of reproducibility when SNPs are high correlated.

Credit should also be given to this study, not only regarding its large sample size, but also for its prospective nature and disease representativeness, for the homogeneous methods applied to collect information and biosamples by the participating centers, for the integration of different type of information (sociodemo-graphics, epidemiological, genetic, clinical and pathological, and molecular), and for the comprehensive and innovative statistical approaches applied to assess UCB susceptibility associated with a highly candidate pathway.

In conclusion, using a comprehensive analysis accounting different models and different approaches, we found no strong evidence that common variants in the *TP53* pathway are associated with UCB risk. However, specific members of the pathway, *TP63* and *SERPINB5* deserve of further exploration in extended studies. On the other hand, our study suggests that it is unlikely that *TP53* Arg72Pro is implicated in the UCB in white Europeans.

While biological sound, candidate pathway analysis have throw limited acknowledge in the genetic susceptibility field of many diseases. The reasons of this relative poor efficiency may be, among others, the still lack of knowledge of all key components of a given pathway, the introduction of noise by considering many genes/variants without showing association, and the lack of coverage of rare variants not tagged through this approach, in addition to methodological explanations such as an impaired statistical power. Scientists should review whether it is time to dismiss this approach towards a more comprehensive strategy such whole genome/exome sequencing in dissecting the genetic architecture of complex diseases.

Supporting Information

File S1 Combined Supporting Information file containing: Table S1, Location and function of the selected genes. Table S2, Heterogeneity in single nucleotide polymorphism (SNP) risk estimates among bladder cancer subphenotypes defined according to stage and grade in the Spanish Bladder Cancer Study. Table S3, Heterogeneity in single nucleotide polymorphism (SNP) risk estimates among bladder cancer subphenotypes defined by p53 expression in the Spanish Bladder Cancer Study.

Acknowledgments

We acknowledge the coordinators, field and administrative workers, technicians and patients of the Spanish Bladder Cancer/EPICURO Study.

Author Contributions

Conceived and designed the experiments: SP RLM NR MK DTS FXR NM. Performed the experiments: SJC JL AGN. Analyzed the data: SP RLM MLC ELdM JH LTG EB. Contributed reagents/materials/analysis tools: AN AC AT MM DTS NR MK MGC FXR NM. Wrote the paper: SP RLM NM.

References

1. Ferlay JSH, Bray F, Forman D, Mathers C, Parkin DM (2010) GLOBOCAN 2008 v1.2, Cancer Incidence and Mortality Worldwide: IARC CancerBase No. 10. Lyon, France: International Agency for Research on Cancer.

2. Samanic C, Kogevinas M, Dosemeci M, Malats N, Real FX, et al. (2006) Smoking and bladder cancer in Spain: effects of tobacco type, timing, environmental tobacco smoke, and gender. Cancer Epidemiol Biomarkers Prev 15: 1348–1354.

3. Malats N (2008) Genetic epidemiology of bladder cancer: scaling up in the identification of low-penetrance genetic markers of bladder cancer risk and progression. Scand J Urol Nephrol Suppl: 131–140.

4. Rothman N, Garcia-Closas M, Chatterjee N, Malats N, Wu X, et al. (2010) A multi-stage genome-wide association study of bladder cancer identifies multiple susceptibility loci. Nat Genet 42: 978–984.

5. Luis NM, Lopez-Knowles E, Real FX (2007) Molecular biology of bladder cancer. Clin Transl Oncol 9: 5–12.

6. Wu XR (2005) Urothelial tumorigenesis: a tale of divergent pathways. Nat Rev Cancer 5: 713–725.

7. Guey LT, Garcia-Closas M, Murta-Nascimento C, Lloreta J, Palencia L, et al. (2010) Genetic susceptibility to distinct bladder cancer subphenotypes. Eur Urol 57: 283–292.

8. Real FX, Malats N (2007) Bladder cancer and apoptosis: matters of life and death. Lancet Oncol 8: 91–92.

9. Mitra AP, Hansel DE, Cote RJ (2012) Prognostic value of cell-cycle regulation biomarkers in bladder cancer. Semin Oncol 39: 524–533.

10. Malkin D, Friend SH, Li FP, Strong LC (1997) Germ-line mutations of the p53 tumor-suppressor gene in children and young adults with second malignant neoplasms. N Engl J Med 336: 734.

11. Malkin D, Li FP, Strong LC, Fraumeni JF Jr, Nelson CE, et al. (1990) Germ line p53 mutations in a familial syndrome of breast cancer, sarcomas, and other neoplasms. Science 250: 1233–1238.

12. Whibley C, Pharoah PD, Hollstein M (2009) p53 polymorphisms: cancer implications. Nat Rev Cancer 9: 95–107.

13. Jiang DK, Ren WH, Yao L, Wang WZ, Peng B, et al. (2010) Meta-analysis of association between TP53 Arg72Pro polymorphism and bladder cancer risk. Urology 76: 765 e761–767.

14. Klug SJ, Ressing M, Koenig J, Abba MC, Agorastos T, et al. (2009) TP53 codon 72 polymorphism and cervical cancer: a pooled analysis of individual data from 49 studies. Lancet Oncol 10: 772–784.

15. Liu KJ, Qi HZ, Yao HL, Lei SL, Lei ZD, et al. (2012) An updated meta-analysis of the p53 codon 72 polymorphism and gastric cancer risk. Mol Biol Rep 39: 8265–8275.

16. Qiao Q, Hu W (2013) The Association Between TP53 Arg72Pro Polymorphism and Lung Cancer Susceptibility: Evidence from 30,038 Subjects. Lung 191: 369–377.

17. Yang ZNS, Zhu H, Wu X, Jia S, Luo Y, et al. (2013) Association of p53 Arg72Pro polymorphism with bladder cancer: a meta-analysis. Gene 512: 408–413.

18. Zhang Z, Wang M, Wu D, Tong N, Tian Y (2009) P53 codon 72 polymorphism contributes to breast cancer risk: a meta-analysis based on 39 case-control studies. Breast Cancer Res Treat 120: 509–517.

19. Epstein JI, Amin MB, Reuter VR, Mostofi FK (1998) The World Health Organization/International Society of Urological Pathology consensus classification of urothelial (transitional cell) neoplasms of the urinary bladder. Bladder Consensus Conference Committee. Am J Surg Pathol 22: 1435–1448.

20. Lorente-Galdos B, Medina I, Morcillo-Suarez C, Heredia T, Carreno-Torres A, et al. (2012) Select your SNPs (SYSNPs): a web tool for automatic and massive selection of SNPs. Int J Data Min Bioinform 6: 324–334.

21. Browning SR, Browning BL (2007) Rapid and accurate haplotype phasing and missing-data inference for whole-genome association studies by use of localized haplotype clustering. Am J Hum Genet 81: 1084–1097.

22. Tibshirani R (1996) Regression Shrinkage and Selection via the Lasso. Journal of the Royal Statistical Society Series B (Methodological) 58: 267–288.

23. Friedman J, Hastie T, Thibshirani R (2001) The Elements of statistical learning: Data mining, inference and prediction. Springer Series in Statistics 533 214–216.

24. Efron B (1979) Bootstrap Methods: Another Look at the Jackknife. Annals of Statistics 7: 1–26.

25. Goeman JJ (2010) L1 penalized estimation in the Cox proportional hazards model. Biom J 52: 70–84.

26. Zhou Y, Li N, Zhuang W, Liu GJ, Wu TX, et al. (2007) P53 codon 72 polymorphism and gastric cancer: a meta-analysis of the literature. Int J Cancer 121: 1481–1486.

27. Yan L, Zhang D, Chen C, Mao Y, Xie Y, et al. (2009) TP53 Arg72Pro polymorphism and lung cancer risk: a meta-analysis. Int J Cancer 125: 2903–2911.

28. Naccarati A, Polakova V, Pardini B, Vodickova L, Hemminki K, et al. (2012) Mutations and polymorphisms in TP53 gene-an overview on the role in colorectal cancer. Mutagenesis 27: 211–218.

29. Lin HY, Yang MC, Huang CH, Wu WJ, Yu TJ, et al. (2013) Polymorphisms of TP53 are markers of bladder cancer vulnerability and prognosis. Urol Oncol 31: 1231–1241.

30. Kiemeney LA, Thorlacius S, Sulem P, Geller F, Aben KK, et al. (2008) Sequence variant on 8q24 confers susceptibility to urinary bladder cancer. Nat Genet 40: 1307–1312.

31. Lichtenstein P, Holm NV, Verkasalo PK, Iliadou A, Kaprio J, et al. (2000) Environmental and heritable factors in the causation of cancer–analyses of cohorts of twins from Sweden, Denmark, and Finland. N Engl J Med 343: 78–85.

32. Gibson G (2011) Rare and common variants: twenty arguments. Nat Rev Genet 13: 135–145.

33. Hoh J, Ott J (2003) Mathematical multi-locus approaches to localizing complex human trait genes. Nat Rev Genet 4: 701–709.

34. Wu TT, Chen YF, Hastie T, Sobel E, Lange K (2009) Genome-wide association analysis by lasso penalized logistic regression. Bioinformatics 25: 714–721.

35. Zhou H, Sehl ME, Sinsheimer JS, Lange K (2010) Association screening of common and rare genetic variants by penalized regression. Bioinformatics 26: 2375–2382.

36. Louhelainen JP, Hurst CD, Pitt E, Nishiyama H, Pickett HA, et al. (2006) DBC1 re-expression alters the expression of multiple components of the plasminogen pathway. Oncogene 25: 2409–2419.

27

Ultrasound-Guided Intramural Inoculation of Orthotopic Bladder Cancer Xenografts: A Novel High-Precision Approach

Wolfgang Jäger[1,2], **Igor Moskalev**[1], **Claudia Janssen**[1,2], **Tetsutaro Hayashi**[1], **Shannon Awrey**[1], **Kilian M. Gust**[1,3], **Alan I. So**[1], **Kaixin Zhang**[1], **Ladan Fazli**[1], **Estelle Li**[1], **Joachim W. Thüroff**[2], **Dirk Lange**[1], **Peter C. Black**[1]*

1 The Vancouver Prostate Centre and Department of Urologic Sciences, University of British Columbia, Vancouver, BC, Canada, 2 Department of Urology, Johannes Gutenberg University, Mainz, Germany, 3 Department of Urology, Johann Wolfgang Goethe University, Frankfurt, Germany

Abstract

Orthotopic bladder cancer xenografts are essential for testing novel therapies and molecular manipulations of cell lines *in vivo*. Current xenografts rely on tumor cell inoculation by intravesical instillation or direct injection into the bladder wall. Instillation is limited by the lack of cell lines that are tumorigenic when delivered in this manner. The invasive model inflicts morbidity on the mice by the need for laparotomy and mobilization of the bladder. Furthermore this procedure is complex and time-consuming. Three bladder cancer cell lines (UM-UC1, UM-UC3, UM-UC13) were inoculated into 50 athymic nude mice by percutaneous injection under ultrasound guidance. PBS was first injected between the muscle wall and the mucosa to separate these layers, and tumor cells were subsequently injected into this space. Bioluminescence and ultrasound were used to monitor tumor growth. Contrast-enhanced ultrasound was used to study changes in tumor perfusion after systemic gemcitabine/cisplatin treatment. To demonstrate proof of principle that therapeutic agents can be injected into established xenografts under ultrasound guidance, oncolytic virus (VSV) was injected into UM-UC3 tumors. Xenograft tissue was harvested for immunohistochemistry after 23–37 days. Percutaneous injection of tumor cells into the bladder wall was performed efficiently (mean time: 5.7 min) and without complications in all 50 animals. Ultrasound and bioluminescence confirmed presence of tumor in the anterior bladder wall in all animals 3 days later. The average tumor volumes increased steadily over the study period. UM-UC13 tumors showed a marked decrease in volume and perfusion after chemotherapy. Immunohistochemical staining for VSV-G demonstrated virus uptake in all UM-UC3 tumors after intratumoral injection. We have developed a novel method for creating orthotopic bladder cancer xenograft in a minimally invasive fashion. In our hands this has replaced the traditional model requiring laparotomy, because this model is more time efficient, more precise and associated with less morbidity for the mice.

Editor: Xiaolin Zi, University of California Irvine, United States of America

Funding: Grant funding was provided through DFG (WJ; www.dfg.de/en; JA 2117/1–1:1), the Canadian Cancer Society Research Institute (PCB; www.cancer.ca/Research.aspx; 2010-700527) and a Mentored Physician Scientist Award from Vancouver Coastal Health Research Institute (PCB; http://www.vch.ca/about_us/awards_&_recognition; F08-04967). The ultrasound imaging platform was funded by the Canadian Foundation for Innovation (PCB; www.innovation.ca; 27255). The funders had no role in study design, data collection and analysis, decision to publish, or preparation of the manuscript.

Competing Interests: The authors have declared that no competing interests exist.

* E-mail: pblack@mail.ubc.ca

Introduction

Bladder cancer is the fourth most common cancer in men and the ninth most common cancer in women in developed countries [1]. In 2010 there were 70,530 incident cases and 14,680 deaths from bladder cancer in the U.S. [2]. Approximately three quarters of cases are non-muscle invasive [3]. These have a high propensity for recurrence and a subset is at risk for progression to invasive disease [4]. The remaining one quarter of cases present as muscle invasive bladder cancer. Despite optimal multimodal therapy, approximately one half of patients with muscle invasive bladder cancer will succumb to their disease [5]. No significant breakthroughs have been made in the past two decades to enhance the systemic therapy of this patient population [6].

Murine models of human cancer using cell lines derived from patient tumors (xenografts) are an essential tool in cancer research.

They allow us to interrogate tumor biology with molecular manipulation, to identify relevant diagnostic and predictive biomarkers, and to test antineoplastic effects of novel therapies. For bladder cancer, inoculation of human cell lines into the mouse bladder (orthotopic xenograft) is the reference standard [7,8]. This inoculation can be achieved either by intravesical instillation of tumor cells ("intravesical model") [9] or direct injection into the bladder wall ("intramural model") [10]. Alternative models include the inoculation of murine bladder cancer cells in immunocompetent mice (syngeneic model) [11] as well as transgenic models [12]. Similar models are also possible in rats [13,14].

Each orthoptic xenograft model has its shortcomings. Intravesical instillation leads to the formation of tumors on the urothelial surface of the bladder that are amenable to subsequent intravesical instillation of novel drugs. However, it has proven to be extraordinarily challenging using this method to achieve reliable tumor take with any cell lines other than KU7 [9], which we have recently demonstrated to be HeLa [15]. Furthermore, intravesical cell inoculation is time consuming and can lead to uncontrolled tumor growth in adjacent organs (urethra, ureter, renal pelvis) [16]. Finally, tumor location within the bladder is unpredictable, such that growth around the ureteral orifices can cause severe upper tract obstruction before mice reach therapeutic endpoints.

Direct injection of tumor cell into the bladder wall leads to the formation of invasive bladder tumors that are suitable for systemic treatments [10]. Although several cell lines grow reliably as xenografts in this model, the application is limited by the morbidity inflicted on the mice by the need for laparotomy and mobilization of the bladder [17]. It is also technically challenging to ensure adequate injection into the bladder wall, and this method is associated with a significant learning curve.

We have developed a novel approach to address these limitations of the intramural inoculation of bladder cancer xenografts, and thereby potentially enhance the accuracy and reproducibility of this model. We have optimized the percutaneous, ultrasound-guided injection of bladder cancer cells into the anterior bladder wall. In addition, we are able to monitor xenograft growth and perfusion in vivo longitudinally during therapy [18,19], and we are able to inject therapeutic agents directly into the tumor under ultrasound guidance. Here we demonstrate the feasibility and reproducibility of ultrasound-guided intramural inoculation of orthotopic bladder cancer xenografts as well as subsequent image guided manipulation and monitoring.

Materials and Methods

Animals

Fifty 10-week-old female athymic nude mice were purchased from Harlan (Indianapolis, IN, USA). All animal procedures were performed according to the guidelines of the Canadian Council on Animal Care (CCAC). The protocol was approved by the Animal Care Committee of the University of British Columbia (Protocol Number: A10-0192).

Tumor Cell Lines

The human bladder cancer cell lines UM-UC1, UM-UC3 and UM-UC13 were kindly provided by the Pathology Core of the Bladder Cancer SPORE at MD Anderson Cancer Center (Houston, TX, USA) [20–22]. Cell line identities were confirmed by DNA fingerprinting using the AmpFlSTR® Identifiler® Amplification protocol (Applied Biosystems, Carlsbad, CA, USA) [23]. All cell lines were cultured for less than 3 months in Dulbecco's modified Eagle's medium (DMEM) with 10% fetal bovine serum (FBS) at 37°C in a humidified 5% CO_2 atmosphere.

For in vivo studies, the cell lines underwent transduction with a lentiviral construct carrying the luciferase firefly gene for in vivo imaging [9]. The luciferase plasmid contained a blasticidin resistance gene enabling positive selection with 10 µg/mL blasticidin (Invitrogen, Life Technologies Inc., Burlington, ON, Canada). Cell lines were controlled for in vitro luciferase activity and cell number was correlated with bioluminescence (R>0.99; data not shown), using the Xenogen IVIS Spectrum (Caliper Lifesciences, Hopkinton, MA, USA). For xenograft studies the cells were harvested at 70% confluence and suspended in Matrigel® (BD Biosciences, Mississauga, ON, Canada). The cell concentration was modified based on previously established growth kinetics of the three different cell lines (UM-UC1 luc

9×10^6/mL; UM-UC3 luc 12×10^6/mL; UM-UC13 luc 11×10^6/mL).

Percutaneous Tumor Inoculation

Tumor inoculation was performed with the Vevo 770® small animal imaging platform (Visual Sonics, Toronto, ON, Canada). A high frequency RMV 706 ultrasound scanhead (20–60 MHz), which allowed a lateral resolution of 30 micron and frame rates up to 240 fps, was used.

The mice were anesthetized with isoflurane and mounted on the imaging table with continuous monitoring of vital signs [Fig. 1A]. The abdomen was disinfected with alcohol and sterile ultrasound gel was applied. The bladder was visualized on the screen [Fig. 1B] and the bladder lumen was filled with sterile, warm phosphate-buffered saline (PBS) through a 24 gauge angiocatheter to a desired volume of 50–100 µL.

A 1.0 mL syringe filled with PBS and connected to a 30 gauge, ¾ inch needle (Kendall, Mansfield, MA, USA) was brought to the skin just above the pubic bone at an angle of 30° with the bevel directed anteriorly. After detection of the needle on the ultrasound screen [Fig. 2A], it was passed through the skin and the abdominal wall muscles [Fig. 2B]. The bevel of the needle was turned 180° (directed posteriorly) before the tip was inserted into the bladder wall without penetration of the mucosa [Fig. 2C]. PBS (50 µL) was injected between the muscular layer and the mucosa to create a space [Fig. 2D] and the needle was withdrawn. A second 1.0 mL syringe (filled with cancer cells suspended in Matrigel®, (BD Biosciences)) with a 30 gauge, ¾ inch needle was guided into the same space [Fig. 2E]. 40 µL (UM-UC1 luc) or 50 µL(UM-UC3 luc, UM-UC13 luc) of the cell suspension were injected into this space [Fig. 2F].

In two additional mice agarose was injected in a similar fashion in order to establish the exact location of xenograft inoculation within the bladder wall. The mice were immediately sacrificed and their bladders were removed for histologic analysis.

Xenograft Growth Monitoring

Tumor growth was monitored by bioluminescence imaging (BLI) and ultrasound every third day starting 4 days after tumor inoculation. The Xenogen IVIS system was used for BLI and mice were imaged 10 and 15 minutes after intraperitoneal injection of D-Luciferin (150 mg/kg bodyweight; Firefly, Caliper Life Science). 3D ultrasound was performed in anesthetized mice with scanning of the bladder as a whole in 0.1 mm steps. The tumor volume was determined using the Visual Sonics imaging software package by analysis of every fifth picture according to the user manual [24].

Microbubble Contrast-Enhanced Ultrasound Analysis of Tumors

To visualize the perfusion status of the xenograft tumors, a cine loop was recorded as the reference. A second cine loop (1000 frames at 30 Hz) was recorded 10 seconds after injection of 120 µL non-targeted microbubbles (Visual Sonics) into the tail vein of anesthetized mice. The point at which microbubbles entered the plane was determined and the background reference was subtracted. The tumor was selected as the contrast region and Reference Subtracted Mean Data were used. Changes of the Contrast Percent Area over time were documented and 2D images were recorded in which any pixel was marked green when a microbubble passed [24].

A.

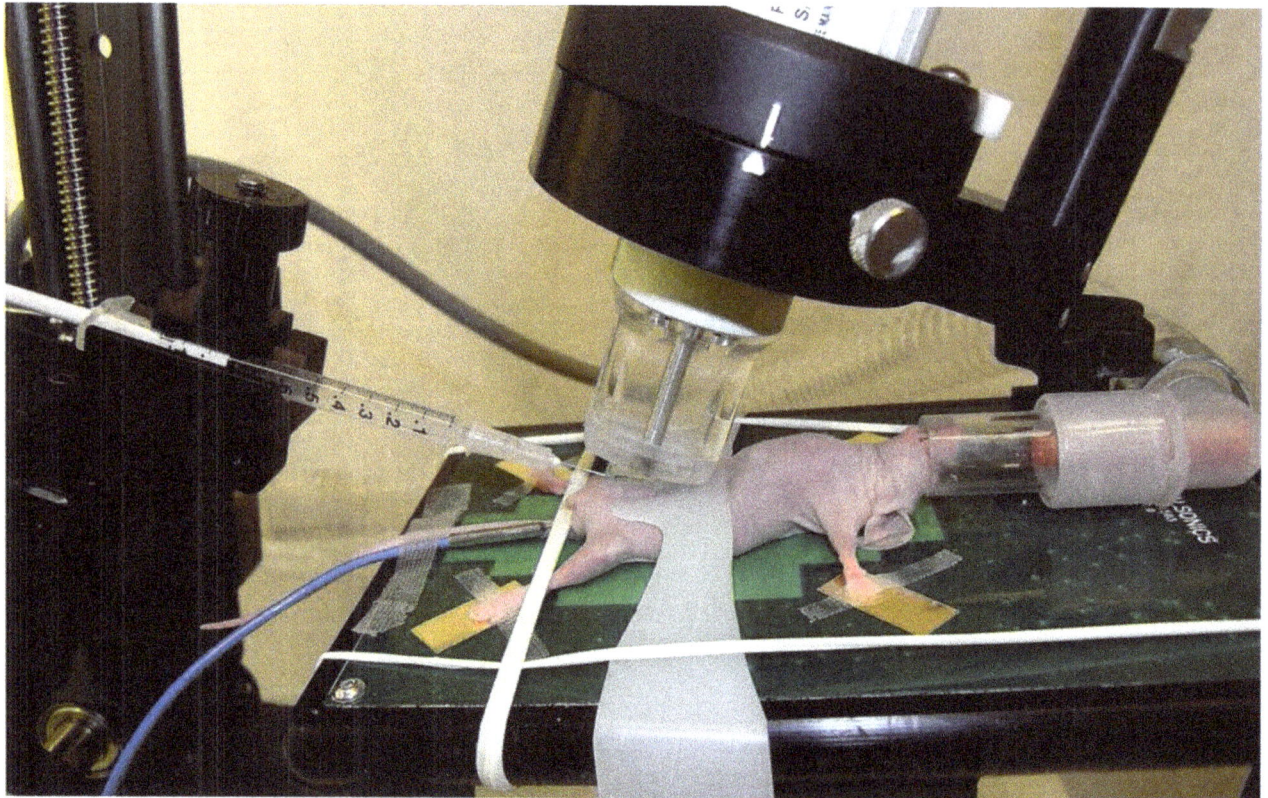

B.

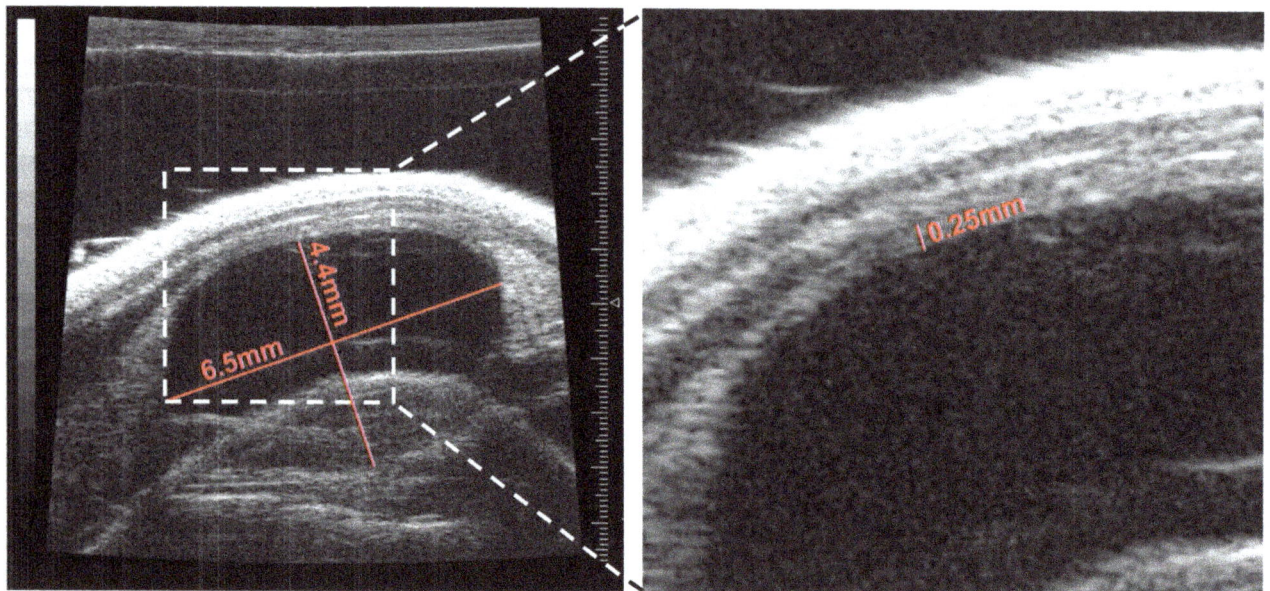

Figure 1. Ultrasound imaging. A. The mice were anesthetized with isoflurane and mounted on the heated imaging table with continuous monitoring of vital signs. After visualization of the bladder with the Vevo 700® small animal imaging platform the skin was perforated with a 30G needle. B. Ultrasound visualisation of normal mouse bladder in sagittal section with typical dimensions indicated (lumen dimensions 4.4×6.5 mm; wall thickness 0.25 mm).

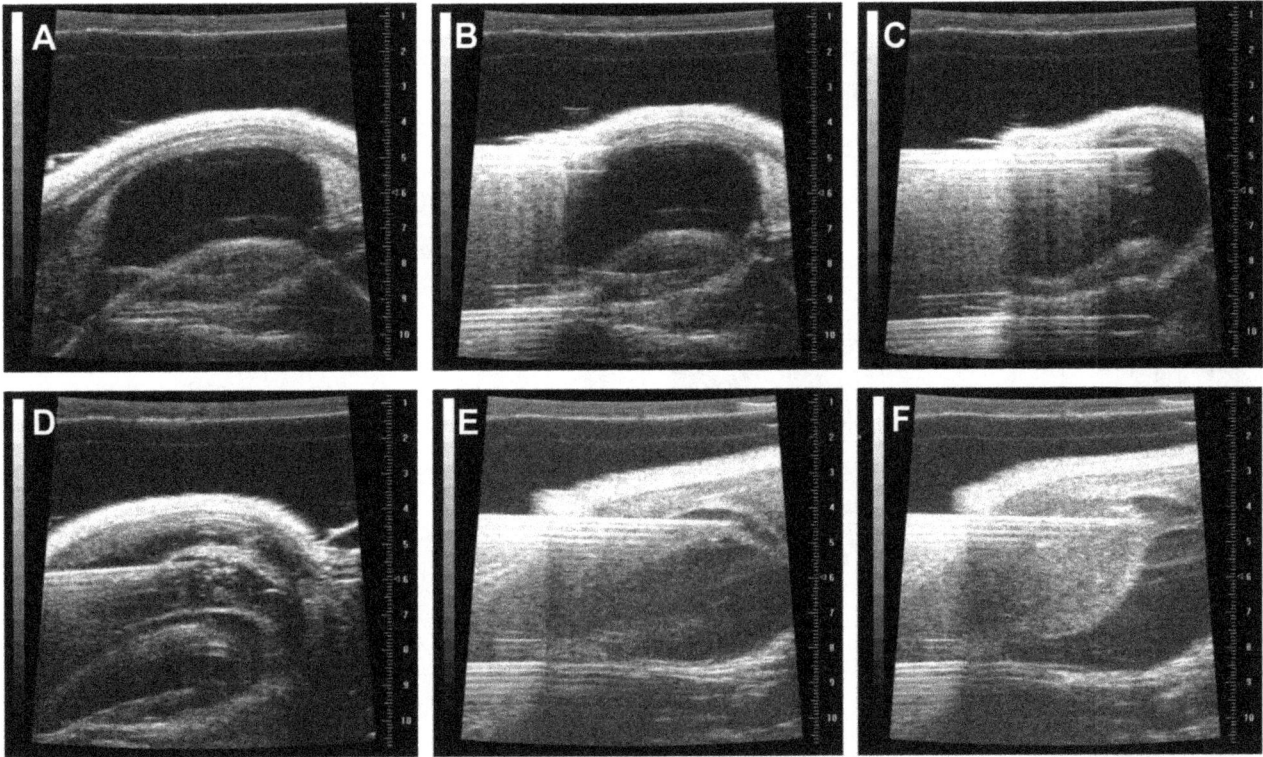

Figure 2. Inoculation of tumor cells. A. Detection of the needle on the ultrasound screen. B. Perforation of the skin and abdominal wall muscles. C. Needle insertion into the bladder wall without penetration of the mucosa. D. Injection of PBS (50 µl) between the muscular layer and the mucosa. E. Guidance of second needle into the artificially created space. F. Injection of tumor cells suspended in Matrigel®.

Treatment

Intratumoral virus-injection. To demonstrate the potential for ultrasound guided percutaneous intratumoral injection of treatment agents into established xenografts, we injected oncolytic virus (VSV) into UM-UC3 luc xenografts on day 22 after inoculation. Tumor burden as determined by BLI and ultrasound was used to divide the animals into two relatively equal groups. The tumors were visualized longitudinally by ultrasound and a 30G needle was inserted in the center of the tumor [Fig. 3A]. VSV (1.05×10^7 pfu) suspended in 25 µL PBS was injected in 7 mice, and PBS alone was injected in the control group (n = 7).

Systemic chemotherapy. To demonstrate the potential for *in vivo* real-time monitoring of xenograft perfusion, we treated UM-UC13 luc tumor-bearing mice with cytotoxic chemotherapy. On day 28 after inoculation, the mice were divided into two equal groups based on tumor burden determined by ultrasound and BLI. Eight animals received intraperitoneal gemcitabine (120 mg/kg bodyweight; SANDOZ, Boucherville, QC, Canada) on day 30 and 35 as well as cisplatin (2.5 mg/kg bodyweight; Hospira, Saint-Laurent, QC, Canada) on day 31 and 36. An equivalent volume of PBS was injected at the same time points in the control animals (n = 7).

Histology

UM-UC3 luc, UM-UC1 luc and UM-UC13 luc xenografts were harvested after 24, 28 and 37 days, respectively. At necropsy, the pelvis, retroperitoneum, liver and lungs were carefully inspected for possible metastasis, and any suspicious tissue was removed. This tissue and the whole bladders were fixed in formalin, embedded in paraffin and cut in 4-µm

sections which were stained with haematoxylin and eosin (H&E). Depth of tumor invasion was determined by a pathologist (LF). For UM-UC3 tumors a T stage was applied according to 7th edition of the American Joint Committee on Cancer/International Union Against Cancer (AJCC/UICC) TNM classification [25].

Detection of apoptotic cells by the TUNEL (Terminal deoxynucleotidyl transferase dUTP nick end labeling) technique was performed using Terminal transferase (#03333566001, Roche Applied Science, Indianapolis, IN, USA), dATP (D4788, Sigma-Aldrich, St. Louis, MO, USA) and DIG-11-dUTP (#1558706, Roche Applied Science). Using polyclonal rabbit antibody against the G protein of VSV (VSV-G; 1:300, ab1874, Abcam, Cambridge, MA, USA) immunohistochemical staining was conducted by the Ventana autostainer model Discover XT (Ventana Medical System, Tuscon, AZ, USA) with an enzyme-labeled biotin streptavidin system and solvent-resistant 3,30-diaminobenyidine Map kit. All samples were subsequently analysed by a pathologist (LF) and the percentage of immunoexpression for VSV-G and staining for TUNEL was detected at 200× magnifications.

Statistical Analysis

For statistical analyses, the mean bioluminescence and tumor volumes with their standard deviations were determined. The significance of differences was measured by Student's t test (GraphPad Software Inc., San Diego, CA, USA) and $P<0.05$ was considered significant. Regression plots were used to describe the correlation between bioluminescence and volume.

A.

B.

H&E   VSV-G   TUNEL

C.

H&E   VSV-G   TUNEL

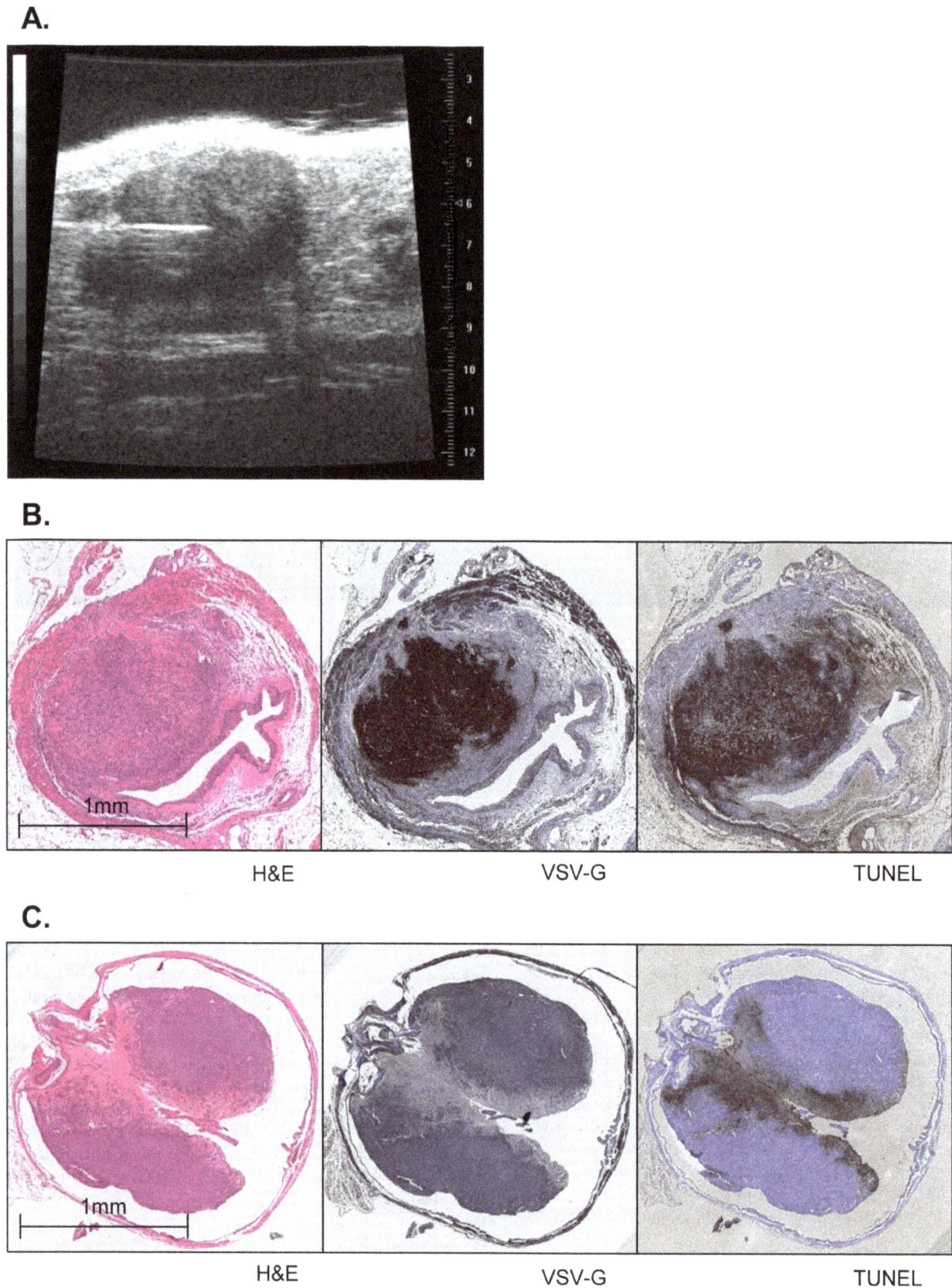

Figure 3. Ultrasound-guided intratumoral injection of treatment agents. A. The xenografts were visualized by ultrasound and either VSV (1.05×10^7 pfu) dissolved in 25 µl PBS or PBS alone was injected through a 30G needle into the center of the tumor. B. 48 h after injection of VSV, all xenograft tumors showed positive staining for VSV-G around the injection site which correlated to TUNEL staining. C. VSV-G and TUNEL staining were negative after PBS injection alone.

Table 1. Percutaneous tumor cell injection – procedure, complications and growth.

Inoculated cell line		UM-UC1 luc	UM-UC3 luc	UM-UC13 luc
Number of mice		50		
		20	15	15
Anesthesia		Isoflurane	Isoflurane	Isoflurane
Time per animal, min		3.4 (+/−1.6)	7.7 (+/−3.7)	6.8 (+/−2.9)
Anesthesia related deaths		0	0	0
Volume injected, μL		40	50	50
Cell count, absolute		3.6×10^5	6×10^5	5.5×10^5
Tumor incidence		49 (98%)		
		20 (100%)	14 (93%)	15 (100%)
Extravesical tumor growth		2 (10%)	–	–
Intraperitoneal dissemination		–	1 (7%)	–
Lymph node metastasis		–	3 (20%)	9 (60%)
Follow up (days)		28	22 [before treatment]	28 [before treatment]
Tumor volume (μL)	day 4	11.6 ($\pm$1.3)	12.5 ($\pm$1.7)	14.4 ($\pm$1.3)
	end of follow up	394.6 ($\pm$72.4)	288.7 ($\pm$66.1)	78.3 ($\pm$13.4)
Tumor luminescence (Photons/sec)	day 4	4.6×10^8 ($\pm 9.4 \times 10^7$)	2.0×10^8 ($\pm 3.7 \times 10^7$)	5.8×10^8 ($\pm 1.3 \times 10^8$)
	end of follow up	1.9×10^{10} ($\pm 4.0 \times 10^9$)	1.4×10^{10} ($\pm 2.3 \times 10^9$)	1.5×10^{10} ($\pm 1.9 \times 10^9$)

Results

Tumor Cell Inoculation

Ultrasound-guided tumor cell inoculation was successfully performed in 50 animals (UM-UC1 luc 20 animals, UM-UC3 luc 15 animals and UM-UC13 luc 15 animals) [Table 1]. The typical experimental set-up and representative ultrasound images and dimensions of the murine bladder are depicted in Fig. 1. The steps of inoculation are shown in Fig. 2. The mean time per procedure (mounting of mice on the table until finished injection) could be decreased from 7.7$\pm$3.7 min for the first group (UM-UC3 luc) to 3.4$\pm$1.6 min for the third group (UM-UC1 luc). None of the animals suffered any complication during the procedure. Injection of agarose gel demonstrated that the inoculation was strictly located between the lamina propria and the tunica muscularis [Fig. 4].

Xenograft Growth Monitoring

All 50 animals showed detectable tumor in the anterior bladder wall on ultrasound on the 4th day after inoculation. The start and

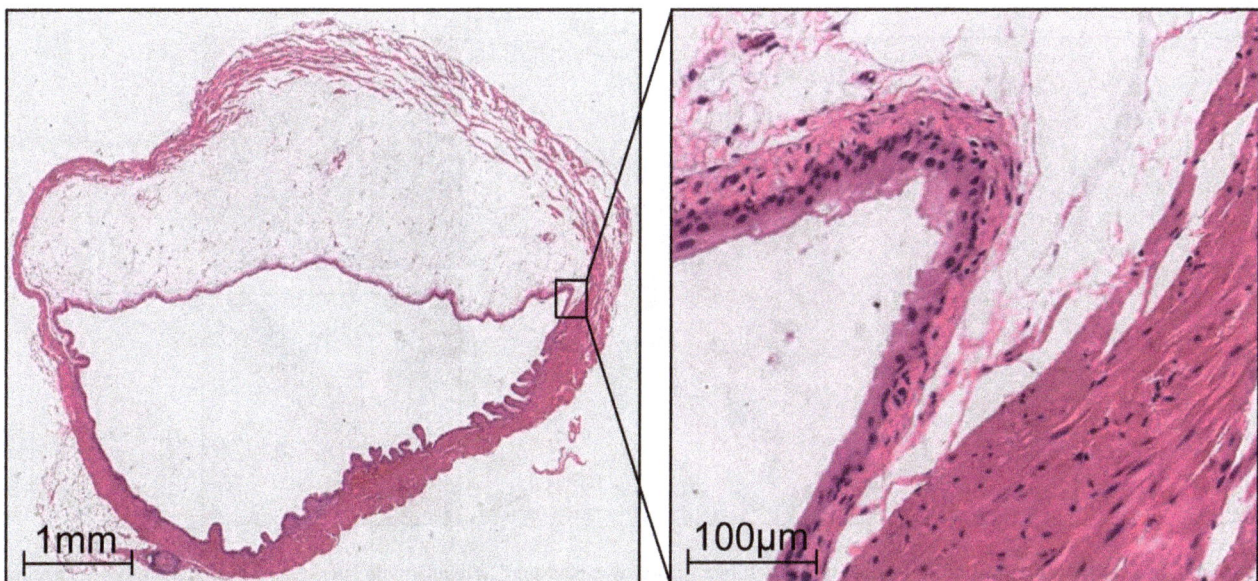

Figure 4. Intramural injection of agarose. The sagittal H&E section of a whole murine bladder demonstrates a layer of gel strictly in the lamina propria between mucosa and the muscularis propria.

A.

B.

C.

UM-UC1 luc (D28)   UM-UC3 luc (D19)   UM-UC13 luc (D34)

D.

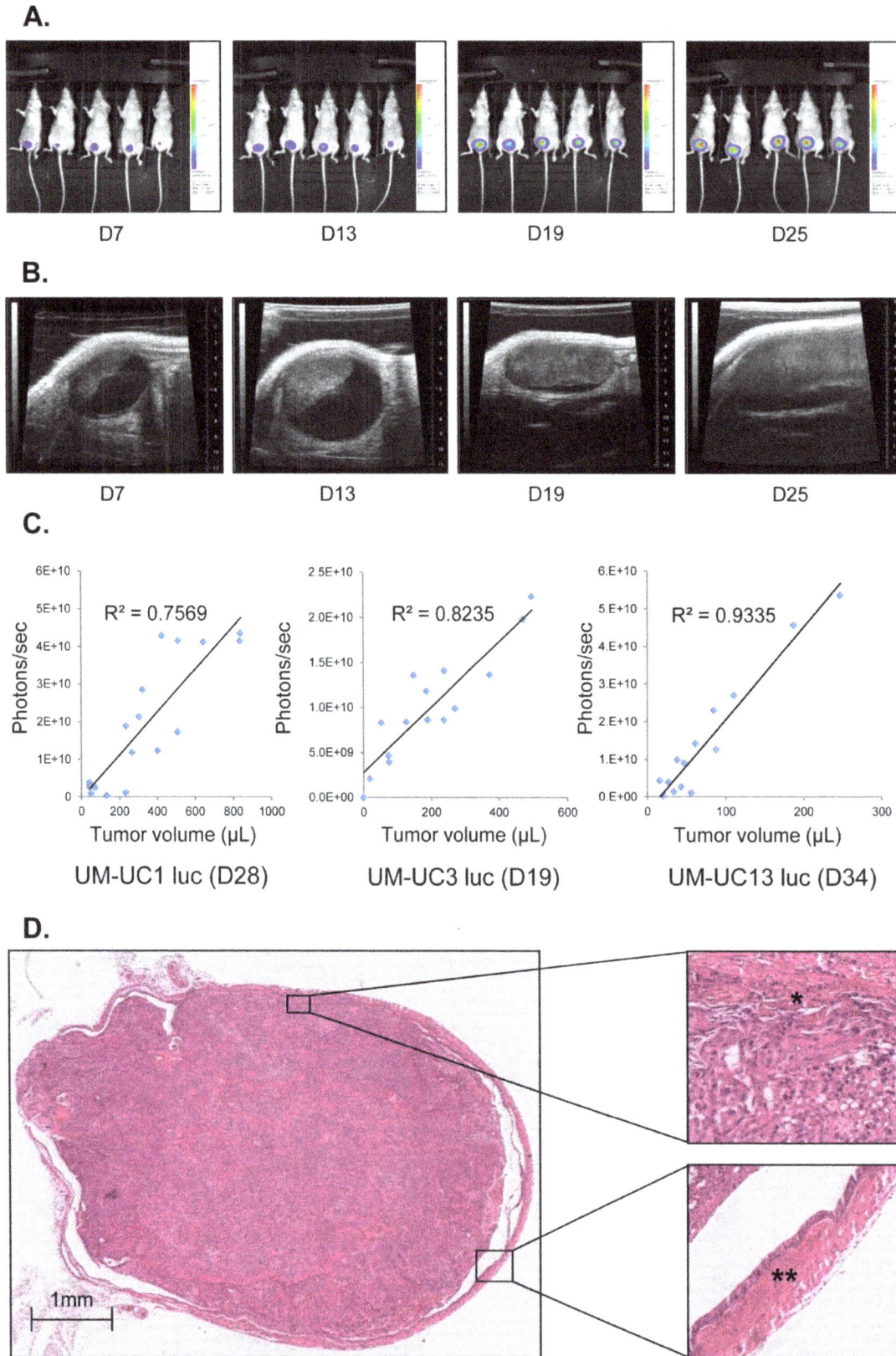

Figure 5. Longitudinal imaging of xenograft growth. Tumor growth was measured at regular time intervals by: A. bioluminescence imaging, and B. ultrasound. C. Correlation of bioluminescence and xenograft volume for all three cell lines. D. H&E section of a representative UM-UC1 luc xenograft demonstrating invasive growth into the muscle (*) without invasion into adjacent organs. All tumors originated from the anterior bladder wall and often occupied most of the bladder lumen without infiltrating the posterior wall (**).

Table 2. TNM Classification of UM-UC3 luc xenograft tumors.

		n	%
T-Stage	pTa	0	(0%)
	pT1	0	(0%)
	pT2a	5	(33%)
	pT2b	5	(33%)
	pT3a	4	(27%)
	pT3b	1	(7%)
	pT4	0	(0%)
Lymph nodes	N+	3	(20%)
	N−	12	(80%)
Metastasis	M+	1	(7%)
	M−	14	(93%)

end tumor volumes are summarized in Table 1. After inoculation of UM-UC3 luc, one mouse showed intraperitoneal tumor dissemination and one tumor involuted after day 7. Similar patterns were seen with BLI. All mice had detectable luminescence on the 4th day, and this increased steadily in all but one mouse. The overall tumor uptake rate was 98%. These findings were confirmed at the time of necropsy.

During tumor growth [Fig. 5A, 5B] the ratio between entire tumor volume and BLI was not stable but variable depending on the time after tumor cell inoculation and the entire tumor volume itself. Although there had been a trend towards better correlation over the time course ($R^2 = 0.75$, 0.82 and 0.92 for UM-UC1 luc at day 16, UM-UC3 luc at day 19 and UM-UC13 luc at day 34 respectively [Fig. 5C]), a drastic decline of the luminescence per mL tumor volume was noticed at high tumor volumes (data not shown). We have previously demonstrated a role for hypoxia and necrosis in this correlation [17].

Three mice (two UM-UC1 luc and one UM-UC3 luc) were sacrificed for humane reasons related to excessive tumor burden before the end of planned follow-up.

Histology

Examination of the xenografts on H&E sections demonstrated that all tumors were invasive into muscle and some into perivesical fat, but there was no evidence of invasion into adjacent organs [Fig. 5D]. None of the tumors grew through the lamina propria into the bladder lumen. Retroperitoneal lymphadenopathy was noted in 60% of UM-UC13 luc and 20% of UM-UC3 luc xenografts. This was confirmed by H&E staining (data not shown). TNM staging was exemplary performed for all UM-UC3 luc tumors by histological analysis of the primary tumors and retroperitoneal lymph nodes, as well as macroscopic analysis of liver and lungs [Table 2].

After intratumoral injection of VSV into UM-UC3 luc xenografts [Fig. 3A], all 7 tumors showed positive staining for VSV-G. The same areas of the tumors staining for VSV-G also demonstrated staining in the TUNEL assay [Fig. 3B]. In contrast, VSV-G staining was negative for xenografts treated with PBS at the negative control [Fig. 3C].

Response to Chemotherapy

The mice bearing UM-UC13 luc tumors showed a remarkable response to the combination of gemcitabine and cisplatin. The median tumor volume significantly decreased from 48.6 µL ($\pm$7.7) to 25.3 µL ($\pm$5.8) after 7 days of therapy, whereas it increased from 48.8 µL ($\pm$14.8) to 114.5 µL ($\pm$26.8) in the control group [Fig. 6A].

The perfusion of the xenograft tumor was measured before and after administration of systemic chemotherapy with non-specific microbubbles. Chemotherapy led to a decrease in the perfusion rate (Contrast Percent Area) from 84% to 66%, whereas the same parameter remained constant after treatment with PBS alone (79% vs. 77%) [Fig. 6B].

Discussion

The existence of reliable animal models is a basic requirement in oncologic research for the in vivo investigation of tumor biology and the testing of novel antineoplastic treatment strategies. Despite the existence of reproducible syngeneic [11] and transgenic [12] orthotopic tumor models of bladder cancer, they are not widely used due to both inherent limitations (e.g. questionable applicability of syngeneic models of murine bladder cancer to human disease) and complexity of the models, as well as the intensity of associated resource utilization. Orthotopic xenograft models have proven to offer the most flexibility (in terms of selection of cell lines) and have the most practical utility, and therefore remain the gold standard for in vivo modeling of bladder cancer [7,8].

In this work, we have generated a novel in vivo model of orthotopic bladder cancer xenografts via the inoculation of human bladder cancer cells into the murine bladder and have shown it to be highly reproducible. Tumors were established in 98% of inoculated mice using three different human cell lines. Due to excellent optical resolution, the tumor cells can be inoculated by high precision strictly into the anterior bladder wall, thus reducing the rate of obstructive complications and allowing longer growth and treatment periods. Furthermore, the time per inoculation is short in comparison to existing models, and decreases rapidly with additional experience. The single observed complication was an intraperitoneal tumor cell dissemination which occurred in one of the first animals injected and can be attributed to the injection of too large a volume relative to the size of the animal. This was supported by the fact that reducing the volume of injection from 50 to 40 µL resulted in no further complications.

Our model is a modification of the orthotopic model previously described by Dinney et al. [10]. We believe that ultrasound-guided tumor inoculation enhances this model due to its ease, rapidity, accuracy and decreased degree of invasiveness. The latter factor is not only one of animal welfare, but may also contribute to reproducibility of experiments by decreasing confounding surgical complications. The accuracy of the standard intramural injection through a laparotomy is limited by the ability to determine exact needle placement at the time of injection. The shape and distribution of the bleb in the bladder wall after injection will often confirm correct location, but there is no a priori confirmation before the cells are injected. This means that a certain proportion of mice will have cells injected into the lumen of the bladder or spilled on the serosal surface of the bladder. With the ultrasound technique, a space is created submucosally in the bladder wall with saline, which carries no risk of spillage, and the subsequent tumor cell inoculation easily follows into the same space under direct visualization.

Monitoring tumor volume by ultrasound augments the information gained by BLI in the orthotopic xenograft model. While BLI has become an integral component of tumor detection and growth analysis, it does not always correlate well with tumor volume. We have previously shown in the orthotopic xenograft

A.

B.

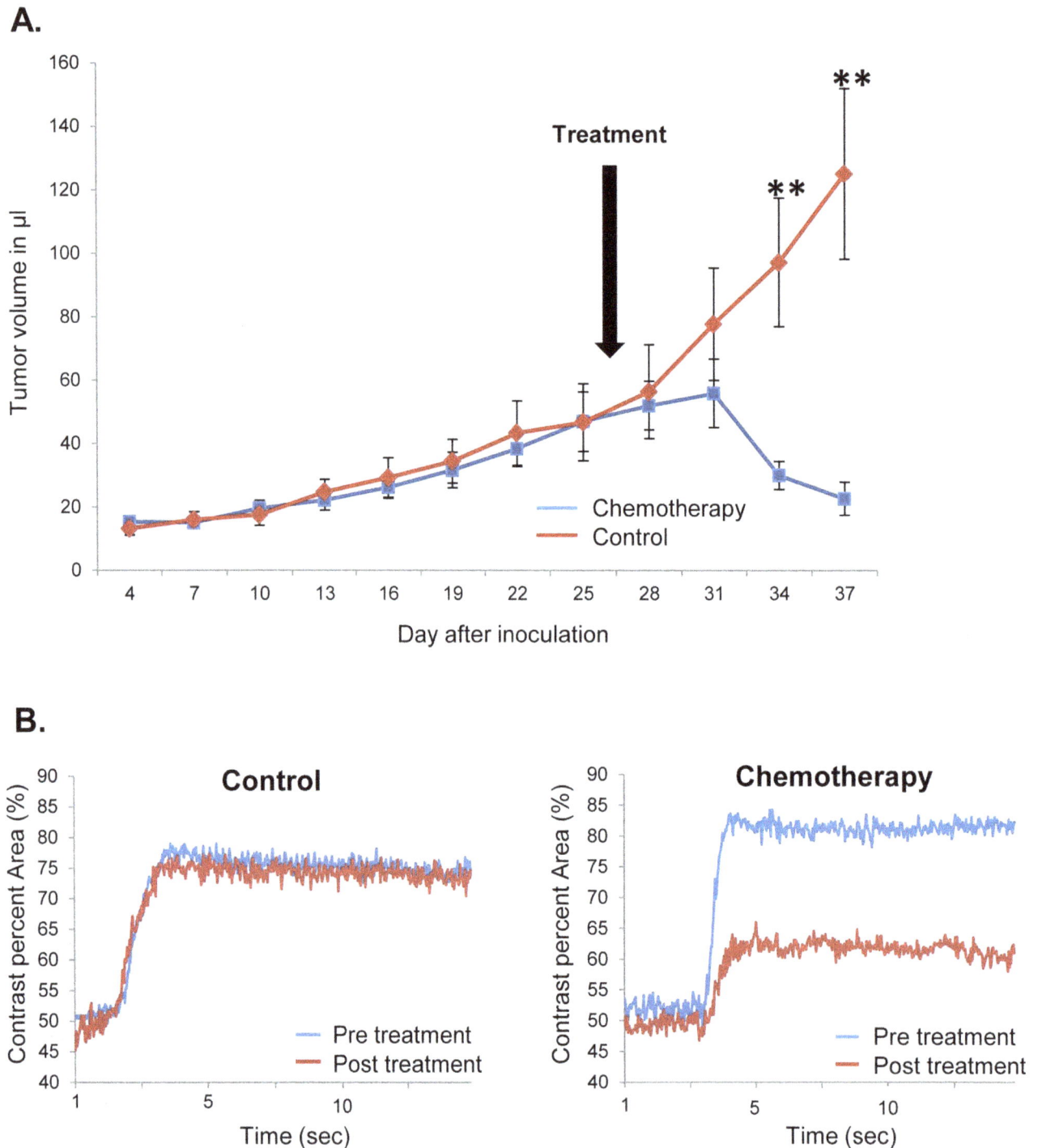

Figure 6. Treatment of xenograft tumors by chemotherapy. A. Mice bearing UM-UC13 luc tumors showed a remarkable decrease in tumor volume after systemic therapy with a combination of gemcitabine and cisplatin starting on day #28 after inoculation, compared to PBS control (** = P<0.01). B. Xenograft perfusion was measured by injection and ultrasound imaging of non-targeted microbubbles in UM-UC13 luc xenografts before and 5 days after administration of control agent (PBS; left panel) or systemic chemotherapy (gemcitabine/cisplatin; right panel). Perfusion was quantified as contrast percent area. Representative single results out of 4 measured animals per group are shown.

model that tumor perfusion and hypoxia confound the relationship between volume and luminescence [17], and the same is presumably responsible for the disparities shown here. This is particularly true in larger tumors [26], whereas early after inoculation ultrasound size may be inaccurate due to the volume of injected fluid, the surrounding tissue edema, and the fact that only a proportion of injected cells survive and grow.

An additional advantage of the ultrasound is the ability to inject novel treatment agents directly into the tumor. Here we have demonstrated the feasibility of intratumoral delivery of oncolytic

VSV. The same technique would be amenable to other treatment strategies for bladder cancer such as gene therapy or the application of nanoparticles [27,28]. As an example of the relevance of intratumoral injection in the treatment of human cancers, the intratumoral injection of DNA plasmid has recently been tested in the therapy of unresectable pancreatic cancers [29].

We have also demonstrated the ability to monitor tumor vascularity during drug treatment, in this case traditional cytotoxic chemotherapy. This ability will be particularly useful when evaluating the response of tumors to novel therapeutics including the development of resistance which may be reflected by a failure to diminish vascularity.

The principal limitation of ultrasound-guided tumor inoculation is the dependence on the ultrasound imaging platform, which may not be readily accessible to many researchers. Furthermore, this model requires familiarity with ultrasound imaging. On the other hand, complex animal modeling of human cancers, just like complex surgery on human patients, may best be performed by centers of excellence through scientific collaborations.

Our model does not necessarily substitute for the intravesical instillation of bladder cancer cell lines [9,30]. The intramural model is superior to the intravesical model for most applications because of the ability to use multiple different cell lines. The intramural model, however, has no utility for testing novel therapies delivered intravesically because the tumors do not disrupt the urothelial surface (lamina propria) in the bladder lumen, and drugs therefore do not easily penetrate into the tumor. These tumors grow expansively away from the lumen of the bladder so that drugs administered into the lumen of the bladder cannot penetrate the full depth of the tumor. Furthermore, the intramural model represents muscle invasive disease, which is never treated with intravesical therapy in clinical practice. In the intravesical tumor model, on the other hand, the tumor surface is exposed in the bladder lumen and the tumor generally does not grow beyond the lamina propria for several weeks [9], so that drugs administered into the bladder lumen can adequately penetrate the tumor. The most significant limitation to the intravesical model, however, is its restriction to very few cell lines which, even in the most experienced hands, grow in only an unreliable fashion.

Conclusions

We have successfully developed a technique for ultrasound-guided inoculation of orthotopic bladder cancer xenografts that significantly enhances pre-existing models of bladder cancer. The major advantages of this model lie in the rapidity and ease of tumor inoculation as well as in the accuracy and reproducibility of the model. Furthermore, we are able to monitor tumor volume longitudinally with ultrasound, to measure in vivo tumor perfusion with microbubble contrast agents, and to inject therapeutic agents into the tumor under ultrasound guidance.

Acknowledgments

We would like to thank Ben Deeley for his assistance in the ultrasound imaging and Eliana Beraldi for her assistance with viral transduction of cell lines.

Author Contributions

Conceived and designed the experiments: WJ IM DL JWT PCB. Performed the experiments: WJ IM TH. Analyzed the data: WJ IM CJ LF EL PCB. Contributed reagents/materials/analysis tools: AS KZ DL PCB SA KMG. Wrote the paper: WJ IM CJ DL PCB.

References

1. Ploeg M, Aben KK, Kiemeney LA (2009) The present and future burden of urinary bladder cancer in the world. World J Urol 27: 289–293.
2. Siegel R, Naishadham D, Jemal A (2012) Cancer statistics, 2012. CA Cancer J Clin. 62: 10–29.
3. Babjuk M, Oosterlinck W, Sylvester R, Kaasinen E, Böhle A, et al. (2011)EAU guidelines on non–muscle-invasive urothelial carcinoma of the bladder, the 2011 update. Eur Urol 59: 997–1008.
4. Sylvester RJ, van der Meijden AP, Oosterlinck W, Witjes JA, Bouffioux C, et al. (2006) Predicting recurrence and progression in individual patients with stage Ta T1 bladder cancer using EORTC risk tables: a combined analysis of 2596 patients from seven EORTC trials. Eur Urol 49: 466–477.
5. Shariat SF, Karakiewicz PI, Palapattu GS, Lotan Y, Rogers CG, et al. (2006) Outcomes of radical cystectomy for transitional cell carcinoma of the bladder: a contemporary series from the bladder cancer research consortium. J Urol 176: 2414–2422.
6. Von der Maase H, Sengelov L, Roberts JT, Ricci S, Dogliotti L, et al. (2005) Long-term survival results of a randomized trial comparing gemcitabine plus cisplatin, with methotrexate, vinblastine, doxorubicin, plus cisplatin in patients with bladder cancer. J Clin Oncol 23: 4602–4608.
7. Chan E, Patel A, Heston W, Larchian W (2009) Mouse orthotopic models for bladder cancer research. BJU Int 104: 1286–1291.
8. Kubota T (1994) Metastatic models of human cancer xenografted in the nude mouse: the importance of orthotopic transplantation. J Cell Biochem 56: 4–8.
9. Hadaschik BA, Black PC, Sea JC, Metwalli AR, Fazli L, et al. (2007) A validated mouse model for orthotopic bladder cancer using transurethral tumour inoculation and bioluminescence imaging. BJU Int 100: 1377–1384.
10. Dinney CP, Fishbeck R, Singh RK, Eve B, Pathak S, et al. (1995) Isolation and characterization of metastatic variants from human transitional cell carcinoma passaged by orthotopic implantation in athymic nude mice. J Urol 154: 1532–1538.
11. Summerhayes IC, Franks LM (1979) Effects of donor age on neoplastic transformation of adult mouse bladder epithelium in vitro. J Natl Cancer Inst 62: 1017–1023.
12. Zhang ZT, Pak J, Shapiro E, Sun TT, Wu XR (1999) Urothelium-specific expression of an oncogene in transgenic mice induced the formation of carcinoma in situ and invasive transitional cell carcinoma. Cancer Res 5914: 3512–3517.

13. Xiao Z, McCallum TJ, Brown KM, Miller GG, Halls SB, et al. (1999) Characterization of a novel transplantable orthotopic rat bladder transitional cell tumour model. Br J Cancer 81: 638–646.
14. Iinuma S, Bachor R, Flotte T, Hasan T (1995) Biodistribution and phototoxicity of 5-aminolevulinic acid-induced PpIX in an orthotopic rat bladder tumor model. J Urol 153: 802–806.
15. Jäger W, Horiguchi Y, Shah J, Hayashi T, Awrey S, et al. (2013) Hiding in plain view: Genetic profiling reveals decades old cross-contamination of bladder cancer cell line KU7 with HeLa. J Urol: in press.
16. Horiguchi Y, Larchian WA, Kaplinsky R, Fair WR, Heston WD (2000) Intravesical liposome-mediated interleukin-2 gene therapy in orthotopic murine bladder cancer model. Gene Ther 7: 844–851.
17. Black PC, Shetty A, Brown GA, Esparza-Coss E, Metwalli AR, et al. (2010) Validating bladder cancer xenograft bioluminescence with magnetic resonance imaging: the significance of hypoxia and necrosis. BJU Int 106: 1799–1804.
18. Patel AR, Chan ES, Hansel DE, Powell CT, Heston WD, et al. (2010) Transabdominal micro-ultrasound imaging of bladder cancer in a mouse model: a validation study. Urology 75: 799–804.
19. Rychak JJ, Graba J, Cheung AM, Mystry BS, Lindner JR, et al. (2007) Microultrasound molecular imaging of vascular endothelial growth factor receptor 2 in a mouse model of tumor angiogenesis. Mol Imaging 6: 289–296.
20. Grossman HB, Wedemeyer G, Ren L (1984) UM-UC-1 and UM-UC-2: characterization of two new human transitional cell carcinoma lines. J Urol 132: 834–837.
21. Grossman HB, Wedemeyer G, Ren L, Wilson GN, Cox B (1986) Improved growth of human urothelial carcinoma cell cultures. J Urol 136: 953–959.
22. Sabichi A, Keyhani A, Tanaka N, Delacerda J, Lee IL, et al. (2006) Characterization of a panel of cell lines derived from urothelial neoplasms: genetic alterations, growth in vivo and the relationship of adenoviral mediated gene transfer to coxsackie adenovirus receptor expression. J Urol 175: 1133–1137.
23. Choi W, Shah JB, Tran M, Svatek R, Marquis L, et al. (2012) p63 Expression Defines a Lethal Subset of Muscle-Invasive Bladder Cancers. PLoS ONE 7(1): e30206.
24. Olson P, Chu GC, Perry SR, Nolan-Stevaux O, Hanahan D (2011) Imaging guided trials of the angiogenesis inhibitor sunitinib in mouse models predict efficacy in pancreatic neuroendocrine but not ductal carcinoma. Proc Natl Acad Sci U S A. 108: 1275–1284.

25. American Joint Committee on Cancer (2010) AJCC cancer staging manual. Springer, New York London.

26. Klerk CP, Overmeer RM, Niers TM, Versteeg HH, Richel DJ, et al. (2007) Validity of bioluminescence measurements for noninvasive in vivo imaging of tumor load in small animals. Biotechniques 43: 7–13.

27. Adam L, Black PC, Kassouf W, Eve B, McConkey D, et al. (2007) Adenoviral mediated interferon-alpha 2b gene therapy suppresses the pro-angiogenic effect of vascular endothelial growth factor in superficial bladder cancer. J Urol 177: 1900–1906.

28. Cho EJ, Yang J, Mohamedali KA, Lim EK, Kim EJ, et al. (2011) Sensitive angiogenesis imaging of orthotopic bladder tumors in mice using a selective magnetic resonance imaging contrast agent containing VEGF121/rGel. Invest Radiol 46: 441–449.

29. Hanna N, Ohana P, Konikoff FM, Leichtmann G, Hubert A, et al. (2012) Phase 1/2a, dose-escalation, safety, pharmacokinetic and preliminary efficacy study of intratumoral administration of BC-819 in patients with unresectable pancreatic cancer. Cancer Gene Ther 19: 374–381.

30. Cheon J, Moon DG, Cho HY, Park HS, Kim JJ, et al. (2002) Adenovirus-mediated suicide-gene therapy in an orthotopic murine bladder tumor model. Int J Urol 9: 261–267.

28

Platelet-Derived Growth Factor Receptor Beta: A Novel Urinary Biomarker for Recurrence of Non-Muscle-Invasive Bladder Cancer

Jiayu Feng[1⊙], Weifeng He[2⊙], Yajun Song[1], Ying Wang[2], Richard J. Simpson[3], Xiaorong Zhang[2], Gaoxing Luo[2], Jun Wu[2]*, Chibing Huang[1]*

1 Department of Urology, Xinqiao Hospital, The Third Military Medical University, Chongqing, China, 2 Chongqing Key Laboratory for Disease Proteomics; State Key Laboratory of Trauma, Burns and Combined Injury, Institute of Burn Research, Southwest Hospital, Third Military Medical University, Chongqing, China, 3 Department of Biochemistry, La Trobe Institute for Molecular Science, La Trobe University, Bundoora, Victoria, Australia

Abstract

Non-muscle-invasive bladder cancer (NMIBC) is one of the most common malignant tumors in the urological system with a high risk of recurrence, and effective non-invasive biomarkers for NMIBC relapse are still needed. The human urinary proteome can reflect the status of the microenvironment of the urinary system and is an ideal source for clinical diagnosis of urinary system diseases. Our previous work used proteomics to identify 1643 high-confidence urinary proteins in the urine from a healthy population. Here, we used bioinformatics to construct a cancer-associated protein-protein interaction (PPI) network comprising 16 high-abundance urinary proteins based on the urinary proteome database. As a result, platelet-derived growth factor receptor beta (PDGFRB) was selected for further validation as a candidate biomarker for NMIBC diagnosis and prognosis. Although the levels of urinary PDGFRB showed no significant difference between patients pre- and post-surgery (n = 185, P>0.05), over 3 years of follow-up, urinary PDGFRB was shown to be significantly higher in relapsed patients (n = 68) than in relapse-free patients (n = 117, P<0.001). The levels of urinary PDGFRB were significantly correlated with the risk of 3-year recurrence of NMIBC, and these levels improved the accuracy of a NMIBC recurrence risk prediction model that included age, tumor size, and tumor number (area under the curve, 0.862; 95% CI, 0.809 to 0.914) compared to PDGFR alone. Therefore, we surmise that urinary PDGFRB could serve as a non-invasive biomarker for predicting NMIBC recurrence.

Editor: Hari K. Koul, Louisiana State University Health Sciences center, United States of America

Funding: This work was supported by the Chongqing Key Laboratory for Disease Proteomics Project. The funders had no role in study design, data collection and analysis, decision to publish, or preparation of the manuscript.

Competing Interests: The authors have declared that no competing interests exist.

* E-mail: junwupro1@aliyun.com (JW); huangchibing@medmail.com.cn (CH)

⊙ These authors contributed equally to this work.

Introduction

Bladder cancer is the seventh most prevalent cancer worldwide, and approximately 80% of cases are non-muscle-invasive bladder cancer (NMIBC), while the remaining 20% are muscle-invasive bladder cancer (MIBC)[1–3]. Of all newly diagnosed cases of transitional cell carcinomas, approximately 80% present as non-muscle-invasive tumors (Ta–T1)[3]. For NMIBC, 50–70% of patients will develop disease recurrence within two years of their initial diagnosis[4]. Current clinical and conventional histopathological parameters such as tumor stage, grade and size of tumors, are well studied in terms of providing prognostic information regarding progression to muscle invasion and recurrence. However, none of these factors have proven to be sufficient to predict the diverse behavior of NMIBC. Thus, biomarkers for NMIBC recurrence, which are non-invasive, are urgently required for clinical treatment.

Human urine is one of the major body fluids and is an ideal source for clinical diagnosis, especially for urinary system diseases, as urine can be obtained non-invasively in large quantities[5].

Urinary proteins should be regarded as potential sources of biomarkers for several diseases. Over the past few years, great technological advances have occurred in proteomics, and a large number of proteins in the urinary proteome of healthy people have been identified[6–10]. However, the application of such a urinary protein databases to facilitate identification of biomarkers for diseases has experienced limited progress. Thus far, protein–protein interaction (PPI) data has been widely used for the identification of biomarkers with the assumption that interaction proteins significantly reflect disease status because proteins do not function in isolation, but rather interact with one another. Additionally, they can provide hypotheses such as signaling pathways and other mechanisms that impact the disease outcome. Construction of a PPI network could highlight the disease-associated proteins that have biological function. In this study, we sought to screen potential biomarkers for NMIBC diagnosis and prognosis by constructing a cancer-associated PPI network based on the healthy human urinary proteome, and we revealed that PDGFRB could serve as a prognostic biomarker for NMIBC recurrence.

Table 1. Patient demographics and clinical parameters.

	Relapse	No relapse
Number of patients	68	117
Age ($\leq$ 60/>60)	28/40	52/65
Gender (male/female)	57/11	103/14
Pathological stage Ta/T1	25/43	49/68
Grade (I/II)	24/44	43/74
Unifocal/Multifocal	30/38	75/42
Tumor size ($\leq$ 3 cm/>3 cm)	43/25	96/21
Time to relapse (months)	11.2$\pm$4.3	N/A

Materials and Methods

Ethics statement

The study was approved by the Ethics Committee of the Xinqiao Hospital, Chongqing and adhered to the tenets of the Declaration of Helsinki. In addition, written informed consent was obtained by the patients in this study.

High abundance urinary proteins dataset

Our previous study identified 1641 high-confidence urinary proteins in the healthy population [11]. The definition of a high-abundance protein was arbitrarily set as one with >4 unique peptides and a spectra number in the database of >10. A total of 592 high-abundance urinary proteins were obtained for further bioinformatics analysis (File S2).

Extracellular and plasma membrane proteins were obtained by GO analysis

We used the BiNGO plug-in to find statistically over-represented GO categories in the biologic data as a tool for enrichment analysis of the high-abundance urinary protein dataset. For enrichment analysis, we needed a test dataset (which contained 592 high-abundance urinary proteins) and a reference set of GO annotations for the complete human proteome. The analysis was performed using a "hyper-geometric test", and all GO terms that were significant with P<0.0001 (after correcting for multiple testing using the Benjamini and Hochberg false discovery rate corrections) were selected as over-represented. Then, the proteins that were annotated as "extracellular" and "plasma membrane" were selected for PPI network construction.

PPI network construction

Protein-protein interactions were predicted using the Search Tool for the Retrieval of Interacting Genes/Proteins (STRING) database v9.0 (http://www.string-db.org/). Proteins were linked based on the following six criteria; neighborhood, gene fusion, co-occurrence, co-expression, experimental evidence and existing databases[12].

Cancer-associated proteins in the PPI network were analyzed by KEGG pathway enrichment

We used ClueGO, an easy-to-use Cytoscape plug-in[13], to integrate Gene Ontology (GO) terms as well as the Kyoto encyclopedia of genes and genomes (KEGG)/BioCarta pathways to create a functionally organized GO/pathway term network for the protein network in urine. The enrichment tests for terms and

groups were two-sided (Enrichment/Depletion) tests based on the hyper-geometric distribution, and all cancer-associated terms that were significant with P<0.05 (after correcting for multiple testing using the Benjamini and Hochberg false discovery rate corrections) were selected for further analysis. The Kappa Score Threshold was set to 0.5. ClueGO visualizes the selected terms in a functionally grouped annotation network that reflects the relationships between the terms based on the similarity of their associated proteins.

Study participants

A total of 185 histologically demonstrated NMIBC cases were selected from January 2007 to January 2010. The criteria for study enrollment were as follows: histopathological diagnosis of transitional cell carcinoma of the bladder that was newly diagnosed and untreated, no history of other tumors, and the ability to conduct follow-up. The patients included 160 men and 25 women from 32 to 83 years (mean age, 62.1 years). All patients underwent transurethral resection of bladder tumor (TURBT). All patients with NMIBC received intravesical mitomycin C (MMC) or pirarubicin (THP) instillations once weekly for the first 8 weeks and then monthly up to 1 year. We defined recurrence as the recurrence of primary NMIBC with an equal or lower pathologic stage. Other clinical and pathological features of the enrolled patients are summarized in Table 1. The grade and stage of the patients were defined according to the WHO 1973 criteria for grade and the 2002 TNM classification system.

Urine sample preparation

Morning urine samples were collected daily over the 3 days before primary surgery and over the 3 days after the surgery. The urine samples were stored at −80°C until all samples were collected. Ten milliliters of urine was taken from each sample before surgery and after surgery and pooled together. The urine samples were centrifuged at 10,000 × g for 30 min at 4°C to remove any cellular debris, and the supernatant was concentrated and desalted by using a membrane with a cutoff of 10 kDa. The protein amount in the urine concentrates was measured using a Coomassie Protein Assay Kit (Pierce, Rockford, IL, USA). Soon after, the urine concentrates were frozen at −80°C.

PDGFRB expression analysis on NMIBC tissues

The NMIBC tissues from relapse and relapse-free patients were selected for immunohistochemical validation. All tissues were fixed with 10% formaldehyde and paraffinembedded. The tissues were cut at 4µm in thickness. The antibody for PDGFRB was purchased from Abcam. A two-step immunohistochemical technique was

A.

B.

C.

D.

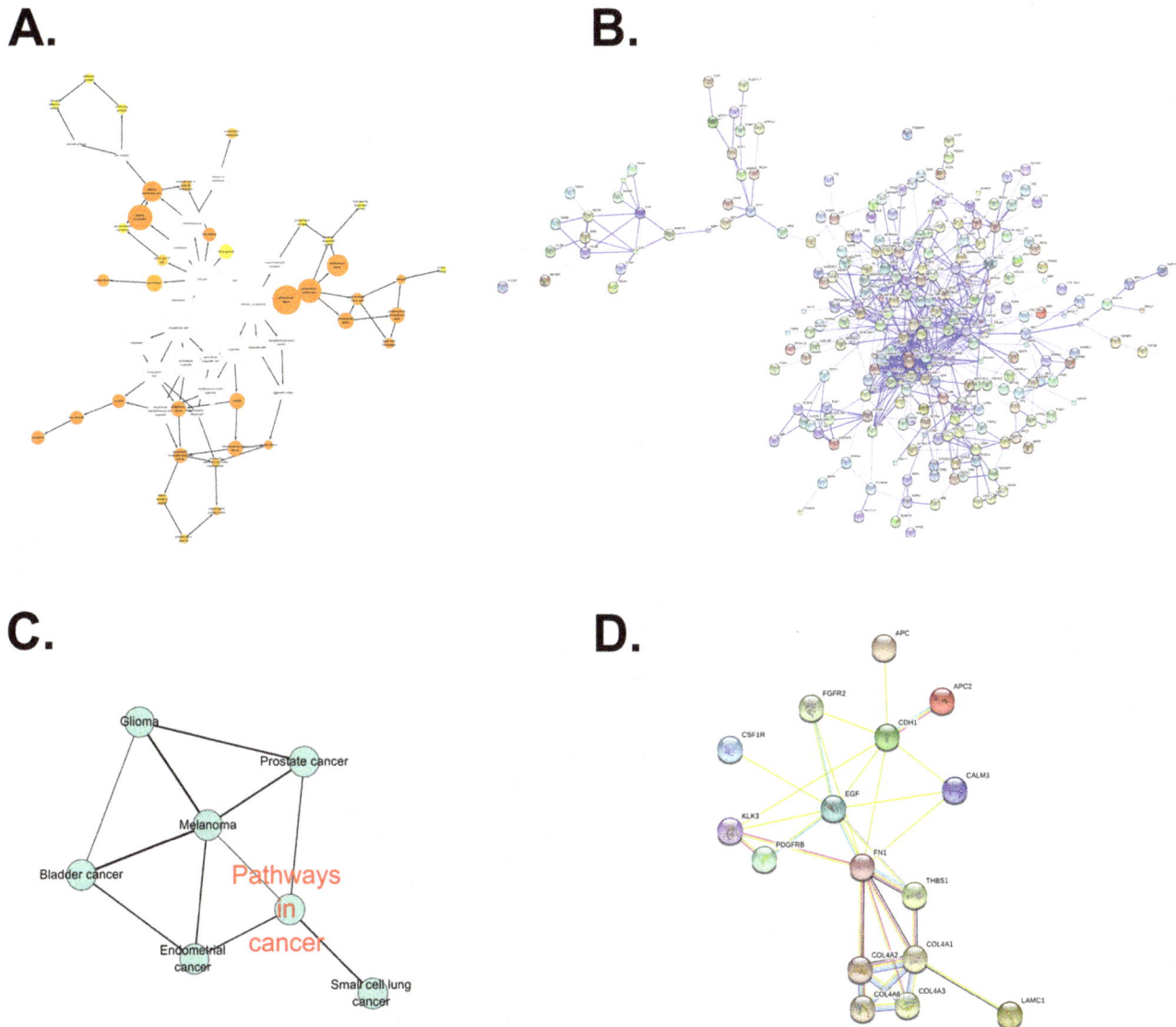

Figure 1. A cancer-associated PPI network in urine was constructed using a bioinformatics approach. (A) A total of 592 high-abundance urinary proteins in our urinary proteome database were selected according to the criteria of having >4 unique peptides and a spectra number >10. Those proteins were analyzed using the BinGO plug-in in Cytoscape software, and 373 proteins were annotated as being "extracellular region" and "plasma membrane." A map of the cellular component is shown. (B). The protein-protein interaction networks of the 373 proteins were constructed by STRING. A PPI network, which was composed of 312 nodes and 1779 interactions with removal of single nodes, was obtained. (C) The PPI network was analyzed by Cytoscape software with the ClueGO+Cluepedia plug-in. Six cancer-associated enriched KEGG terms were obtained and shown. (D) A cancer-associated urinary PPI network comprised of 15 urinary proteins that were associated with the 6 cancer-associated terms were constructed by STRING.

used. Briefly, the sections were dewaxed and hydrated, and then boiled in 10 mM citrate buffer, pH 6.0 for 10 min. Blocking was performed with nonspecific binding with 5% (v/v) bovine serum albumin (BSA) for 10 min. The sections were incubated with PDGFRB Ab (1:200 working dilution) at 4°C for 12 h in a moist chamber. After washing with 0.02M phosphate buffer saline (PBS) pH 7.4 three times, the sections were incubated with secondary antibody conjugated with HRP-labeled polymer (Abcam) at 37 °C for 30 min. The sections were then incubated with liquid DAB substrate-chromogen for 10 min at room temperature, rinsed in distilled water, and counterstained with hematoxylin.

Validation by Western Blot

Approximately 20 μg urinary protein was separated by 12% SDS-PAGE, then transferred to a PVDF membrane (Millipore, USA), and probed with polyclonal rabbit anti-human PDGFRB proteins antibody (1:2000, Abcam, USA), respectively. The blots were labeled with horseradish peroxidase-conjugated secondary antibodies (1:10000), and visualized with enhanced chemiluminescence (ECL) detection system (Pierce Biotech Inc., Rockford, IL).

ELISA

The protein amount in the urine concentrates was measured using a Coomassie Protein Assay Kit (Pierce, Rockford, IL, USA).

Table 2. Cancer-associated KEGG/GO terms.

GOTerm	Nr. Genes	Term P value	Group P value	Associated genes found
Pathways in cancer	15	2.9 E-2	2.0 E-11	[APC, APC2, CDH1, COL4A1, COL4A2, COL4A3, COL4A6, SF1R, CTNNA3, EGF, FGFR2, FN1, KLK3, LAMC1, PDGFRB]
Endometrial cancer	5	1.2 E-2	2.0 E-11	[APC, APC2, CDH1, CTNNA3, EGF]
Glioma	3	2.5 E-1	2.0 E-11	[CALM3, EGF, PDGFRB]
Prostate cancer	4	2.1 E-1	2.0 E-11	[EGF, FGFR2, KLK3, PDGFRB]
Melanoma	3	2.9 E-1	2.0 E-11	[CDH1, EGF, PDGFRB]
Bladder cancer	3	8.1 E-2	2.0 E-11	[CDH1, EGF]
Small cell lung cancer	6	2.7 E-2	2.0 E-11	[COL4A1, COL4A2, COL4A3, COL4A6, FN1, LAMC1]

Human PDGFRB protein was quantified with ELISA kits from Uscn Life Science Inc. (Wuhan, China) according the manufacturer's instructions.

Statistical analysis

An unpaired t-test and one-way ANOVA were used to analyze the correlation between the groups. A stepwise model selection process was used to arrive at a parsimonious model. The logistic regression modeling was employed to describe the relationship between levels of urinary PDGFRB and the risk of breast cancer recurrence and other clinical observations. Receiver operating characteristic (ROC) curves were plotted to evaluate the sensitivity and specificity of the biomarker measurements in predicting the recurrence of NMIBC. Two-tailed P values less than 0.05 were considered significant. Continuous variables are expressed as the mean ± the standard deviation unless otherwise indicated.

Results

Construction of a cancer-associated urinary PPI network based on our previous urinary proteome database

We previously reported that 1641 high-confidence urinary proteins were identified in a healthy human population by four fractionation techniques (in-gel, 2DLC, OFFGEL and mRP) coupled with HPLC-CHIP-MS/MS[11]. Herein, we sought to find non-invasive prognostic biomarker candidates for NMIBC recurrence through bioinformatics analysis of the healthy population urinary proteome. To find urinary protein biomarkers that are suitable for routine clinical examination methods, we first screened for high-abundance urinary proteins in the urinary proteome database, which by our definition had >4 unique peptides and had a spectra number >10. A total of 592 high-abundance urinary proteins were obtained from the urinary proteome database for further analysis (File S2).

To avoid contamination with cellular debris, the proteins that were annotated as "extracellular" and "plasma membrane" among the total urinary proteins were selected by the BiNGO analysis. In total, 544 proteins were linked to at least one annotation term within the GO cellular component. In total, 37 terms exhibited significance (P<0.0001) as being over-represented and under-represented terms compared with the entire list of International Protein Index (IPI) entries. More detailed information regarding the GO analysis is available as File S2. As shown in Figure 1A, in the cellular component category, GO terms related to extracellular proteins such as the extracellular region (269 proteins found), the extracellular space (140), the extracellular matrix (68), and the plasma membrane (197) were over-represented, as

was expected. A total of 373 urinary proteins that were annotated as "extracellular region" and "plasma membrane" were obtained for further PPI network construction (File S2). Because the PPI network is significant to reflect the disease status compared with single proteins, the 373 proteins were used to construct a PPI network through STRING analysis. Single nodes and small components of the PPI network that were initially assembled were removed, and only the largest component was saved as a new PPI network, which was composed of 312 nodes and 1779 interactions (Figure 1B). The PPI network information is described in detail as File S2. To further investigate cancer-associated proteins in this sub-network, the 312 encoded proteins were analyzed using the Cytoscape plug-in ClueGO+CluePedia. An annotation network based on KEGG pathways was created as a group of functionally organized GO/pathway terms network (Figure S1 in File S1). The term network information is described in detail as File S2. Among these term networks, a functionally grouped cancer-associated network is shown in figure 1C. It comprises 6 specific significantly overrepresented terms such as "pathways in cancer", "endometrial cancer", "prostate cancer", "glioma", "melanoma", "bladder cancer" and "small cell lung cancer". The information regarding the cancer terms in the associated KEGG network is described in detail in Table 2. Furthermore, a total of 15 proteins, which were associated with all 6 cancer terms (Table 3), were used to construct a cancer-associated urinary PPI network (Figure 1D). It was further observed that EGF and CDH1 in the PPI network were annotated as being bladder cancer-associated proteins, and both receptor FGFR2 and PDGFRB could interact with EGF (Table 3). Because PDGFRB/EGFR heterodimers were reported to express on bladder cancer cells[14], and the EGF/EGFR pathway played an important role in bladder cancer development[15,16], PDGFRB was selected for further validation as a candidate biomarker of bladder cancer.

There were no significant differences of urinary PDGFRB between patients pre- and post-surgery

To confirm the preliminary informatics result, urine samples from 185 subjects who were confirmed to have NMIBC (Table 1) were collected before and after surgery. The urinary PDGFRB levels were examined by ELISA. The results showed that the levels of urinary PDGFRB decreased (300.1 ng/mg before surgery vs. 287.23 ng/mg after surgery), but the difference was not significant (P = 0.0607) (Figure 2). This indicated that urinary PDGFRB could not be majorly derived from NMIBC tissue and could not serve as a good early diagnosis biomarker for NMIBC.

Table 3. Cancer-associated urinary PPI network.

#node1	node2	cooccurence	homology	coexpression	experimental	knowledge	textmining	combined_score
COL4A1	THBS1	0	0	0.104	0.62	0	0.29	0.724
COL4A3	COL4A1	0.525	0.936	0	0	0.9	0.66	0.907
FGFR2	EGF	0	0	0	0	0.8	0.528	0.899
COL4A1	COL4A2	0.525	0.927	0.776	0.999	0.9	0.87	0.999
COL4A6	COL4A2	0.525	0.933	0	0	0.9	0.675	0.907
FN1	KLK3	0	0	0	0.621	0	0.374	0.746
CSF1R	EGF	0	0	0	0	0	0.43	0.43
EGF	THBS1	0	0.442	0	0	0	0.885	0.521
FGFR2	FN1	0	0	0	0	0	0.43	0.43
COL4A1	COL4A6	0.525	0.925	0	0	0.9	0.672	0.908
COL4A3	COL4A6	0.525	0.92	0	0	0.9	0.791	0.909
CDH1	APC	0	0	0	0	0	0.67	0.669
COL4A3	COL4A2	0.525	0.917	0	0	0.9	0.718	0.909
COL4A1	LAMC1	0	0	0.215	0	0	0.34	0.447
CDH1	APC2	0	0	0	0.769	0.72	0.176	0.939
COL4A3	FN1	0	0	0	0.62	0	0.341	0.732
EGF	CDH1	0	0	0	0	0	0.927	0.927
COL4A1	FN1	0	0	0.18	0.62	0	0.379	0.779
EGF	PDGFRB	0	0	0	0	0.8	0.412	0.874
FN1	THBS1	0	0.406	0.13	0.846	0.72	0.917	0.98
COL4A2	FN1	0	0	0.163	0.62	0	0.275	0.737
KLK3	CDH1	0	0	0	0	0	0.469	0.469
FN1	EGF	0	0	0	0	0.9	0.946	0.994
FN1	CDH1	0	0	0	0	0	0.752	0.752
KLK3	EGF	0	0	0	0	0	0.463	0.462
FGFR2	CDH1	0	0	0	0	0	0.467	0.467
KLK3	PDGFRB	0	0	0	0.621	0	0.068	0.623
COL4A6	FN1	0	0	0	0.62	0	0.148	0.654

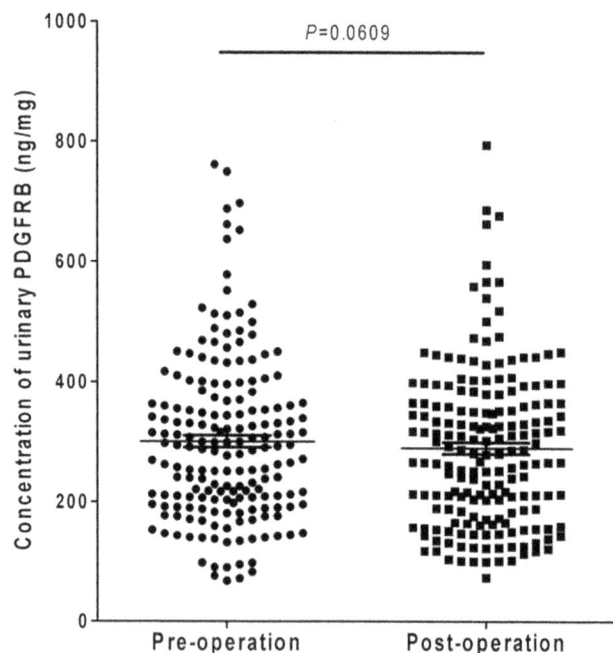

Figure 2. Determination of urinary PDGFRB concentrations in NMIBC patients pre- and post-surgery by ELISA. There was no significant difference between the levels of urinary PDGFRB in NMIBC patients pre-surgery and post-surgery (n = 185) (P = 0.067).

Correlation of the levels of urinary PDGFRB and recurrence of NMIBC

To know whether urinary PDGFRB could be associated with a relapse of NMIBC, a 3-year follow-up study on the 185 NMIBC patients was conducted. The follow-up data showed that among the 185 NMIBC patients, 68 (36.8%) were later found to have recurrence after primary surgery (Table 1). In the relapsed group, the median level of urinary PDGFRB was 395.3 ng/mg (inter-quartile range 306.65 to 440.01 ng/mg total urinary protein), while it was 245 ng/mg (interquartile range 175.12 to 307.16 ng/mg total urinary protein) for the relapse-free group (Figure 3A, P< 0.0001).Indeed, the PDGFRB expression in urine of patient with relapse was confirmed to be significantly increased than that without relapse in 3 years follow-up by Western Blot (Figure S2A in File S1). However, there were no significant differences of the PDGFRB expression on cancer tissue between the patients with relapse and relapse-free in 3 years follow-up by IHC (Figure S2B and S2C in File S1).

A logistic regression model was used to estimate the relationship between urinary PDGFRB and other clinical observations. Significant positive associations were observed between urinary PDGFRB levels and tumor size (P = 0.03) and age (P = 0.019) (Table 4). However, there were no significant associations between urinary PDGFRB and gender, pathological stage, or grade (Table 4). The relationship between urinary PDGFRB and the risk of breast cancer recurrence was further estimated. The result showed that the correlation between urinary PDGFRB levels and the risk of breast cancer recurrence was statistically significant (Table 5, coefficient factor was −1.274, P<0.001). Tumor size (coefficient, −1.193; P = 0.009) and tumor number (coefficient, −0.986; P = 0.022) were also associated with an increased risk of NMIBC recurrence (Table 5). However, other clinical observations such as age, gender, pathological stage, and grade

were not significantly associated with the risk of NMIBC recurrence (Table 5).

ROC curves were constructed for the clinical factors and PDGFRB. The area under the curve (AUC) of the ROC curve for PDGFRB alone was 0.826 (95% CI, 0.768 to 0.884) (Figure 3B). The AUC of age, tumor size, and tumor number combined was 0.636 (95% CI, 0.552 to 0.721) (Figure 3C). Inclusion of PDGFRB in this model increased the AUC to 0.862 (95% CI, 0.809 to 0.914) (Figure 3D). Using a threshold of 324.12 ng/mg, the sensitivity was 70.6%, while the specificity was 81.2%. When PDGFRB, age, tumor size, and tumor number were combined, the sensitivity increased to 82.7%, and the specificity increased to 88.5%.

Discussion

The urinary proteome could reflect the urinary system microenvironment, which might play a very important role in urinary system tumor development and progression. Screening the urine for non-invasive biomarkers for bladder cancer is promising. Here, we constructed a cancer-associated PPI network comprised of 15 high-abundance urinary proteins using informatics approach to analyze the urinary proteome of a healthy population (11). Interestingly, of the 15 proteins, 9 (CTNNA3, COL4A6, KLK3, APC, APC2, FGFR2, PDGFRB, EGF, and COL4A2) were identified as being high-abundance proteins in the urinary proteome, but these were not detected or identified as being low abundance proteins in the plasma proteome[17]. This indicates that these proteins were majorly derived from the urinary system cell secretion rather than from plasma and could reflect the characteristic microenvironment of urinary system, which in turn could provide valuable information about the prognosis of a urinary system tumor. Among the 9 proteins, EGF, FGFR2, KLK3, and PDGFRB were associated with urinary system cancer according to the KEGG pathway analysis. Indeed, EGF/ EGFR[18], FGFR2 [4,19], KLK3[20–23], and PDGFRB[14] were reported to play important roles in urinary system cancer development and progression. It is well known that the EGF/ EGFR pathway plays a critical role in bladder cancer development, progression and recurrence. Although urinary EGFR could serve as a promising prognostic biomarker candidate for bladder cancer, it was identified as a low abundance urinary protein (1 unique peptide and <10 spectrums) and in practice was hard to measure by ELISA (data not shown). Similar to EGFR, FGFR2 and PDGFRB could have the ability to bind EGF (Table 3, STRING database) and transduce the PI3K and MAPK signal pathways[24,25]. Moreover, PDGFRB rather than FGFR2 could form a heterodimer with EGFR on bladder cancer cells, and this could induce resistance to anti-EGFR therapy for bladder cancer[14]. Together, it is reasonable to assume that PDGFRB is an important receptor for bladder cancer biological progression, and it should serve as a potential biomarker for NMIBC diagnosis and/or prognosis.

The urine is derived from the plasma that is ultrafiltrated by the kidney to eliminate waste products. Unlike serum protein, urinary protein concentration varies with urine dilution. Moreover, the urinary protein from the same individual varies at different times due to the effect of exercise, diet, lifestyle and other factors[10,26–28]. In this study, the variation from urine dilution was eliminated through normalization to total protein, and the variation over time was sufficiently controlled for by using pooled morning urine samples from an individual patient over 3 days before and 3 days after primary surgery (samples were collected once per day). It is known that urinary protein differs by gender and age[26]. Urinary

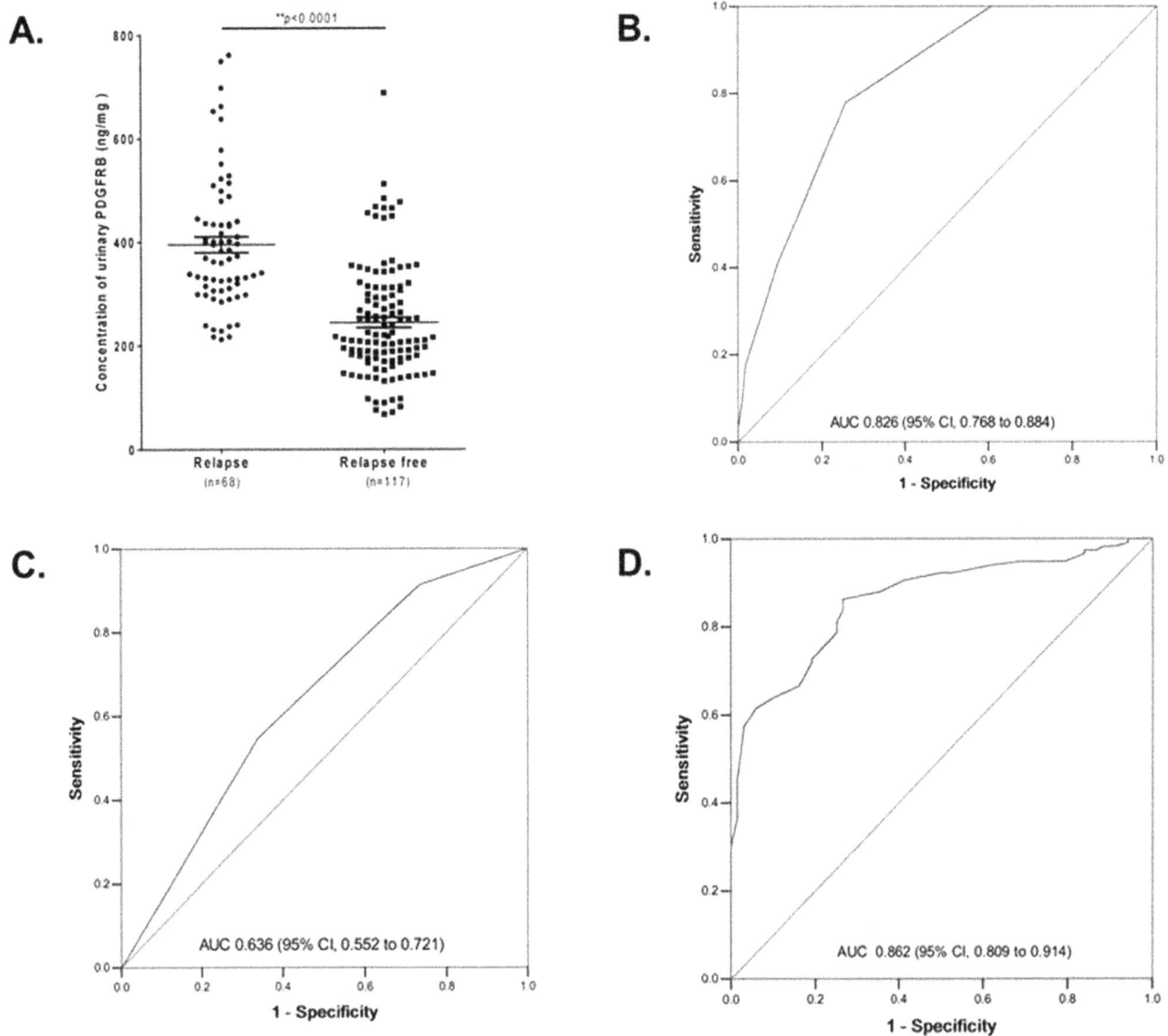

Figure 3. Pre-validation of urinary PDGFRB as a biomarker for predicting the recurrence of NMIBC. (A) Comparison of the level of urinary PDGFRB in relapsed (n = 68) and relapse-free (n = 117) patients with NMIBC. The level of urinary PDGFRB was significantly lower in the patients with recurrence than those without recurrence (P<0.001). (B) The receiver operating characteristics (ROC) curve of urinary PDGFRB. The AUC was 0.826 (95% CI, 0.768 to 0.884). (C) The AUC of age, tumor size, and tumor number combined was 0.636 (95% CI, 0.552 to 0.721). (D) Inclusion of PDGFRB in this model increased the AUC to 0.862 (95% CI, 0.809 to 0.914).

PDGFRB was observed to be significantly associated with age rather than gender in this study (Table 4). In addition, urinary PDGFRB was significantly positively associated with tumor size (Table 4). In 183 NMIBC patients, the level of urinary PDGFRB was increased in patients with a large tumor size (>3 cm; 329.6 ± 22.10 ng/mL, n = 46) compared with those with a small tumor size (≤3 cm; 290.4 ± 11.08 ng/mL, n = 139) (Figure S3 in File S1, P = 0.0907). This suggests that levels of urinary PDGFRB increase with tumor size. Furthermore, there was no significant difference between pre- and post-surgery NMIBC patients (Figure 2, P = 0.0607), which indicates that urinary PDGFRB could not serve as an effective early diagnostic biomarker for NMIBC. In an additional follow-up study, it was observed that the levels of urinary PDGFRB in subjects with relapse were

significantly higher than those without recurrence (Fig 3A), and these were also correlated to the risk of 3-year cancer recurrence. The corresponding AUC was 0.826 (Figure 3B; 95% CI, 0.768 to 0.884). Moreover, along with clinical characteristics such as age, tumor size, and tumor number, the AUC increased to 0.862 (Figure 3D; 95% CI, 0.809 to 0.914), which suggests that urinary PDGFRB is a risk factor for NMIBC recurrence and could serve as potential non-invasive biomarker for predicting the recurrence of NMIBC.

Conclusion

In summary, we for the first time showed that urinary PDGFRB could serve as a non-invasive biomarker for prediction of NMIBC

Table 4. Correlation between PDGFRA expression and clinicopathologic factors.

Variables	Case	PDGFRB levels (ng/mg total urinary protein)									P value
		0–99	100–199	200–299	300–399	400–499	500–599	600–699	700–799	
Gender		9	37	56	44	25	7	5	2	0.205
Female	25	0	6	10	3	5	1	0	0	
Male	160	9	31	46	41	20	6	5	2	
Age (years)										0.030
≤60	81	1	17	25	18	15	5	0	0	
>60	104	8	20	31	26	10	2	5	2	
Tumor size (cm)										0.019
≤3	139	7	34	38	30	22	4	4	0	
>3	46	2	3	18	14	3	3	1	2	
Tumor number										0.235
Unifocal	105	6	25	30	23	12	6	3	0	
Multifocal	80	3	12	26	21	13	1	2	2	
Grade										0.837
I	67	4	13	18	14	12	4	1	1	
II	118	5	24	38	30	13	3	4	1	
T stage										0.717
Ta	74	3	18	24	14	10	3	1	1	
T1	111	6	19	32	30	15	4	4	1	
Recurrence										<0.01
Positive	68	0	0	15	25	16	6	4	2	
Negative	117	9	37	41	19	9	1	1	0	

NOTE: A logistic regression model was used to estimate the odds of PDGFRB adjusted for all of the variables listed in the table.

Table 5. Relationship between the biomarker, clinical characteristics and the risk of NMIBC recurrence.

Variable	Coefficient	SE	P
Level of urinary PDGFRB	−1.274	.213	<0.001
Gender	−.836	.547	.127
Age	−.548	.402	.172
Tumor size	−1.193	.456	.009
Grade	.042	.476	.930
Pathological stage	.594	.484	.220
Tumor number	−.986	.431	.022

NOTE: A logistic regression model was used to estimate the odds of NMIBC recurrence adjusted for all of the variables listed in the table.

recurrence. Validation by multiple clinical centers is required for further application in clinical settings.

Supporting Information

File S1 Contains Supporting Figures. Figure S1 Example of network. Figure S2 Validation of relapse. Figure S3 Determination of urinary PDGFRB. **Figure S1. The PPI network was analyzed by Cytoscape software with the ClueGO+Cluepedia plug-in.** The enriched KEGG terms were shown. **Figure S2. Validation of PDGFRB expression in urine and on tumor tissues of NMIBC patients with relapse and relapse-free.** The expression of PDGFRB in urine of NMIBC patients with relapse and relapse-free was analyzed by Western Blotting (A). The expression of PDGFRB on tumor tissue of NMIBC patients with relapse (B) and relapse-free (C) was analyzed by IHC. A total of 50 cancer tissues from 27 relapsed and 23 relapse-free patients were evaluated through immunohistochemistry. There were no significant differences of PDGFR expression

on cancer tissues between relapsed and relapse-free groups. The representative 6 samples from relapsed and relapse-free patients were showed in 3A and 3B, respectively. **Figure S3. Determination of urinary PDGFRB concentrations in NMIBC patients with a large and small tumor size by ELISA.** In 183 NMIBC patients, the level of urinary PDGFRB was increased in patients with a large tumor size (>3 cm) compared with those with a small tumor size (≤3 cm)(P = 0.0906).

File S2 Supplemental Data.

Author Contributions

Conceived and designed the experiments: WFH JW CBH. Performed the experiments: JYF YJS YW XRZ. Analyzed the data: JYF WFH GXL YJS. Contributed reagents/materials/analysis tools: JYF WFH JW CBH RJS. Wrote the paper: WFH CBH JW RJS.

References

1. Cheung G, Sahai A, Billia M, Dasgupta P, Khan MS (2013) Recent advances in the diagnosis and treatment of bladder cancer. BMC Med 11: 13.
2. Smith ZL, Christodouleas JP, Keefe SM, Malkowicz SB, Guzzo TJ (2013) Bladder preservation in the treatment of muscle-invasive bladder cancer (MIBC): a review of the literature and a practical approach to therapy. BJU Int 112: 13–25.
3. Fauconnet S, Bernardini S, Lascombe I, Boiteux G, Clairotte A, et al. (2009) Expression analysis of VEGF-A and VEGF-B: relationship with clinicopathological parameters in bladder cancer. Oncol Rep 21: 1495–1504.
4. Proctor I, Stoeber K, Williams GH (2010) Biomarkers in bladder cancer. Histopathology 57: 1–13.
5. Decramer S, Gonzalez de Peredo A, Breuil B, Mischak H, Monsarrat B, et al. (2008) Urine in clinical proteomics. Mol Cell Proteomics 7: 1850–1862.
6. Adachi J, Kumar C, Zhang Y, Olsen JV, Mann M (2006) The human urinary proteome contains more than 1500 proteins, including a large proportion of membrane proteins. Genome Biol 7: R80.
7. Marimuthu A, O'Meally RN, Chaerkady R, Subbannayya Y, Nanjappa V, et al. (2011) A comprehensive map of the human urinary proteome. J Proteome Res 10: 2734–2743.
8. Li QR, Fan KX, Li RX, Dai J, Wu CC, et al. (2010) A comprehensive and non-prefractionation on the protein level approach for the human urinary proteome: touching phosphorylation in urine. Rapid Commun Mass Spectrom 24: 823–832.
9. Kentsis A, Monigatti F, Dorff K, Campagne F, Bachur R, et al. (2009) Urine proteomics for profiling of human disease using high accuracy mass spectrometry. Proteomics Clin Appl 3: 1052–1061.
10. Nagaraj N, Mann M (2011) Quantitative analysis of the intra- and inter-individual variability of the normal urinary proteome. J Proteome Res 10: 637–645.
11. He W, Huang C, Luo G, Dal Pra I, Feng J, et al. (2012) A stable panel comprising 18 urinary proteins in the human healthy population. Proteomics 12: 1059–1072.
12. Franceschini A, Szklarczyk D, Frankild S, Kuhn M, Simonovic M, et al. (2013) STRING v9.1: protein-protein interaction networks, with increased coverage and integration. Nucleic Acids Res 41: D808–815.
13. Bindea G, Mlecnik B, Hackl H, Charoentong P, Tosolini M, et al. (2009) ClueGO: a Cytoscape plug-in to decipher functionally grouped gene ontology and pathway annotation networks. Bioinformatics 25: 1091–1093.
14. Black PC, Brown GA, Dinney CP, Kassouf W, Inamoto T, et al. (2011) Receptor heterodimerization: a new mechanism for platelet-derived growth factor induced resistance to anti-epidermal growth factor receptor therapy for bladder cancer. J Urol 185: 693–700.
15. Mason RA, Morlock EV, Karagas MR, Kelsey KT, Marsit CJ, et al. (2009) EGFR pathway polymorphisms and bladder cancer susceptibility and prognosis. Carcinogenesis 30: 1155–1160.
16. Theodorescu D, Laderoute KR, Gulding KM (1998) Epidermal growth factor receptor-regulated human bladder cancer motility is in part a phosphatidylinositol 3-kinase-mediated process. Cell Growth Differ 9: 919–928.
17. Farrah T, Deutsch EW, Omenn GS, Campbell DS, Sun Z, et al. (2011) A high-confidence human plasma proteome reference set with estimated concentrations in PeptideAtlas. Mol Cell Proteomics 10: M110 006353.
18. Neal DE, Marsh C, Bennett MK, Abel PD, Hall RR, et al. (1985) Epidermal-growth-factor receptors in human bladder cancer: comparison of invasive and superficial tumours. Lancet 1: 366–368.
19. Marzioni D, Lorenzi T, Mazzucchelli R, Capparuccia L, Morroni M, et al. (2009) Expression of basic fibroblast growth factor, its receptors and syndecans in bladder cancer. Int J Immunopathol Pharmacol 22: 627–638.
20. Thompson IM, Goodman PJ, Tangen CM, Lucia MS, Miller GJ, et al. (2003) The influence of finasteride on the development of prostate cancer. N Engl J Med 349: 215–224.
21. Risk MC, Lin DW (2009) New and novel markers for prostate cancer detection. Curr Urol Rep 10: 179–186.
22. Laxman B, Morris DS, Yu J, Siddiqui J, Cao J, et al. (2008) A first-generation multiplex biomarker analysis of urine for the early detection of prostate cancer. Cancer Res 68: 645–649.

23. Roobol MJ, Haese A, Bjartell A (2011) Tumour markers in prostate cancer III: biomarkers in urine. Acta Oncol 50 Suppl 1: 85–89.

24. Tamborini E, Virdis E, Negri T, Orsenigo M, Brich S, et al. (2010) Analysis of receptor tyrosine kinases (RTKs) and downstream pathways in chordomas. Neuro Oncol 12: 776–789.

25. Ranzato E, Martinotti S, Burlando B (2013) Honey exposure stimulates wound repair of human dernal fibroblasts. Burn Trauma 1:32–38.

26. Shao C, Wang Y, Gao Y (2011) Applications of urinary proteomics in biomarker discovery. Sci China Life Sci.

27. Thongboonkerd V, Chutipongtanate S, Kanlaya R (2006) Systematic evaluation of sample preparation methods for gel-based human urinary proteomics: quantity, quality, and variability. J Proteome Res 5: 183–191.

28. Sun W, Chen Y, Li F, Zhang L, Yang R, et al. Dynamic urinary proteomic analysis reveals stable proteins to be potential biomarkers.

Permissions

The contributors of this book come from diverse backgrounds, making this book a truly international effort. This book will bring forth new frontiers with its revolutionizing research information and detailed analysis of the nascent developments around the world.

We would like to thank all the contributing authors for lending their expertise to make the book truly unique. They have played a crucial role in the development of this book. Without their invaluable contributions this book wouldn't have been possible. They have made vital efforts to compile up to date information on the varied aspects of this subject to make this book a valuable addition to the collection of many professionals and students.

This book was conceptualized with the vision of imparting up-to-date information and advanced data in this field. To ensure the same, a matchless editorial board was set up. Every individual on the board went through rigorous rounds of assessment to prove their worth. After which they invested a large part of their time researching and compiling the most relevant data for our readers.

The editorial board has been involved in producing this book since its inception. They have spent rigorous hours researching and exploring the diverse topics which have resulted in the successful publishing of this book. They have passed on their knowledge of decades through this book. To expedite this challenging task, the publisher supported the team at every step. A small team of assistant editors was also appointed to further simplify the editing procedure and attain best results for the readers.

Apart from the editorial board, the designing team has also invested a significant amount of their time in understanding the subject and creating the most relevant covers. They scrutinized every image to scout for the most suitable representation of the subject and create an appropriate cover for the book.

The publishing team has been an ardent support to the editorial, designing and production team. Their endless efforts to recruit the best for this project, has resulted in the accomplishment of this book. They are a veteran in the field of academics and their pool of knowledge is as vast as their experience in printing. Their expertise and guidance has proved useful at every step. Their uncompromising quality standards have made this book an exceptional effort. Their encouragement from time to time has been an inspiration for everyone.

The publisher and the editorial board hope that this book will prove to be a valuable piece of knowledge for researchers, students, practitioners and scholars across the globe.

List of Contributors

Moniek M. Vedder, Esther W. de Bekker-Grob and Ewout W. Steyerberg
Department of Public Health, Erasmus Medical Centre, Rotterdam, the Netherlands

Mirari Márquez and Nuria Malats
Genetic and Molecular Epidemiology Group, Spanish National Cancer Research Centre (CNIO), Madrid, Spain

Malu L. Calle
Systems Biology Department, University of Vic, Vic, Barcelona, Spain

Lars Dyrskjøt and Torben F. Ørntoft
Department of Molecular Medicine, Aarhus University Hospital, Aarhus, Denmark

Manoils Kogevinas
Centre for Research in Environmental Epidemiology, Municipal Institute of Medical Research, Barcelona, Spain

Ulrika Segersten and Per-Uno Malmström
Department of Surgical Sciences, Uppsala University, Uppsala, Sweden

Ferran Algaba
Department of Pathology, Fundació Puigvert-University Autonomous, Barcelona, Spain

Willemien Beukers and Ellen Zwarthoff
Department of Pathology, Erasmus Medical Centre, Rotterdam, the Netherlands

Francisco X. Real
Epithelial Carcinogenesis Group, Spanish National Cancer Research Centre (CNIO), Madrid, Spain
Department of Experimental and Health Sciences, Universitat Pompeu Fabra, Barcelona, Spain

Cherith N. Reid, Mark W. Ruddock and John V. Lamont
Molecular Biology, Randox Laboratories, Crumlin, Northern Ireland

Michael Stevenson
Department of Epidemiology and Public Health, Queens University Belfast; Belfast, Northern Ireland

Funso Abogunrin, Frank Emmert-Streib and Kate E. Williamson
Centre for Cancer Research and Cell Biology, Queens University Belfast, Belfast, Northern Ireland

Nadine Ratert and Klaus Jung
Department of Urology, University Hospital Charité, Berlin, Germany
Berlin Institute for Urologic Research, Berlin, Germany

Hellmuth-Alexander Meyer
Department of Urology, University Hospital Charité, Berlin, Germany
Institute of Physiology, University Hospital Charité, Berlin, Germany

Monika Jung, Kurt Miller and Steffen Weikert
Department of Urology, University Hospital Charité, Berlin, Germany

Hans-Joachim Mollenkopf and Ina Wagner
Max Planck Institute for Infection Biology, Berlin, Germany

Ergin Kilic
Institute of Pathology, University Hospital Charité, Berlin, Germany

Andreas Erbersdobler
Institute of Pathology, University Rostock, Rostock, Germany

Tadeusz Majewski, Jolanta Bondaruk and Bogdan Czerniak
Department of Pathology, The University of Texas MD Anderson Cancer Center, Houston, Texas, United States of America

Philippe E. Spiess, Peter Black, Herbert Barton Grossman and Colin P. Dinney
Department of Urology, The University of Texas MD Anderson Cancer Center, Houston, Texas, United States of America

Charlotte Clarke
Ciphergen Biosystems, Inc., Fremont, California, United States of America

William Benedict
Department of Genitourinary Medical Oncology, The University of Texas MD Anderson Cancer Center, Houston, Texas, United States of America

Kuang S. Tang
Department of Biostatistics and Applied Math, The University of Texas MD Anderson Cancer Center, Houston, Texas, United States of America

Yong Wang, He Wang, Wei Zhang, Mei Li, Qiang Fu, Wei Xue, Yong Hua Lei, Jing Yu Gao, Juan Ying Wang and Xiao Ping Gao
Department of Urology, Tangdu Hospital, Fourth Military Medical University, Xi'an, Shaanxi, China

Chen Shao, Jian Lin Yuan and Yun Tao Zhang
Department of Urology, Xijing Hospital, Fourth Military Medical University, Xi'an, Shaanxi, China

Peng Xu
Department of Medical and Training Department, Tangdu Hospital, Fourth Military Medical University, Xi'an, Shaanxi, China

Chang Hong Shi
Department of Experimental Animal, Fourth Military Medical University, Xi'an, Shaanxi, China

Jian Guo Shi
Department of Cancer Research Institute, Fourth Military Medical University, Xi'an, Shaanxi, China

Jin Qing Li
Department of Plastic Surgery, Tangdu Hospital, Fourth Military Medical University, Xi'an, Shaanxi, China

Jun Lin, Yi Lu and Yichen Zhu
Department of Urology, Beijing Friendship Hospital Affiliated to Capital Medical University, Beijing, P.R China

Qiang Zhang, Wenrui Xue, Yue Xu and Xiaopeng Hu
Department of Urology, Beijing Chao-Yang HospitalAffiliated to Capital Medical University, Beijing, P.R China

Jonathan A. Ewald, Tracy M. Downs and William A. Ricke
Department of Urology, University of Wisconsin School of Medicine and Public Health, Madison, Wisconsin, United States of America
America University of Wisconsin Carbone Cancer Center, Madison, Wisconsin, United States of America

Jeremy P. Cetnar
Department of Medicine, Hematology/Oncology Unit, University of Wisconsin School of Medicine and Public Health, Madison, Wisconsin, United States of America University of Wisconsin Carbone Cancer Center, Madison, Wisconsin, United States of America

Maciej J. Czachorowski, André F. S. Amaral and Núria Malats
Genetic and Molecular Epidemiology Group, Spanish National Cancer Research Centre (CNIO), Madrid, Spain

Santiago Montes-Moreno
Servicio de Anatomía Patológica, Hospital Universitario Marqués de Valdecilla, Santander, Spain

Josep Lloreta
Institut Municipal d'Investigació Mèdica – Hospital del Mar, Barcelona, Spain
Departament de Patologia, Hospital del Mar – Parc de Salut Mar, Barcelona, Spain
Departament de Ciències Experimentals i de la Salut, Universitat Pompeu Fabra, Barcelona, Spain

Alfredo Carrato
Hospital General Universitario de Elche, Elche, Spain
Hospital Ramon y Cajal, Madrid, Spain

Adonina Tardón
Universidad de Oviedo, Oviedo, Spain

Manuel M. Morente
Tumor Bank Unit, Spanish National Cancer Research Centre (CNIO), Madrid, Spain

Manolis Kogevinas
Centre de Recerca en Epidemiologia Ambiental (CREAL), Barcelona, Spain

Francisco X. Real
Departament de Ciències Experimentals i de la Salut, Universitat Pompeu Fabra, Barcelona, Spain
Epithelial Carcinogenesis Group, Spanish National Cancer Research Centre

Jose Joao Mansure, Roland Nassim, Simone Chevalier, Konrad Szymanski, Joice Rocha, Saad Aldousari and Wassim Kassouf
McGill Urologic Oncology Research, Division of Urology, McGill University Health Center, Montreal, Quebec, Canada

Junhua Luo, Wang He, Hao Yu and Jian Huang
Department of Urology, Sun Yat-sen Memorial Hospital, Sun Yat-sen University, Guangzhou, China

Qingqing Cai
Department of Internal Medicine, Cancer Center, Sun Yat-sen University, Guangzhou, China

Wei Wang
Department of Urology, Guangzhou General Hospital of Guangzhou Military Command (Guangzhou Liuhuaqiao Hospital), Guangzhou, China

Hui Huang
Department of Cardiology, Sun Yat-sen Memorial Hospital, Sun Yat-sen University, Guangzhou, China

Hong Zeng
Department of Pathology, Sun Yat-sen Memorial Hospital, Sun Yat-sen University, Guangzhou, China

Weixi Deng
Lin Bai-xin Research Center, Sun Yat-sen Memorial Hospital, Sun Yat-sen University, Guangzhou, China

Eddie Chan and Chi-fai NG
Division of Urology, Department of Surgery, The Chinese University of Hong Kong, Hong Kong, China

Tianxin Lin
Department of Urology, Sun Yat-sen Memorial Hospital, Sun Yat-sen University, Guangzhou, China
Lin Bai-xin Research Center, Sun Yat-sen Memorial Hospital, Sun Yat-sen University, Guangzhou, China

Valérie M. Laurent and Claude Verdier
Univ. Grenoble Alpes, LIPHY, F-38000, Grenoble, France
CNRS, LIPHY, F-38000, Grenoble, France

Alain Duperray and Vinoth Sundar Rajan
INSERM, IAB, F-38000, Grenoble, France
Univ. Grenoble Alpes, IAB, F-38000, Grenoble, France
CHU de Grenoble, IAB, F-38000, Grenoble, France

Xin Xu, Jian Wu, Yeqing Mao, Yi Zhu, Zhenghui Hu, Xianglai Xu, Yiwei Lin, Hong Chen, Xiangyi Zheng, Jie Qin and Liping Xie
Department of Urology, First Affiliated Hospital, Zhejiang University, Hangzhou, Zhejiang Province, China

Marco Genua, Shi-Qiong Xu, Leonard G. Gomella and Andrea Morrione
Endocrine Mechanisms and Hormone Action Program, Department of Urology, Kimmel Cancer Center, Thomas Jefferson University, Philadelphia, Pennsylvania, United States of America

Simone Buraschi, Stephen C. Peiper and Renato V. Iozzo
Cancer Cell Biology and Signaling Program, Department of Pathology, Anatomy and Cell Biology, Kimmel Cancer Center, Thomas Jefferson University, Philadelphia, Pennsylvania, United States of America

Antonino Belfiore
Endocrinology, Department of Health, University of Catanzaro, Catanzaro, Italy

Li Jiang, Xiao Xiao, Jin Ren, YongYong Tang, HongQing Weng, Qi Yang and Wei Tang
Department of Urology, The First Affiliated Hospital of Chongqing Medical University, Chongqing, China

MingJun Wu
Institute of Life Science, Chongqing Medical University, Chongqing, China

Laura Grau and Marta Sánchez-Carbayo
Tumor Markers Group, Spanish National Cancer Research Center, Madrid, Spain

Jose L. Luque-Garcia
Department of Analytical Chemistry, Complutense University of Madrid, Madrid, Spain

Pilar González-Peramato
Pathology Department, Hospital Universitario La Paz, Madrid, Spain

Dan Theodorescu
Mellon Urologic Cancer Institute, University of Virginia, Charlottesville, Virginia, United States of America

Joan Palou
Urology Department, Fundacio Puigvert, Barcelona, Spain

Jesus M. Fernandez-Gomez
Urology Department, Hospital Central de Asturias, Oviedo, Spain

Maturada Patchsung, Chanchai Boonla, Thasinas Dissayabutra and Piyaratana Tosukhowong
Department of Biochemistry, Faculty of Medicine, Chulalongkorn University, Bangkok, Thailand

Passakorn Amnattrakul
Department of Surgery, Faculty of Medicine, Chulalongkorn University, Bangkok, Thailand

Apiwat Mutirangura
Department of Anatomy, Faculty of Medicine, Chulalongkorn University, Bangkok, Thailand

Yasuyoshi Miyata, Shin-ichi Watanabe, Yuji Sagara, Kensuke Mitsunari, Tomohiro Matsuo, Kojiro Ohba and Hideki Sakai
Department of Nephro-Urology, Nagasaki University Graduate School of Biomedical Sciences, Nagasaki, Japan

Stefano Porru, Angela Carta and Cecilia Arici
Department of Medical-Surgical Specialties, Radiological Sciences and Public Health, Section of Public Health and Human Sciences, University of Brescia, Brescia, Italy

Sofia Pavanello and Giuseppe Mastrangelo
Department of Cardiac, Thoracic, and Vascular Sciences, Unit of Occupational Medicine, University of Padova, Padova, Italy

Claudio Simeone
Department of Medical-Surgical Specialties, Radiological Sciences and Public Health, Section of Surgical Specialties, University of Brescia, Brescia, Italy

Alberto Izzotti
Department of Health Sciences, University of Genoa, Italy/Mutagenesis Unit, IRCCS Hospital-University San Martino Company – IST National Institute for Cancer Research, Genoa, Italy

Anne J. Grotenhuis
Department for Health Evidence, Radboud University Medical Center, Nijmegen, The Netherlands

Aleksandra M. Dudek, Gerald W. Verhaegh and J. Alfred Witjes
Department of Urology, Radboud University Medical Center, Nijmegen, The Netherlands

Katja K. Aben
Department for Health Evidence, Radboud University Medical Center, Nijmegen, The Netherlands
Comprehensive Cancer Center The Netherlands, Utrecht, The Netherlands

Saskia L. van der Marel
Department of Human Genetics, Radboud University Medical Center, Nijmegen, The Netherlands

Sita H. Vermeulen
Department for Health Evidence, Radboud University Medical Center, Nijmegen, The Netherlands
Department of Human Genetics, Radboud University Medical Center, Nijmegen, The Netherlands

Lambertus A. Kiemeney
Department for Health Evidence, Radboud University Medical Center, Nijmegen, The Netherlands
Department of Urology, Radboud University Medical Center, Nijmegen, The Netherlands

Shufang Zhang, Zhenxiang Liu, Chong Zhang, Hui Cao, Shunlan Wang, Ying'ai Zhang, Sifang Xiao, Peng Yang, Jindong Li and Zhiming Bai
Affiliated Haikou Hospital, Xiangya School of Medicine Central South University, Haikou Municipal People's Hospital, Haikou, China

Yanxuan Liu
Department of Genetic Disease, the First Affiliated Hospital of Xinxiang Medical University, Xinxiang, China

Yongqing Ye
Department of Shanghai Claison Bio-Technology, Shanghai, China

Jiahua Pan, Wei Xue, Jianjun Sha, Hu Yang, Fan Xu, Hanqing Xuan, Dong Li and Yiran Huang
Department of Urology, Renji Hospital, Affiliated to Shanghai Jiao Tong University, School of Medicine, Shanghai, China

Won Jun Lee, Seul Ji Lee, Jeong Hill Park and Sung Won Kwon
College of Pharmacy and Research Institute of Pharmaceutical Sciences, Seoul National University, Seoul, Republic of Korea

Sang Cheol Kim
Samsung Genome Institute, Samsung Medical Center, Seoul, Republic of Korea

Jeongmi Lee
School of Pharmacy, Sungkyunkwan University, Suwon, Republic of Korea

Kyung-Sang Yu
Seoul National University College of Medicine and Hospital, Seoul, Republic of Korea

Johan Lim
Department of Statistics, Seoul National University, Seoul, Republic of Korea

Hanwei Zhang and Arnold I. Chin
Department of Urology, Broad Stem Cell Research Center, Jonsson Comprehensive Cancer Center, University of California Los Angeles, Los Angeles, California, United States of America

Sumanta K. Pal, Sergio Villegas, Mark Chang and Kara DeWalt
Department of Medical Oncology and Experimental Therapeutics, City of Hope Comprehensive Cancer Center, Duarte, California, United States of America

Nora Ruel
Division of Biostatistics, Department of Information Science, City of Hope Comprehensive Cancer Center, Duarte, California, United States of America

Timothy G. Wilson and Bertram E. Yuh
Division of Urology, Department of Surgery, City of Hope Comprehensive Cancer Center, Duarte, California, United States of America

Nicholas J. Vogelzang
US Oncology Research, Comprehensive Cancer Centers, Las Vegas, Nevada, United States of America

Patrícia M. R. Pereira
QOPNA and Department of Chemistry, University of Aveiro, Aveiro, Portugal

Laboratory of Pharmacology and Experimental Therapeutics, Institute for Biomedical Imaging and Life Sciences (IBILI), Faculty of Medicine, University of Coimbra, Azinhaga de Santa Comba, Coimbra, Portugal

Sandrina Silva and José A. S. Cavaleiro
QOPNA and Department of Chemistry, University of Aveiro, Aveiro, Portugal

Carlos A. F. Ribeiro
Laboratory of Pharmacology and Experimental Therapeutics, Institute for Biomedical Imaging and Life Sciences (IBILI), Faculty of Medicine, University of Coimbra, Azinhaga de Santa Comba, Coimbra, Portugal

João P. C. Tomé
QOPNA and Department of Chemistry, University of Aveiro, Aveiro, Portugal
Department of Organic Chemistry, Ghent University, Gent, Belgium

Rosa Fernandes
Laboratory of Pharmacology and Experimental Therapeutics, Institute for Biomedical Imaging and Life Sciences (IBILI), Faculty of Medicine, University of Coimbra, Azinhaga de Santa Comba, Coimbra, Portugal
Center of Investigation in Environment, Genetics and Oncobiology, Coimbra, Portugal
Center of Ophthalmology and Vision Sciences, IBILI, Faculty of Medicine, University of Coimbra, Coimbra, Portugal

Silvia Pineda, Roger L. Milne, Evangelina López de Maturana, Jesús Herranz, Mirari Márquez, Lin T. Guey, Erin Baum and Anna Gonzá lez-Neira
Spanish National Cancer Research Center (CNIO), Madrid, Spain

M. Luz Calle
Systems Biology Department, University of Vic, Vic, Spain

Nathaniel Rothman, Stephen J. Chanock, Montserrat García-Closas and Debra T. Silverman
Division of Cancer Epidemiology and Genetics, National Cancer Institute, Department of Health and Human Services, Bethesda, Maryland, United States of America

Manolis Kogevinas
Centre for Research in Environmental Epidemiology (CREAL), Barcelona, Spain
Institut Municipal d'Investigació Mèdica – Hospital del Mar, Barcelona, Spain

Adonina Tardón
Department of Preventive Medicine, Universidad de Oviedo, Oviedo, Spain

Josep Lloreta
Institut Municipal d'Investigació Médica – Hospital del Mar, Barcelona, Spain
Departament de Patologia, Hospital del Mar – IMAS, Barcelona, Spain

Alfredo Carrato
Servicio de Oncología, Hospital Universitario de Elche, Elche, Spain
Servicio de Oncología, Hospital Universitario Ramon y Cajal, Madrid, Spain

Arcadi Navarro
Departament de Ciéncies Experimentals i de la Salut, Universitat Pompeu Fabra, Barcelona, Spain
Institut de Biologia Evolutiva (UPF-CSIC), Barcelona, Spain
Institució Catalana de Recerca i Estudis Avançats (ICREA), Barcelona, Spain
Instituto Nacional de Bioinformática, Barcelona, Spain

Francisco X. Real
Spanish National Cancer Research Center (CNIO), Madrid, Spain
Departament de Ciéncies Experimentals i de la Salut, Universitat Pompeu Fabra, Barcelona, Spain

Wolfgang Jäger and Claudia Janssen
The Vancouver Prostate Centre and Department of Urologic Sciences, University of British Columbia, Vancouver, BC, Canada
Department of Urology, Johannes Gutenberg University, Mainz, Germany

Igor Moskalev, Tetsutaro Hayashi, Shannon Awrey, Alan I. So, Kaixin Zhang, Ladan Dirk Lange, Fazli, Estelle Li and Peter C. Black
The Vancouver Prostate Centre and Department of Urologic Sciences, University of British Columbia, Vancouver, BC, Canada

Kilian M. Gust
The Vancouver Prostate Centre and Department of Urologic Sciences, University of British Columbia, Vancouver, BC, Canada
Department of Urology, Johann Wolfgang Goethe University, Frankfurt, Germany

Joachim W. Thüroff
Department of Urology, Johannes Gutenberg University, Mainz, Germany

Jiayu Feng, Yajun Song and Chibing Huang
Department of Urology, Xinqiao Hospital, The Third Military Medical University, Chongqing, China

Weifeng He, Ying Wang, Xiaorong Zhang, Gaoxing Luo and Jun Wu
Chongqing Key Laboratory for Disease Proteomics; State Key Laboratory of Trauma, Burns and Combined Injury, Institute of Burn Research, Southwest Hospital, Third Military Medical University, Chongqing, China

Richard J. Simpson
Department of Biochemistry, La Trobe Institute for Molecular Science, La Trobe University, Bundoora, Victoria, Australia

Index

www.ingramcontent.com/pod-product-compliance
Lightning Source LLC
Chambersburg PA
CBHW061331190326
41458CB00011B/3965